Program Evaluation Theory and Practice

Program Evaluation Theory and Practice

A COMPREHENSIVE GUIDE

Donna M. Mertens
Amy T. Wilson

THE GUILFORD PRESS
New York   London

© 2012 The Guilford Press
A Division of Guilford Publications, Inc.
72 Spring Street, New York, NY 10012
www.guilford.com

Printed in the United States of America

This book is printed on acid-free paper.

Last digit is print number: 9   8   7   6   5   4   3   2   1

The authors have checked with sources believed to be reliable in their efforts to provide information that is complete and generally in accord with the standards of practice that are accepted at the time of publication. However, in view of the possibility of human error or changes in behavioral, mental health, or medical sciences, neither the authors, nor the editor and publisher, nor any other party who has been involved in the preparation or publication of this work warrants that the information contained herein is in every respect accurate or complete, and they are not responsible for any errors or omissions or the results obtained from the use of such information. Readers are encouraged to confirm the information contained in this book with other sources.

Library of Congress Cataloging-in-Publication Data

Mertens, Donna M.
      Program evaluation theory and practice : a comprehensive guide / Donna M. Mertens and Amy T. Wilson. — 1st ed.
            p. cm.
      Includes bibliographical references and index.
      ISBN 978-1-4625-0315-5 (pbk. : alk. paper) — ISBN 978-1-4625-0324-7 (hardcover : alk. paper)
      1. Evaluation research (Social action programs).   2. Social sciences—Research—
Methodology.   I. Wilson, Amy T.   II.   Title.
      H62.M42317 2012
      361.2072—dc23

                                                            2011042703

Preface

Program evaluation is a relatively young discipline in the formal sense of systematically collecting data for the purpose of informing decision making. However, because program evaluation builds on many other disciplines (e.g., social science, statistics), evaluators have a long history of scholarship and practice to inform their work. This text explores the philosophical and theoretical roots of evaluation, and builds a bridge between those roots and evaluation practice. The text is divided into four major sections: Part I, "The Landscape of Evaluation"; Part II, "Historical and Contemporary Evaluation Paradigms, Branches, Theories, and Approaches"; Part III, "Planning Evaluations"; and Part IV, "Implementation in Evaluation: Communication and Utilization of Findings, Management, Meta-Evaluation, and Challenges."

The four parts provide a logical and somewhat linear flow, in that they start with an explanation of the meaning of evaluation and its historical roots; move to philosophical and theoretical orientations that provide guidance for thinking about evaluation; and then cover the specifics of planning, implementing, and using evaluations. You can use Part I to get an overview of the field, Part II to get an understanding of historical and contemporary philosophical and theoretical perspectives and to take the initial steps for planning an evaluation, Part III to engage in detailed planning of an evaluation, and Part IV to gain specific insights into the implementation and use of evaluations. Thus the text is intended to provide a broad understanding of the evaluation field, as well as to provide the tools necessary to engage in planning and implementing evaluations.

The principal themes illustrated in Part I include the diversity of evaluation's historical roots, as well as the dynamic state of the field because of its interdisciplinary nature. Evaluation is an evolving field of study that is enriched by the various perspectives represented in its roots and in its current configuration. This evolution is enhanced by the situating of evaluation in real-world conditions confronting real-world challenges. Hence this text relies heavily on examples of evaluation from different sectors, nations, populations, and disciplines. These examples illustrate the realistic conditions that evaluators encounter in their work. Evaluators are called upon to evaluate a wide range of entities; they have developed a variety of strategies for depicting what is being evaluated. Examples of these strategies illustrate how theory is used to inform an understanding of the program, policy, or other entity that is being evaluated, and the advantages and challenges associated with these different strategies. We provide you with practical guidance in applying these strategies to depict a program, policy, or other entity of your choosing.

In Part II, the focus shifts from the broad evaluation landscape and the evaluand to the philosophical and theoretical positions that have developed within the evaluation community. The prominence given to these perspectives is supported by the influence of philosophical and theoretical assumptions on ways evaluators think about their work, how evaluators are perceived in the wider communities they serve, decisions about practice, and consequent use of findings. Hence this section of the text seeks to blend the philosophical and theoretical with the practical implications by means of discussions and examples illustrating various theoretical positions in practice. Personal reflections from selected evaluation theorists provide unique insights from their different points of view. We encourage you to examine your own assumptions about evaluation, and to derive implications for evaluation practice from your own philosophical and theoretical beliefs.

Part III concerns the part of evaluation planning that overlaps most with applied research methods. Hence the level of detail here reflects current thinking about design, data collection, sampling, and data analysis. Specific web-based resources are provided to enhance your abilities to plan these aspects of the evaluation. It should be noted that in this section of the text, these topics are discussed in the specific context of evaluation. In addition, issues of culture are highlighted throughout Part III, as these have surfaced as critical concerns in terms of validity and ethics in evaluation. We provide you with practical guidance in this section that will allow you to prepare a plan for an evaluand of your choice.

Part IV moves from a planning focus to an implementation focus. This includes a detailed explanation of the topics of reporting and using evaluations. Practical topics such as how to plan for managing an evaluation are addressed, along with a discussion of challenges associated with this part of an evaluator's work. Examples illustrate the real-world challenges that evaluators encounter and strategies they use to address these challenges. Issues that are relevant throughout the evaluation process are revisited in this final section of the text, to encourage deeper reflection on politics, values, ethics, reporting, human relations, use of evaluation findings, and the quality of evaluation work.

Intended Audience

We perceive this book's primary audience as including graduate students (or advanced undergraduates) and faculty in program evaluation, social sciences, education, health, and international development; professionals undertaking evaluations; and interdisciplinary readers (as reflected in the membership of the American Evaluation Association [AEA] and other national, regional, and international evaluation organizations). We see its secondary audience as including people who commission evaluations, issue requests for proposals for evaluations, and review proposals for evaluations.

Pedagogical Features

- Each chapter begins with reflective questions to prepare you for reading the chapter and to serve as a guide as you move through the chapter.

- Chapters include sections entitled "Extending Your Thinking" that include questions and activities to enable you to go beyond the information given in the chapter.

■ Examples of evaluations are included from many sectors and disciplines. The evaluators for many of the evaluations offer reflective commentary based on their experiences. Their commentary is designed to provide direction to those of you who are novice evaluators.

■ You can use this book as a guide to develop an evaluation plan for a specific project or program.

■ A glossary of terms is included at the end of the book. Terms that are specific to the evaluation field are given in **boldface** when they first appear in the text. These are the terms that can also be found in the glossary.

Personal Notes

The two of us represent different stances with regard to evaluation. Donna M. Mertens has been immersed in the field of evaluation since her early days in graduate school at the University of Kentucky College of Medicine, followed by several years working with the Appalachian Regional Commission on the evaluation of professional development programs that used one of the first National Aeronautics and Space Administration (NASA) satellites as a delivery mechanism for residents of the Appalachian Mountains, stretching across a 13-state region from New York to Alabama. She moved from there to Ohio State University when that institution hosted the National Center for Research in Vocational Education. While at Ohio State, she conducted a good deal of policy research and a few evaluation studies for different agencies, such as the Peace Corps. She then did a short stint at Xerox International Training Center, evaluating its sales training program. Finally, she found a professional home at Gallaudet University in Washington, D.C., the only university in the world with the mission to serve deaf and hard-of-hearing students at the undergraduate and graduate levels. During her almost four decades of work in evaluation, she has had many opportunities to conduct and consult on evaluations, as well as to contribute to the development of evaluation capacity in many communities around the world. Given her lengthy experiences in the world of evaluation, you should assume that when the text uses the pronoun "I" in referring to an evaluation experience, this pronoun refers to Mertens.

Amy T. Wilson, on the other hand, taught deaf high school students for 12 years; the programs in which she taught were evaluated by the state, the county special education evaluation office, and the school administrators. In turn, she continually evaluated her students' coursework and participated in administering standardized tests and developing Individual Evaluation Plans for the students. Wilson then volunteered in an economically deprived neighborhood in northeast Brazil, acting as an advocate and community development worker with deaf children and adults who, because of their deafness, were marginalized by society. When Wilson returned to the United States to study for her PhD, Mertens became her mentor and introduced her to the transformative world of evaluation. Since that time, she has been fortunate to engage in international program development, with opportunities to conduct evaluations in various venues around the world. She brings the dual perspectives of program developers and users of evaluation to this work.

Acknowledgments

We wish to thank our students and colleagues at Gallaudet and around the world who have allowed us to partner with them in the pursuit of better ways to conduct evaluations and develop programs. They have challenged us, taught us, and helped us extend our own thinking about evaluation. We also want to thank C. Deborah Laughton, Publisher, Methodology and Statistics, at The Guilford Press, as well as other Guilford staff members who have supported the production of this book (particularly Anna Brackett, Editorial Project Manager, and Marie Sprayberry, Copyeditor). As we recognize that evaluation is a continually developing field, we express appreciation for the comments of reviewers who provided us with ideas for making this text more responsive to readers' needs, including Linda Schrader, Wendy Hicks, Joseph Nichols, John C. Thomas, Steven Rogg, and Mark Hopper. A large number of evaluators provided us with invaluable comments about their own work that they believe would be helpful for the reader; this has enriched our relationships with them and allowed us to offer a broad base of wisdom in this book. Finally, we wish to thank our friends and families for their support as we engaged in preparing to write this book—both over our lifetimes and during the period of time in which the writing actually occurred.

Brief Contents

PART IV

IMPLEMENTATION IN EVALUATION: 473
COMMUNICATION AND UTILIZATION OF FINDINGS,
MANAGEMENT, META-EVALUATION, AND CHALLENGES

Extended Contents

THE LANDSCAPE OF EVALUATION

Part I is designed to give you an overview of the field of program evaluation, exploring definitions, purposes, and ethical issues in the field. Evaluation is situated in a broad landscape in terms of its diverse meanings in different disciplines, sectors, nations, and venues. The hallmarks of the evaluation field are its interdisciplinary roots and the ways in which the resultant conversations around the meaning of evaluation have benefited from this diversity of perspectives. We introduce you to the historical evolution of the field, as well as to current issues around ethics and rigor in evaluation. The beginning stages of evaluation planning are enhanced by a discussion of the role of the evaluator and the focus of the evaluation in terms of the nature of the evaluand (the entity that is to be evaluated). Multiple purposes of evaluation are explored, as well as strategies for identifying and working with stakeholders. Part I includes these chapters:

■ Chapter 1. Introduction to Evaluation: Defining Terms and Ethical Considerations
  • Looking at the World through the Eyes of an Evaluator
  • Definitions of Evaluation
  • Distinguishing Research and Evaluation
  • Evaluation Terms
  • Scale as a Dimension of Relevance in Evaluations
  • The U.S. Government and Evaluation
  • International Development and Evaluation
  • Brief Historical Overview of Evaluation
  • Evaluation Standards and Ethical Guidelines

■ Chapter 2. Framing Evaluation: Philosophy, Branches, and Theories
  • Paradigms and Theories
  • Paradigms
  • Evaluation Theory
  • Models and Approaches
  • Social Science Theory
  • Program Theory
  • Evaluators' Roles

Preparing to Read Chapter One

As you prepare to read this chapter, think about these questions:

1. What is an "evaluation"? Where are evaluations done and why?

2. How does evaluation differ from research?

3. What professional and personal characteristics would you hope to find in an effective evaluator?

4. Have you ever been on the receiving end of an evaluation? What do you remember about your feelings of being evaluated?

5. How has participating in an evaluation helped you at school, at work, or in your daily life?

6. Evaluators can find themselves in ethical dilemmas because evaluations are associated with expenditure of resources and provision of services. What kinds of dilemmas do you think might arise in an evaluation study?

CHAPTER ONE

Introduction to Evaluation

Defining Terms and Ethical Considerations

Looking at the World through the Eyes of an Evaluator

Evaluators focus on real-world issues of importance to themselves and the people with whom they share the planet. What does it mean to look at the world through the eyes of an evaluator? What distinguishes evaluators from others with whom we share living spaces? In some ways, nothing at all: For example, we all use evaluative thinking when someone asks us how we liked our dinner or what we thought of a movie. In other ways, evaluators' ways of thinking are different from ordinary daily decision making, because they engage in a process of figuring out what is needed to address challenges through the systematic collection and use of data. Thus looking over an evaluator's shoulder as she/he reads the newspaper with morning coffee can be an opportunity to catch a glimpse into the ways evaluators look at the world. For example, the following stories appeared in *The Washington Post* within the span of a few weeks:

▨ Gang-related crime is higher in some Washington, D.C., neighborhoods than in others, and a trend toward increasing violence is evident (Velazquez, 2009). District Council members propose to address the gang problem by issuing a "gang injunction," which is "a judicial order that prevents people identified as gang members from congregating in public spaces within certain areas and that creates additional restrictions on otherwise legal activities" (p. C7). An evaluator reading this article thinks: What is the current research on prevention of gang-related violence? How does that correspond with the use of injunctions as a strategy? If prevention programs that focus on summer programs and employment for youth worked elsewhere, what is the likelihood that they would have a similarly positive effect in Washington, D.C.? What is the possibility that the gang injunction would unfairly target minority youth? What are the long-term implications of the use of such an injunction on the life chances of youth who are identified as gang members?

▨ Many Iraqi Arabs have left Baghdad after witnessing the burning of their homes and brutal slayings of their family members at the hands of masked gunmen; they have set up roadside camps in the Kurdish autonomous region in northern Iraq (Bakri, 2009). When they try to help, humanitarian agencies encounter difficulties because of the sectarian violence. The people living in the camps have no electricity; water is trucked in; garbage is everywhere; latrines are nonexistent; and employment is almost impossible, except for occasional day laborer opportunities. An evaluator asks: Who needs to be involved in discussions of solutions to this crisis? What alternatives could be considered to address the basic human needs of the displaced Iraqi Arabs? If intervention strategies are developed, what can be done to monitor their implementation and determine their effectiveness? What is the situation with regard to women and/or people with disabilities? How are they differentially affected by this displacement and lack of basic services?

▓ The National Center for Education Statistics has issued a report revealing increasing diversity in the population of U.S. students: 44% of these students are now from minority groups (Planty et al., 2009). This report is cited in an article in *The Washington Post*, along with commentary about the relationship between poverty and quality of educational experiences (Strauss, 2010). In another article in *The Washington Post*, Anderson (2011) writes about an initiative to develop national standards for education. As an evaluator, one might go to the original source of the report (Planty et al., 2009) and begin to wonder about what interventions might be used to address the appropriate educational needs of diverse students and about ways to reduce poverty as a possible strategy to improve educational experiences. Also, one might wonder about the relationship between having national standards and these issues of diversity, poverty reduction, and quality of education. How could an evaluation be designed that would take into account the diversity of the study body, the national standards, the need to improve educational experiences, and the goal of poverty reduction?

▓ In 1973, the mayor of Washington, D.C.; the governors of Virginia, Maryland, and Pennsylvania; and the head of the Environmental Protection Agency signed the Chesapeake Bay Agreement, making a commitment to clean up the bay (Winegrad & Ernst, 2009). In the period between 1973 and today, the bay's conditions have worsened: more frequent fish kills; diminishing populations of blue crabs and oysters; rockfish contaminated with mercury; catfish with cancerous lesions; male bass with female egg sacs; and swimmers who contract serious infections. An evaluator reading this story asks: What are the contextual variables that serve as barriers to cleaning up the bay? What programs could be put in place that might have a chance of reversing this environmental and economic disaster? Which **stakeholders** (those who have a stake in the health of the bay) need to be engaged in order to address these problems, and what are appropriate strategies for engaging with them? How can data be brought to bear in a way that accurately assesses the current conditions, contributes to the development of interventions, measures the progress toward established goals, and determines whether changes are needed in those interventions? How are current policies either contributing to or detracting from the ability to solve these problems?

▓ Chandler (2009) reports:

Federal data show the proportion of special education teachers who transfer to other teaching jobs or leave the profession is higher than the rate in almost any other area of teaching. Nearly every school system reports a short supply of certified special education candidates. The high turnover means special education students are far more likely to be taught by uncertified or inexperienced teachers. (p. PW16)

An evaluator might wonder: What are the federal data that are referred to in this article? What is it about the special education teacher's job that leads to low retention?

What can schools do to support special educators so they will stay in their positions longer and provide much-needed services for students with disabilities?

As these examples illustrate, evaluation is situated in the challenges of everyday life; yet it differs from everyday ways of responding to such issues by focusing on a systematic process that is known as program evaluation. Next, we explore various definitions of "evaluation" that have arisen in different sectors of the evaluation community.

Definitions of Evaluation

Going beyond Everyday Usage

Trochim (1998) highlighted differences between the everyday-use concept of evaluation and program evaluation by pointing out that the latter "is a *profession* that uses *formal methodologies* to *provide useful empirical evidence* about *public entities* (such as programs, products, performance) *in decision-making contexts* that are inherently *political* and involve multiple often-conflicting *stakeholders*, where *resources* are seldom sufficient, and where *time-pressures* are salient" (p. 248; emphasis in original). How does this translate into the actual work of an evaluator? Here is how it plays out: My (A. T. W.) most recent job as an evaluator is to use surveys and interviews to provide data about the effectiveness of the HIV/AIDS Outreach Center's workshops teaching adults about the female condom. Before the fiscal year ends, city monies must be budgeted and the city council needs to decide whether to continue to support the Center's workshops or move the last of this year's fiscal funding to Metropolitan Churches United, a vocal faith-based coalition, and their proposed project, Action Plan on Abstinence (Wilson, 2008).

How does this example illustrate Trochim's definition of evaluation? Wilson works as a *professional evaluator*; she has chosen to use the *formal methodologies* of surveys and interviews. The *empirical evidence* has been used to gather data about the Outreach Center's HIV/AIDS program (a *public entity*). The City Council will use the information for *making decisions* about how to allocate funds to prevent HIV/AIDS in the coming year; the Outreach Center staff and the faith-based coalition (*stakeholders*) have different ideas about what should be done (*political context*). The decision has to be made within *time constraints* for the next year's budget to be approved.

Definitions Emphasizing Values, Merit, and Worth

Evaluators have developed other definitions of evaluation that emphasize different aspects of the process. Fournier (2005) and Scriven (1967b) provide definitions of evaluation that highlight the importance of values in defining this term. Fournier (2005, pp. 139–140) provided this as a general definition of evaluation:

> Evaluation is an applied inquiry process for collecting and synthesizing evidence that culminates in conclusions about the state of affairs, value, merit, worth, significance, or quality of a program, product, person, policy, proposal, or plan. Conclusions made in evaluations encompass both an empirical aspect (that something is the case) and a normative aspect (judgment about the value of something). It is the value feature that distinguishes evaluation from other types of inquiry, such as basic science research, clinical epidemiology, investigative journalism, or public polling.

In evaluation's early days, Scriven (1967b) defined evaluation as a method of determining the merit or worth of an **evaluand** (the project, program, or other entity that you are evaluating), arguing that the placement of value on something should be appraised based on these two dimensions. The terms **merit** and **worth** are defined in the *Encyclopedia of Evaluation* (Mathison, 2005), and we summarize these definitions as follows.

Merit is the absolute or relative quality of something, either intrinsically or in regard to a particular criterion. For example, other doctors may hold Dr. Letitia Jones, a cardiologist, in high esteem and judge her merit based on her excellent surgical skills and technique. These admired *intrinsic* characteristics would be brought with her wherever she practiced medicine. To determine the merit of an evaluand in regard to a *particular criterion*, it is necessary to collect relevant performance data and to explicitly ascribe value to it. The merit of the evaluand is then determined by the criterion noted as being valuable or not. Therefore, Dr. Jones's merit may also be judged by determined criteria, such as having patients who experience fewer cardiac episodes and decreased hospitalizations, or having a good bedside manner. To determine the overall merit of the evaluand, the merit question asks about the intrinsic value of the evaluand (surgical technique, scholarliness, or renown in the field of cardiology). A further step in judging merit is the synthesis of performances with multiple criteria: How good is the entity (in this example, Dr. Jones) when compared to a set of criteria (e.g., communication skills, patient care)? According to Davidson (2005, p. 247), "Merit determination and synthesis are two of the core methodological tasks that distinguish evaluation from the collection and reporting of descriptive data for interpretation by others."

Whereas merit can be judged on the evaluand's *intrinsic* value, **worth** is an outcome of an evaluation and refers to the evaluand's value *in a particular context*. Worth and merit are not dependent on each other, and an evaluand (e.g., Dr. Jones) may have intrinsic merit (she is a highly skilled cardiologist) but may have little worth (the hospital needs an anesthesiologist). The opposite is also the case (the hospital has found an anesthesiologist [high worth] but not a very good one [little merit]). "The worth of an evaluand requires a thorough understanding of the particular context as well as the qualities and attributes of the evaluand" (Mathison, 2005, p. 452). The particular context may be the needs that exist in an individual hospital, and the evaluand may be the type of services that the doctors provide in relation to that need.

Scriven (2009) extends this distinction with an example of how you might evaluate a car. It might be a great car (high quality/merit), but was it worth what it cost?, thus making the point that worth involves consideration of different types of costs, both monetary and nonmonetary. Can a person who lives in the flat land of sunny central Florida appreciate the $25,000, five-speed, 4 × 4 Jeep Wrangler that handles any road or weather condition? (There is no correct answer to this question; the merit and worth of something are judged according to the criteria specific to that context. The "cool" factor may outweigh the utility features of the car designed to handle rough terrain.)

Michael Patton (2008) makes a further distinction between merit and worth:

> Merit refers to the intrinsic value of a program, for example, how effective it is in meeting the needs of those it is intended to help. Worth refers to extrinsic value to those outside the program, for example, to the larger community or society. A welfare program that gets jobs for recipients has merit for those who move out of poverty and worth to society by reducing welfare costs. (p. 113)

If we return to the example of the evaluation of a program to promote the use of female condoms within this discussion of merit or worth, merit could be determined on the basis of criteria such as ease of use, affordability, and willingness to make use of these condoms. Worth might be determined in terms of the need to reduce sexually transmitted diseases (STDs) and the effectiveness of the intervention toward that end. As an evaluator, my (A. T. W.) colleagues and I collected and synthesized the data from the interviews and surveys at the HIV/AIDS Center and in the community. We concluded that the workshops were taught well and women found the condoms useful and reliable to prevent STDs; however, negative attitudes toward the use of the condoms prevailed. The women considered the condoms to be expensive, and they would only use them if they were given to them for free. Even then, use was low because the women said that the condoms interfered with the pleasure of love making (Wilson, 2008). Thus the female condom program satisfies the worth aspect, in that they are needed and they do prevent the spread of STDs. However, the program does not meet the merit criteria in terms of cost and women's willingness to use them.

Further discussion of the ideas of merit and worth are provided by Ernie House (1990) as he questions the relationship between values and the determination of merit and worth. He asks these important questions: Whose values should be used to establish the meanings of merit and worth in a particular evaluation study? And what methodologies are best suited to address the question of values. (His remarks are displayed in Box 1.1.)

Box 1.1. Merit, Worth, and Values: House's Views

The increasing social conflict of the past two decades throws the problem of values into prominence. Where do the values come from in an evaluation? The act of public evaluation requires that some criteria of merit be established and that these criteria be justified. Typically, the stated program goals have served as the source of criteria, with the evaluator assessing whether the program has met its goals. Furthermore, by taking the program manager as the client for the evaluation, the evaluator could act on what was important to the manager.

However, several theorists challenged this acceptance of managerial goals as the essence of evaluation. Scriven in particular worked out the logic of evaluation in general terms, contending that the question Is *x* good (bad, indifferent)? and its variants (How good is *x*? Is *x* better than *y*?) are the prototypical evaluative questions, and that answering these questions requires identifying and validating standards of merit for *x* and discovering *x*'s performance on dimensions that are merit-related (Scriven, 1980). According to this reasoning, the program goals themselves must be assessed. For example, a responsible evaluator would not accept General Motors' contention that the best car is the one that earns the highest profit as the criterion for evaluating cars.

This general logic still leaves open the question of where the particular criteria of merit come from. One can say in general that criteria are derived from what is appropriate for things of its kind. For example, one would not say that an educational program which warped personality and retarded intellectual growth was a good edu-

(cont.)

Box 1.1 (*cont.*)

cational program, regardless of whether the developers wanted this effect. Given a particular entity in a particular context, criteria of merit which are not arbitrary can be justified. The fruit of this reasoning is that evaluative judgments are not arbitrary any more than is a descriptive statement that an elephant is large compared to other animals, but small compared to an office building.

Of course, the social world is not simple. For complex entities like educational programs, there are multiple and often conflicting criteria of merit. There is immediate retention versus long-term recall, knowledge of facts versus critical thinking, more history versus more math. Furthermore, people do not always want the same things from public programs. Their values, and in fact their interests, differ. A program good for one group may not be good for another. Yet for the practicing evaluator, there is no choice but to make a choice of criteria of merit.

Many choose the traditional measures of educational achievement, believing that those best reflect overall interests.

Source: House (1990, p. 26).

· · · · · · · · · · · E X T E N D I N G   Y O U R   T H I N K I N G · · · · · · · · · · ·

Merit and Worth

Using the chart below, discuss with others the merit and worth of each evaluand. For example, what are the merit and worth of scuba gear? In judging merit, what would be the intrinsic value of scuba gear, and what criteria would be used to determine its merit? What would the worth of the scuba gear be in the context of a dive boat? In Washington, D.C.? In Mongolia? Discuss how individuals in your discussion group may value one evaluand differently from another and why. Whose values should you use in establishing the definitive merit and worth of each evaluand?

The Merit and Worth of Evaluands

	Dive boat	Washington, D.C.	Mongolia
Scuba gear	Merit? Worth?	Merit? Worth?	Merit? Worth?
Kiswahili teacher	Merit? Worth?	Merit? Worth?	Merit? Worth?
Fur coat	Merit? Worth?	Merit? Worth?	Merit? Worth?
$10 bill	Merit? Worth?	Merit? Worth?	Merit? Worth?

Definitions in Applied Social Research

Some evaluation scholars frame their definitions of evaluation more within the realm of applied social research. For Rossi, Lipsey, and Freeman (2004), program evaluation (or, as they suggest, "evaluation research" as an interchangeable term) is "defined as a social science activity directed at collecting, analyzing, interpreting, and communicating information about the workings and effectiveness of social programs" (p. 2). Shadish, Cook, and Leviton (1991) also framed their definition of evaluation as applied social research.

Definitions in Political Contexts

Other evaluators—such as Weiss (1972), Greene (2006), Schwandt (2008), House and Howe (1999), MacDonald (1976), and Mertens (2009)—situate their work more explicitly within the political contexts in which evaluations are conducted. Their concepts of evaluation place emphasis on values that reflect social justice and human rights as goals for evaluators. For example, if the evaluation of the program to promote the use of female condoms (Wilson, 2008) had revealed that the condoms had been donated by a pharmaceutical company and the community was not asked about their desire to use them, then this would bring the program's politics into play. The community might have interests related to the prevention of HIV/AIDS and other STDs. However, they might lobby their City Councilman and the Board of the Metropolitan Churches United for assistance in obtaining free HIV/AIDS testing, HIV/AIDS counseling, and HIV/AIDS programs in the middle and high schools in the neighborhoods.

Definitions in International Development

Monitoring is differentiated from **evaluation** in international development communities. The United Nations Development Programme (UNDP, 2002, p. 6) provides the following definition, which is relevant in evaluations undertaken in international development:

> [Monitoring is] a continuing function that aims primarily to provide the management and main stakeholders of an ongoing intervention with early indications of progress, or lack thereof, in the achievement of results. An ongoing intervention might be a project, programme or other kind of support to an outcome.

The U.S. Agency for International Development (USAID, 2009) gives this definition: "**Monitoring** focuses on whether a program is achieving its objectives; these objectives are expressed as measurable performance standards."

Here is an example of monitoring. During its intentional design and monitoring stages, outcome mapping (described in Chapter 7) allows certain questions to be posed within the intervention's community of inquiry: For example, do we "see" the changes or outcomes that we want? To what degree? What can boundary partners (such as counselors, action researchers, and the core team) do to enhance the intervention? (Buskens & Earl, 2008). In the wider evaluation world, monitoring is most akin to **process evaluation**.

The UNDP (2002, p. 6) defines evaluation in international development as a

> selective exercise that attempts to systematically and objectively assess progress towards and the achievement of an outcome. Evaluation is not a one-time event, but an exercise involving

assessments of differing scope and depth carried out at several points in time in response to evolving needs for evaluative knowledge and learning during the effort to achieve an outcome.

The USAID (2009) provides this definition for evaluation:

> Program, project, or policy performance **evaluations** typically examine a broader range of information on program, project, or policy performance and its context than is feasible to monitor on an ongoing basis. Evaluations may examine aspects of program operations, such as in a process evaluation; process evaluations focus primarily on how an intervention has been carried out and use indicators such as how many people have been trained, how many community discussions have been held, or how many women have been counseled in exclusive breastfeeding. Process evaluations also examine financial systems, reporting systems, and other aspects of project implemenation management. Evaluations may also examine factors in the program environment that may impede or contribute to the program's success, to help explain the linkages between program inputs, activities, outputs, and outcomes. Alternatively, evaluations may assess the program's effects beyond its intended objectives, or estimate what would have occurred in the absence of the program, in order to get an objective sense of the program's net impact. Additionally, program, project, or policy evaluations may systematically compare the effectiveness of alternative programs aimed at the same assistance objective.

Marra (2000) describes her study of the World Bank's efforts to decrease corruption as evaluation rather than monitoring:

> The mid-term evaluation of the WBI's [World Bank Institute's] anti-corruption activities in Tanzania and Uganda was commissioned in 1997 to shed light on the strengths, weaknesses and impacts of the activities as they had unfolded. The evaluation was requested by WBI management in view of the pending expansion of the program to at least 15 other countries, especially in Central and Eastern Europe, where task managers will need to address corruption in a region with totally different historical, political, economic and social characteristics. (p. 24)

· · · · · · · · · · **E X T E N D I N G   Y O U R   T H I N K I N G** · · · · · · · · · · ·
Definitions of Evaluation

Each definition of evaluation has different implications for the types of issues that are likely to be salient.

1. Contrast everyday, informal ideas of evaluations with formal definitions of program evaluation. Discuss examples of each and how they differ.

2. Discuss the use of "merit" and "worth" within the context of evaluation work. Provide examples of these terms from your own experience or from the scholarly literature.

3. Review the definitions of evaluation provided in this chapter and/or definitions of evaluation from other sources.

- The American Evaluation Association [AEA] website (***www.eval.org***) has many resources.

- Gene Shackman has assembled a broad range of resources (***gsociology. icaap.org/methods***). The "Basic guides" link on this page is useful for beginners.

- Bill Trochim has compiled the Research Methods Knowledge Base (***www. socialresearchmethods.net/kb/index.php***).

- *The Evaluation Exchange* on the Harvard Family Research Project website (***www.hfrp.org/evaluation/the-evaluation-exchange***) is a helpful online peri- odical.

- USAID's website for evaluators (***www.usaid.gov/policy/evalweb***) is very use- ful.

4. Contrast two definitions of evaluation; explain why issues of power are important in determining which definition is used in a study.

Distinguishing Research and Evaluation

Given the definitions of evaluation already discussed, you may already have an inkling of how research and evaluation differ. Although there is much overlap between the world of research and evaluation, evaluation occupies some unique territory (Mertens, 2009). Greene (2000) writes about the commonalities that demarcate evaluation contexts and distinguish program evaluation from other forms of social inquiry (such as research). She argues, based on the writings of Patton (1987), Cronbach et al. (1980), and Weiss (1987), that what distinguishes evaluation from other forms of social inquiry is its political inher- ency; that is, in evaluation, politics and science are inherently intertwined. Evaluations are conducted on the merit and worth of programs in the public domain, which are them- selves responses to prioritized individual and community needs that resulted from politi- cal decisions. Program evaluation "is thus intertwined with political power and decision making about societal priorities and directions" (Greene, 2000, p. 982).

Trochim (2006) also argues that evaluation is unique because of the organizational and political contexts in which it is conducted, which require skills in management, group processes, and political maneuvering that are not always needed in research. Mathison (2008) makes a strong claim that evaluation needs to be considered as a distinct discipline because of its historical emergence in the 1960s as a mechanism to examine valuing as a component of systematic inquiry, as well as the ensuing development of methodological approaches that focus on stakeholder input and use of defined criteria. (See AEA, 2004, and Joint Committee on Standards for Educational Evaluation, 2011, both of which are discussed later in this chapter.)

Scriven (2003) gives a thoughtful turn to this train of thought by describing evalu- ation as a "transdiscipline" because it is used in so many other disciplines. He writes: "Evaluation is a discipline that serves other disciplines even as it is a discipline unto itself, thus its emergent transdisciplinary status" (p. 42). He adds that evaluation is like such disciplines as statistics and ethics, which have unique ways of approaching issues but are also used in other areas of inquiry (such as education, health, and social work).

Mertens (2009; see also Ginsberg & Mertens, 2009) recognizes the uniqueness of evaluation, as well as its overlap with applied research in education and the social sciences. While evaluation has contributed to our understanding of how to bring people together to address critical social issues, parallel developments have also been occurring in applied social research. Hence "there is a place at which research and evaluation intersect—when research provides information about the need for, improvement of, or effects of programs or policies" (Mertens, 2009, p. 2). Thus this provides an additional rationale for framing evaluation as a major genre of systematic inquiry that both borrows from and enhances the methodologies developed in the research community.

· · · · · · · · · · · **EXTENDING YOUR THINKING** · · · · · · · · · · ·

Characteristics of Evaluation (as Compared to Research)

1. Locate an evaluation study. You could use any of the studies cited so far in this book or by searching in evaluation journals such as these:

   - *American Journal of Evaluation*
   - *Gender, Technology and Development*
   - *Educational Evaluation and Policy Analysis*
   - *Evaluation and Program Planning*
   - *Evaluation and the Health Professions*
   - *Evaluation Review*
   - *Indian Journal of Gender Studies*
   - *New Directions for Evaluation*
   - *Studies in Educational Evaluation*

2. What evaluation terms (e.g., those that are defined and illustrated in this chapter) are included in the studies that reflect the specific technical jargon used by evaluators?

3. What characteristics of the study convey to you that this is distinctively evaluation (as opposed to applied research)?

Evaluation Terms

Like professionals in most fields, evaluators have a specialized vocabulary that takes on specific meanings when used in this context. Definitions of several important terms are provided along with illustrative examples. Other relevant vocabulary for evaluators can be found in the *Encyclopedia of Evaluation* (Mathison, 2005) or other resources (such as those found at ***www.eval.org***).

Evaluand

Evaluand, a generic term coined by Michael Scriven, may apply to any object of an evaluation. It may be a person, program, idea, policy, product, object, performance, or any other entity being evaluated (Mathison, 2005, p. 139). Examples of evaluands are provided in Box 1.2. (We should note that personnel evaluation is not a topic that is included in this text.)

Box 1.2. Examples of Evaluands

■ **Program:** The Native American community in North Carolina wanted a program to reduce the number of teenagers who smoked tobacco. The Not on Tobacco intervention was designed to help American Indian teens stop smoking (Horn, McCracken, Dino, & Brayboy, 2008).

■ **Project:** The W. K. Kellogg Foundation (WKKF) funded a project to determine how to improve the accessibility of courts for deaf and hard-of-hearing people across the United States (Mertens, 2000).

■ **Policy:** The Los Angeles Unified School District wanted an evaluation of its Title I[1] Achieving Schools initiative, which was implemented in the K–12 school system to support the use of promising school-level practices in elementary schools in high-poverty areas (Barela, 2008).

■ **Product:** An evaluation proved that portable music players, such as Apple's iPod, do not interfere with cardiac pacemakers (BioMed Central, 2008).

■ **Idea:** The United Nations Foundation–Vodafone Foundation Partnership (2009) evaluated the idea of improving the health of people in the developing world by sending them crucial health information through mobile technology, such as smart-phones, personal digital assistants (PDAs), laptops, and tablet PCs.

■ **Program:** A comprehensive reading reform model called Success for All was evaluated in 35 schools over a 3-year period (Borman et al., 2007).

■ **Program:** Mertens, Harris, Holmes, and Brandt (2007) conducted an evaluation of a master's program in one university to prepare teachers who are deaf or hard of hearing and/or from ethnic/racial minority groups to teach children who are deaf and who have an additional disability.

■ **Program:** A midsized Midwestern city implemented a local program to reduce and prevent homelessness and chronic unemployment (Coryn, Schröter, & Hanssen, 2009).

■ **Program:** A program for people with developmental disabilities was in place for 5 years and had centers in multiple locations across one state. The program was designed to provide individualized services for people with developmental disabilities in order to improve their quality of life (Fredericks, Deegan, & Carman, 2008).

(cont.)

Box 1.2 (*cont.*)

■ **Program:** The World Bank initiated an evaluation of a program to reduce corruption in Uganda and Tanzania (Marra, 2000).

■ **Program:** Mareschal, McKee, Jackson, and Hanson (2007) conducted an evaluation of a program to reduce youth violence in four communities.

■ **Project:** The Infant Feeding Research Project was evaluated to determine its effectiveness in reducing the rate of pediatric HIV/AIDS in southern Africa via interventions to enhance infant feeding by counseling the mothers of at-risk babies (Buskens & Earl, 2008).

■ **Program:** Hovey, Booker, and Seligman (2007) measured the impact of a theatrical program on knowledge and attitudes about HIV/AIDS among an audience of Mexican farm workers who were at elevated risk for contracting HIV/AIDS and were in need of HIV/AIDS-related education.

Internal and External Evaluators

An **external evaluator** is someone who conducts an evaluation who is not an employee of the organization that houses the object of the evaluation (e.g., a program) (Barrington, 2005, p. 151). Here is an example of external evaluation. The program serving individuals with developmental disabilities (see Box 1.2) made this statement indicating that an external evaluation team was used: "A comprehensive evaluation of the ... project was conducted by outside consultants in collaboration with a Steering Committee comprised of representatives from a state agency that provides funding for programs that serve people with developmental disabilities and from the participating implementation agency sites" (Fredericks et al., 2008, p. 254).

Internal evaluators are employees of the organization in which the evaluation is conducted. For example, Barela (2008), who works in the research and planning division of the Los Angeles Unified School District, served as an internal evaluator for the Title I Achieving Schools initiative (again, see Box 1.2).

· · · · · · · · · · E X T E N D I N G   Y O U R   T H I N K I N G · · · · · · · · · ·

External and Internal Evaluators

Read this passage about the advantages and disadvantages of using either an external or internal evaluation:

> The trade-offs between external and internal are roughly as follows. The internal evaluator knows the program better and so avoids mistakes due to ignorance, knows the people better and hence can talk to them more easily, will be there after the evaluation is finished and hence can facilitate implementation, probably knows the subject matter better,

costs less, and is sure to know of some other comparable projects for comparison. The external evaluator is less likely to be affected by personal or job benefit considerations, is often better at evaluation, has often looked closely at comparable programs, can speak more frankly because there is less risk of job loss or personal attribution/dislike, and carries some cachet from externality. (Scriven, 1991, p. 61)

1. What do you see as the advantages and disadvantages of external versus internal evaluations?

2. How can evaluators address the disadvantages of each position?

Formative and Summative Evaluation

Formative evaluation has been defined as follows:

> Evaluation is considered to be *formative* when it is conducted during the development or delivery of a program or product with the intention of providing feedback to improve the evaluand. Formative evaluation may also focus on program plans or designs. (Mathison, 2005, p. 160)

Here is an example of formative evaluation. The problem of reducing youth violence does not have an easy solution. The Federal Mediation and Conciliation Service's Youth Initiative recognized that different communities might have different needs and thus require different interventions. Hence they allowed communities to develop their own youth violence prevention programs. A formative evaluation was conducted to "document the different approaches to program development and implementation across cases and provide feedback to policy makers and program stakeholders that can be used to make future improvements" (Mareschal et al., 2007, p. 168).

Summative evaluation has been defined thus:

> A *summative evaluation* is one that is done at the end of or on completion of a program. Summative evaluations may be done internally or externally and typically for the purpose of decision making. Michael Scriven, the originator of the terms formative and summative evaluation, distinguishes summative evaluation's aim as reporting "on" the program rather than "to" the program. (Mathison, 2005, p. 402)

For example, the World Bank instituted a program to decrease corruption in Uganda and Tanzania, at the request of the national governments. The evaluation was both formative and summative. Marra (2000) explained it as follows:

> The study had both summative and formative objectives. The study was summative to the extent that it addressed questions of accountability, impacts and outcomes. Of special concern was what the program did or did not accomplish—whether objectives were met, and whether the implementation strategies were successful in moving the program in the desired direction. The study also played a formative role when looking at what kinds of mid-course corrections needed to be made to keep the program on track. The retrospective data gathered during the various stages of the program lifecycle met the task managers' continuing need for information. As the task managers report, their collaborative interactions with the evaluation team helped clarify aspects of the program design and implementation. (p. 28)

Stakeholders

Here is a definition of **stakeholders:**

> *Stakeholders* are people who have a stake or a vested interest in the program, policy, or product being evaluated (hereafter referred to as "the program") and therefore also have a stake in the evaluation. Stakeholders are usefully clustered into four groups: (a) people who have decision[-making] authority over the program, including other policy makers, funders, and advisory boards; (b) people who have direct responsibility for the program, including program developers, administrators in the organization implementing the program, program managers, and direct service staff; (c) people who are the intended beneficiaries of the program, their families, and their communities; and (d) people disadvantaged by the program, as in lost funding opportunities. (Greene, 2005, p. 398)

Clearly, there can be many different types of stakeholders. In the prevention of youth violence study (see Box 1.2), for instance, the stakeholders were identified as the commissioner of the local Federal Mediation and Conciliation Service's Youth Initiative, "the youth officer from the local police department, members of the city human resources department, a high school teacher, and a middle school teacher" (Mareschal et al., 2007, p. 174).

In the World Bank anticorruption study, the stakeholders were identified as "the task managers directly involved in the design and management of anticorruption activities; then moved to the WBI at large, which has an explicit mandate to combat corruption; and then to the Bank's operational sectors, who are involved in lending operations and consulting with governments in developing countries; to client governments that benefited from anti-corruption activities; and finally to civil society as a whole" (Marra, 2000, p. 26).

Gender Analysis

Gender analysis is used in domestic and international contexts where evaluations are conducted. Resources called "gender analysis tools" have emerged from the international development community, to address the findings in several studies that development projects often increase the "feminization of poverty, gender-based violence, and the incidence of human trafficking, sex work, and sexually transmitted infections" (Rooke & Limbu, 2009, p. 3).

For example, Ghertner (2006) conducted a gender analysis of the impact of a cookstove improvement program in India. The stoves were made by women masons in the community, and they were designed to decrease the need for biomass fuel (e.g., wood, charcoal), the time women spent searching for fuel, and cooking time. However, the stoves cost money to buy, and the women in the community did not control expenditure of funds; they had to convince their husbands to buy the stoves. The gender analysis also revealed that the cookstove improvement project had unintended consequences, in that the women engaged in negotiations with their husbands to buy the stoves, albeit sometimes resorting to trickery related to the stove's full cost. Ghertner interpreted this as a strategic gain for women in that they were finding a voice through the negotiation process. Interestingly, the government decided to provide a full subsidy for the new stoves made by people outside of the community, so purchase became a nonissue. Husbands almost universally accepted having the new stoves when they did not have to pay for them. Although the full subsidy might at first appear to have solved a problem, it created several others. The women masons in the community lost income from sales; the women who represented potential buyers lost the opportunity to negotiate; and the men had different ideas about how to use the new stoves. "In particular, the chimneys were made of sheet metal and had alternative uses for which the men dismantled the *chulhas*. The men thus appropriated the stoves for non-cooking related activities, clearly removing any material benefit that would have gone to women" (Ghertner, 2006, p. 295). Thus use of a gender analysis method allowed for the examination of the impact of well-meaning innovations in projects that further serve to subordinate women.

Scale as a Dimension of Relevance in Evaluations

Evaluators sometimes describe their work as "large-scale" or "small-scale." There is no specific quantitative measure that determines whether an evaluation is large- or small-scale. However, the evaluation of a single program housed in a single university would probably provide the "small" anchor for a continuum from large to small. The Barela (2008) evaluation that included the entire Los Angeles Unified School District would be appropriately categorized as large-scale, as would evaluations encompassing entire countries.

The theme of the purposes of evaluation surfaces at different levels of complexity throughout this text. In this initial chapter, many examples of evaluations have been used to provide a practice-grounded understanding of what evaluation is. These examples have been chosen to reflect not only multiple disciplines, but also various levels of evaluation work (i.e., large-scale vs. small-scale, national vs. international).

· · · · · · · · · · E X T E N D I N G   Y O U R   T H I N K I N G · · · · · · · · · ·
Scaling Up

Read the following description of an evaluation project that attempted to take a small-scale project to a wider area. Then answer the questions that follow.

The British government hoped to increase the economic prosperity of Gambian farmers by increasing the production and variety of crops in The Gambia, through a project that trained farmers how to use oxen in cultivating their dry fields (Mettrick, 2004). Traditionally the farmers used animals for plowing their groundnut (peanut) fields, but not for other crops, such as maize and rice. The British supplied the necessary capital equipment needed to train the farmers on using oxen for cultivating all of their dry crops throughout the country. Women, whose economic income is essential for family survival, do the majority of their agricultural work in swampy rice fields. They were left out of the training, as oxen are used in cultivating crops on dry land where men work. Evaluators made field visits to only observe the program and evaluated the impact of the program on the rural economy and the inputs needed.

There was a "possible improvement" of 10–20% in the family income of those

(cont.)

receiving the equipment and training, but the nonavailability of credit to other farmers in the rural areas to purchase oxen and equipment prohibited economic gains in rural communities. Farmers reported that the British equipment was complicated to use, was expensive, and did not fit local conditions. A hoe that was developed in the neighboring country of Senegal and was being used by some farmers was adopted instead of the British oxen scheme. The oxen program did not increase yields as hoped, although groundnut fields have increased in acreage.

1. What was the evaluand?
2. Who were the stakeholders?
3. Was this evaluation summative, formative, or both?
4. What effects did the program have on Gambian farmers other than "possible" economic growth?
5. A gender analysis was completed, as we see that women were not included in the oxen program, since rice cultivation does not use animals in The Gambia (although it does in other countries). Did the British oxenization program "increase the feminization of poverty"?
6. If you were the evaluator of this project, what recommendations might you make for further projects meant to increase the economic prosperity of Gambian farmers?

The U.S. Government and Evaluation

According to the home page of its website (*www.gao.gov*), the U.S. Government Accountability Office (GAO) "supports the Congress in meeting its constitutional responsibilities and helps improve the performance and accountability of the federal government for the benefit of the American people." Evaluators are interested in the U.S. GAO's auditing standards, which are published in its "Yellow Book" webpage (*www.gao.gov/yellowbook*); these were revised in 2011. The U.S. GAO holds to consistent, principled standards for auditors throughout the Yellow Book: accountability (auditors actions are explainable), transparency (nothing is hidden or obscured), competence (auditors should have education and experience), and service (the auditor is doing its work for the tax-paying public).

The AEA directs its members to the following chapters of the Yellow Book, as they may have lessons applicable to the work of evaluators:

- Chapter 1. Ethical Principles
- Chapter 2. Section on Performance Audits
- Chapter 3. General Standards
- Chapter 6. Field Work Standards for Performance Audits (paragraphs 6.15, 6.37–6.75)
- Chapter 7. Reporting Standards for Performance Audits
- Appendix I. Additional Information for Chapters 1 and 2

International Development and Evaluation

Picciotto (2007) explains that the global community views the goals of international development as emanating from the United Nations' framing of international development in "the Millennium Declaration endorsed by all heads of state in New York in December 2000," which "defined development as a global partnership for poverty reduction" (p. 509). The recent history of international development evaluation has involved a shift from donor-agency-controlled evaluations to partnership evaluations and even country-led evaluations. This shift has brought with it a change in the types of evaluations conducted, from project-based evaluations focused on assessment of outcomes to a broader focus on the Millennium Development Goals (MDGs) and the measurement of results (Conlin & Stirrat, 2008). Box 1.3 summarizes the MDGs.

Box 1.3. The Millennium Development Goals of the United Nations

Goals	Performance indicators
1. Eradicate extreme poverty and hunger	Halve the proportion of people with incomes of less than $1 a day between 1990 and 2015
	Halve the proportion of people who suffer from hunger between 1990 and 2015
2. Achieve universal primary education	Ensure that boys and girls everywhere complete primary schooling by 2015
3. Promote gender equality and empower women	Eliminate gender disparity at all levels of education by 2015
4. Reduce child mortality	Reduce by two-thirds the younger-than-5 mortality rate between 1990 and 2015
5. Improve maternal health	Reduce by three-fourths the maternal mortality ratio
6. Combat HIV/AIDS, malaria, and other diseases	Halt and reverse the spread of HIV/AIDS, malaria, and other major diseases by 2015
7. Ensure environmental sustainability	Integrate sustainable development into country policies and programs, and reverse the loss of environmental resources
	Halve the proportion of people without sustainable access to safe drinking water and basic sanitation by 2015
	Achieve a significant improvement in the lives of at least 100 million slum dwellers by 2020

(cont.)

Box 1.3 (*cont.*)	
Goals	**Performance indicators**
8. Develop a global partnership for development	Increase aid levels and improve aid quality
	Develop an open, rule-based, predictable, nondiscriminatory trading and financial system
	Deal comprehensively with developing countries' debt
	Implement strategies for youth employment
	Make available the benefits of new technologies

Source: United Nations (2006; based on Picciotto, 2007, p. 511).

Country-led evaluations are becoming more common because of the current practices of international financial institutions such as the World Bank and the International Monetary Fund, whose members come from the world's wealthiest countries. These two institutions make loans and offer technical assistance to middle- and lower-income countries, with the aim of reducing poverty and achieving the MDGs; however, the countries must agree to specific economic programs. The Independent Evaluation Group of the World Bank conducts country assistance evaluations (CAEs) to assess the Bank's work, the effectiveness of its development projects, the long-term impact on development of the countries they assist, and lessons that can be learned from their evaluations. Some nongovernmental organizations (NGOs) believe that national governments and aid agencies must follow the demands of those who lend them money, and become more focused on attempting to achieve the MDGs than on evaluating the reality on the ground. Easterly (2006) asserts that "Collective responsibility for the Millennium Development Goals or any other goals does not work. Hold aid agencies individually responsible for what their own programs achieve, not for global goals" (pp. 204–205).

Top-down CAEs miss the complex, diverse realities of the in-country beneficiaries and focus more on the World Bank's evaluation tools than on the accomplishments of the program objectives (World Bank Independent Evaluation Group, 2009). Chambers (2005) states that poor people have a remarkable capacity to analyze their own reality, to inform development agencies on what they need and how they need it, and to participate in the assessment of development programs. However, poor people are rarely asked to participate in any phase of these evaluations, even though the purpose of CAEs is to reduce the number of people living in poverty.

Picciotto (2009) describes a micro–macro paradox in the international development evaluation community, with country-level evaluations at the macro level and program- or project-level evaluations at the micro level. Chambers (2005) argues for micro-level evaluations on the basis of valuing the local experience and enabling the voices of diverse groups to be present in the evaluations. A macro-level program evaluation may determine that decreasing Thailand's rice and palm oil production with increased tapioca production could improve the country's per capita income. Yet a micro-level evaluation may discover that the social, cultural, and historical ties rural farmers have to the land would be disrupted if the government takes the land to expand tapioca farming. Such individuals' voices are lost when data are aggregated at a country level. Picciotto (2009) states that micro-level evaluations appeal to social scientists who believe that "the transformation processes associated with development are local phenomena that take place at the community level where social relationships are forged" (p. 42). However, he argues that the real impact of aid needs to be measured at the country level, because the policy goal is improvement at the country level rather than at the project level.

Box 1.4 describes resources created by two international aid agencies for international development evaluation.

Box 1.4. International Development Evaluation Players and Actions

The Organisation for Economic Co-operation and Development (OECD) is an international body that works at the level of governments in countries committed to democracy, to support sustainable economic growth. The Development Assistance Committee (DAC) is the principal body through which the OECD deals with issues related to cooperation with developing countries. The OECD DAC (2006a) developed five criteria to evaluate international development interventions: relevance of objectives, effectiveness of programs to fulfill those objectives, efficiency, impact, and sustainability.

The OECD's Paris Declaration on Aid Effectiveness (OECD, 2005) posed an important challenge both to the world of development cooperation in general and to the field of development evaluation in particular. Compared with previous joint statements on aid harmonization and alignment, it provided a practical, action-oriented roadmap, with specific targets to be met by 2015 and definite review points in the years between. The number of countries and international organizations participating in the 2005 High Level Forum and putting their signature to the joint commitments contained in the Declaration was unprecedented, reflecting a progressive widening of the range of voices included in major meetings convened by the OECD DAC.

The evaluation of the implementation of the Paris Declaration is an integral part of the Declaration itself. In addition, ministers of developing and donor countries responsible for promoting development, and heads of multilateral and bilateral development institutions, endorsed a statement in Accra, Ghana on September 4, 2008 to accelerate and deepen implementation of the Paris Declaration on Aid Effectiveness (OECD, 2008). The first part of the implementation evaluation, which was also presented at the High Level Forum in Accra, was an early evaluation and focused on ways of improving and enhancing implementation, rather than giving any definite judgment about effectiveness. The second part of the evaluation was completed in 2011 (Woods et al., 2011) and indicates mixed results in the delivery and effectiveness of aid.

A different agency, the International Fund for Agricultural Development (IFAD) Office of Evaluation (2009), developed an evaluation manual that is specific to planning and conducting evaluations funded by IFAD across the globe. It is an interesting portrayal of one organization's roadmap for evaluations.

· · · · · · · · · · **E X T E N D I N G   Y O U R   T H I N K I N G** · · · · · · · · · ·
International Development

The international development community is undergoing a transformation from donor-controlled interventions and evaluations toward more country-led evaluations. What are the advantages and disadvantages associated with these two different approaches?

Brief Historical Overview of Evaluation

The origins of evaluation can be traced back to the 1800s, when the U.S. government first asked for external inspectors to evaluate public facilities such as prisons, schools, hospitals, and orphanages (Stufflebeam, Madaus, & Kellaghan, 2000). However, most writers peg the beginning of the profession of evaluation as we now know it to the 1960s, with the start of Lyndon Johnson's Great Society initiatives (e.g., Head Start programs and the Elementary and Secondary Education Act) that mandated evaluations as a part of the programs. The history of evaluation is also complicated by its pluralistic disciplinary roots, with educational evaluators coming from a testing-, assessment-, and objectives-based evaluation background, and psychologists more closely aligned with applied social research traditions (Mark, Greene, & Shaw, 2006).

Only a brief history of evaluation is presented here, with the intent of providing an overview of the historical origins and current status of evaluation. The history of evaluation, like histories on many topics, differs depending on who is telling the story. These differences are in part due to the disciplinary backgrounds of the writers. Primarily from the perspective of education, Guba and Lincoln (1989) conceptualized four generations of evaluation:

- First generation: Measurement—testing of students
- Second generation: Description—objectives and tests (Tyler's work, cited in Stufflebeam et al., 2000)
- Third generation: Judgment—the decision-based models, such as Stake (1983), Scriven (1967a), and Stufflebeam (1982)
- Fourth generation: Constructivist, heuristic evaluation

From a social science perspective, Rossi et al. (2004) note that social scientists were conducting studies of major social programs related to education, public health, and employment as early as the years preceding World War I. Program evaluation rooted in social sciences expanded in the 1950s to encompass studies of delinquency prevention, public housing, and international initiatives. By the 1960s, the War on Poverty fueled the need for a systematic approach to evaluating the social programs that were part of that era.

In 1976, two professional associations related to evaluation were founded in the United States: the Evaluation Research Society and Evaluation Network. In 1986, these two organizations merged to become the AEA, which at this writing has a membership of nearly 6,000 (*www.eval.org*) from all 50 U.S. states and over 80 foreign countries. Members work in universities, private corporations and consulting firms, government agencies, and educational and social organizations, among other settings. It holds an annual conference, hosts a listserv (EvalTalk), and publishes two journals: the *American Journal of Evaluation* and *New Directions for Evaluation*.

Before 1995, there were only five regional and/or national evaluation organizations in the world (Mertens, 2005). After 7 years in planning and development, an international organization was inaugurated in March 2003 at a meeting with representatives from Latin America, Europe, Africa, Australasia, North America, and the former Soviet Union. The International Organisation for Cooperation in Evaluation (IOCE; *ioce.net*) is an alliance of evaluation networks and associations focused on providing a venue for capacity building and sharing of evaluation experience and expertise across these organizations. The IOCE website now lists almost 70 regional, international, or national evaluation associations, so clearly there has been an increase in the presence of formally acknowledged bodies whose mission it is to enhance evaluation theory and practice around the world.

Evaluation Standards and Ethical Guidelines

An important part of this first chapter is the introduction of the standards and ethical guidelines for the field of evaluation. National, regional, and international evaluation organizations' standards are discussed, with an acknowledgment of recent revisions to enhance focus on cultural competency.

Standards for Critically Evaluating Programs

The Program Evaluation Standards (referred to hereafter as the *Standards*; Joint Committee on Standards for Educational Evaluation, 2011) were developed by a joint committee with members from three organizations: the American Educational Research Association (AERA), the American Psychological Association (APA), and the National Council on Measurement in Education. The representatives of these three organizations were joined by members of 12 other professional organizations (e.g., the American Association of School Administrators, the Association for Assessment in Counseling, and the National Education Association) to develop a set of standards that would guide the evaluation of educational and training programs, projects, and materials in a variety of settings. The *Standards* have not yet been adopted as the official standards for any of these organizations; however, they do provide one comprehensive (albeit not all-encompassing) framework for examining the quality of an evaluation.

The *Standards* are organized according to five main attributes of an evaluation:

- Utility—how useful and appropriately used the evaluation is
- Feasibility—the extent to which the evaluation can be implemented successfully in a specific setting
- Propriety—how humane, ethical, moral, proper, legal, and professional the evaluation is

■ Accuracy—how dependable, precise, truthful, and trustworthy the evaluation is

■ Meta-evaluation—the extent to which the quality of the evaluation itself is assured and controlled

Each of the main attributes is defined by standards relevant to that attribute. Box 1.5 contains a summary of the standards organized by attribute. Guidelines and illustrative cases are included in *The Program Evaluation Standards* text (Joint Committee, 2011) itself. The illustrative cases are drawn from a variety of educational settings, including schools, universities, the medical/health care field, the military, business/industry, the government, and law.

Box 1.5. A Summary of *The Program Evaluation Standards*

Utility

U1 Evaluator Credibility

Evaluations should be conducted by qualified people who establish and maintain credibility in the evaluation context.

U2 Attention to Stakeholders

Evaluations should devote attention to the full range of individuals and groups invested in the program and affected by its evaluation.

U3 Negotiated Purposes

Evaluation purposes should be identified and continually negotiated, based on the needs of stakeholders and intended users.

U4 Explicit Values

Evaluations should clarify and specify the individual and cultural values underpinning purposes, processes, and judgments.

U5 Relevant Information

Evaluation information should serve the identified and emergent needs of evaluation users.

U6 Meaningful Processes and Products

Evaluations should construct activities, descriptions, findings, and judgments in ways that encourage participants to rediscover, reinterpret, or revise their understandings and behaviors.

U7 Timely and Appropriate Communication and Reporting

Evaluations should attend in a continuing way to the information needs of their multiple audiences.

U8 Concern for Influence and Consequences

Evaluations should promote responsible and adaptive use, while guarding against unintended negative consequences and misuse.

Feasibility

F1 Practical Procedures

Evaluations should use practical procedures that are responsive to the customary way programs operate.

F2 Contextual Viability

Evaluations should recognize, monitor, and balance the cultural and political interests and needs of individuals and groups.

F3 Resource Use

Evaluations should use resources efficiently and effectively.

F4 Project Management

Evaluations should use effective project management strategies.

Propriety

P1 Responsive and Inclusive Orientation

Evaluations should include and be responsive to stakeholders and their communities.

P2 Formal Agreements

Evaluations should be based on negotiated and renegotiated formal agreements, taking into account the contexts, needs, and expectations of clients and other parties.

P3 Human Rights and Respect

Evaluations should protect human and legal rights, and should respect the dignity and interactions of participants and other stakeholders.

P4 Clarity and Balance

Evaluations should be complete, understandable, and fair in addressing stakeholder needs and purposes.

P5 Transparency and Disclosure

Evaluations should make complete descriptions of findings, limitations, and any resulting conclusions available to all stakeholders, unless doing so would violate legal and propriety obligations.

(cont.)

Box 1.5 (cont.)

P6 Conflicts of Interests

Evaluations should identify, limit, and if necessary play a mediating role in situations where conflicts of interest may compromise processes and results.

P7 Fiscal Responsibility

Evaluations should account for all expended resources, comply with sound fiscal procedures and processes, and ensure that clients are knowledgeable about fiscal resources expended.

Accuracy

A1 Trustworthy Conclusions and Decisions

Evaluation conclusions and decisions should be trustworthy in the cultures and contexts where they have consequences.

A2 Valid Information

Evaluation information should have sufficient validity and scope for the evaluation purposes.

A3 Reliable Information

Evaluation information should be precise, dependable, and consistent.

A4 Explicit Evaluand and Context Descriptions

Evaluations should document evaluands and their contexts with appropriate detail and scope for the evaluation purposes.

A5 Sound Qualitative and Quantitative Methods

Evaluations should employ sound information selection, collection, and storage methods.

A6 Sound Designs and Analyses

Evaluations should employ technically adequate designs and analyses that are appropriate for the evaluation purposes.

A7 Explicit Evaluation Reasoning

Evaluation reasoning leading from information and analyses to findings, interpretations, conclusions, and judgments should be clearly documented without omissions or flaws.

A8 Valid Communication and Reporting

Evaluation communications should be truthful in detail and scope and as free as possible from misconceptions, distortions, and errors.

Meta-Evaluation

MI Purposes

Meta-evaluations should be responsive to the needs of their intended users.

M2 Standards of Quality

Meta-evaluations should identify and apply appropriate standards of quality.

M3 Documentation

Meta-evaluations should be based on adequate and accurate documentation.

Source: Joint Committee on Standards for Educational Evaluation (2011).

The African Evaluation Association's Guidelines

Evaluation organizations in several countries have developed sets of standards or guidelines. The AEA's guidelines are discussed in the next section; the evaluation associations in Canada, France, Germany, Switzerland, the United Kingdom, Australia, and New Zealand have also developed evaluation standards or guidelines. The development of a set of guidelines for use in Africa is used to illustrate issues that arise in different contexts.

When the African Evaluation Association (AfrEA, 2000) developed guidelines for African evaluators, it used the American *Standards* as a guide; however, it did not adopt them wholesale. In these guidelines, AfrEA discusses culturally based differences between the African and American contexts. The guidelines include important modifications, particularly in regard to the attributes of utility and propriety. Hopson (2001, p. 378) explains:

> Pertaining to utility guidelines, our African evaluation colleagues were particularly sensitive to evaluation findings being not only operational but *owned by* stakeholders, and that these same findings should be responsive to stakeholder concerns and needs. In short, an evaluation that purports to serve the needs of intended users inextricably involves maximum stakeholder ownership and feedback. With regard to legal and ethical evaluation standards, our African evaluation colleagues have modified several propriety guidelines, especially as they relate to respect for the cultural values of those affected by evaluation results. Moreover, the African evaluation guidelines serve not only to protect those affected by evaluation results but also to protect the communities that they serve and of which they are members. (emphasis in original)

Two examples from the AfrEA guidelines illustrate the differences between these and the American *Standards*:

> *Utility*—The utility guidelines are intended to ensure that an evaluation will serve the information needs of intended users and be owned by stakeholders ...
> > *U1. (modified) Stakeholder Identification.*
> > Persons and organizations involved in or affected by the evaluation (with special attention to beneficiaries at community level) should be identified and included in the evaluation

process, so that their needs can be addressed and the evaluation findings can be operational and owned by stakeholders, to the extent this is useful, feasible and allowed.

> ***U4. (modified) Values Identification.***
>
> The perspectives, procedures, and rationale used to interpret the findings should be carefully described, so that the bases for value judgments are clear. The possibility of allowing multiple interpretations of findings should be transparently preserved, provided that these interpretations respond to stakeholders' concerns and needs for utilization purposes. (AfrEA, 2000, pp. 3–4; emphasis in original)

Ethics and Evaluation: The AEA's Guiding Principles

Another important resource for designing high-quality evaluations is the AEA's (2004) *Guiding Principles for Evaluators*. There are five guiding principles:

- *Systematic inquiry.* Evaluators should conduct systematic data-based inquiries about the program being evaluated.

- *Competence.* Evaluators provide competent performance in the design, implementation, and reporting of the evaluation, including demonstration of cultural competence.

- *Integrity/honesty.* Evaluators need to display honesty and integrity in their own behavior and attempt to ensure the honesty and integrity of the entire evaluation process.

- *Respect for people.* Evaluators must respect the security, dignity, and self-worth of the respondents, program participants, clients, and other stakeholders with whom they interact.

- *Responsibilities for general and public welfare.* Evaluators should articulate and take into account the diversity of interests and values that may be related to the general and public interests and values.

The Program Evaluation Standards and the *Guiding Principles for Evaluators* are both useful tools for evaluators in developing and implementing evaluation studies. Conducting a **meta-evaluation** (i.e., a critical study of the evaluation itself) at the design stage provides a mechanism to determine the worth of an evaluation in terms of its likelihood of producing information needed by stakeholders, and can also increase the confidence of those associated with the evaluation. Conducting the meta-evaluation across the life cycle of the evaluation will enable the evaluators to make needed changes throughout the process.

· · · · · · · · · · E X T E N D I N G   Y O U R   T H I N K I N G · · · · · · · · · ·
Ethical Dilemmas

Several useful sources allow novice evaluators to practice responding to ethical dilemmas. The *American Journal of Evaluation* publishes ethical dilemmas with responses from experienced evaluators in each issue, as well as articles that explore such dilemmas.

Dilemma 1

One such example is drawn from McDonald and Myrick's (2008) description of an evaluation conducted by student evaluators under the mentoring of a professor of evaluation. The students conducted an evaluation of a series of workshops offered by their university's diversity center. When they analyzed their data, they were surprised to find that one of the workshop leaders used derogatory language about a specific minority group. They debated what to do with this finding, finally agreeing to present it to their client (the diversity center's director) without providing the name of the offending individual. The center director subsequently contacted the mentoring professor and asked for the individual's name. The professor offered to discuss it with the students and get back to the director. The students perceived conflicts in the directives found in the *Guiding Principles for Evaluators,* in that the principle "respect for people" says that evaluators should "abide by current professional standards ... regarding confidentiality, informed consent, and potential risks or harms to participants" (AEA, 2004). Yet the principle "responsibilities for general and public welfare" states: "Evaluators should maintain a balance between the client needs and other needs" (AEA, 2004).

> How would you suggest that the professor and students should respond to the director? Are there any other standards or guidelines that you would see as relevant to responding to this dilemma? You might want to consider your answer to this question before you continue reading about possible solutions in the next few paragraphs.
>   McDonald and Myrick (2008, p. 350) provide the following solution to this ethical dilemma:

> Our analysis leads to a solution that we feel supports the indicated change while also avoiding violations of professional ethics: The evaluation team should decline to identify the workshop leader to the director and instead work with the Diversity Center to constructively address the problem. Our reflections also shed light on lessons that we can learn from this situation, including the need for evaluators to educate clients and consumers on our ethical codes, having written agreements, anticipating controversial findings and working to proactively address their eventual emergence, creating a team with considerable cultural awareness, and carefully examining conflicts of interest before engaging in an evaluation.

Perry (2008) provides another perspective on the solution proposed by McDonald and Myrick (2008). She praises the students for adhering to Propriety guidelines P4 and P5 in the *Standards,* which relate to a complete and fair assessment and reporting of findings. However, she also identifies the specific principles that may have been violated in the evaluation during the early discussions with the program staff:

(cont.)

The development process provides an opportunity to identify any obstacles that could be problematic to the evaluation of the program. These obstacles could be issues of feasibility (such as the practicality of procedures, standard F1) or propriety (such as the rights of human subjects, standard P3). As there was no reference to the conversations between the student evaluators, the DC director, and the advisory board members, it is not clear whether any concerns that suggested potential, practical, or ethical issues were raised. If this discussion did not occur, it represents a missed opportunity to plan for potential challenges. (p. 353)

Perry continues her analysis of the response to the dilemma by praising the professor's first response to the advisory board (i.e., that he could not reveal the name of the individual leader, based on the ethical principle to protect the rights of the human subjects). However, she is perplexed as to why the professor would equivocate when the director calls him the next day to ask for the name. Perry writes:

> *Professor ... , why would your response change overnight? The standards that address propriety do not change with the position of the inquirer. Of course, I know you will remember this and give the appropriate response to the director, as you also explain your desire to be helpful and not a hindrance.* (p. 355; italics in original)

Perry contends that there is no ethical dilemma in determining the appropriate response to the diversity center director. The name of the leader cannot be revealed. However, she does suggest that evaluations need to be more explicitly framed with the relevant guidelines and principles, so that all stakeholders understand their implications from the beginning of the project.

What do you think of these two solutions?

Dilemma 2

Morris (2008) edited a book in which case study scenarios that illustrate ethical dilemmas were analyzed by leading evaluators, based on their experiences, the *Standards,* and the *Guiding Principles for Evaluators.* In one of the scenarios, an evaluator is hired to conduct a process evaluation and inadvertently comes upon information about the potential firing of the project director. The ethical dilemma concerns whether to include this information in the final evaluation for public consumption, or to disregard it and protect the project director. In response, Hendricks (2008) cites the AEA (2004) integrity/honesty principle, which states that evaluators must "negotiate honestly with clients and relevant stakeholders concerning the ... tasks to be undertaken," to reach the conclusion that personnel evaluation is outside the scope of the agreed-upon tasks. Therefore, he asserts that mention of the director's firing would violate his contractual agreement.

In contrast, Davis (2008) also cites the same principle, but reaches an opposite conclusion. She provides the full text of the principle:

> Evaluators should negotiate honestly with clients and relevant stakeholders concerning the costs, tasks to be undertaken, limitations of methodology, scope of results likely to

be obtained, and uses of data resulting from a specific evaluation. It is primarily the evaluator's responsibility to initiate discussion and clarification of these matters, not the client's. (AEA, 2004)

She then states that "the Guiding Principles clearly compel the evaluator to disclose knowledge of her discovery to all stakeholders, first to the funders and then to the other stakeholders associated with the project" (p. 106). Her rationale is based on her interpretation of this principle as a directive to avoid misleading evaluation information by communicating concerns and the reasons for those concerns with the stakeholders.

What is your reaction to these two interpretations of the *Guiding Principles* and the recommended course of action?

Dilemma 3

To protect the innocent, the names of the parties in this real ethical dilemma will not be mentioned. An intern worked in a developing country in a participatory evaluation that involved many stakeholder groups. She was very careful to share drafts of the evaluation report, hold meetings to engage stakeholders in the review of the draft, and interview individuals who could not attend meetings. Overall, the report indicated that the program had been viewed very positively and that the service recipients had made several recommendations to improve the program. However, when she submitted the final report to the person in authority in the agency, he said that he could not allow the report to be released, because it contained information that was critical of the program.

What are the ethical issues that arise in this scenario? How would you recommend that the intern proceed? How might use of the *Guiding Principles* and *Standards* contribute to resolving this problem?

 ## Moving On to the Next Chapter

Chapter 2 is an introduction to the philosophical and theoretical frameworks that are associated with different evaluation approaches. It provides the foundation for entering Part II of this text, in which specific philosophies, theories, and approaches are explained.

Note

1. Title I is part of the Elementary and Secondary Education Act, which was passed in 1965 specifically to target schools in high-poverty areas.

Preparing to Read Chapter Two

As you prepare to read this chapter, think about these questions:

1. Is your experience of the world the same as mine? Can you ever really understand me, or I you? Is it really possible to be objective?

2. Do the three blindfolded evaluators in the photo below know the bison in the same way?

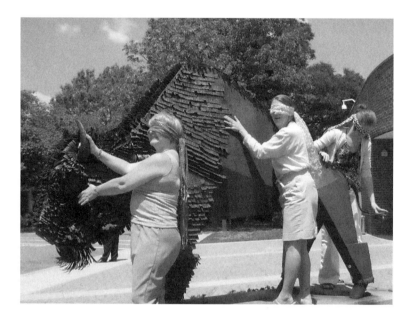

3. How is it that when hot issues are discussed in the mass media, research from one "expert" will differ greatly from what was found by another "expert"?

4. What skills do you think you will need to develop to become an effective evaluator?

Framing Evaluation

Paradigms, Branches, and Theories

If you do not know much about evaluation theory, you are not an evaluator. You may be a great methodologist, a wonderful philosopher, or a very effective program manager. But you are not an evaluator. To be an evaluator, you need to know that knowledge base that makes the field unique. That unique knowledge base is evaluation theory.

— W. R. SHADISH, Presidential Address at the American Evaluation Association (1998, pp. 6–7)

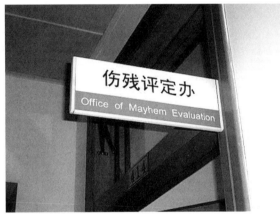

Copyright 2010 by Simon Cousins. Used by permission.

One might assume that an evaluation begins when an evaluand is identified. However, an evaluand can be identified in many ways, and decisions about appropriate strategies begins with the evaluators' beliefs about themselves and their roles, as well as their world-views. Evaluators naturally construct explanations for everything that exists, and they live with their own preconceptions about how the world works. They can believe that others perceive life experiences in the same way as they do, or (ideally) they can appreciate that people make claim to different realities from their own. Evaluators can step back and broaden their worldviews by learning from previously published research and practice. For example, in planning an evaluation for an after-school program teaching middle school children about using social media, evaluators might find some relevant information and guidance about how other middle schools have used similar strategies (e.g., antibullying education, education on appropriate information to share, managing time online, etc.). Program theory or social science theory can enhance evaluators' planning as they discern in which paradigm they will work and which evaluation model or approach they will use.

Paradigms as sets of philosophical assumptions, and theories of evaluation, programs, and social science, are discussed in this chapter as ways of framing more extensive discussion of theorists and their approaches. (See Figure 2.1.)

Paradigms and Theories

In this chapter, the discussion of historical and contemporary approaches to evaluation is framed as an extension of Guba and Lincoln's (1989, 2005) framework for understanding major worldviews (or paradigms). Paradigms are broad metaphysical constructs that include sets of logically related philosophical assumptions. Theories provide frameworks for thinking about the interrelationships of constructs and are more limited in scope than paradigms. Hence a variety of theoretical perspectives can be associated with a particular paradigm.

Theory plays multiple roles in evaluation (Donaldson & Lipsey, 2006). There are theories of evaluation, program theories, and social science theories that inform our work. The concept of evaluation theory is discussed in this section as an exploration of what we say we do when we do an evaluation. Social science theories are inclusive of such areas as motivation; social change; and feminist, queer, and critical race theories. These are used both to inform decisions about evaluation practice and to inform programmatic decisions. Program theories help explain the mechanisms believed to influence the achievement of the desired program outcomes.

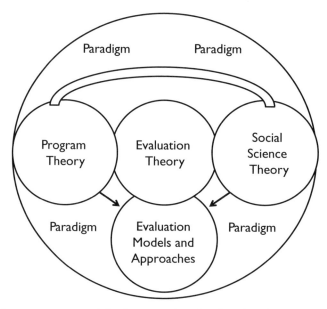

Figure 2.1. Paradigms; program, social science, and evaluation theories; and evaluation models and approaches.

"Paradigm" in Plain English

Through your life experiences, you have constructed a worldview that leads you to understand reality differently from the way I do. What you think is true may not be true for me. What you think is ethical, I may not. Neither of us is wrong (although each of us may think the other is). For example, Lisa lives in a state with the highest capital punishment rate in the United States. She might argue that it's appropriate if a court decides to sentence a woman to death for murdering her boyfriend. To her, it's black and white: If you murder someone, you should die, too. Martina is from a country that does not have capital punishment; to her, an important variable to consider would be the fact that the woman's boyfriend was beating her. Finally Kent, who is of the same minority group as the accused woman, might argue that she was not given the appropriate protection from the police or social services when she contacted them about her fears of violence. Lisa's, Martina's, and Kent's ethical principles are a type of metaphysical construct. We can see philosophical assumptions that we can frame into specific paradigms in the different ways that each person thinks.

We can see how the different ethical principles that guide these individuals philosophically provide a logical connection to what they accept as real and how they each understand what is real. For Lisa, it's real to her that the woman is guilty of murder. Martina believes that extenuating circumstances need to be considered before guilt or innocence can be determined, but that the death sentence is not an ethical punishment. And Kent believes that larger societal forces need to be considered to interpret what really happened. Paradigms are made up of four sets of philosophical assumptions related to the nature of ethics, reality, knowledge, and systematic inquiry, which we'll continue discussing in the text.

Box 2.1. Four Sets of Philosophical Assumptions in Paradigms

Philosophical assumption	Guiding question	As experienced in life
Axiology	What is the nature of ethics?	We all have moral standards and values that characterize what we believe is right or wrong, as well as norms that allow us to judge whether our actions are right or wrong. Ethics, then, is an area of philosophy that we use to judge our moral standards and values and how they apply to our lives. For example, if your morals tell you that all people are equal, is it ethical to vote against gay marriage? If your moral standards say that stealing is wrong, is it ethical to say

(cont.)

		Box 2.1 (*cont.*)
Philosophical assumption	*Guiding question*	*As experienced in life*
		nothing when you learn that the boss is keeping some project money for personal use?
Ontology	What is the nature of reality?	Is there one reality that I can discover? Or are there multiple realities that differ, depending on the experiences and conditions of the people in a specific context? Do I, a white, hearing, American upper-middle-class woman, understand the life of a Ugandan, deaf, low-income immigrant? Whose reality is real?
Epistemology	What is the nature of knowledge, and what is the relationship between the knower and that which would be known?	Another wording for the epistemological question might be: How should the evaluator relate to the stakeholders? Do you as the evaluator objectively stand apart from the stakeholders, or do you engage with them in deep conversation and in their activities?
Methodology	What are the systematic approaches to gathering information about what would be known?	Do you need to compare two groups, or can you document progress by intensively studying one group? Should you use quantitative, qualitative, or mixed methods approaches?

Paradigms

Guba and Lincoln (1989, 2005) use the term "paradigm" somewhat differently than Thomas Kuhn (1962) did in his book *The Structure of Scientific Revolutions,* in order to bring clarity of thinking to the assumptions that underlie research and evaluation. They have characterized paradigms within this context as metaphysical constructs made up of four sets of philosophical assumptions (see Box 2.1). Shadish (1998) notes that many of the fundamental issues in evaluation reflect differences in basic philosophical assumptions: Most debates in the evaluation field are "about epistemology and ontology, about what assumptions we make when we construct knowledge, about the nature of many fundamental concepts that we use in our work like causation, generalization, and truth" (p. 3).

Four paradigms provide a useful structure for examining different worldviews that are functioning in today's evaluation world: the **postpositivist, constructivist, transformative,** and **pragmatic.** Each paradigm is described in Box 2.2 (later in this chapter), and is explained with approaches and sample studies in Part II. The boundaries between these paradigms and the evaluation approaches associated with them are not clear-cut. Rather, each paradigm can be regarded as placing different emphasis on different philosophical assumptions, but overlap among the paradigms through the permeable boundaries that define them is still possible.

One quirky thing about evaluation history is that evaluators do not seem to leave their past behind. Rather, they seem to hold on to the various paradigms, theories, and approaches that served them in the early years, despite their recognition of developments and evolutions in these paradigms, theories, and approaches. For example, postpositivists are still in business and advocating for **randomized controlled trials;** pragmatists continue to write about strategies to increase the utilization of evaluation findings; constructivists add to the discussion about use of qualitative methods to capture the complexity of reality; and transformative evaluators bring to light the voices of those who were not included in the earlier history of evaluation.

Evaluation Theory

Shadish (1998) has described evaluation theory as "who we are" (p. 5), in the sense that it gives us the language we use in this transdiscipline to describe what we do uniquely as evaluators. The uniqueness of evaluation is "our willingness to attack value questions by studying merit and worth, our understanding about how to make results more useful than most other social scientists can do, or the strategies we have developed to help us choose which methods for knowledge construction to use depending on the needs of the evaluation client" (p. 5).

Smith (2008) centers his description of evaluation theory on the purposes of evaluation. Evaluation theory is that aspect that reflects "our thinking about how and why we engage in evaluation. Is the purpose of evaluation validation, accountability, monitoring, or improvement and development?" (p. 3). Theories provide guidance in determining the purposes for evaluations, as well as in defining what we consider to be acceptable evidence for making decisions in an evaluation.

Elements of an Evaluation Theory: Scriven's Scheme

Scriven (1998) tells us that a good evaluation theory should provide criteria of demarcation between evaluation and other types of investigations such as prediction or data analysis. He has proposed a minimalist theory of evaluation that includes nine elements.

First,

> The discipline of evaluation undertakes the systematic, objective, determination of the extent to which any of three properties are attributable to the entity being evaluated: merit, worth, or significance. (Merit is roughly equivalent to quality; worth is roughly equivalent to value or cost-effectiveness; significance is roughly equivalent to importance.) Each of these concepts is context-dependent, especially significance, and understanding the difference between context dependence and arbitrariness is part of understanding the logic of evaluation. (Scriven, 1998, p. 65)

Second, evaluation conclusions are expressed in terms of ranking, grading, scoring, or apportioning. A different design is needed for each of these to determine the relative importance of outcomes (ranking), how performance compares to a standard (grading), how outcomes compare (scoring), and how resources should be distributed (apportioning).

Third, in order to move from recommendations or explanations, additional knowledge beyond the evaluative data is needed (e.g., contextual variables, organizational culture; political considerations).

Fourth,

> The general outline of an evaluative investigation will normally involve determining some and often all of the following: (i) the nature of the questions, assumptions, and context (e.g., client, audiences, stakeholders, history, reasons for the evaluation) that define the entry point to the evaluation; (ii) the nature of the entity being evaluated (the evaluand); (iii) the sources and validation of values that will be used in order to generate answers to the evaluative questions (e.g., via needs assessment, existing codes, standards, principles, strategies, law, ethics, management or employee preferences, competitor performance, generalizability, costs, objectives, conceptual analysis); (iv) the criteria of merit (or worth or significance) for an entity of this kind in this context (e.g., access, outcomes, reduction of alcohol use), and their justification; (v) the relative importance or weight of each of the criteria, and their justification; (vi) the identification of standards ("cutting scores") on the (qualitative or quantitative) scales on which these criteria run (if grading is required—standards are not required for ranking, scoring, and apportioning) and the justification for these standards; (vii) the empirical or analytical determination of the achievements of the evaluand on each of these scales (using measurement, observation, experimentation, expert testimony, logical analysis, etc.); (viii) the integration (internal synthesis) of the achievements and weights into an overall conclusion about the merit (etc.) of the evaluand (this step is dispensable in a few special types of evaluation); (ix) the conversion of the results into an appropriate report or set of reports, which may be verbal, written, or graphical. (Scriven, 1998, pp. 65–66)

Fifth, evaluation is a "transdiscipline," meaning that it serves as a tool for other disciplines while at the same time having uniqueness as a discipline, much like statistics, measurement, or logic.

Sixth, there are several fields of evaluation, including program evaluation, personnel evaluation, performance evaluation (educational testing), and product evaluation/ technology assessment.

Seventh, evaluators need to evaluate their own theories and methods. As noted in Chapter 1, the evaluation of evaluation is called "meta-evaluation." It can be carried out through the use of checklists such as those available from the Western Michigan University Evaluation Center (see Chapter 14 for further details). It is useful to have an independent evaluator assess the quality of an evaluation at different stages of the evaluation's life, such as in the planning stage, in the middle, and at the end.

Eighth, evaluators work across disciplines; hence a wide knowledge of those fields that overlap with evaluation helps evaluators to avoid "reinventing the wheel."

And, finally, evaluation skills are used in many different types of activities. According to Scriven (1998), "These include planning, designing, needs assessment, goal-clarifying, diagnosing, recommending, auditing, mentoring, explaining, mediating, decision making, selecting, trouble-shooting, leading, and the formulation of regulations and legislation" (p. 67).

Trochim (1998) suggests that Scriven's minimalist theory does not sufficiently provide a demarcation between the types of evaluation that we all do in everyday life and the profession of evaluation. Hence he offers the definition of evaluation we have quoted at the beginning of Chapter 1: "Evaluation is a *profession* that uses *formal methodologies* to *provide useful empirical evidence* about *public entities* (such as programs, products, performance) *in decision-making contexts* that are inherently *political* and involve multiple often-conflicting *stakeholders,* where resources are seldom sufficient, and where *time-pressures* are salient" (p. 248; emphasis in original).

Criteria for a Good Evaluation Theory

Shadish et al. (1991) have suggested that evaluation theories need to meet the following criteria:

- Knowledge: What do we need to do to produce credible knowledge?
- Use: How can we use the knowledge we gain from an evaluation?
- Valuing: How do we construct our value judgments?
- Practice: What do we evaluators actually do in practice?
- Social programming: What is the nature of social programs and their roles in solving societal problems?

Stufflebeam and Shinkfield (2007) state that a program evaluation theory should have six components: "overall coherence, core concepts, tested hypotheses on how evaluation procedures produce desired outcomes, workable procedures, ethical requirements, and a general framework for guiding program evaluation practice and conducting research on program evaluation" (pp. 63–64). The evaluation profession has many core concepts and ethical principles, which are discussed in Chapter 1. Theorists in evaluation have also developed many different approaches that provide guidance for the conduct of evaluations. However, the evaluation field has not yet produced a core body of research on evaluation to support suggestions that specific use of particular procedures leads to desired outcomes. Stufflebeam and Shinkfield conclude that the evaluation profession

> has far to go in developing overarching, validated theories to guide the study and practice of program evaluation. The program evaluation literature's references to program evaluation theories are numerous, but these references are often pretentious. They usually denote as theories conceptual approaches or evaluation models that lack the comprehensiveness and validation required of sound theories. (p. 68)

Models and Approaches

Alkin (2004), in agreement with Stufflebeam and Shinkfield, has acknowledged that many descriptions of evaluation "theory" would be better labeled as evaluation "approaches" or "models," because they do not strictly meet the test for being theories. He writes that what are commonly referred to as "evaluation theories do not fully qualify for that status" (p. 5). We agree with him on that point, and therefore we discuss models and approaches developed by theorists. Models can be thought of as "a set of rules, prescriptions, and prohibitions and guiding frameworks that specify what a good or proper evaluation is and how it should be done" (Alkin, 2004, p. 5).

The historical roots of evaluation have been depicted in many different ways, due in part to the interdisciplinary nature of the field.[1] Alkin (2004, 2007) uses a metaphor of a tree, with its roots represented as social accountability, fiscal control, and social inquiry. To illustrate the historical and contemporary theoretical perspectives in evaluation, he depicts method-, use-, and values-based theories (approaches/models) as three major branches of the tree. This tree is useful in some respects; however, it is limited in that it primarily reflects the work of American, white, male evaluation theorists[2] and is not inclusive of evaluation theorists who are feminists, people of color, persons with disabilities, members of the lesbian/gay/bisexual/transgender/queer (LGBTQ) community, or members of indigenous groups. See Figure 2.2 as an example of a tree that includes four branches of evaluation.

In a rough way, Alkin and Christie's (2004) three branches can be mapped onto three of the major paradigms listed earlier in this chapter (and described further in Part II of this book): postpositivist (Chapter 3), pragmatic (Chapter 4), and constructivist (Chapter 5). The Methods Branch maps onto the postpositivist paradigm, the Use Branch onto the pragmatic paradigm, and the Values Branch onto the constructivist paradigm. We propose Social Justice as a fourth branch that maps onto the transformative paradigm (Chapter 6). As its name indicates, this branch focuses on furthering social justice, and it includes evaluators who develop theoretical frameworks based on cultural responsiveness, race/ethnicity, human rights, feminist, disability rights, deafness, postcolonial/indigenous, and queer theories.

The depiction of evaluation models can thus be linked to our earlier discussion of paradigms. Box 2.2 contains lists the four paradigms introduced at the beginning of this chapter and shows their relationship to the major evaluation branches: Methods, Use, Values, and Social Justice.

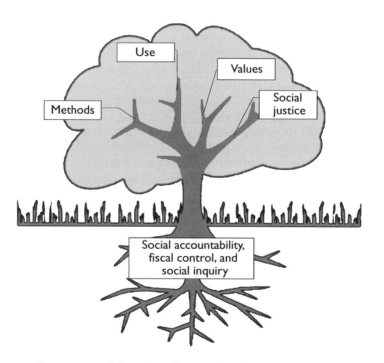

Figure 2.2. A four–branch tree of evaluation approaches.

Box 2.2. Major Paradigms in Evaluation

Paradigm	Branch	Description
Postpositivist	Methods	Focuses primarily on quantitative designs and data
Pragmatic	Use	Focuses primarily on data that are found to be useful by stakeholders; advocates for the use of mixed methods
Constructivist	Values	Focuses primarily on identifying multiple values and perspectives through qualitative methods
Transformative	Social justice	Focuses primarily on viewpoints of marginalized groups and interrogating systemic power structures through mixed methods to further social justice and human rights

Critics have wondered whether a tree is the best metaphor for depicting the theoretical perspectives in evaluation. Patton (2004) has suggested that instead of tree branches, the various perspectives in evaluation should be depicted as branches in a river, where the water flows over the banks and opportunities exist for intermingling of ideas. We think that a water metaphor might be even more inclusive; perhaps the streams that lead into rivers and rivers that flow into oceans would provide a complex enough metaphor to capture evaluation's rich history and current status. There are places where freshwater and saltwater mix, and these are indicators of the permeable borders of theories and approaches. The major theoretical perspectives might be thought of as ocean currents. An ocean current is a movement of water created by the force of the wind, temperature, salinity, tides, the magnetic pull of the sun and moon, depth contours, and shoreline configurations (National Oceanic and Atmospheric Administration [NOAA], 2009). The ocean's currents flow vast distances and play a large role in determining climate differences in the world. The ocean currents flow at a shallow level; however, there is another deep water circulation system that is called the "Global Conveyor Belt." Its route covers most of the world: It travels through the Atlantic Basin around South Africa, into the Indian Ocean, and on past Australia into the Pacific Ocean Basin. (See Figure 2.3.)

This metaphor not only allows for intermingling of waters; it also demonstrates that many forces come into play to determine the nature and effects of different ocean currents. Although we do not want to push this metaphor too far, we do suggest that it is useful to demonstrate the complexity of evaluation theories, methods, and approaches.[3] Now we are going to add another piece of the puzzle: the role of social science theory in the development of the evaluand and the evaluation plan.

Social Science Theory

Social scientists have generated theories to explain human development, learning, motivation, literacy development, and changing behaviors, among others. Evaluators can use

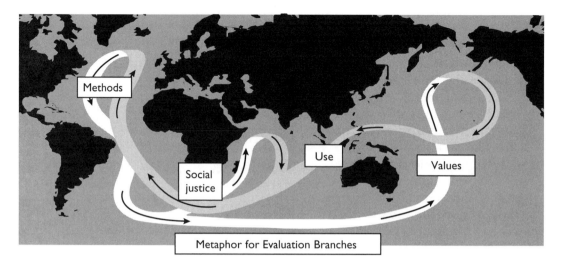

Figure 2.3. The Global Conveyor Belt as a metaphor for evaluation branches. *Source:* Adapted from NOAA (2009).

these theories to help guide program developers. Donaldson and Lipsey (2006) suggest that the use of social science theories can contribute to the development of interventions that reflect collective wisdom, and hence can reduce wasted time on treatments already known to be ineffective. A caveat that must be mentioned is the difficulty of transferring social science theories across cultures. As obvious as it seems, evaluators must be cognizant of unique cultural factors that might limit their ability to generalize from a theory developed on a white, middle-class group of people from the United States to other populations and contexts.

Bledsoe and Graham (2005) evaluated a family literacy program based on child development and cognitive learning theories, which postulated that parent–child bonding provides an opportunity for cognitive stimulation through reading and interactive activities. Thus the program included several components, such as the use of literature and music to support preliteracy and reading readiness skills; provision of health services and parent education programs; and a family literacy component that encouraged in-home reading between parents and children. Seigart (2007) used feminist theory to evaluate school-based health services in Canada, Australia, and the United States. The use of a feminist theoretical framework allowed her to uncover systemic power inequities in the provision of such services on the basis of gender, nationality, and religion.

Program Theory

Program theory began with the work of Chen and Rossi (1983), which is discussed in more detail in Chapter 3. In its early days, it was largely based on attempts to identify and quantify those variables that would have an impact on program outcomes. Through the years, other evaluators have used program theory to develop ways of describing the evaluand, known as **logic models** or **log frames** (discussed in Chapter 7). These are graphic depictions of the inputs, resources, assumptions, activities, outcomes, outputs, and impacts of a program being evaluated. Donaldson and Lipsey (2006) have contributed greatly to the use of program-theory-driven evaluation by extending this approach to different methodologies in evaluation. Bledsoe and Graham (2005) demonstrate this mixing of program theory and multiple approaches in their combination of the program-theory-driven approach with an inclusive, transformative approach that also has elements of a utilization approach and empowerment evaluation. Program-theory-based approaches are discussed further in Chapters 3 and 6.

Trochim (1998) believes that evaluators rely too much on social science theory and too little on the perceptions of stakeholders who are closest to the programs. Social science theory can be useful to provide broad guidance on such areas as literacy development or motivation; however, it does not reflect the specific contextual needs of stakeholders. He has developed mechanisms to help elicit the program theory that the stakeholders have about what is needed for a program to be successful. He calls these the "implicit theories" that the people closest to the program hold.

Evaluators' Roles

Ryan and Schwandt (2002) connect evaluation theory with evaluators' roles quite directly: "The concept of the 'role of the evaluator' is central to the theory and practice of evaluation" (p. vii). If we accept the description of evaluation theory as what we do and who we are as evaluators, then this connection seems important as part of the theoretical explorations in this chapter. Each major branch of evaluation theorists and approaches within those branches discuss roles of the evaluator that emphasize different aspects of what evaluators do and the roles they assume.

Skolits, Morrow, and Burr (2009) suggest that linking evaluators' roles with specific approaches does not do justice to the complexity and dynamic nature of the roles that evaluators play in practice. They argue that during the course of an evaluation, evaluators play many different roles, depending on the stage of the evaluation and the demands of the situation. They examine what they consider to be a generic list of activities that most evaluators are called upon to pursue in an external evaluation, and then describe dominant and supportive roles for an evaluator. Although these roles change from the beginning to the middle to the end of an evaluation, one role is dominant throughout: the role of manager. Evaluators need to be able to manage the complex process of planning an evaluation, implementing it, and bringing it to closure. Skolits et al. also identify specific roles that occur more commonly during the planning, implementation, and postevaluation phases. (See Figure 2.4.)

· · · · · · · · · · E X T E N D I N G   Y O U R   T H I N K I N G · · · · · · · · · ·

Evaluators' Roles

1. Which evaluators' roles have you had experience in doing in your life?

2. Which roles do you think you will do well in?

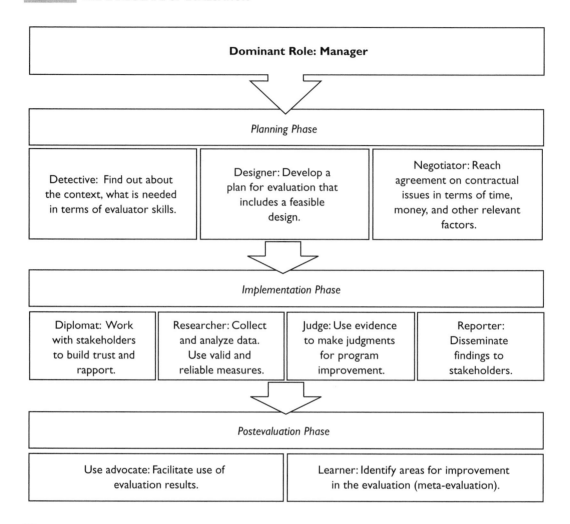

Figure 2.4. Evaluators' roles throughout the course of an evaluation. *Source:* Based on Skolits, Morrow, and Burr (2009, pp. 282–283).

This generic depiction of evaluators' roles is useful to see how evaluators adopt different roles throughout the course of a study. Theorists associated with different branches of evaluation emphasize different aspects of these roles. Hence in the discussion of these branches in Part II, the roles of evaluators are examined in specific theoretical contexts. The different paradigms offer food for thought in terms of concepts that provide a more nuanced picture of evaluators' roles, such as values, political contexts, objectivity, distance from or involvement with stakeholders, bias, and advocacy.

Because evaluation occurs in political contexts, the roles of evaluators necessitate attention to the social relations that occur in an evaluation study (Abma & Widdershoven, 2008). Skolits et al.'s (2009) model suggests the importance of political context in an evaluator's role as diplomat. Abma and Widdershoven (2008) emphasize the pervasive need for evaluators to be aware of their roles in terms of social relations with stakeholders. The quality of the relations established and maintained throughout the study determines, in part, the quality of the results. Skolits et al. extend the discussion of evaluators' roles with these points:

▦ Part of an evaluator's role is to establish social relations with stakeholders and monitor those relations throughout a study. This includes being aware of and responsive to possible power differences that might result in conflicts. Conflict is not necessarily bad; it can be an opportunity to address important issues if it is handled appropriately.

▦ An evaluator is often called upon to play a leadership role in terms of making possible conflicts visible and providing space for discussions about the situation to occur.

▦ Evaluators also play an important role as communicators throughout the life of the study. They need to be effective communicators not just when they write the final report, but from their first contacts with clients and through the many interim contacts with various stakeholders.

▦ Evaluators work as facilitators of change, especially if a project includes a phase of formative evaluation in which the intent is to improve the program during the course of the study.

▦ Evaluators also provide insights in terms of the program's context and the constraints and opportunities that the evaluation encounters. For example, if there are limited funds or negative stereotypes that need to be addressed in the discussion of program changes, an evaluator can propose these as variables to be included, in addition to evaluation data on process or outcomes.

Abma and Widdershoven (2008) summarize the roles of the evaluators for the four major evaluation branches. A graphic version of their summary is displayed in Figure 2.5.

Method Evaluator as objective, neutral party	**Use** Social relations manager to facilitate use
Values Communicator who engages in meaningful dialogue	**Social Justice** Relationship builder based on trust and cultural respect; investigator of structural inequities

Figure 2.5. Evaluators' roles by major evaluation branches. *Source:* Based on Abma and Widdershoven (2008).

In Part II

This chapter's summary of the status of philosophy, theory, approaches, methods, and roles prepares you for Part II of this book, in which specific branches of evaluation are examined in more detail. In particular, you will be using the terms and asking the questions listed below for the remainder of the book. Figure 2.6 is an illustration of this list; it will be a helpful guide as you read Part II.

1. The axiological belief system asks: What is the nature of ethics?

2. The ontological belief system asks: What is the nature of reality?

3. The epistemological belief system asks: What is the nature of knowledge, and what is the relationship between the knower and that which would be known?

4. The methodological belief system asks: What are the systematic approaches to gathering information about what would be known?

Part II also addresses the philosophy, theories, and approaches of the four major evaluation branches: Methods, Use, Values, and Social Justice. Specific approaches that are commensurate with the philosophical assumptions associated with each branch are explained. In addition, extensive examples of the components of evaluation studies are provided to give you a context in which to place the discussion of theoretical

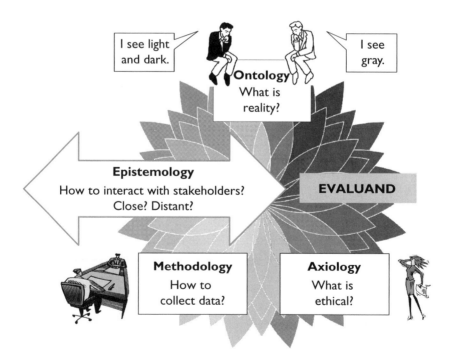

Figure 2.6. The four philosophical belief systems in evaluations, and the questions associated with them.

positions. Thus each chapter presents examples of evaluation studies in summary form, with the various components identified. Many of the evaluators who conducted these studies also provide commentary on the process they used and the challenges they faced in the conduct of the study.

Notes

1. Fitzpatrick, Sanders, and Worthen (2004) describe five major approaches to evaluation (objectives-oriented, management-oriented, consumer-oriented, expertise-oriented, and participant-oriented). Stufflebeam and Shinkfield (2007) focus on eight recommended approaches that they situate in four categories: questions and methods (objectives-based evaluations, experimental design, and case study); improvement and accountability (context input–process product model and consumer-oriented evaluations); social agenda and advocacy (responsive/client-centered evaluations and constructivist evaluations); and eclectic (utilization evaluations). We have chosen to use an adaptation of Alkin's roots model because it fits more comfortably with the concept of paradigms which enable evaluators to clarify the assumptions that guide their work.

2. Critics of Alkin and Christie's (2004) evaluation tree have also mentioned the lack of attention given to evaluators who work in private industry and nonprofits, such as the Brookings Institute, the Rand Corporation, the Urban Institute, and Westat. The evaluators on the original tree are primarily academic sociologists and psychologists. Few, if any, economists or statisticians are listed on the tree.

3. If you want to know more about the ocean's currents, you can consult the NOAA website in the References. There are five major ocean currents: in the North Atlantic, South Atlantic, North Pacific, South Pacific, and Indian Oceans (NOAA, 2009). The Gulf Stream in the North Atlantic is the largest and most powerful, and it is fed by a current from North Africa to the West Indies. When the Gulf Stream reaches South America, it splits into the Caribbean Current (which goes into the Caribbean Sea and the Gulf of Mexico) and the Antilles Current (which flows to the West Indies). The Caribbean Current flows up the eastern coast of the United States. It turns off south of Newfoundland, producing eddies that flow toward the United Kingdom and Norway.

HISTORICAL AND CONTEMPORARY
EVALUATION PARADIGMS, BRANCHES,
THEORIES, AND APPROACHES

Part II is organized to provide a detailed examination of the major evaluation paradigms, branches, and theorists' approaches. It includes four chapters, one for each of the major paradigms:

- Chapter 3. The Postpositivist Paradigm and the Methods Branch
  - The Postpositivist Paradigm
  - Methods Branch Theorists
  - Theory to Practice
  - Critiques of the Methods Branch
  - Your Evaluation Plan: Your Philosophical Stance

- Chapter 4. The Pragmatic Paradigm and the Use Branch
  - The Pragmatic Paradigm
  - Use Branch Theorists
  - Theory to Practice
  - Critiques of the Use Branch
  - Your Evaluation Plan: Your Philosophical Stance

- Chapter 5. The Constructivist Paradigm and the Values Branch
  - The Constructivist Paradigm
  - Values Branch Theorists
  - Theory to Practice
  - Your Evaluation Plan: Your Philosophical Stance

- Chapter 6. The Transformative Paradigm and the Social Justice Branch
  - The Transformative Paradigm
  - Social Justice Branch Theorists
  - Theory to Practice
  - Your Evaluation Plan: Your Philosophical Stance

Dividing the world of evaluation into four separate paradigms is one way of organizing the major influences that have affected the evolution of this transdiscipline. Some of the differences among the various paradigms are fundamental and lead to very different approaches. If you are a novice evaluator, remember that evaluators who might situate themselves more strongly in one of the paradigmatic positions than in the others share a common desire to see effective interventions that work toward social betterment (Christie, 2007; Henry & Mark, 2003; Mark & Henry, 2004; Mark, Henry, & Julnes, 2000).

Paul and Marfo (2001, p. 532) provide this historical glimpse into the concept of paradigm in evaluation:

> Guba (1990) provided one of the most useful analyses of alternative paradigms and their relevance to education. In an edited collection of papers presented at a conference on the paradigm dialog, Guba distinguished among paradigms of positivism, postpositivism, constructivism, and critical theory.[1] He and his colleagues, who contributed papers, analyzed the paradigms along three dimensions: ontological, epistemological, and methodological. They also considered the ethical meaning and implications of various paradigmatic orientations. This and other works addressing the larger paradigm issues in research offer two overarching messages for educators. The first is that paradigms differ in their assumptions about what is real, the nature of the relationship between the one who knows and what is known, and how the knower goes about discovering or constructing knowledge. The second is that paradigms shape, constrain, and enable all aspects of educational inquiry.

Sample studies are used in this section to illustrate the differences in evaluation planning, implementation, and use that reflect differences in evaluators' underlying assumptions. The sample studies were chosen in part to provide pictures of evaluation within each of the four major branches that characterize historical and contemporary views of evaluation.

Evaluation studies typically include a number of elements. The typical elements of an evaluation study—along with information about each element, and the chapters of this book in which is each is covered—appear below. It should be noted that information about each element may not be reported in all the sample studies included in this text. Therefore, we have included as much detail about the sample studies as was available from the published versions. We have also contacted the authors of many of the studies to ask them to correct our summaries, add details that they feel are relevant, and provide reflective commentary that they think will be useful for novice evaluators.

■ *The evaluators:* Who are the evaluators? What are their disciplinary backgrounds? What is the nature of their experience in evaluation? What are the skills and competencies needed for this evaluation? (Chapters 2, 3, 4, 5, and 6)

■ *Philosophical and theoretical lenses:* Through what philosophical and theoretical lenses do the evaluators view their work? What values do the evaluators hold? What is the nature of the relationship between the evaluators and the community in which the evaluation is conducted? (Chapters 2, 3, 4, 5, and 6)

▨ *The evaluand and its context:* What was the entity being evaluated? How did the evaluator depict the evaluand? What contextual variables were relevant in this evaluation? (Chapter 7)

▨ *Method:* How was the evaluand evaluated? What design was used? What were the evaluation purposes and questions? Who were the stakeholders and participants, and how were they selected (sampling strategies)? What methods of data collection were used? What indicators were used to determine achievement of goals? How did the evaluators analyze the data? How were the evaluation results used? (Chapters 2, 7, 8, 9, 10, 11, and 12)

▨ *Management and budget:* How did the evaluators implement the evaluation plans in terms of time and resources? (Chapter 14)

▨ *Meta-evaluation:* How did the evaluators evaluate the evaluation? (Chapters 8 and 14)

▨ *Reports and utilization:* How were the evaluation processes and outcomes used? What reports were generated from the evaluation? (Chapter 13)

A Word about Evaluands

Evaluators evaluate many different types of things. As mentioned in Chapter 1, members of the evaluation community use the term "evaluand" to indicate the generic object of their work. The evaluand can be a program, project, policy, climate, or product.[2] Evaluation plans are often developed for long-standing programs, but sometimes evaluators are engaged before there is a program to evaluate, in order to determine what type of program is needed (needs assessment). Sometimes they are asked to focus on specific aspects of a program and conduct studies such as cost analysis. On other occasions, they are asked to develop evaluation plans based on a description of a potential program that appears in a proposal for funding before that program is actually developed or implemented. This gives evaluators many opportunities to be creative in their work.

Box II.1 displays the sample studies used throughout this text and shows how they relate to the various evaluation branches. These studies represent the various branches of philosophy and theory in evaluation. The studies discussed in separate boxes in Chapters 3–6 are associated with specific icons.

Box II.1. Sample Studies, Evaluation Approaches, and Topical Areas for Each Theoretical Branch

Sample study	Evaluation approach	Topical area
Φ4Σ8Ω≤pμ **Methods Branch**		
Brady and O'Regan (2009)	Mixed methods with randomized controlled design (also, theory-based evaluation; logic model)	Youth mentoring in Ireland
Duwe and Kerschner (2008)	Quasi-experimental design; cost analysis	Preventing return to prison in the United States
Fredericks, Deegan, and Carman (2008)	Theory-based evaluation	Demonstration program for people with developmental disabilities
Busch, O'Brien, and Spangler (2005)	Training evaluation using Kirkpatrick's model	School leadership
Coryn, Schröter, and Hanssen (2009)	Time series with success cases method	Homelessness and unemployment
Donaldson and Gooler (2002)	Participatory theory-based evaluation	Employment and mental health in the United States
French et al. (2000)	Cost analysis	Addiction program cost benefit analysis in the United States
Bloom and Riccio (2005)	Quasi-experimental design; cost analysis	Job programs and public housing in the United States
Borman et al. (2007)	Quasi-experimental design	Reading reform: Success for All
Planty et al. (2009)	Surveys	U.S. schools, poverty, and quality of education
Fredericks et al. (2008)	Theory-based evaluation; logic model; external evaluation	Developmental disabilities
Johnson, Young, Suresh, and Berbaum (2002)	Randomized experiment	Drug abuse treatment training in Peru
Moss and Yeaton (2006)	Regression discontinuity	Developmental English at a community college

Sample study	Evaluation approach	Topical area
Use Branch		
Stufflebeam, Gullickson, and Wingate (2002)	Context, input, process, product (CIPP) evaluation	Housing for poor people in Hawaii
Walden and Baxter (2001)	Utilization-focused evaluation (UFE)	Condom use among sex workers
Sutherland (2004)	Learning organization evaluation	School reform in high-poverty areas in the United States
Fetterman (2009)	Empowerment evaluation	Improving clerkships for medical students
Sharma and Deepak (2001)	Practical participatory evaluation	Community-based rehabilitation (CBR) with disabled persons
Chinman, Imm, and Wandersman (2004)	Empowerment evaluation	Alcohol, tobacco, and drug use in the United States
Marra (2000)	Utilization-focused formative and summative evaluation, not monitoring	Corruption in Uganda and Tanzania
Values Branch		
Stufflebeam, Gullickson, and Wingate (2002)	Goal-free evaluation	Housing for poor people in Hawaii
Barela (2008)	Case study	Los Angeles Unified School District case study
Trotman (2006)	Connoisseurship evaluation	Imagination and creativity
Abma (2005)	Responsive evaluation	Injury prevention in a dance academy in the Netherlands
Greene and Lee (2006)	Qualitative, responsive evaluation	School reform in the United States
Mareschal, McKee, Jackson, and Hanson (2007)	Case study: Formative evaluation and stakeholders	Using technology to prevent youth violence

(cont.)

	Box II.1 *(cont.)*	
Sample study	*Evaluation approach*	*Topical area*
	Social Justice Branch	
House (2004)	Deliberative democratic evaluation (DDE)	Denver bilingual program
Pennarz, Holicek, Rasidagic, and Rogers (2007)	Country-led evaluation (CLE)	Bosnia-Herzegovina poverty reduction study
Fierro (2006)	Critical race theory (CRT) evaluation	Welfare-to-work program in Philadelphia
Cross, Earle, Echo-Hawk Solie, : Manness (2000)	Indigenous evaluation	Mental health services in Indian country
Zulli and Frierson (2004)	Culturally responsive evaluation	Upward Bound program in North Carolina
Mertens, Harris, Holmes, and Brandt (2007)	Disability- and deaf-rights-based evaluation	Teacher preparation in deaf education at Gallaudet University
Seigart (2007)	Feminist evaluation	School health issues in Australia, the United States, and Canada
Buskens and Earl (2008)	Transformative participatory evaluation	Breast feeding to prevent HIV/AIDS in infants in Africa
Rosenstein and Ganem (2008)	Participatory and cyclical evaluation	Kindergarten teaching in Israel
Ghertner (2006)	Gender analysis	Cookstove program in India
Horn, McCracken, Dina, and Brayboy (2008)	Indigenous evaluation	Cessation of tobacco smoking among American Indian teens

Notes

1. Guba labels the fourth paradigm "critical theory." As explained in Chapter 2, we use the term "transformative" for the fourth paradigm, in order to maintain consistency in the level of abstraction from paradigm to theory.

2. As noted in Chapter 1, personnel evaluation is not the focus of this book.

Preparing to Read Chapter Three

The following table appears at the beginning of each chapter in Part II, with the evaluation branch covered in that chapter and its associated paradigm highlighted. For example, the Methods Branch and the postpositivist paradigm are highlighted for this chapter. This table can serve as a map to help you find your way through Part II.

Branch	Paradigm	Description
Methods Φ4Σ8Ω≤pμ	**Postpositivist**	**Focuses primarily on quantitative designs and data**
Use	Pragmatic	Focuses primarily on data that are found to be useful by stakeholders; advocates for the use of mixed methods
Values	Constructivist	Focuses primarily on identifying multiple values and perspectives through qualitative methods
Social justice	Transformative	Focuses primarily on viewpoints of marginalized groups and interrogating systemic power structures through mixed methods to further social justice and human rights

As you prepare to read this chapter, think about these questions:

1. What are the characteristics of the postpositivist paradigm?

2. How do those characteristics influence the practice of evaluation?

3. Which of the major thinkers have contributed to the approaches associated with the Methods Branch?

4. How did the ideas grow from the early days to the present in this theoretical context?

CHAPTER THREE

The Postpositivist Paradigm
and the Methods Branch

The Postpositivist Paradigm

Weiss (1998) asserted that the traditional and still dominant role conceptualization of evaluators is methods-based and representative of a neutral, detached social scientist: "The traditional role of the evaluator has been one of detached objective inquiry.... She puts her trust in methodology" (p. 98) ... Mark (2002) cited Campbell's (1969) view of an evaluator's role as a "technical servant" to an experimenting society as an example of the traditional methods-based understanding of an evaluator's role. (Skolits et al., 2009, p. 277)

The Methods Branch reflects evaluation's roots in applied social research involving the use of rigorous methods of inquiry, largely based in the assumptions of the positivist and postpositivist paradigms. The origins of the positivist paradigm can be traced back to the writings of Sir Francis Bacon (1561–1626), in which he articulated the principles of the scientific method (Turner, 2001). In the 1800s, Comte and Spencer contributed to the development of the positivist paradigm in the social sciences, seeing it as a means of improving society by applying scientific methods to discover laws about human behavior. Under this philosophical banner, social research was viewed as the search for general laws of human organization through the conduct of empirical observations.

In the 1950s in the United States, positivism became associated with **quantitative research,** measurement, and statistical analysis as a way of testing hypotheses about the general laws applied to human behavior. Positivists hold the ontological belief that one reality exists and that it is independent of the observer (Fielding, 2009). Their epistemological belief is that distance from the object of study contributes to avoiding bias. The positiv-

In U.S. schools, many people have early experiences with the scientific method. Do you remember your elementary-school science class where you wrapped a bean in a wet paper towel and then wrote up your "experiment"? The scientific method includes a problem statement, hypothesis, experiment (materials and method), results, and conclusion. Did your bean grow? The results were pretty black and white, weren't they? Either the bean grew, or it didn't.

ist paradigm's methodological belief is associated with an approach prioritizing the use of true experiments, which require random selection of subjects and random assignment to interventions—conditions that can be very difficult to satisfy in the world of social research and evaluation.

Campbell (1991) envisioned the role of researchers in terms of an "experimenting society," which would make use of social science research methods to test theories to improve society. He offered a way for researchers to adapt the principles of positivism by the development of **quasi-experimental methods** (i.e., designs sharing many characteristics with experimental designs, but adapted for use with human populations) (Shadish & Cook, 1998). This topic is discussed at great length in Chapter 9. Hence the research and evaluation world came to operate more under the belief systems of the postpositivist paradigm than of the positivist paradigm. Postpositivists still hold to the methodological belief in quantitative approaches; however, they have reframed their ontological view of reality to take into account the complexity of human behavior. The ontological belief continues to be that there is one reality; postpositivists have added the notion that reality can be known within a certain level of probability. Distance from the object of study continues to be a hallmark of the epistemological belief system in postpositivism. Researchers strive to be "objective" by limiting their contact or involvement with people in the study. Campbell did not view experimental and quasi-experimental approaches as the only possible methods for conducting social research and evaluation; however, he did hold that true experiments are superior to other approaches because of their potential to control for bias.

Postpositivism is a major paradigm that guides many evaluators in their work. The axiological assumption of this paradigm is intertwined with the methodological assumption, in that the conduct of "good research" is a fundamental requirement for ethical conduct. Good research is described as that which reflects "intellectual honesty, the suppression of personal bias, [and] careful collection of empirical studies" (Jennings & Callahan, 1983; cited in Christians, 2005, p. 159).

The postpositivist paradigm axiological assumption is closely aligned with the ethical principles articulated by the National Commission for the Protection of Human Subjects of Biomedical and Behavioral Research (1979) in its Belmont Report (see Sieber, 1992, pp. 18–19). This report identifies three ethical principles and six norms that should guide scientific research:

Ethical Principles

1. *Beneficence:* Maximizing good outcomes for science, humanity, and the individual research participants and minimizing or avoiding unnecessary risk, harm, or wrong.

2. *Respect:* Treating people with respect and courtesy, including those who are not autonomous (e.g., small children, people who are intellectually challenged or senile).

3. *Justice:* Ensuring that those who bear the risk in the research are the ones who benefit from it; ensuring that the procedures are reasonable, nonexploitative, carefully considered, and fairly administered.

Norms of Scientific Research

1. A valid research design must be used. Faulty research is not useful to anyone and not only is a waste of time and money, but also cannot be described as ethical, in that it does not contribute to the well-being of participants.

2. The researcher must be competent to conduct the research.

3. Consequences of the research must be identified: Procedures must respect privacy, ensure confidentiality, maximize benefits, and minimize risks.

4. The sample selection must be appropriate for the purposes of the study, representative of the population to benefit from the study, and sufficient in number.

5. The participants must agree to participate in the study through voluntary informed consent—that is, without threat or undue inducement (voluntary), knowing what a reasonable person in the same situation would want to know before giving consent (informed), and explicitly agreeing to participate (consent).

6. The researcher must inform the participants whether harm will be compensated.

These principles and norms apply to all evaluators, no matter what their philosophical or theoretical beliefs. However, evaluators who hold different paradigmatic beliefs typically interpret these principles and norms differently, as will be seen in subsequent chapters.

·········· **EXTENDING YOUR THINKING** ··········
Ethical Principles and Norms

1. Goode (1996) created personal ads in a newspaper in order to gather data to learn more about courtship through personal advertisements. He did not respond to any of the men and women who answered his ads, and their identities remained anonymous. Do you think that this kind of research follows ethical principles and norms of scientific inquiry as described above? Explain.

2. Locate and review one website or article about unethical practices in evaluation. Why are ethics needed in the world of evaluation?

Situated in the postpositivist paradigm, Mark and Gamble (2009) suggest that the methodological choice of a randomized experimental design is ethically justified when the purpose of the study is to establish a cause-and-effect relationship and there is uncertainty about the effect of a particular intervention, because this design provides greater value in terms of demonstrating the effects of a treatment than do other approaches. According to Mark and Gamble, "a case can be made that good ethics justifies the use of research methods that will give the best answer about program effectiveness as this may increase the likelihood of good outcomes especially for those initially disadvantaged" (2009, p. 205).

········· E X T E N D I N G   Y O U R   T H I N K I N G ·········

Philosophical Assumptions of the Postpositivist Paradigm and the Methods Branch

Using the table below, answer the following questions:

1. Can you imagine what a postpositivist evaluation would look like?

2. How would the evaluator set up the evaluation?

3. Would the evaluator be involved with the stakeholders or not?

4. How would the evaluator's assumptions guide his/her decisions?

The Postpositivist Paradigm and the Methods Branch

Description	Axiological assumption	Ontological assumption	Epistemological assumption	Methodological assumption
Focuses primarily on quantitative designs and data	• Respect • Justice • Beneficence	One reality knowable within a certain level of probability	• Distant • Objective	• Scientific method • Hypothesis • Quantitative methods

Methods Branch Theorists

Methods Branch theorists have had and continue to have a great deal of influence on what is considered to be good evaluation. This brief history provides you with the necessary building blocks to proceed with the planning of evaluations that are reflective of lessons learned by eminent evaluators. Alkin (2004) identifies the following evaluation theorists in the Methods Branch: Tyler, Campbell, Cook, Shadish, Cronbach, Rossi, Chen, Henry, Mark, and Boruch.[1] We add Lipsey and Donaldson as contributors to the Methods Branch, especially as it is envisioned in a theory-based evaluation. And we add Kirkpatrick as another contributor to this branch, because of his model of the evaluation of training. These theoretical positions are explained briefly and used to build a composite picture of current views of "methods" as a theoretical basis for evaluation practice. Advantages and challenges associated with approaches that reflect this branch are discussed. Examples of studies that reflect the Methods Branch illustrate how these theoretical perspectives are manifested in practice.

Methods Branch Theorists

Ralph Tyler
Donald Campbell
Thomas Cook
William Shadish
Robert Boruch
Lee Cronbach
Peter Rossi
Gary Henry
Mel Mark
Huey-Tsyh Chen
Mark Lipsey
Stuart Donaldson
Donald Kirkpatrick
Robert Brinkerhoff

Specific emphasis is placed on those aspects of these approaches that lead to designs addressing issues of causality.

Early Theorists and Theories

Ralph Tyler used the term "educational evaluation" back in the 1930s, making him one of the earliest scholars in this field (Fitzpatrick, Worth, & Sanders, 2004; Stufflebeam & Shinkfield, 2007). His approach to evaluation consisted primarily of establishing educational objectives and then determining whether those objectives had been met. An evaluator met with educators to determine broad goals and the desired student behaviors that the teachers hoped to see following instruction (the "objectives," now more commonly known as "student outcomes"). Then the educators were supposed to design the curriculum to teach what was needed in order to achieve the objectives. The evaluator gave advice on the development of measures to determine whether the objectives were achieved. The results of the assessment were compared with the desired results to reach a judgment about the effectiveness of the instruction. Tyler is perhaps best known for his evaluation study known as the Eight-Year Study, which involved evaluation of the effectiveness of educational initiatives across the nation (Smith & Tyler, 1942). Although he did not employ experimental and control groups, he did posit that establishment of clear objectives and rigorous measurement of outcomes were key components of educational evaluation.

Donald Campbell's work in the early years of evaluation is discussed in the opening to this chapter: his contribution to the use of experimental and quasi-experimental designs and their role in controlling for extraneous variables in determining causal relationships. He did identify himself with the experimental approach and to quantification, but at the same time realized that other approaches could contribute to increased understanding of program effects (Campbell, 1991; Shadish & Cook, 1998).

Thomas Cook, William Shadish, and **Robert Boruch** extended the evaluation community's understanding of the Methods Branch. Boruch (1997) published an early book that explained how randomized designs could be used in evaluation; he continues to contribute to the conversations on that topic (Boruch, 2007). Cook published a book with Donald Campbell that expanded on the topic of quasi-experiments (Cook & Campbell, 1979); then Shadish partnered with Thomas Cook and Laura Leviton (Shadish et al., 1991) to write about the foundations of program evaluation. Cook, Campbell, and Boruch were faculty members at Northwestern University when Shadish accepted a postdoctoral position there. This set the stage for Cook and Shadish to work together to further understandings of the use of experimental approaches in evaluation. Connections with Northwestern University are evident for a number of theorists in the Methods Branch.

Lee Cronbach also focused on the role of evaluation in addressing social problems. He believed that an evaluator needs to work as an educator to inform stakeholders and policy makers about the methods and findings of evaluation. He served as Ralph Tyler's assistant during his early years in Chicago. Cronbach is well known for his contributions to measurement theory, particularly the development of Cronbach's alpha as a reliability indicator, as well as improved understandings of validity (Shavelson, 2002). Cronbach agreed with Tyler on the need for specific objectives and good measurement; he also agreed with Cook and Shadish on the importance of using experimental designs. Moreover, he acknowledged that not all evaluations would be conducive to the use of such designs. One of his contributions consisted of suggesting that giving information to teachers or students at the end of a school year (or intervention cycle) did not give the teachers or students a chance to improve their learning. Hence he suggested opportunities for feedback at frequent intervals.

Peter Rossi contributed his thinking to evaluation from the perspective of evaluation research in the form of survey methods and social science experiments. He began writing about the connection between evaluation and social policy in the early 1970s. He continued making contributions along this line through his multiple books, the last of which was published in 2004 with coauthors Mark Lipsey and Howard Freeman (Rossi et al., 2004). The strength of his contribution is in the explanation of how randomized controlled designs and quasi-experimental designs could be used in evaluation, and how evaluation findings could be tied to national policy in education and human services.

Gary Henry and Melvin Mark (Mark was also a student at Northwestern) extended theories of evaluation in the context of the use of causal modeling for evaluation, with particular attention to ethical issues (Mark & Gamble, 2009; Mark & Henry, 2006). They also presented extensions of a theory of evaluation that Pawson and Tilley (1997) discussed, known as "emergent realist evaluation" (ERE) theory (Henry, Julnes, & Mark, 1998). For Henry et al., ERE is a theoretical position based on the philosophy of neorealism, which holds that a reality exists independently of the observer and that regularities in the patterns of events can be explained by generative mechanisms (e.g., you can observe a tree falling and infer that gravity is a generative mechanism that pulls the tree to earth). ERE reflects earlier Methods Branch theorists' views in these terms, as well as in the view that evaluation has a role to play in making sense of what is going on in the world. However, ERE offers an additional twist on these earlier views:

> Emerging realist (ER) evaluators explicitly recognize that different individuals and groups assign varying levels of importance to different values, and that choices made in the evaluation process can serve some value perspectives and the parties that hold them over others. In addition, ER evaluators believe that the value positions surrounding social programs can and should be directly studied, and it is this belief that differentiates the ERE position on values from many other approaches to evaluation. (Henry et al., 1998, p. 6)

Theory–Based Evaluation

"Theory-based evaluation" is an approach that focuses on the theories people have about what it takes to have a successful program. In simple terms, you could think about how people learn or how they change their behavior. What conditions need to be in place for that to happen?

Huey-Tsyh Chen (1994, 2005; Chen & Rossi, 1980, 1983) worked with Peter Rossi to develop the concept of theory-based evaluation as the logical extension of quantitative models that permit identification of variables contributing to the outcomes of a program. The "theory" part of this approach consists of the social science theories and stakeholders' beliefs (theories) about what is necessary for a program to succeed. Lipsey (2007) describes Chen and Rossi's early arguments as follows:

Methods Branch Theorists

Ralph Tyler
Donald Campbell
Thomas Cook
William Shadish
Robert Boruch
Lee Cronbach
Peter Rossi
Gary Henry
Mel Mark
Huey-Tsyh Chen
Mark Lipsey
Stuart Donaldson
Donald Kirkpatrick
Robert Brinkerhoff

Each social program embodies a theory of sorts—an action theory that reflects the assumptions inherent in the program about the nature of the social problem it addresses and the way it expects to bring about change in that problem. Chen and Rossi argued that evaluators should bring that theory to the surface and, if necessary, draw on other sources to further differentiate it. (p. 200)

One approach to theory-based evaluation involves the use of sophisticated statistical analyses such as path analysis and structural equation modeling (discussed in Chapter 12) to determine the significant contributions of theoretically derived variables to the outcomes. Interestingly, Chen (1994) saw theory-based evaluation as a move *away* from methods-driven evaluation. He argued that if evaluators started with a method (e.g., experimental design), then that would lead them to specific directives for how to conduct the evaluation. However, if the evaluators started with the theory of what was supposed to make the program work, then they would consider different methodological options. He recommends the use of both quantitative and qualitative methods in evaluation; however, for outcome evaluations he supports the use of randomized experimental designs in order to control threats to validity. Because he divorces himself from method as the determinant factor for evaluation decisions, his work provides a bridge to other branches in the evaluation tree.

Mark Lipsey is another notable theorist who has contributed to the development of theory-based evaluation. He justified the need to add attention to the theory of programs by writing:

Conventional treatment effectiveness research, speaking generally, is based on constructs that substantially underrepresent the complexity of the causal processes at issue; it is theoretically impoverished and yields little knowledge of practical value; it is crudely operationalized and rarely meets even minimal standards for quality of design and measurement; it is largely insensitive to the very treatment effects it purports to study; and its results and conclusions are largely a matter of chance and have little to do with the efficacy of the treatments under consideration. (Lipsey, 1988, p. 6)

He went on to suggest that evaluators need to develop strategies to determine the underlying theory of programs, identify mediating variables that influence outcomes, and develop designs reflecting more real-world conditions.

Stewart Donaldson (2007; Donaldson & Lipsey, 2006) offers a change in labeling for evaluations that have program theory at their core. He defines "program-theory-driven evaluation science" as "the systematic use of substantive knowledge about the phenomena under investigation and scientific methods to improve, to produce knowledge and feedback about, and to determine the merit, worth, and significance of evaluands such as social, educational, health, community, and organizational programs" (Donaldson, 2007, p. 9). The rationale for this label is that evaluators use the program theory to define and prioritize evaluation questions. The evaluators build a program theory with stakeholders by reviewing documents, prior research, talking with stakeholders, and observing the program in operation. They then use scientific methods to answer the evaluation questions.

Evaluation of Training Programs

The "**Kirkpatrick** model" for evaluation of training programs dominated human resource development evaluations for many decades (Kirkpatrick, 1975, 1998; Nickols, 2005). It essentially has four levels of evaluation: participant reactions, learning, behavior, and results. This model was extended to consider the financial return on investment (ROI) of training by Phillips (1997). Reaction evaluation is probably a familiar format for most of you who have participated in training programs. At the end of the program, your reactions are evaluated by means of a questionnaire that asks whether you found the training relevant, interesting, worthwhile, and appropriately conducted. Learning is evaluated in terms of the knowledge or skills gained or changes in attitudes from the training. Behavior changes refer to changes in performance on the job or in a simulated situation. Results refer to the impact of the training on the organization in terms of its effectiveness of successful achievement of its mission. ROI measures how the results of the training affect the organization's bottom line. A list of resources for evaluations of training programs is found in Box 3.1.

Russ-Eft and Preskill (2005) criticize the Kirkpatrick model and ROI because these are based on an assumption that if people like the training (i.e., have a positive reaction), this will affect the bottom-line results. A model for evaluation of training that is situated in the Use Branch is discussed in Chapter 4.

Brinkerhoff (2003) also developed an impact model for training evaluations called the "success case method," which includes both quantitative and qualitative data. He recommends its use in contexts in which a full experimental study is not feasible. This method has six steps:

1. Create a focus for the evaluation and develop a plan.

2. Develop an impact model for the intervention that depicts how it will achieve its results (akin to a logic model).

Methods Branch Theorists

Ralph Tyler
Donald Campbell
Thomas Cook
William Shadish
Robert Boruch
Lee Cronbach
Peter Rossi
Gary Henry
Mel Mark
Huey-Tsyh Chen
Mark Lipsey
Stuart Donaldson
Donald Kirkpatrick
Robert Brinkerhoff

Box 3.1. Resources for Evaluating Training Programs

■ A section of the Business Performance website updates the Kirkpatrick model (*www.businessperform.com/workplace-training/evaluating_training_effectiven.html*).

■ A National Staff Development and Training Association (NSDTA) publication by Parry and Berdie (1999) is very useful.

■ The NSDTA journal, *Training and Development in Human Services*, published a special issue on training evaluation in 2007. This issue, and the proceedings of the annual National Human Services Training Evaluation Symposium, are available at NSDTA's website (*nsdta.aphsa.org*).

■ The American Society for Training and Development website (*www.astd.org*) is another valuable resource.

■ Finally, Phillips (1997) provides a detailed review of this area.

3. Conduct a survey with all participants to identify those who were successful and those who were not.

4. Select a random sample from each group, and interview these individuals to get their stories.

5. Prepare a report with the findings, conclusions, and recommendations; these sometimes take the form of "success stories."

6. Report on ROI in terms of the benefit to the company; divide the benefit (a performance measure) by the cost of the training to obtain the ratio of ROI.

Theory to Practice

This section of the chapter is divided into three parts. The first part looks at practice based on the work of Methods Branch theorists who prioritize the use of experimental and quasi-experimental designs (e.g., Brady & O'Regan, 2009; Duwe & Kerschner, 2008). The second part looks at practice based on the work of Methods Branch theorists who prioritize theory-based evaluation approaches (e.g., Donaldson & Gooler, 2002). The third part contains examples of the evaluation of training programs via methods-based approaches. Here is a "map" of this section, showing that we begin with looking at experimental and quasi-experimental approaches to evaluation.

Theory to Practice: Methods Branch

1. **Experimental** and quasi-experimental approaches

2. Theory-based evaluation

3. Evaluation of training programs

Experimental and Quasi-Experimental Approaches

Independent and Dependent Variables; Experimental and Control Groups

Experimental and quasi-experimental studies have an intervention designed to create change in knowledge, behavior, attitudes, aptitude, or some other construct. The **independent variable** is the program (or policy or process) that is implemented in hopes of seeing a change in knowledge, behavior, attitude, aptitude, or some other relevant construct (the **dependent variable**).

One application of this approach is embodied in the U.S. government's What Works Clearinghouse (WWC; *ies.ed.gov/ncee/wwc*), which was established to identify effective programs in human service areas. The WWC is a product of the U.S. Department of Education's Institute of Education Sciences. The Institute has established standards for the review of methods used to indicate the effectiveness of programs funded by the Department of Education, including programs for reading, dropout prevention, early childhood education, elementary school math, English language learners, and middle school math. Each intervention is rated on the degree to which it meets the WWC standards as having either strong evidence ("meets evidence standards"), weaker evidence ("meets evidence standards with reservations"), or insufficient evidence ("does not meet evidence standards"). The standards are defined on the WWC website as follows:

> Currently, only well-designed and well-implemented randomized controlled trials (RCTs) are considered strong evidence, while quasi-experimental designs (QEDs) with equating [our note: this means that the researchers compared the experimental and control groups to show their equivalence] may only meet standards with reservations; evidence standards for regression discontinuity and single-case designs are under development.

The Brady and O'Regan (2009) youth mentoring study of the effects of having a Big Brother or Big Sister is summarized in Box 3.2; this is an example of a Methods Branch study that used randomized controlled trials or an experimental design. Another sample study is presented later (in Box 3.3): Duwe and Kerschner's (2008) "boot camp" study used a quasi-experimental design to evaluate the effects of a program to reduce recidivism for people who had spent time in jail.

An Example of an Experimental Design

In the Brady and O'Regan (2009) study, the independent variable was the mentoring program, with two levels: participation in the mentoring program and nonparticipation. The group that received the mentoring program is called the **experimental group**; the group that did not receive the program is the **control group**. The dependent variables included risky behaviors for the youth's health (e.g., use of alcohol and drugs), socially appropriate behaviors (e.g., nonviolent resolution of conflicts), attitudes toward schoolwork, and peer and family relationships.

Box 3.2. Sample Study with an Experimental (Randomized Controlled) Design: The Youth Mentoring Study

Sample study	Evaluation approach	Document title
Brady and O'Regan (2009)	Mixed methods with randomized controlled design (also, theory-based evaluation; logic model)	"Meeting the Challenge of Doing an RCT Evaluation of Youth Mentoring in Ireland: A Journey in Mixed Methods"

The Evaluators

Bernadine Brady is a Social Science Researcher and Connie O'Regan is a Doctoral Fellow in the Child and Family Research Centre, National University of Ireland, Galway.

Philosophical and Theoretical Lenses

This study is situated in the Methods Branch and illustrates the use of a randomized controlled design, thus exemplifying the approach most closely linked with the postpositivist paradigm. However, the evaluators describe their initial philosophical stance as reflective of the pragmatic paradigm, in that they used both quantitative and qualitative approaches. As they progressed through the study and began to use both types of data, they describe a shift from a pragmatic to a dialectical stance, because they contrasted the findings from the quantitative impact study with the inductive findings of the qualitative data. The dialectical stance allowed them to compare and contrast the quantitative and qualitative approaches to the exploration of youth mentoring.

The evaluators are part of a small evaluation team headed by Professor Pat Dolan, Principal Investigator. The role of the evaluation team encompasses study design, data collection, and analysis.

The Evaluand and Its Context

Big Brothers Big Sisters (BBBS) is an international youth mentoring program. The evaluand in this study was a BBBS program in the western part of Ireland that had been in operation for 5 years. When the study began, the program supported 60 pairs of adult mentors and youth. Box Figure 3.1 displays the underlying theory that guided the program.

Method

Design

The evaluation team used a concurrent embedded mixed methods design that included randomized controlled trials as well as collection of qualitative data. Again, Box Figure

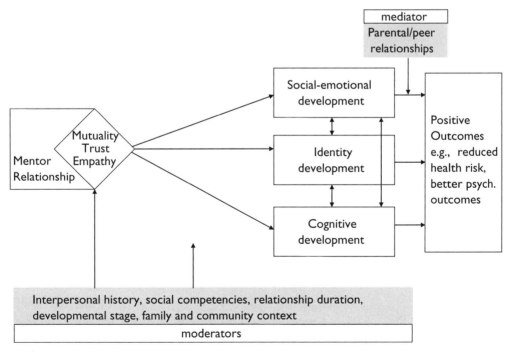

Box Figure 3.1. Rhode's model of mentoring. *Source*: Du Bois and Karcher (2005). Copyright 2005 by Sage Publications. Reprinted by permission.

(cont.)

Box 3.2 (cont.)

3.1 illustrates the theoretical model the evaluators tested to discover whether the treatment (the BBBS mentoring program) decreased the teens' risky health behaviors and improved their socially appropriate behaviors, attitudes toward schoolwork, and peer/family relationships. Youth were randomly assigned either to participate in the BBBS program or not to participate. Given the integration of a theoretical model for youth mentoring programs, this evaluation could also be described as a theory-based evaluation.

Evaluation Purposes

The study aimed to measure the impact of the BBBS mentoring program on the development of youth in the community. The evaluation started from a point of view of uncertainty about the effectiveness of mentoring as a policy intervention in an Irish context, and randomized controlled trials are deemed to be valuable in terms of exploring the impact (be it positive or negative) of interventions about which there is uncertainty (Oakley, 2000). Furthermore, it was decided that the randomized controlled trials should be undertaken in conjunction with a qualitative study to examine implementation and stakeholder perspectives.

Evaluation Questions

1. What is the impact of the BBBS program on the participating youth?
2. How is the program experienced by stakeholders?
3. How is the program implemented?
4. From comparing the outcome data from the impact study with the case study data from the mentoring pairs, what results emerge regarding the potential of this youth mentoring program?

Stakeholders and Participants

Stakeholders included the agency funding the evaluation—the Atlantic Philanthropies, which strongly supported the use of randomized controlled trials in evaluations. The host agency for the BBBS program is the Irish national youth organization, Foroige. An expert advisory group (EAG) was formed of leading researchers and academics to guide the research team. Youth in the evaluation study ranged in age from 10 to 14, although youth in the entire program ranged in age from 10 to 18. Project staff included BBBS managers and project workers.

Data Collection

The evaluators used a survey-based methodology to answer the first evaluation question, concerning the impact of the program on the youth. The second question, concerning the experiences of the stakeholders, was addressed by means of "interviews conducted with key program participants, including youth, mentors, parents, and staff" (p. 275). Data for the third question about program implementation were collected by means of reviewing documents from case files and focus groups conducted with staff.

Data were collected at baseline and at 12, 18, and 24 months. An integrated analysis based on both quantitative and qualitative data was used for the fourth question.

The sample for the first question consisted of 164 youth representing all those who were available in the western region's program. Parents, mentors, and teachers also completed survey data. The interviews were conducted with a purposive sample of 10 mentoring pairs who were selected to reflect "differences in age, gender, and location [i.e., rural or urban]" (p. 275).

For the focus groups, the research team approached the BBBS caseworkers seeking an opportunity sample of matches within the study who would be willing to participate. The staff identified matches that were established and that would be willing to participate in a series of interviews with the research team. A total of 21 matches agreed to participate. The research team then reviewed this sample and selected a purposive sample representing a balance across characteristics of age, gender, location, family situation, and reason for referral. As the team members rolled out the design, they decided to reduce the number from 12 to 10 mentoring pairs, as this would provide them with a spread of participants across the characteristics of interest and would be more feasible for the research team to follow over two time periods: (1) when the match was established but less than 6 months old, and (2) once the pairs had been meeting for 1 year. Interviews were conducted separately at both time periods with each young person and with his/her mentor, parent, and caseworker.

Once off-focus groups were conducted with members of the Foroige staff to review their attitudes about the program and gain their perspective on the potential of youth mentoring. Three such focus groups were held, involving 12 project staffers. An additional 12 individual interviews were held with BBBS caseworkers and line managers.

Management

The study covered a 3-year period. Its EAG was chaired by the Foroige CEO and was composed of representatives of the study funders, the Atlantic Philanthropies, and international experts in the area of mentoring research and research methodology. Meetings of the EAG were convened at critical times to advise the research team on design, implementation, and analysis issues and to provide feedback on draft reports. At the local level, the research team held regular meetings with Foroige and BBBS staff, to ensure that the study was implemented as planned and to troubleshoot in relation to any issues that arose. Good working relationships with all stakeholders greatly facilitated the successful implementation of the research. The research team consisted of the Principal Investigator, Researcher, and Doctoral Fellow, with additional support brought in as required.

Meta-Evaluation

Evaluations of social interventions in Ireland have rarely drawn upon randomized controlled trials. This study was the first of its kind, so there was naturally a sense of apprehension among the research team and the study commissioner regarding the task of designing and implementing such a study. The support of the EAG was critical, therefore, in terms of ensuring that advice was provided at key stages of the study design and

(cont.)

Box 3.2 (cont.)

implementation. The process was a transparent one, in which the study commissioner, funder, research team, and experts were all aware of the issues and challenges encountered and could collaborate in addressing them.

Reports and Utilization

The full study findings will be used by Foroige to inform the ongoing development of the BBBS mentoring program in Ireland. It is envisaged that the findings will also be of interest to mentoring programs in other countries.

REFLECTIONS FROM THE EVALUATORS

- *It is useful to see a study design as a framework, the finer details of which will evolve as you encounter challenges and develop a greater understanding of the program context. In this study, we had to constantly reflect on progress and change our plans to respond to the realities of the program's constraints and ethical issues. Our experience was a "journey," as the title of our 2009 article suggests. The study design can change even during the implementation stage. For example, recruitment of the sample took longer than anticipated. Once recruited and randomized, matching of intervention group youth also took longer than planned. As a result of these issues, the overall study's time frame was extended.*

- *Good working relationships with program staff are absolutely critical. If we had attempted to impose a study design, devised in the ivory tower of academia, without ongoing consultation with staff on the ground, it would have been a failure. Instead, we had to work with staff on all levels, acknowledging different ways of working, to try to ensure that the study could be implemented as consistently as possible across the 10 sites in which we were evaluating the program. It took some time to get the lines of communication clear and ensure that all staff members felt included and up to date with what was expected of them in the study. At the same time, we had to be careful not to overload them with too much complexity or detract from their ability to do their job. The time required for planning and relationship building is usually underestimated in studies of this nature, which is why flexibility in timescale is important.*

- *It's important to be aware that responding to ethical concerns can have implications for the study design. For example, in our case, one implication of the ethical protocols was a reduction in the study sample size, due to a compressed target age range and requirements for full consent from both young people and parents. The evaluators and other stakeholders must jointly agree on what compromises must be made.*

- *Having a theoretical model upon which to base the study was important in terms of facilitating the selection of relevant measures and guiding analysis of findings through testing a series of hypotheses.*

- *The input of an expert group is very valuable. In our case, the fact that the evaluand and study funder were also represented on the EAG ensured that there was direct communication and transparency between all key stakeholder groups. It is our belief that the communication process was more seamless as a result.*

- *There is scope to be creative regarding how qualitative and quantitative methods can work together to enhance understanding of the issue under study. In our case, the same team members were involved in both qualitative and quantitative work, which helped in terms of allowing a **dialectical approach** to emerge. [The dialectical approach is explained further in Chapter 9; essentially, this means that the evaluators were able to compare results from the quantitative and qualitative parts of their study and reach conclusions based on an integration of these two methods.]*

- *We came to the mixed methods literature as a way of resolving our concerns with implementing the experimental design within the limitations of the real-world setting. We had been concerned that incorporating qualitative elements would result in an evaluation with two separate parts that did not "speak" to each other, either epistemologically or methodologically. However, we were much heartened to discover that many of these arguments had been developed throughout the mixed methods literature. This provided us with useful frameworks and design options from which to integrate the study design into a coherent, "whole" evaluation design.*

· · · · · · · · · · E X T E N D I N G   Y O U R   T H I N K I N G · · · · · · · · · ·
Experimental Design

Φ4Σ8Ω≤pμ **Methods Branch**

Sample study	Evaluation approach	Topical area
Brady and O'Regan (2009)	Mixed methods with randomized controlled design (also, theory-based evaluation; logic model)	Youth mentoring in Ireland

Using the description of the Brady and O'Regan (2009) study in Box 3.2, answer the following questions:

1. What was the theory that drove this evaluation?

2. Which parts of this study were the quantitative and which were qualitative?

3. What data were the evaluators able to gather by using concurrent mixed methods, rather than a purely positivist, quantitative, pre–post survey (using only evaluation question 1)?

4. Explain how this study moved from a pragmatic to a dialectical stance and why.

(cont.)

5. What do you think the evaluators mean when they say that a mixed method design allowed them to use a "coherent, 'whole' evaluation design"?

6. Do you think the random assignment was the best way to decide which teens would be in the experimental group? What concerns would you have about this method?

7. In Box 3.2, the evaluators state: "We came to the mixed methods literature as a way of resolving our concerns with implementing the experimental design within the limitations of the real-world setting." What does this statement illustrate about modifications the evaluators felt were needed instead of doing a straightforward experimental design?

Theory to Practice: Methods Branch

1. Experimental and **quasi-experimental approaches**

2. Theory-based evaluation

3. Evaluation of training programs

An Example of a Quasi-Experimental Design

Quasi-experimental designs are used when evaluators are not able to assign participants randomly to treatment groups. Duwe and Kerschner (2008) used a quasi-experimental design for their evaluation of an alternative "boot camp" program for nonviolent drug and property offenders. They could not randomly assign individuals to be in the experimental program or the existing program, because when they started the evaluation study, the experimental and control treatments had already been implemented with large groups. Therefore, they had to use a quasi-experimental approach, which does not require randomly assigning participants to groups. (See Box 3.3.)

Box 3.3. Sample Study with a Quasi-Experimental Design: The Boot Camp Study

Sample study	Evaluation approach	Document title
Duwe and Kerschner (2008)	Quasi-experimental design; cost analysis	"Removing a Nail from the Boot Camp Coffin: An Outcome Evaluation of Minnesota's Challenge Incarceration Program"

The Evaluators

Grant Duwe is a Senior Research Analyst with the Minnesota Department of Corrections. Deborah Kerschner is a Senior Program Manager for the Minnesota Department of Corrections.

Philosophical and Theoretical Lenses

The evaluators work within the postpositivist paradigm. In this study, they adhered to the beliefs of objectivity by distance from the program, lack of interaction with the offenders to prevent bias, and the use of a quasi-experimental design as their methodology. The two evaluators worked independently from the program staff. They analyzed extant data on characteristics of offenders and outcomes after release from the program or the traditional incarceration facilities.

The Evaluand and Its Context

In 1972, the state of Minnesota opened an alternative incarceration program for non-violent drug and property offenders called the Challenge Incarceration Program (CIP), which included 6 months of chemical dependency treatment combined with a physically demanding program (called "boot camp"), followed by two 6-month phases of community service with intensive supervision.

Method

Design

The evaluators used a retrospective quasi-experimental design with two groups. The experimental group participated in CIP; the control group was incarcerated in a Minnesota correctional facility, but did not participate in CIP. Individuals were not randomly assigned to their groups; hence this was a quasi-experimental study.

Evaluation Purposes and Questions

"The present study evaluates CIP since its inception, focusing on two main questions: (a) Does CIP significantly reduce offender recidivism? and (b) Does CIP reduce costs?" (Duwe & Kerschner, 2008, p. 616).

Stakeholders and Participants

The evaluators do not explicitly discuss the stakeholders and participants, although they do provide an extensive discussion of the offenders from whom the data were collected.

Data Collection

This study used "four different measures—rearrest, reconviction, reincarceration for a new crime, and any return to prison (for either a new offense or a technical violation)" (Duwe & Kerschner, 2008, p. 619). "Recidivism was operationalized as a rearrest, a felony reconviction, a return to prison for a new criminal offense (i.e., reimprisonment), and any return to prison (i.e., reincarceration because of a new crime or technical violation). It is important to emphasize that the first three recidivism measures contain only

(cont.)

Box 3.3 (cont.)

new criminal offenses, whereas the fourth measure is much broader in that it includes new crimes and supervised release violations" (p. 622).

The sample consisted of an experimental group and a control group. The experimental group included "all offenders who entered CIP from the time it opened, October 1992, through the end of June 2002. During this time, there were 1,347 offenders (1,216 male and 131 female) who entered CIP" (p. 621). The control group included "offenders who were released from a Minnesota Correctional Facility within a similar timeframe, January 1, 1993, to December 31, 2002" (p. 621). Violent offenders were eliminated because they would not have been eligible for the CIP program. The evaluators randomly sampled from the remaining individuals to end up with a control group of 1,555 people who were similar to the experimental group on a number of defined variables, such as sex, age, race, and prior arrests.

Management and Budget

The evaluation was conducted retrospectively; that is, the data used were already collected, and the evaluators conducted the analysis independently of the implementation of the program. No mention is made of the management plan or budget.

Reports and Utilization

The results revealed that the experimental program participants stayed out of prison longer than control group participants. Also, even when experimental group participants returned to prison, they spent significantly less time there than did the control group participants, because their crimes were less serious. Finally, the CIP saved the state of Minnesota $6.2 million because of the reduced costs associated with early release. Duwe and Kerschner suggest that their findings can be used to justify the use of a boot camp approach if it is combined with drug treatment and is followed up with intensive supervision over a year.

Meta-Evaluation

The evaluators do not mention meta-evaluation strategies.

· · · · · · · · · · E X T E N D I N G   Y O U R   T H I N K I N G · · · · · · · · · ·
Quasi–Experimental Design

| Φ4Σ8Ω≤pμ | **Methods Branch** |

Sample study	Evaluation approach	List the distinguishing characteristics
Duwe and Kerschner (2008)	Quasi-experimental design; cost analysis	

Using the description of the Duwe and Kerschner (2008) study in Box 3.3, please respond to the following questions:

1. The authors used a quasi-experimental design because the groups had already been chosen, so they could not be randomly assigned (as is required with an experimental design). Do you think there are any ethical concerns that those in the control group did not receive the alternative program?

2. What was the independent variable? The dependent variable?

3. What was the theory that drove this evaluation?

4. What were the results, and what was concluded from the results, of this study?

5. Were you expecting different results than those reported by the authors? If so, what results were you expecting?

6. The authors state that the CIP reduced costs for the state of Minnesota. Do you think that there may have also been other variables at play instead of or concurrently with the CIP program? If yes, how would you investigate what those variables might have been?

Theory–Based Evaluation

Theory to Practice: Methods Branch

1. Experimental and quasi-experimental approaches

2. Theory-based evaluation

3. Evaluation of training programs

This second part of the "Theory to Practice" section looks at practice based on the work of methods theorists who prioritize theory-based evaluation approaches. The waters that flow through the evaluation landscape took a distinctive turn when Lipsey and Chen first introduced the concept of theory-based evaluation. Building a program theory involves first identifying those elements that the stakeholders believe are necessary to achieve their desired results, and then developing a model that shows how the elements relate to each other in that process. As mentioned briefly in Chapter 2, theory-based evaluations sometimes result in tables, charts, or diagrams that are called "logic models," "log frames," or "program theory models." The Brady and O'Regan (2009) youth mentoring study summarized in Box 3.2 provides a diagram that represents the theory underlying the BBBS program in western Ireland. Fredericks et al.'s (2008) quality-of-life study used a theory-based approach to evaluate a program designed to provide individualized services for people with developmental disabilities, with an improved quality of life as the desired result. They used a logic model as a way to represent the program theory. A summary of this study appears in Box 3.4.

Box 3.4. Sample Study Using Theory-Based Evaluation: The Quality-of-Life Study

Sample study	Evaluation approach	Document title
Fredericks, Deegan, and Carman (2008) **D**Ⓓ	Theory-based evaluation	"Using System Dynamics as an Evaluation Tool: Experience from a Demonstration Program"

The Evaluators

The evaluation was conducted under contract with a local university. Members of the team included three doctoral students studying public administration: Kimberly Fredericks, Joanne Carman, and Michael Deegan. Kimberly Fredericks is Assistant Professor and Coordinator of the Graduate Health Services Administration Program at the Sage Colleges in Albany, New York. Michael Deegan is a policy analyst and is Postdoctoral Research Fellow at the National Academies of Science in Alexandria, Virginia. Joanne Carman is an Assistant Professor and Coordinator of the Graduate Certificate Program in Nonprofit Management at the University of North Carolina at Charlotte.

Philosophical and Theoretical Lens

The evaluators situated their work in the social science theoretical framework known as the systems dynamic approach, which involves building a model to capture "the dynamic structures and processes of complex systems" (Fredericks et al., 2008, p. 252). Their overarching philosophical beliefs are in accord with the postpositivist paradigm, in that their goal is to develop a mathematical relationship between the variables in a system that influences the outcomes of a program. The first step in the process was to identify relevant variables and create a conceptual model that shows their relationships to each other and the desired results. The second step involved creating a mathematical model for examining the variables over time in order to capture the structure and processes as they relate to outcome variables.

The Evaluand and Its Context

The evaluand was a demonstration program for people with developmental disabilities being delivered by six nonprofit agencies over 5 years. The goal of the program was to provide individualized services to these people that would lead to improved quality of life. The project had three primary goals: to provide individualized service in response to a person's specific needs (rather than services delivered to a group), to provide flexible funding for service providers, and to streamline regulatory and administrative processes.

Services provided by agencies included evaluation and assessment; early childhood development; day care and universal PreK; school-age education; adult day programs (including day habilitation and day treatment); vocational and supported employment programs; after-school and weekend recreation programs; summer day camp; assistive technology resources; health care (including medical care, rehabilitation, dental care, audiology, and augmentative communication); residential programs (ranging from community residences to supported apartments to independent living); and family support services (including service coordination, family reimbursement, recreation, after-school and overnight respite, and housing and accessibility assistance). Most consumers received residential habilitation services, day habilitation services, or both (Fredericks, 2005; cited in Fredericks et al., 2008, p. 254).

The evaluand was represented by a logic model capturing the inputs (what resources are needed?); the process (activities); the outputs and short-term outcomes (evidence that the project is accomplishing its goals in the short term); and the long-term outcomes and impacts (the goals in the long term). This logic model is the portrayal of the program theory; that is, what needs to occur in order to achieve the desired effects? The logic model for this study appears in Chapter 7.

Method

Design

This evaluation used a theory-based approach. The evaluators worked with the project's Steering Committee to develop a comprehensive evaluation for the project. The Steering Committee consisted of members of the evaluation team, directors from the agencies, and representatives from the state agency that funded the project.

Evaluation Purposes and Questions

The evaluation was organized around four primary evaluation questions: (1) Who was served during the project? (2) What services did they get, and how much? (3) What were the outcomes? How did they relate to the project's goals of increases in individualized service planning and delivery; increases in person-centered planning; increases in consumer choice; increases in community integration; and improved quality of life for consumers in terms of home, relationships, personal life, work/school, and community? (4) How much did the services cost?

Data Collection

Data collection consisted of review of case records for demographic and disability diagnosis; Medicaid billing and expenditure data; site visits to the agencies that provided the services; and interviews. An outcome survey was also used to collect data from project staff, families, and participants each year. Service providers (direct care, supervisory, and support staff) were also interviewed anonymously about their attitudes and perceptions about the services they provided. Data were compiled and analyzed each year by site and in the aggregate.

(cont.)

Box 3.4 (cont.)

Management and Budget

The evaluation was staffed by two doctoral students working 20 hours a week. The students were responsible for managing the data collection, data analysis, and report writing, with additional support provided by the evaluation team's director (as well as members of the Steering Committee, as needed). The annual budget for the evaluation was approximately $90,000.

Meta-Evaluation

The evaluation team met with the Steering Committee periodically to discuss the progress of the evaluation. The content and discussions that emerged from these meetings helped the evaluators to realize they needed to add another component to the evaluation, which is described in the next section of this summary.

Reports and Utilization

The evaluation information was reported back to the sites on a regular basis. The sites received multiple copies of detailed reports, as well as one- to two-page executive summaries that were intended to be distributed to front-line staff, board members, and other interested stakeholders.

The evaluators noted that data from the fourth year of the evaluation revealed discrepancies from site to site in implementation of the various program components, and that sites were experiencing challenges that limited their ability to provide services as specified in the logic model. They shared these findings with the Steering Committee and recommended that the evaluation team use a qualitative system dynamics approach to see whether it could identify implementation problems and ways to ameliorate these problems. This involved three meetings between the evaluators and the stakeholders to develop a diagram that captured how the project worked in practice (not in theory). Through this process, they were able to "identify and conceptualize several issues that may have been hindering the success of the program, including competing goals, capacity limitations in the agencies, community constraints, and time-management problems for employees. Specifically, the model identified the pressures that were inhibiting the project's ability to increase individualized services and to improve certain aspects of the consumer's quality of life" (Fredericks et al., 2008, p. 257). The evaluators provide a detailed description of the various diagrams that were developed and how they enhanced the project's ability to gain knowledge about its effectiveness.

REFLECTIONS FROM THE EVALUATORS

During the course of this evaluation, we learned several valuable lessons. The first lesson has to do with how the stakeholders in an evaluation can have different understandings of specific concepts and terms. For example, the funder approached the evaluation team and asked us to design a "comprehensive evaluation." As evaluators, we took this to mean exactly that—developing an evaluation that looks at the project's implementation, outcomes, program theory, and answer some efficiency and effectiveness questions. We collected the baseline data during the first year of the project, and a few months into the second year of the project, we presented our first report summarizing the baseline data to the Steering Committee. We described the population being served at each of the sites, as well as a summary of the baseline measures for the outcome data that we would be tracking for the next 4 years.

In spite of the project's being somewhat participatory in nature—in that we asked for input from the Steering Committee at every stage of the evaluation design (they approved the survey instruments, data collection plans, etc.)—the report was not very well received. Immediately following the presentation, the committee members started asking us, "Where are the recommendations?" As the evaluators, we were a bit surprised by this. We asked, "What do you mean by recommendations? We are only in the second year of the program. We don't even have any outcome data to report." They responded by explaining that they wanted us to tell them what was working well so far, what wasn't, and what changes they should be making to improve the implementation of the program. It was very clear, by the end of this meeting, what the group had really wanted was for us to design a "formative evaluation." In hindsight, this made sense, given that this was a demonstration program. Yet, when the funder and the sites approached the evaluators, they used the phrase "comprehensive evaluation." This was the language that ended up in the evaluation contract. Whereas we interpreted the phrase "comprehensive evaluation" in terms of evaluation design, the funder and the sites used the phrase so that it would give them great flexibility over what they could ask us to deliver over time.

Not surprisingly, after this meeting, we evaluation team members had to regroup and change our data collection strategies, change the way we allocated resources, and find money in the budget to visit all of the sites. We added a person to the evaluation team, and traveled to each of the six sites to conduct personal and group interviews with different levels of staff (i.e., direct care workers, supervisors, financial administrators, etc.) to find out how implementation of the project was going. We tape-recorded the interviews, transcribed the data, and wrote a new report answering the questions that they were most interested in—what was working so far and what could be improved.

Another lesson that we learned has to do with the assumptions that well-intended and presumably informed stakeholders can make about the population being targeted by an evaluation. In designing the evaluation, we had a meeting where the subject of attrition came up. Given that this was going to be a 5-year project, we knew that tracking people over time might be difficult. The members on the Steering Committee who represented the agencies, however, assured us that attrition would not be a problem, in that this was not a transient group of people. In analyzing the data during second and third years of the evaluation, we began to realize that attrition was indeed a problem at some of the program sites. Follow-up interviews confirmed that at some of the program sites, consumers dropped in and out of the program on a fairly regular basis. Typically, this occurred at the smaller sites that had collaborative relationships with other service providers. As the consumers' needs changed, they were being referred to other providers to meet those needs.

The final lesson that we learned has to do with the importance of the political and institutional support for demonstration projects and their evaluations. The project was originally created in response to political and institutional fears that the Medicaid funding stream might be converted to a block grant (just as Aid to Families with Dependent

(cont.)

Box 3.4 *(cont.)*

Children was converted to Temporary Assistance for Needy Families). By the end of the third year of the project, there had been a shift in the larger political environment, and the funder and agencies were no longer worried that this was going to happen. This realization had profound effects on the momentum of the evaluation. Data collection for the evaluation was no longer a priority for most of the sites. Evaluation team members had to expend considerably more time and effort to ensure that data were being collected, and interest in the evaluation reports declined markedly. In fact, when the final report was delivered, it was emailed to the funder. There was no Steering Committee meeting, no official presentation, and no feedback.

········· E X T E N D I N G Y O U R T H I N K I N G ·········
Theory–Based Evaluation

Φ4Σ8Ω≤pμ **Methods Branch**

Sample study	Evaluation approach	List the distinguishing characteristics
Fredericks, Deegan, and Carman (2008)	Theory-based evaluation	

Using the description of the Fredericks et al. (2008) study in Box 3.4, please answer the following questions:

1. Building a program theory involves identifying those elements that the stakeholders believe are necessary to achieve their desired results. Name three elements or variables that Fredericks et al. believed were necessary to improve the quality of life for people with developmental disabilities.

2. Building a program theory involves developing a model that shows how the elements relate to each other in that process. What do you call the kind of model Fredericks et al. developed to illustrate their program?

3. Return Box 3.4, and note the questions the evaluators asked and then how the data were collected. Do you think they missed collecting data from any group that might have wanted to give their input? Was everything and everyone covered, in your opinion?

4. Why couldn't the evaluators continue using exclusively quantitative methods

for the study during the fourth year? What happened to make them include qualitative methods to the study?

5. The evaluators were quite kind in sharing with us, the authors and readers of this book, three major problems they encountered in the study. Select one of the three and explain how you think the evaluators could have avoided the problem, or explain why you believe none of the problems could have been avoided.

6. The findings were emailed to the funder. How else could the findings from this evaluation been disseminated and to whom? How do you think the final report was eventually used? After the amount of time and money placed in this project, and the findings that might improve the demonstration program, do you feel this is ethical? What power do evaluators have in this situation?

Evaluation of Training Programs

Theory to Practice: Methods Branch

1. Experimental and quasi-experimental approaches

2. Theory-based evaluation

3. **Evaluation of training programs**

This final part of the "Theory to Practice" section includes early theoretical approaches to the evaluation of training programs. One of the earliest approaches to training evaluation, and one that continues to be used in many organizations, was developed by Kirkpatrick (1975). As mentioned previously in this chapter, the Kirkpatrick model has four levels or stages (see Box 3.5). A sample study that used the Kirkpatrick model to evaluate training is presented in Box 3.6. Busch et al. (2005) conducted a study of school leadership that illustrates Kirkpatrick's four-level model of evaluation.

Box 3.5. Kirkpatrick's Model of Evaluation

1	Reaction stage	Measuring how much the participants enjoyed the training
2	Learning stage	Looking at what skills or information were absorbed by the participants during and immediately after the training

(cont.)

Box 3.5 (cont.)

| 3 | Behavior stage | Testing the transfer of learning and the application of knowledge and skills by the participants after training, back in the workplace |
| 4 | Results stage | Attempting to capture the effect of a training program on the organization's performance |

Source: Based on O'Toole (2009).

Box 3.6. Training Evaluation of School Leadership Using Kirkpatrick's Model

Sample study		*Evaluation program*	*Document title*
Busch, O'Brien, and Spangler (2005)		Training evaluation using Kirkpatrick's model	"Increasing the Quantity and Quality of School Leadership Candidates through Formation Experiences"

The Evaluators

Joseph R. Busch is an associate dean at the Fielding School of Psychology, Thomas P. O'Brien is the principal at Brentwood High School on Long Island, NY, and William D. Spangler teaches at the School of Management, Binghamton University in New York.

Philosophical and Theoretical Lenses

The evaluators situate their work in the postpositivist paradigm, and they use the Kirkpatrick model of evaluation. They also make use of a leadership theory postulating that leadership development requires recognition of an individual's leadership style, the development of a plan for enhancing leadership skills, and mentoring and reflection.

The Evaluand and Its Context

A leadership development program was implemented through a collaborative effort with the state department of education, the university, and local school superintendents. It was not a certificate- or degree-granting program; rather, it was designed to encourage potential leaders to consider pursuing leadership positions. It had several components: assessments of individuals' leadership styles and competencies; workshops on leadership theory and practice; mentoring by school administrators; and opportunities for individual and group reflection.

Method

Design

Kirkpatrick's four-level model was used to design the evaluation approach (reaction, learning, behavior, results; see Box 3.5).

Stakeholders and Participants

The participants in the training program were teachers who showed promise as leaders. The evaluation reported on the experiences of three cohorts who completed the 8-month training (n's = 25, 10, and 22 for these cohorts).

Data Collection

The evaluators used both quantitative and qualitative measures, including two reaction surveys; a quantitative assessment of learning and behavior through role plays and an in-basket scenario; the Multifactor Leadership Questionnaire (also for measuring learning and behavior); and a survey on the participants' educational and career plans (results). Qualitative data included responses to open-ended questions in the reaction surveys, the mentors' and superintendents' written conclusions about the program, and participant journals.

Management and Budget

No information is included in the article about this topic.

Meta-Evaluation

The evaluators do not directly address meta-evaluation; however, they do offer commentary about the unreliability of some of their measures and suggest that these might be changed in future evaluations of this type.

Reports and Utilization

No specific uses of the evaluation are mentioned, but the evaluators do conclude that their study's overall findings support the use of this type of program to identify potential leaders for school systems and to help program participants determine whether they should pursue administrative positions.

········· **E X T E N D I N G   Y O U R   T H I N K I N G** ·········
Evaluation of Training Programs

$\Phi4\Sigma8\Omega\leq p\mu$ **Methods Branch**

Sample study	Evaluation approach	List the distinguishing characteristics
Busch, O'Brien, and Spangler (2005)	Training evaluation using Kirkpatrick's model	

Using the description of the Busch et al. (2005) study in Box 3.6, please respond to the following questions:

1. What are the characteristics that illustrate Busch et al.'s use of the Kirkpatrick Model of evaluation?

2. What do you identify as the strengths and weaknesses of this model in terms of the type of data that were collected by the evaluators?

3. What would you suggest modifying in this study to improve the usefulness of the results?

The school leadership study illustrates the Kirkpatrick four-level model as follows: The evaluators (1) used two reaction surveys to determine how much the participants enjoyed the training (the reaction stage); (2) tested the transfer of learning and changes in behavior through the use of role plays, a questionnaire, and an in-basket scenario (the learning and behavior stages); and (3) obtained information about the participants' educational and career plans (the results stage). Other studies to be discussed in later chapters demonstrate additional approaches that are commensurate with the postpositivist paradigm and the Methods Branch.

Critiques of the Methods Branch

Lack of Applicability in the "Real World"

Some criticisms of the approaches associated with the Methods Branch provide a transition to Chapter 4 on the Use Branch. For example, Stufflebeam (2003, p. 27) has critiqued the theory-based approach to evaluation, saying that it makes little sense because it "assumes that the complex of variables and interactions involved in running a project in the complicated, sometimes chaotic conditions of the real world can be worked out and used a priori to determine the pertinent evaluation questions and variables." He continues:

> Many evaluation plans that appeared in proposals were true to the then current evaluation orthodoxy, i.e., evaluations should determine whether valued objectives had been achieved and met requirements of experimental design and post hoc, objective measurement. This

conceptualization was wrong for the situations I found in Columbus classrooms. At best, following this approach could only confirm schools' failures to achieve (dubious) objectives. Such evaluations would not help schools get projects on track and successfully meet the education needs of poor kids. (Stufflebeam, 2003, p. 30)

Pros and Cons of Experimental Approaches

A portion of the evaluation community agrees that well-conducted randomized experiments are best suited for assessing effectiveness when multiple causal influences create uncertainty about what caused results. However, they are often difficult (and sometimes impossible) to carry out. An evaluation must be able to control exposure to the intervention and to ensure that treatment and control groups' experiences remain separate and distinct throughout the study.

Several rigorous alternatives to randomized experiments are considered appropriate for other situations: quasi-experimental comparison group studies, statistical analyses of observational data, and (in some circumstances) in-depth case studies. The credibility of their estimates of program effects relies on how well the studies' designs rule out competing causal explanations. Collecting additional data and targeting comparisons can help rule out other explanations (Kingsbury, Shipman, & Caracelli, 2009).

· · · · · · · · · · EXTENDING YOUR THINKING · · · · · · · · · ·
Methods Branch Evaluations

1. On the U.S. Department of Education's What Works Clearinghouse website (*ies.ed.gov/ncee/wwc*), go to "Publications and Reviews" and then "Intervention Reports." You will see a list of different topics, which all lead to summaries of program evaluations done by the U.S. government. After you find a study that is interesting to you, answer these questions:

   a. Did the study use randomized controlled trials, or did it use a quasi-experimental design?

   b. What was the independent variable?

   c. What was the experimental group?

   d. What was the control group?

   e. What were the dependent variables?

   f. Who were the stakeholders?

   g. What was the methodology used?

   h. What did the study find?

   i. What branch of our tree does this study illustrate and why?

2. As noted above, Stufflebeam (2003) has written: "This conceptualization was wrong for the situations I found in Columbus classrooms. At best, following this

(cont.)

approach could only confirm schools' failures to achieve (dubious) objectives" (p. 30). Do you agree with Stufflebeam that discovering failures is a "dubious objective"? Why or why not?

3. Describe the similarities and differences among an experimental approach, a quasi-experimental approach, a theory-based approach, and training programs.

4. From your perspective, what do you think are some of the pros and cons of working in the Methods Branch?

Your Evaluation Plan: Your Philosophical Stance

Begin writing your understandings of the postpositivist paradigm and the Methods Branch as a way of clarifying your own thinking about your philosophical beliefs and how they might influence the way you conduct an evaluation. This can become part of your evaluation plan later, when you decide which approach you will use.

▶ *Moving On to the Next Chapter*

Evaluators expressing concerns with a narrow focus on methods have proposed that evaluators begin to give more attention to their interactions with stakeholders and to how those interactions influence the use of the evaluation findings. The Use Branch is the topic of Chapter 4. The chapter explores those theorists who have focused on the need to be responsive to the stakeholders in order to improve the probability that their findings will be used to improve programs and for other uses that are appropriate.

*   *   *

Remember the studies below, as we refer to them again in later chapters.

Φ4Σ8Ω≤pμ **Methods Branch**		
Sample study	*Evaluation approach*	*Topical area*
Brady and O'Regan (2009)	Mixed methods with randomized controlled design (also, theory-based evaluation; logic model)	Youth mentoring in Ireland
Duwe and Kerschner (2008)	Quasi-experimental design; cost analysis	Preventing return to prison in the United States
Fredericks, Deegan, and Carman (2008) **D**ⅅ	Theory-based evaluation	Demonstration program for people with developmental disabilities

Φ4Σ8Ω≤pµ Methods Branch		
Sample study	**Evaluation approach**	**Topical area**
Busch, O'Brien, and Spangler (2005)	Training evaluation using Kirkpatrick's model	School leadership

Note

1. Alkin included Carol Weiss in the Methods Branch, but we think she belongs in the Use Branch, because much of her work has focused on how to improve the use of evaluation findings.

Preparing to Read Chapter Four

Branch	Paradigm	Description
Methods	Postpositivist	Focuses primarily on quantitative designs and data
Use	**Pragmatic**	**Focuses primarily on data that are found to be useful by stakeholders; advocates for the use of mixed methods**
Values	Constructivist	Focuses primarily on identifying multiple values and perspectives through qualitative methods
Social justice	Transformative	Focuses primarily on viewpoints of marginalized groups and interrogating systemic power structures through mixed methods to further social justice and human rights

As you prepare to read this chapter, think about these questions:

1. What are the characteristics of the pragmatic paradigm?

2. How do those characteristics influence the practice of evaluation?

3. Which major thinkers have contributed to the approaches associated with the Use Branch?

4. How did the ideas grow from the early days to the present in this theoretical context?

CHAPTER FOUR

The Pragmatic Paradigm

and the Use Branch

When I (Donna M. Mertens) entered the evaluation field in the early 1970s, my work in evaluation was centered on collection of data and writing reports for the "feds" (i.e., the U.S. federal government). This statement is telling in a number of ways. First, I have been doing evaluation since I was very young. Second, we evaluators of that era rarely spent much time thinking about who the stakeholders were for evaluation reporting. Third, we generally believed that our work was completed if we could produce a report of our findings and ship it off to the funder. I suppose most of us felt a bit dissatisfied if our reports were never read, but we continued to produce them nonetheless.

However, some evaluation theorists from that era felt a great deal of dissatisfaction and took action to change this situation, so that evaluators became more conscious of the importance of getting people to pay attention to and use evaluation findings to inform their decisions, instead of filing them away unused. These theorists also thought that allowing the beneficiaries to decide for themselves what to include in an evaluation, as well as how to plan and implement the evaluation, would put them in a better position to use the results.

In this chapter, we begin with a description of the pragmatic paradigm, because its assumptions align closely with the idea of use of evaluation findings as a priority. We then explain the use theorists' positions and approaches, as well as the advantages and challenges associated with their approaches. Examples of studies that reflect the Use Branch illustrate how these theoretical perspectives are manifested in practice. Specific emphasis is placed on those aspects of these approaches that facilitate use of evaluation findings.

The Pragmatic Paradigm

The history of the pragmatic paradigm began in the second half of the 19th century, William James, John Dewey, George Herbert Mead, and Arthur F. Bentley. They rejected the claim that "truth" could be discovered through the use of scientific methods. (Early pragmatists resemble the ontological assumption of the constructivist paradigm [discussed in Chapter 5] in this way.) A neopragmatic period emerged around 1960 and continues to this day (Maxcy, 2003). Neopragmatists of note include Abraham Kaplan, Richard Rorty, and Cornel West. These philosophers have distinguished themselves from the early pragmatists by their emphasis on common sense and practical thinking.

The pragmatic paradigm has been adopted by some mixed methods researchers as being reflective of the assumptions that underlie their work (Morgan, 2007; Teddlie & Tashakkori, 2009). Morgan (2007) borrows from Dewey, James, and Mead to explain what researchers (evaluators) do in pragmatic terms. As the word "pragmatic" comes from the Greek word meaning "to act," it makes sense that evaluators test the workability (effectiveness) of a line of action (intervention) by collecting results (data collection) that provide a warrant for assertions (conclusions) about the line of action.

Axiology (Ethics)

Early pragmatists emphasized the ethics of caring as their axiological assumption. However, contemporary pragmatists' ethical assumption is more closely aligned with the utilitarian theory of ethics, which holds that the value of something is a function of its consequences (Christians, 2005). Morgan (2007) describes the ethical stance of pragmatism as gaining knowledge in the pursuit of desired ends. Rather than doing an evaluation for the sake of an evaluation, pragmatists see the value of the evaluation as *how it is used and the results of that use.* My reports for the "feds" might have had little value under this theory, as the consequences of the reports were hard to see. The specific consequence was not seen in the use of any particular findings, but more as an indicator that we had completed the scope of work. Hard as it is to admit, I fear that many of the reports were simply put on a shelf or into a file cabinet (or, God forbid, into the wastebasket) and never referred to again.

All evaluators adhere to the ethical principles outlined in Chapter 3 on the Methods Branch; therefore, they are not repeated here. This chapter expands on axiology as it is seen from the pragmatic paradigm.

Ontology (Reality)

Tashakkori and Teddlie (2003) assert that pragmatists avoid spending a great deal of time arguing about metaphysical terms such as truth and reality. They justify this stance by explaining that the value of evaluations is not based on whether they discover the "truth," but on the demonstration that the results "work" with respect to the problem that is being studied. Thus pragmatists do not proclaim that they will discover the truth. Rather, they focus on what difference it makes to believe one thing or another (Morgan, 2007).

Epistemology (Knowledge)

Unlike a postpositivist researcher, who assumes that a detached, neutral observer will collect objective, unbiased data, a pragmatist is "free to study what interests you and is of value to you, study it in the different ways that you deem appropriate, and utilize the results in ways that can bring about positive consequences within your value system" (Tashakkori & Teddlie, 1998, p. 30). The appropriateness of the relationship between you as an evaluator and the stakeholders is judged by how well that relationship allows you to achieve your purpose in the evaluation. If your purpose is to get the results of the evaluation used, then that determines the nature of your relationship with the stakeholders.

Methodology (Systematic Inquiry)

The pragmatic paradigm is identified by some researchers as the philosophical framework that guides their choice of **mixed methods.** (The transformative paradigm, discussed in Chapter 6 can also lead to such a choice.) The underlying methodological assumption of pragmatism is that the method should match the purpose of the study (Patton, 2002a). Neopragmatists see mixed methods as a way of addressing the problem of conflicting assumptions that lead to the belief that evaluators had to choose either quantitative (post-positivist; see Chapter 3) or qualitative (constructivist; see Chapter 5) methods. The pragmatic paradigm's methodological assumption gets around that dichotomous way of thinking. The evaluator chooses a method on the basis of what is right for a particular study in a particular context with a particular stakeholder group. Quite often the methods of choice are mixed methods (i.e., both quantitative and qualitative methods used in one study or in a sequence of studies).

· · · · · · · · · · · E X T E N D I N G   Y O U R   T H I N K I N G · · · · · · · · · · ·

Philosophical Assumptions of the Pragmatic Paradigm and the Use Branch

Using the table below, answer the following questions:

1. Can you imagine what a pragmatic evaluation would look like?

2. How would the evaluator set up the evaluation?

3. Would the evaluator be involved with the stakeholders or not?

4. How would the the evaluator's assumptions guide her/his decisions?

The Pragmatism/Neopragmatism and the Use Branch

Description	Axiological assumption	Ontological assumption	Epistemological assumption	Methodological assumption
Scientific method is insufficient to discover truth; use common sense and practical thinking	Gain knowledge in pursuit of desired ends as influenced by the evaluator's values and politics	There is a single reality, and all individuals have their own unique interpretation of reality	Relationships in evaluation are determined by what the evaluator deems as appropriate to that particular study	Match methods to specific questions and purposes of research; mixed methods can be used as evaluators work back and forth between various approaches

Use Branch Theorists

Daniel Stufflebeam (1980) began his career in evaluation in 1965 by using the recommended practice of the time, which involved the development of objectives for educational programs, followed by measurement of outcomes to see whether the objectives were achieved. He quickly came to the conclusion that evaluators should have a more expansive role—one that starts with a critical evaluation of the program's objectives, what is needed to make the program work, the extent to which the program is being implemented as planned, and what the outcomes are. Based on this line of thinking, he developed the **"context, input, process, product"** (CIPP) model of evaluation, which he first presented to the evaluation community in 1968. Shortly thereafter, Phi Delta Kappa, an honors organization that promotes scholarly work, engaged Stufflebeam to chair a Committee on Evaluation. The outcome of this was a book entitled *Educational Evaluation and Decision Making* (Stufflebeam et al., 1971), which elaborated on the CIPP model and established the importance of technical adequacy of method, as well as use of evaluation by decision makers. The following quotation displays his thinking processes as he developed this model, while he was considering program alternatives that would appear to give reasonable hope of success at feasible cost levels.

> **Use Branch Theorists**
>
> Daniel Stufflebeam
> Carol Weiss
> Joseph Wholey
> Eleanor Chelimsky
> Michael Patton
> John Owen
> Hallie Preskill
> Marvin Alkin

> That is basically where[in] the model I began to talk about *context evaluation* to help in setting goals, *process evaluation* to guide implementation, and *product evaluation* to help with the recycling of programs. I tend to like order in my schemes, and I realized I had a gap. I realized there was another crucial decision that gets made in programs that I had not attended to. That is the decision of what procedures, what strategy, what budget, what staffing pattern should be adopted in order to address a set of objectives. So I came up with a horrible label, but, nevertheless, it was aimed at helping people to choose appropriate project designs. It was the label of *input evaluation*. By that I meant that people in the districts ought to search out alternative ways of responding to students' needs and to objectives. They ought to evaluate those alternative responses and formulate projects that appear to have some good prospect for success at some kind of a feasible cost level. (Stufflebeam, 1980, p. 87)

The Phi Delta Kappa Committee changed the focus of evaluation from the measurement of objectives to "a process for identifying and judging decision alternatives" (Stufflebeam, 1982, p. 16). Stufflebeam's work was geared toward the provision of information that would be useful for decision makers. Hence use of evaluation was primarily framed in terms of policy makers and upper-level administrators. Stufflebeam (2003) suggested specifically that the evaluator's overall focus should be on a process of creating information to support managerial decisions.

Carol Weiss also began her career in evaluation in the 1960s—in her case, by evaluating a program that was a precursor to the War on Poverty initiative. She too used the evaluation strategies of the time (objectives, measurement) and was quickly disillusioned because she did not see policy makers using the evaluation findings as a basis for decision making. In contrast to Stufflebeam, who began his work in education, Weiss worked from a social science perspective. She explored the connection between evaluation and policy making in a paper she presented in 1965 at the American Sociological Association's meeting, entitled "Utilization of Evaluation: Toward Comparative Study." She also published one of the earliest textbooks (in which the 1965 paper was included), *Evaluation Research: Methods of Assessing Program Effectiveness* (Weiss, 1972). Her contributions are many, but three of these in the early days of evaluation stand out. First, she recognized the complexity of decision making at the policy level and acknowledged that evaluation was only one source of information used by policy makers. Second, she researched how policy makers used information and found that they rarely used evaluation findings to make specific decisions; rather, they used them to enlighten their decisions. Third, she began the idea of investigating program theory as an evaluator's responsibility. (Program theory has been discussed in greater detail in Chapter 3.)

Weiss (1998) suggested that evaluators serve roles as critical friends, facilitators, and problem solvers. She also brought evaluators' attention to the different uses that can be made of their findings. "Instrumental" use is direct use of evaluation findings as a basis for decision making. "Conceptual" use is harder to link directly to the evaluation findings, but is described as changes in the thinking, attitudes, or knowledge of the intended users, without necessarily involving specific actions. Moreover, Weiss recognized that evaluations are sometimes used for political, persuasion, or symbolic reasons. She did not want political uses of evaluation to be looked upon as evil; however, she did not endorse use of evaluation for personal gain or for harmful purposes.

Two other noted evaluators have made significant contributions to evaluation within the federal context: **Joseph Wholey** and **Eleanor Chelimsky**. Wholey (2001) situated his work in the context of public policy making and the culture of results-oriented management practices in public and nonprofit organizations. He suggested the role of the evaluators as facilitating the development of agreed-upon goals and strategies, measuring the intended outcomes, and encouraging the use of their findings. Chelimsky (see Oral History Project Team, 2009) was the first director of evaluation at what was then the U.S. General Accounting Office (GAO). The major stakeholder for U.S. GAO evaluations was and is the U.S. Congress; therefore, Chelimksy had many opportunities to share her wisdom and experience on the use of evaluation findings to influence policy.

In the mid-1970s, **Michael Patton** realized that stakeholders in his evaluation studies did not understand what evaluators were doing and therefore did not find the evaluations useful. Rather than assuming that the stakeholders were in some way inferior to evaluators and continuing doing the same kind of work, Patton did two very interesting things:

1. He offered training programs to educate consumers about what evaluation is and how it can benefit organizations.

2. He did research on what influences the degree of use of evaluation findings, as well as strategies for enhancing that use.

The result of his work is what is now known as **utilization-focused evaluation (UFE)**. In an interview (Oral History Project Team, 2007), Patton remarked that his focus on facilitating thinking about and use of evaluation puts him in a position that keeps him "out of the business of writing reports, which I never much cared for anyway, and which I generally try to avoid" (p. 109). In saying this, he supports multiple ways of communicating with stakeholders throughout the evaluation, and not depending on a final report to be the instrument for providing information for decision making.

Patton has defined UFE as evaluation that provides information to intended users. The major components of UFE include discussion of potential uses of evaluation findings from the very beginning of a project, not only at the end when the data are in hand. Patton realizes that encouraging stakeholders to think about what they want to do with evaluation findings before any data are collected should be an effective strategy for collecting data that has an increased probability of being used. Another key aspect is the identification of the intended users. He calls this the "personal factor" that leads to intended use by intended users. In the following quotation, Patton explains the personal factor in the context of developmental evaluations—an extension of UFE that is discussed more in later chapters.

> People matter. Relationships matter. Evaluation is not just about methods and data. Studies of evaluation use have consistently found that evaluation use is significantly increased when those in a position to make decisions understand the importance of reality-testing and care about using data to inform their decision-making. This is what has come to be called the *personal factor*.... Developmental evaluation, in particular, is relationship-based. No matter how rigorous, systematic, and elegant the methods, if the relationship between the evaluator and those developing an innovation doesn't work, the full potential of developmental evaluation won't be realized. (Patton, 2010, p. xiii)

··········· E X T E N D I N G   Y O U R   T H I N K I N G ···········
Pragmatic versus Postpositivist Paradigms

1. Can you describe how the perspective of a pragmatist working in the Use Branch may differ from that of a postpositivist working in the Methods Branch? What do you think is the most important difference?

2. Consider Fredericks et al.'s (2008) study that you read about in Chapter **D**Ⓓ 3 (see Box 3.4). If it had been a study using a pragmatic paradigm rather than a positivist one, how might the evaluators have proceeded differently?

John Owen is an Australian evaluator who has contributed to the utilization focus of evaluation in his book *Program Evaluation: Forms and Approaches* (Owen, 2006). He views the role of the evaluator as contributing knowledge relevant to decision making, and he describes several ways in which evaluators can do this. "Proactive" evaluations seek to inform planning decisions needed for new programs or for substantial revisions of existing programs. "Clarification" evaluations answer questions about the desired outcomes of a program and about the match between the program design and the desired outcomes. "Monitoring" evaluations compare implementation of programs in different sites at different times as a way to provide evidence for improving program effectiveness. And "impact" evaluations look at the achievement of outcomes for the purposes of funders and program-level stakeholders. Owen's goal in writing this book emanated from his perception of a common misunderstanding by Australian decision makers that evaluation was primarily suitable as a good way to judge program effectiveness. He wanted to influence their thinking to include the idea of using evaluations for broader purposes.

Hallie Preskill began exploring the theory of evaluation use in her doctoral dissertation (Preskill, 1984), based on the evaluation of training programs in the banking industry. She used the work of Alkin and his colleagues (Alkin, Daillak, & White, 1979) on factors that influence evaluation use. Her research revealed that instrumental use (i.e., use for specific decision making) was more common at the local program level and that conceptual use (i.e., use to enlighten thinking) was more common at the policy level. She continued to examine factors associated with evaluation use, primarily within the context of training programs. In 1999, she published a book with Rosalie Torres (*Evaluative Inquiry for Learning in Organizations*), which provides important insights into how the culture of an organization affects its receptivity to the actual use of evaluation findings. In the Preskill and Torres approach, evaluation is seen as an opportunity for continual improvement. The client (user) defines the evaluation purpose. For this to occur, it is helpful if the organization has guidelines for how evaluation can be used as a tool for improving organizational effectiveness, and if it has a pool of evaluators available who can provide the needed customized evaluation services. The evaluators can arrange for activities such as team-building meetings to enhance the organization's ability to participate meaningfully.

Preskill and Torres (1999) have presented a "learning organization evaluation" model and suggested an overarching role for evaluators as facilitators of organizational inquiry. They identify an evaluator's specific roles as those of collaborator, facilitator, interpreter, mediator, coach, and educator. Owen and Lambert (1998; cited in Skolits et al., 2009, p. 278) suggest that the expanding needs of organizational leaders for expertise in organizational development have blurred evaluators' traditional orientations toward an organizational development consultant role.

David Fetterman (1994) has proposed a model of evaluation known as **empowerment evaluation.** This model is based on the premise that program participants who conduct their own evaluations will be more likely to use the information forthcoming from that evaluation. The program participants, coached by the evaluator, develop their own capacity to conduct evaluations; this is designed to increase the likelihood that the evaluation will become institutionalized in the program and will continue to be conducted and used after the evaluator leaves.

Jean King (1998) and **Brad Cousins** (Cousins & Earl, 1995; Cousins & Whitmore, 1998) have explored the relationship between the evaluators and intended users, and have developed participatory approaches to evaluation based on the premise that more active involvement of stakeholders should result in increased use of evaluation findings. In a paper for an issue of *New Directions for Evaluation* (Cousins & Whitmore, 1998), they made the distinction between **practical participatory evaluation** and **transformative participatory evaluation.** In this chapter, the focus is on the former; the latter is discussed in Chapter 6.

There are both similarities and differences between these two types of participatory evaluation. The two approaches are similar in that evaluators work with the stakeholders to build trust and evaluation capacity; recognize the need to build and support local leadership; and work as outside facilitators who need to address complex interpersonal relationships and issues of power (Cousins & Whitmore, 1998). The two approaches are different in terms of how an evaluator views and engages the stakeholders. In practical participatory evaluation, the focus is on decision makers as users. In transformative participatory evaluation, the focus is on engaging all stakeholders, especially those who have traditionally been excluded from evaluations and from the decisions associated with evaluation studies.

Both King and Cousins are more inclined toward the practical participatory evaluation model. King's (2005) description of the role of the evaluator in a study of the Bunche–DaVinci Learning Partnership Academy illustrates the connection between practical participatory evaluation and Patton's UFE:

> The evaluator serves as teacher, the users as students, the evaluation process and results as "curriculum," and the evaluation context as the milieu (Schwab, 1969; King & Thompson, 1983). My goal at Bunche–DaVinci would be instructional: to connect with the principal, faculty, and staff (and others as appropriate) both to teach evaluation processes and facilitate people's use of the results we generate. Once Garcia [the principal investigator of the program] agreed, my goal would be to collaborate with Bunche–DaVinci staff to increase the likelihood that an evaluation process could continue within the school. Evaluation capacity building means using this process not only for its immediate and direct results, but also for the explicit purpose of building participants' personal capacity to evaluate again. (Some may see [this] practice as a branch of the "use" limb of Alkin's evaluation theory tree, that is, a natural extension of [Patton's] utilization-focused evaluation; Patton, 1997.) (p. 87)

Intersecting Branches

Melvin Mark and **Gary Henry** (Henry & Mark, 2003; Mark & Henry, 2004; Mark, Henry, & Julnes, 2000) [who are discussed in Chapter 3 as Methods Branch theorists] have also pushed for broadening the way evaluators conceptualize the consequences of their work. They argue that the goal of evaluation is social betterment and suggest the need to identify the mechanisms through which evaluations lead to this ultimate goal along differing paths of influence and at different levels (i.e., individual, interpersonal, and collective). Mark and Henry map out a logic model for evaluation, focusing on evaluation consequences related to the improvement of social conditions. Just as program theory connects program activities with outcomes while also explaining the processes through which the outcomes are achieved, program theory of evaluation by Mark and Henry identifies evaluation as an intervention with social betterment as its ultimate outcome. They label traditional notions of instrumental, conceptual, and persuasive use more specifically as, for example, skill acquisition, persuasion, or standard setting. These, then, would be the mechanisms through which social betterment can be achieved. (Johnson et al., 2009, p. 378)

· · · · · · · · · E X T E N D I N G   Y O U R   T H I N K I N G · · · · · · · · · ·
Use Branch Theorists

1. Owen thinks it is important for decision makers to understand that evaluations can judge program effectiveness, but that evaluations can be used for other purposes, too. List several other ways that evaluations can be used.

2. Fetterman, King, and Cousins suggest that evaluators train program participants

to conduct their own evaluations and that there should be more of a participatory approach to evaluation. What do you think would be the benefits? What do you foresee as being problematic about conducting evaluations with stakeholder participation?

3. Henry (2005) has said, "Ultimately, we should be concerned with an evaluation's influence on the beneficiaries of a program or policy, and look at whether people are better off as a result of the evaluation." If you were with Henry, what thoughts would you share with him about his belief? Do you agree with him? Explain.

Theory to Practice

In this section, several evaluation approaches based on the Use Branch of evaluation are examined in terms of steps to undertake such an evaluation. Sample studies are used to illustrate these approaches. The approaches include CIPP, UFE, learning organization evaluation, empowerment evaluation, and practical participatory evaluation.

Components of the CIPP Model

Box 4.1 contains an explanation of the meaning of each component of the CIPP model, what is evaluated, and the types of decisions that such evaluations would be designed to inform. Figure 4.1 illustrates the model.

Box 4.1. An Explanation of the CIPP Model

Type of evaluation	What is evaluated	Types of decisions
C: Context	Needs, problems, assets, opportunities	Define goals and priorities and desired outcomes
I: Input	Alternative approaches, competing action plans, participant characteristics, staffing plans, budgets	Determine feasibility and potential cost-effectiveness; choose among competing plans; write funding proposals; allocate resources; assign staff; schedule work
P: Process	Implementation of plans	Help staff make needed revisions in activities; judge performance and interpret outcomes
P: Product	Identification and assessment of intended and unintended outcomes, both short- and long-term	Help staff keep focused on achieving desired outcomes; gauge the success of the program in addressing needs

Source: Based on Stufflebeam (2003).

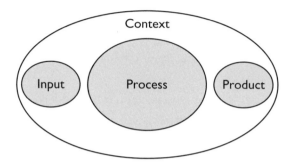

Figure 4.1. An illustration of the CIPP model.

Context Evaluation

Context evaluation is designed to provide the "big picture" into which a program and its evaluation fit. As the evaluation handbook prepared by the W. K. Kellogg Foundation (WKKF, 1998, p. 21) states, the following questions typify context evaluations:

▧ What about our community and our umbrella organization hinders or helps us [in achieving] project goals?

▧ Which contextual factors have the greatest bearing on project successes or stumbling blocks?

Thus context evaluation is often looked upon as a type of needs assessment that can identify the needs, assets, and resources of a community in order to plan programs suitable for that community. It is also used to identify the political climate that could influence the potential success of the program. Box 4.2 explains context evaluation in more detail. (Specific approaches to needs assessment are described in Chapter 9.) Box 4.3 describes an example of a CIPP evaluation conducted by Daniel Stufflebeam and his colleagues at Western Michigan University. This study illustrates that context evaluation can also be conducted throughout a study as a means to documenting any contextual changes that could influence implementation or outcomes, such as changes in leadership, personnel, policies, legislation, or economic conditions.

Box 4.2. Context Evaluation

Context evaluation assesses needs, assets, and problems within a defined environment.

Evaluator activities	*Client/stakeholder activities—Program aims*
▧ Compile and assess background information, especially on the intended beneficiaries' needs and assets.	▧ Use the context evaluation findings in selecting and/or clarifying the intended beneficiaries.

Evaluator activities	Client/stakeholder activities— Program aims
■ Interview program leaders to review and discuss their perspectives on beneficiaries' needs and to identify any problems (political or otherwise) the program will need to solve.	■ Use the context evaluation findings in reviewing and revising, as appropriate, the program's goals to assure they properly target assessed needs.
■ Interview other stakeholders to gain further insight into the needs and assets of intended beneficiaries and potential problems for the program.	■ Use the context evaluation findings in assuring that the program is taking advantage of pertinent community and other assets.
■ Assess program goals in light of beneficiaries' assessed needs and potentially useful assets.	■ Use the context evaluation findings—throughout and at the program's end—to help assess the program's effectiveness and significance in meeting beneficiaries' assessed needs.
■ Engage an evaluator to monitor and record data on the program's environment, including related programs, area resources, area needs and problems, and political dynamics.	
■ Request that program staff [members] regularly make available to the evaluation team information they collect on the program's beneficiaries and environment.	
■ Annually, or as appropriate, prepare and deliver to the client and agreed-upon stakeholders a draft context evaluation report providing an update on program-related needs, assets, and problems, along with an assessment of the program's goals and priorities.	
■ Discuss context evaluation findings in feedback workshops presented annually to the client and designated audiences.	
■ Finalize context evaluation reports and associated visual aids and provide them to the client and agreed-upon stakeholders.	

Source: Stufflebeam (2002, p. 4). Reprinted by permission of Daniel L. Stufflebeam.

Box 4.3. Sample CIPP Study: The Hawaiian Housing Study

Sample study	Evaluation approach	Document title
Stufflebeam, Gullickson, and Wingate (2002)	Context, input, process, product (CIPP) evaluation	"The Spirit of Consuelo: An Evaluation of Ke Aka Ho'ona"

The Evaluators

Daniel Stufflebeam is Director of the Western Michigan University (WMU) Evaluation Center and has made major contributions to the field of evaluation (as described earlier in this chapter). He developed the CIPP model of evaluation and served as the Principal Investigator throughout this study. Arlen Gullickson is Manager of Evaluation Projects at the WMU Evaluation Center. Lori Wingate is Research and Evaluation Specialist at the WMU Evaluation Center.

Philosophical and Theoretical Lenses

Stufflebeam et al. (2002) wrote:

> The evaluation design was based on the CIPP Evaluation Model.... This model presents a comprehensive approach to assessing *context*, including the nature, extent, and criticality of beneficiaries' needs and assets and pertinent environmental forces; *input*, including the responsiveness and strength of project plans and resources; *process*, involving the appropriateness and adequacy of project operations; and *product*, meaning the extent, desirability, and significance of intended and unintended outcomes.
>
> To gain additional insights into project outcomes, the product evaluation component was divided into four parts: (1) impact, regarding the project's reach to the intended target audience; (2) effectiveness, regarding the quality, desirability, and significance of outcomes; (3) sustainability, concerning the project's institutionalization and long-term viability; and (4) transportability, concerning the utility of the project's meritorious features in other settings. (p. 65)

The role of the evaluators was to provide ongoing and continuous feedback to the foundation leaders and staff so they could make decisions about the project's goals and plans, as well as to make modifications to the implementation of the project.

The Evaluand and Its Context

The Consuelo Foundation proposed a self-help housing project called Ke Aka Ho'ona, which started in 1994 and ended in 2002. The foundation wanted to "provide housing for poor people such that they could succeed over the long haul in maintaining their homes, paying for them, and building a safe, healthy community environment for their families" (Stufflebeam et al., 2002, p. vii). Beginning in 1991, the foundation focused this—its first major project—on addressing housing and community development needs in one of Hawaii's most depressed and crime-ridden areas, the Waianae Coast on Oahu. Through this innovative project, the foundation assisted 75 low-income families to construct their own homes and develop a values-based community, with the long-term aim of engaging the families to take over and govern the community. Moreover, these families, over time, were required to pay for and become full owners of their homes through low-interest mortgages and land leases. For each of 7 years, a module of between 6 and 17 families devoted about 10 months, by working on weekends, to constructing their own homes. They were supervised and assisted by Consuelo Foundation staff and licensed contractors. Also, during this period the foundation provided educational and other social services to address needs of involved families, especially the children. By the end of the 7 years, the foundation, families, and support contractors had converted what was once a 14-acre plot of agricultural land to a beautiful, values-based community of 75 homes that included 390 men, women, and children. Moreover, this community was essentially free of crime.

Method

Design

The evaluation as designed used the CIPP model and included both formative and summative evaluation as part of the design. The formative part of the evaluation provided periodic feedback to the foundation leaders and staff on the project's plans and operations. The summative part of the evaluation summarized and evaluated the outcomes.

Evaluation Purposes and Questions

Stufflebeam et al. (2002) wrote:

1. Context: To what extent was the project targeted to important community and beneficiary needs?

2. Input: To what extent were the project's structure and procedural and resource plans consistent with [Consuelo] Foundation values, state of the art, feasible, and sufficiently powerful to address the targeted needs?

3. Process: To what extent were the project's operations consistent with plans responsibly conducted, and effective in addressing beneficiaries' needs?

4. Impact: What beneficiaries were *reached*, and to what extent were they the targeted beneficiaries?

5. Effectiveness: To what extent did the project *meet* the needs of the involved beneficiaries?

6. Sustainability: To what extent was the project institutionalized in order to sustain its successful implementation?

7. Transportability: To what extent could or has the project been successfully adapted and applied elsewhere? (p. 66; emphasis in original)

Stakeholders and Participants

Beneficiaries, program leaders, and staff were interviewed. The funding organization was viewed as the most important stakeholder.

Data Collection

The evaluators used multiple methods of data collection. These included environmental analysis (contextual information available from existing documents and interviews);

(cont.)

Box 4.3 (cont.)

program profile (qualitative data about the project's "mission, goals, plan, constituents, staff, timetable, resources, progress to date, accomplishments, and recognitions" [Stufflebeam et al., 2002, p. 68]); traveling observers (local individuals who collected data in an ongoing manner based on observation, interviews, and newspaper articles about the project); case studies (interviews with families about the quality of the project and how it influenced their lives); and stakeholder interviews (interviews with the builders of the homes about the construction process and community outcomes). In addition, draft evaluation reports were disseminated to staff members in advance of workshops at which the staff could give feedback on the accuracy and clarity of the reports). Finally, the evaluation team synthesized the 7½ years of evaluation findings, reviewed relevant foundation documents, and submitted a draft evaluation report to the foundation leaders and project staff; the draft was discussed in a format similar to that of the feedback workshops. (These data collection methods are explored further in the discussions of data collection and reporting in Chapters 10 and 13.)

Management and Budget

For the full duration of the project, Stufflebeam was the Principal Investigator. Project managers changed three times over that period. Initial funding of the evaluation allowed for comprehensive data collection. Starting in about year 3, the Consuelo Foundation found it necessary to cut the evaluation budget, therefore, some of the evaluation activities were discontinued or reduced (e.g., the environmental analysis was eliminated after year 3). In an unusually frank disclosure of budgeting for an evaluation, the evaluation report includes this information:

> While the full cost budgets negotiated for this evaluation totaled $947,815, at this writing The Evaluation Center has actually billed $509,980. The $947,815 figure should be reduced by approximately $216,788, since the former figure includes two 2-year budgets that were renegotiated after the first year of the budget period. Using this adjustment, the evaluation's budgeted full cost was $731,027, compared with the $509,980 so far expended. At this writing, the evaluators have saved the Foundation approximately $221,047 or 30 percent of the budgeted amount. This savings will be reduced by up to about $50,000 when the Center submits its final bill, but the savings will still be 23 percent or more. (Stufflebeam, 2002, p. 71)

Meta-Evaluation

The evaluators provide an excellent model of how to conduct a meta-evaluation. They used the 1994 edition of *The Program Evaluation Standards* (Joint Committee on Standards for Educational Evaluation, 1994) to document how they addressed these indicators of quality throughout the evaluation process. Their analysis revealed that they had appropriately addressed all of the standards with the exception of disclosure of information, because that was seen as the prerogative of the foundation.

Reports and Utilization

The evaluation findings were used throughout the project. For example, the initial goal of the project was to serve the poorest of the poor. However, early experiences with this population led to the realization that these families could not get mortgages and were therefore not suitable for inclusion in this project. Instead, the foundation decided to focus on the working poor or the "hidden homeless" (i.e., families who were too poor to own their own homes and lived with other family members in overcrowded conditions). The project required that families work with contractors to help build their homes. The evaluation data were used to document the need to train the families in construction skills and home maintenance skills, as well as to improve their physical conditions so they could participate in the building. Evaluation data were also valuable in highlighting issues that needed to be resolved during the project, such as deciding who would get which house by holding a lottery, so everyone working would give adequate effort in the building. The evaluation data also led to more equity in the amount of land that surrounded each house. The final evaluation report summarizes the use of the evaluation findings thus:

> Ultimately, the [Consuelo] Foundation used lessons learned from the experiences of the eight increments of housing development to improve its project design and enrich it with an option for including different types of housing. A stable, key feature of the project plan was its grounding in a clear set of values, enforceable by invocation of pertinent community covenants. (Stufflebeam et al., 2002, p. 79)

REFLECTIONS FROM THE EVALUATORS

A key to the evaluation's success was its client, Ms. Patti Lyons, the Consuelo Foundation's president. She was a creative, decisive, evaluation-oriented leader. In launching the foundation's flagship project, she sought critical evaluative feedback from the project's very beginning. Moreover, she, members of her staff, and the foundation's board used findings both to guide decision making and to inform interested parties concerning the project's nature and progress. Other keys to the evaluation's success were (1) a clear contract from the outset for an independent evaluation; (2) grounding in the Joint Committee Program Evaluation Standards; (3) an up-front agreed-upon design, calling for context, input, process, and product evaluations; (4) a resident observer who kept track of project events and documents and served as a liaison to the outside evaluators; (5) interviews and case studies involving all Ke Aka Ho'ona families and persons in the broad Waianae area; (6) systematic collection and analysis of relevant foundation and Hawaii documents; (7) a photographic record of project activities and events; (8) interim, formative evaluation reports; (9) regular feedback sessions with President Lyons and her staff to discuss interim findings and assist decision making; (10) periodic reports to the foundation's board; (11) a three-part final summative report, divided into "Project Antecedents," "Project Implementation," and "Project Results," à la Stake's countenance evaluation model; (12) photographs at the end of each report section to illustrate the section's key findings; and (13) delineation of product evaluation findings in terms of impact, effectiveness, sustainability, and transportability. Interestingly, upon reviewing the summative evaluation report, Egon Guba remarked that he would not have believed the extent of success in the Ke Aka Ho'ona project had he not seen the confirmatory photographs at the end of each report section.

As with any evaluation, this one had limitations. For whatever reasons, the foundation

(cont.)

Box 4.3 (cont.)

did not and maybe could not provide the evaluators with sufficiently clear and delineated cost data for determining and analyzing the project's costs. Also, the foundation did not implement the external evaluators' recommendation for an independent meta-evaluation of the external evaluation. Nevertheless, the evaluators provided their attestation of the extent to which the evaluation met the requirements of the Joint Committee Program Evaluation Standards. In the main, they judged that the evaluation had met the Standards' requirements for utility, feasibility, propriety, and accuracy. We also commissioned two [reports] by independent evaluators. Their reports definitely added valuable material and perspectives.

One other recollection is that we learned early not to include the traveling observer (TO) in the feedback sessions. Since this person lived in the neighborhood and sometimes provided us with information on project problems and shortfalls, it proved important to insulate [the TO] from cross-examination by foundation leaders and project staff. Otherwise, we saw that the project staff members could become defensive and also press the TO into a defensive posture. Obviously, such face-to-face conflicts could make it difficult for the TO to perform the close-up day-to-day surveillance of project activities and to maintain cooperation from project staff as well as project beneficiaries. It was better that the TO feedback be incorporated into our reports and that we navigate this potentially sensitive territory.

As noted in Box 4.3, the evaluators conducted contextual evaluation activities through several processes. An environmental analysis included review of existing documents and interviews. The evaluators also used the feedback workshops and interim reports as part of the context evaluation processes. The environmental analysis included gathering information about the "economics, population characteristics, related projects and services, and the needs and problems of the targeted population" (Stufflebeam et al., 2002, p. 68). In addition, interviews were conducted with key stakeholders, including "area school teachers and administrators, government officials, Catholic Charities' personnel, department of Hawaiian Home Lands personnel, local social workers, etc." (p. 68). The information was used to gather information about the targeted population and their needs. The evaluation team conducted the context evaluation activities from the beginning of the project (1994) through 1998, when budget cuts resulted in the elimination of this part of the evaluation.

Input Evaluation

According to Stufflebeam et al. (2002), **input evaluation** is a process of collecting information about the project's "mission, goals, plan, constituents, staff, timetable, resources, progress to date, accomplishments, and recognitions" (p. 68). Box 4.4 explains input evaluation in more detail.

Box 4.4. Input Evaluation

Input evaluation assesses competing strategies and the work plans and budgets of the selected approach.

Evaluator activities	*Client/stakeholder activities—* *Program planning*
Identify and investigate existing programs that could serve as a model for the contemplated program.	Use the input evaluation findings to devise a program strategy that is scientifically, economically, socially, politically, and technologically defensible.
Assess the program's proposed strategy for responsiveness to assessed needs and feasibility.	Use the input evaluation findings to assure that the program's strategy is feasible for meeting the assessed needs of the targeted beneficiaries.
Assess the program's budget for its sufficiency to fund the needed work.	Use the input evaluation findings to support funding requests for the planned enterprise.
Assess the program's strategy against pertinent research and development literature.	Use the input evaluation findings to train staff to carry out the program.
Assess the merit of the program's strategy compared with alternative strategies found in similar programs.	Use the input evaluation findings for accountability purposes in reporting the rationale for the selected program strategy and the defensibility of the operational plan.
Assess the program's work plan and schedule for sufficiency, feasibility, and political viability.	
Compile a draft input evaluation report and send it to the client and agreed-upon stakeholders.	
Discuss input evaluation findings in a feedback workshop.	
Finalize the input evaluation report and associated visual aids and provide them to the client and agreed-upon stakeholders.	

Source: Stufflebeam (2002, p. 5). Reprinted by permission of Daniel L. Stufflebeam.

Sidani and Sechrest (1999, p. 233) identify input variables associated with the participants (clients), staff, and setting:

> *Client characteristics* can be classified into three categories: (1) Personal characteristics, including variables related to demographics, personality traits, and/or personal beliefs. Examples of these variables are: age, gender, educational level, trait anxiety, sense of mastery or control, and cultural values and beliefs. (2) Presenting problem characteristics, including variables that indicate the factor(s) leading to and the level of severity of the presenting problem.... (3) Resources available to clients, which consist of internal and external factors that provide them with the support needed to carry out the prescribed treatment(s).
>
> *Characteristics of the program staff/interveners* include personal and professional attributes or qualities of the person(s) delivering the program services, which are necessary for carrying out the specific program services. Examples of such characteristics are: communication, demeanor, educational background, level of competence or expertise in providing the program services, preferences for treatment modalities, and beliefs and attitudes toward the presenting problem/target population.
>
> *Characteristics of the setting* in which the program is being implemented refer to the physical and psychosocial features of the environment. The physical features include convenience of the setting location to potential clients, availability of material resources necessary for delivering the program services, and the physical layout and its attractiveness. The psychosocial features consist of the social, political, and economic context of the program, such as organizational culture, composition and working relationships among program staff, and norms and policies (Beutler, 1991; Costner, 1989; Finney & Moos, 1989).

Stufflebeam et al. (2002) used a program profile strategy as well as feedback workshops and report reviews by stakeholders for their input evaluation for the Consuelo Foundation study. The program profile strategy consisted of periodic recording of the profile of the project as it moved from its initial stages throughout the first 3 years of the project. The evaluators submitted reports to the foundation staff summarizing the project features that remained stable, noting those that changed, and capturing things that were added. This evaluation activity was also cut after the first 3 years because of budget constraints.

Process Evaluation

Process evaluation, sometimes called implementation evaluation, focuses on the appropriateness and quality of the project's implementation. Box 4.5 explains process evaluation in greater detail.

The WKKF evaluation handbook (WKKF, 1998, p. 25) offers these questions to frame a process or implementation evaluation:

▪ What are the critical components/activities of this project (both explicit and implicit)?

▪ How do these components connect to the goals and intended outcomes for this project?

▪ What aspects of the implementation process are facilitating success or acting as stumbling blocks for the project?

Sidani and Sechrest (1999, pp. 233–234) used the process evaluation concept as a way of developing a theory-based approach to their CIPP evaluation:

Box 4.5. Process Evaluation

Process evaluation monitors, documents, and assesses program activities.

Evaluator activities	*Client/stakeholder activities—Managing and documenting*
▓ Engage an evaluation team member to monitor, observe, maintain a photographic record of, and provide periodic progress reports on program implementation.	▓ Use the process evaluation findings to control and strengthen staff activities. ▓ Use the process evaluation findings to strengthen the program design.
▓ In collaboration with the program's staff, maintain a record of program events, problems, costs, and allocations.	▓ Use the process evaluation findings to maintain a record of the program's progress.
▓ Periodically interview beneficiaries, program leaders, and staff to obtain their assessments of the program's progress.	▓ Use the process evaluation findings to help maintain a record of the program's costs.
▓ Maintain an up-to-date profile of the program.	▓ Use the process evaluation findings to report on the program's progress to the program's financial sponsor, policy board, community members, other developers, etc.
▓ Periodically draft written reports on process evaluation findings and provide the draft reports to the client and agreed-upon stakeholders.	
▓ Present and discuss process evaluation findings in feedback workshops.	
▓ Finalize each process evaluation report (possibly incorporated into a larger report) and associated visual aids and provide them to the client and agreed-upon stakeholders.	

Source: Stufflebeam (2002, p. 6). Reprinted by permission of Daniel L. Stufflebeam.

In this framework, process consists of (1) the theoretically-specified components of a program and the processes believed responsible for producing the anticipated effects, and (2) the program-as-delivered variables that represent the actual implementation of the program. The process variables should accurately reflect which client(s) received which component(s) of the program at which dosage, as well as the series of changes that take place after receiving the program services and that lead to the achievement of the program effects.... Amount refers to the quantity (i.e., how much) of the program services/treatments that should be given. Frequency refers to the number of times the program services/treatments are to be given over a specified period of time. Duration refers to the total length of time the services/treatments are to be implemented for the expected effects to take place (Scott & Sechrest, 1989).

Stufflebeam et al. (2002) used several strategies for their process evaluation: environmental analysis, traveling observers, case studies, stakeholder interviews, goal-free evaluation (discussed in Chapter 5), feedback workshops, and report reviews. The traveling observers were people living in Hawaii who were trained to "monitor and assess both project implementation and project outcomes" (p. 69). They were provided with an explicit protocol to guide them in their activities, which were primarily qualitative data collection (as noted in Box 4.3); they interviewed participants, kept newspaper articles about the project, and briefed the university evaluators before each of their visits. In addition, trained interviewers conducted case studies with families in the project in years 2, 4, and 7, with a focus on the collection of process data about the project's quality, successes, challenges, and strategies for overcoming those challenges.

Product Evaluation

The final part of the CIPP model is **product evaluation,** although many evaluators call this outcome, effectiveness, or impact evaluation. The WKKF evaluation handbook (WKKF, 1998, p. 28) uses these questions to focus a product or outcome evaluation:

- What are the critical outcomes you are trying to achieve?

- What impact is the project having on its clients, its staff, its umbrella organization, and its community?

- What unexpected impact has the project had?

These questions bring attention to intended and unintended outcomes of the project. They also indicate that effects can be observed at different levels: participants, staff, organization, and community. Another important dimension of outcomes of importance is the temporal aspect. Outcomes can be short-term, intermediate-term, or long-term; some broader social impacts may even take years to achieve. Box 4.6 explains product or impact evaluation in more detail.

Sidani and Sechrest (1999) discuss outputs as the part of the program theory that is expected to result from the program. Outputs reflect the "expected output" element of a program theory; they consist of the ultimate outcomes of the program. In order to determine program effectiveness, evaluators need to specify particular outcomes within an expected time frame.

> The nature of the outcomes refers to the particular aspect of the clients' life/condition that the program impacts; it is determined by the presenting problem which the program attempts to resolve and/or the goals of the program. The timing refers to the point at which the changes in the outcomes take place after receipt of the program services/treatments. Some changes occur immediately after program implementation while others take some time to appear (Lipsey, 1993). (p. 234)

Box 4.6. Product or Impact Evaluation

Product or impact evaluation assesses a program's effect on or reach to the target audience.

Evaluator activities	*Client/stakeholder activities— Controlling who gets served*
Engage the program's staff and consultants and/or an evaluation team member to maintain a directory of persons and groups served, make notations on their needs, and record program services they received.	Use the impact evaluation findings to assure that the program is reaching intended beneficiaries.
Assess and make a judgment of the extent to which the served individuals and groups are consistent with the program's intended beneficiaries.	Use the impact evaluation findings to assess whether the program is reaching or did reach inappropriate beneficiaries.
Periodically interview area stakeholders, such as community leaders, employers, school and social programs personnel, clergy, police, judges, and homeowners, to learn their perspectives on how the program is influencing the community.	Use the impact evaluation findings to judge the extent to which the program is serving or did serve the right beneficiaries.
Include the obtained information and the evaluator's judgments in a periodically updated program profile.	Use the impact evaluation findings to judge the extent to which the program addressed or is addressing important community needs.
Determine the extent to which the program reached an appropriate group of beneficiaries.	Use the impact evaluation findings for accountability purposes regarding the program's success in reaching the intended beneficiaries.
Assess the extent to which the program inappropriately provided services to a nontargeted group.	
Draft an impact evaluation report (possibly incorporated into a larger report) and provide it to the client and agreed-upon stakeholders.	

(cont.)

Box 4.6 (*cont.*)

Evaluator activities	Client/stakeholder activities— Controlling who gets served
Discuss impact evaluation findings in a feedback workshop.	
Finalize the impact evaluation report and associated visual aids and provide them to the client and agreed-upon stakeholders.	

Source: Stufflebeam (2002, p. 7). Reprinted by permission of Daniel L. Stufflebeam.

Thus the CIPP model of evaluation is a time-tested approach to use-focused evaluation. It has provided a new perspective for evaluators, moving them away from a way of thinking based on applied social science research and toward a recognition of the need to consider the stakeholders and their need for information. One limitation long associated with this approach, and approaches within the Use Branch in general, is that the stakeholders for whom information is provided are the most powerful. The Social Justice Branch, discussed in Chapter 6, shifts the focus from the most powerful stakeholders to those who have traditionally had less power in the evaluation context.

- - - - - - - - - - E X T E N D I N G   Y O U R   T H I N K I N G - - - - - - - - - -

The CIPP Model

 Use Branch

Sample study	Evaluation approach	List the distinguishing characteristics
Stufflebeam, Gullickson, and Wingate (2002) 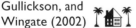	Context, input, process, product (CIPP) evaluation	

Using the description of the Stufflebeam et al. (2002) study in Box 4.3, answer the following questions:

1. What about the Ke Aka Ho'ona community hindered or helped the Consuelo Foundation in achieving its goals?

2. Describe the quantitative and qualitative methods used during the self-help housing project.

3. Since the Consuelo Foundation's evaluation of the Ke Aka Ho'ona community project was done within a pragmatic paradigm, several insights were made that would have been difficult to attain if the evaluation had been done within a postpositivist paradigm. Name several insights attained through this evaluation that were products of this study.

4. According to The Program Evaluation Standards, "Evaluations should account for all expended resources, comply with sound fiscal procedures and processes, and ensure that clients are knowledgeable about fiscal resources expended." Stufflebeam's evaluation team was able to return almost one-fourth of the projected budget for the evaluation of the Consuelo Foundations project. You may not yet be working in the field, but if you were (or if you are), where are areas that you feel that you may be able to be fiscally responsible and be able to cut costs for the funders of the evaluation?

Utilization Focused Evaluation

As stated earlier, Patton (2008) developed the UFE approach as a method of working with "specific intended primary users" (p. 37) to obtain the information they need for specific uses. Box 4.7 describes Walden and Baxter's (2001) "condoms on the waterfront" study, which illustrates the UFE approach, with acknowledgment of borrowing also from the CIPP model.

Box 4.7. Sample UFE Study: The "Condoms on the Waterfront" Study

Sample study	Evaluation approach	Document title
Walden and Baxter (2001)	Utilization-focused evaluation (UFE)	"An Evaluation Model to Assess the HIV/AIDS-Related Behavior Change in Developing Countries"

The Evaluators

Vivien Margaret Walden is an evaluation adviser for Oxfam in the United Kingdom. **David Baxter** is a consultant in Communicable Diseases Control and District Immunisation Coordinator in Stockport, Greater Manchester, United Kingdom; he is also Lecturer in Epidemiology and Health Sciences at Manchester University.

(cont.)

Box 4.7 (cont.)

Philosophical and Theoretical Lenses

The evaluators note that their work was consistent with Patton's UFE approach. This led to the use of a mixed methods approach in order to refine their evaluation questions and to allow for participation of beneficiaries in the evaluation design, implementation, and interpretation of the findings. Thus their theoretical model for evaluation is a participatory mixed methods model that is based on the UFE approach to evaluation. The evaluators' role was to provide data-based information to the project staff throughout the project to establish baseline, make continuous improvements, and measure impact.

The Evaluand and Its Context

The evaluand was a "community-based HIV/AIDS/STD-prevention programme for single women (including sex workers) and their potential partners, especially fishermen and workplace men. The project catchment area is a lakeside border town with fishing and tourism as the two main activities" (Walden & Baxter, 2001, p. 441). Volunteer peer educators were recruited from the sex worker community; they received training and then provided health education and distributed condoms.

Method

Design

The evaluators used a mixed methods approach. The evaluation design was based on UFE and the comprehensive community-oriented evaluation (CCOE) model, which has three components (Walden & Baxter, 2001, p. 441):

> Design evaluation is concerned with the pre-programme data collection such as baseline surveys, feasibility studies and assessment of pilot projects.
>
> Process evaluation (including monitoring) covers the implementation period and was designed to show how the intervention was delivered and how the results were achieved.
>
> Impact evaluation is the term given to an assessment carried out at the end of the project life, mid-term or at [any] other time it is deemed necessary to measure success or failure of achieving project objectives.

During the actual program evaluation carried out by the evaluators, only the process and impact components were used.

Evaluation Purposes and Questions

The evaluation purposes were (1) to determine how the program was being implemented, and (2) to determine the impact of the program on safe sex practices against the baseline. The evaluation questions were not stated in the article, but could be inferred to be these : (1) What factors need to be considered in the ongoing improvement of the program? (2) What is the impact of the program on the two indicator variables?

Stakeholders and Participants

Three levels of stakeholders were identified: the donor, the project staff, and the program participants (beneficiaries).

Data Collection

The initial feasibility study indicated that reliable quantitative baseline measures of condom use and safe sex practices were available for two of the target groups (but not for the men in the workplace). These data were used to measure outcomes during the evaluation.

The implementation evaluation (carried out by program staff) involved having frequent meetings with the peer educators. During these meetings, data about support groups and condom distribution were written on wall charts for everyone to see and discuss. Unfortunately, these data were not always interpreted or acted upon. For example, the evaluators noted that some of the target groups were only sporadically addressed and that condom distribution was at times erratic.

The outcome evaluation focused on the number of condoms distributed and safer sex practices among risk groups. As well as looking at unexpected outcomes and impact (spinoffs), it also attempted to look at attribution of behavior change to the program activities.

These elements—mixed methods, stakeholder involvement, feedback, evaluation audit, and results consensus—were necessary in varying degrees at each stage of the evaluation cycle.

Management and Budget

As this was a PhD dissertation project for one of the evaluators (Walden), costs differed from those of a conventional external program evaluation.

Meta-Evaluation

After the impact evaluation was carried out, the results and methodology were discussed with a representative of the donor agency, the project field staff and managerial team, and the volunteer peer educators, using semistructured interviews and focus group discussions.

Reports and Utilization

The pre- and postintervention data on condom distribution were used to establish the impact of the program. Unfortunately, no design stage data were collected from the beneficiaries about the nature of the project. Hence the beneficiaries were not included in the project planning, and at times they had a very different idea of the project's purpose. The single women thought that the project was also supposed to assist women to get out of prostitution, but the project staff had the objectives of providing education and condoms, reducing STD infections, establishing support groups, and making small loans.

(cont.)

Box 4.7 (cont.)

The beneficiaries (apart from the peer educators) were also not involved in the collection of the data during the implementation phase. As mentioned above in the "Method" section, data were presented at monthly meetings; however, the volunteers did not consistently use this information to change their activities. For example, the lack of qualitative data did not highlight the number of unused and discarded condoms, or the fact that a large number of foreign sex workers had come across the border. After the study was over, the volunteers did indicate that they would have liked to have been trained in better data collection skills.

REFLECTIONS FROM AN EVALUATOR

What have I [Vivien Walden] learned since? I guess the most important thing is that if evaluations are not used to improve programming or to share learning, then they really are a waste of time and resources. I now work for one of the United Kingdom's largest NGOs and carry out numerous evaluations every year across the globe in our humanitarian programs. I do facilitated self-evaluations whereby I facilitate the program team [members] to evaluate their own program. My experience has shown that if people are involved during the process and discover constraints and weaknesses for themselves, they are more likely to "own the process" and to take forward recommendations. My role is often to challenge their actions and assumptions, but together we look for solutions—the results consensus that we used in the CCOE model.

Involving the recipients of the program—in our case, people affected by crisis—also means that whatever we do is contextually sound and is meeting the needs of the population. Everyone has a right to comment on and evaluate a program in which they are involved as either recipients or participants.

The first step in UFE is to identify the specific intended primary users who have the responsibility to act on the evaluation findings. This means that names of specific persons need to be identified and relationships established (as opposed to doing the evaluation for the "feds" or the "deaf" community or "homeless people"). The evaluator's responsibility is to identify who the intended users are, present them with a menu of choices for how evaluations can be used, and adhere to the other standards for a good evaluation (i.e., accuracy, feasibility, and propriety). I usually include an explanation of the standards for a good evaluation in my early meetings with clients, so they can see that my emphasis on utility, accuracy, feasibility, and propriety are criteria that my profession endorses. In this way, I communicate that I am a member of a larger professional community with responsibilities to uphold quality in my work, and that my doing so adds value to the evaluation that I will do for them.

In the Walden and Baxter (2001) study (see Box 4.7), the evaluators identified three groups of stakeholders: the donor, project staff, and beneficiaries. The majority of their provision of information for decision making focused on the donor and the staff. They did not report going through a process of presenting a menu of possible uses of evaluation results with their intended users.

UFE does not prescribe particular methods or models for evaluation; its mission is to be sure that the methods or models are matched to the needs of the intended users. UFE can be used for formative and summative evaluations; in conjunction with program developers; with quantitative, qualitative, or mixed methods; for the purpose of cost analysis, context, input, process, and product evaluations; and for needs assessments. Walden and Baxter (2001) undertook a participatory approach to evaluation by selecting and training members of the community to deliver the services to the beneficiaries. However, they acknowledge that they did not establish a clear set of expectations in terms of the project's mission or of adherence to the program as it was outlined in the proposal. Hence they discovered that the workers were only implementing part of the program (i.e., distribution of condoms and not support groups).

As most evaluators know, evaluations are often commissioned with the best intentions; however, there are times when these intentions are not fulfilled, for a variety of reasons. Perhaps the funding initiative is ending; perhaps staff cuts leave everyone without time for reflective program changes; or perhaps priorities change. Therefore, UFE moves from identifying intended users to educating them about the possible uses of evaluation and establishing the conditions that lead to their commitment to make use of the evaluation findings. Patton (2008) solicits the intended users' perceptions of evaluation (ranging from measuring things to being useless), and then presents his own perspective on evaluation, which includes the ideas that it involves the systematic collection of information about a wide range of possible issues for a variety of possible uses. This sets up subsequent discussion about the types of information uses that are crucial for this particular group of intended users.

Discussions about evaluation should include consideration of possible barriers and resistance to evaluation, as well as a focus on positive constructive uses. Such barriers can include beliefs that nothing will really change; that intended users already know what is good and what is not, that they may lose their jobs if negative findings emerge; that change just upsets things; that money for evaluation is better spent on service delivery; or that "I know it is required, but please do as little as possible so you don't disturb what we are really trying to do" (compliance attitude). Patton (2008) suggests that evaluators directly address this "evaluation anxiety" (p. 46).

I have found that most people who are running programs do not really want to waste time and money. As a caveat, there are dishonest people in programs who want to take the money and not provide the services. (See Box 4.8.) There are also people who are hostile early in the evaluation process, or who have rigid ideas and resent having an evaluation imposed upon them from the outside (e.g., as part of the requirements to get funding). Early in my evaluation career, the first time I came face to face with a specific client, he asked me: "What are you going to do if you get negative findings?" His tone of voice and body language were not congenial. I said, "I expect that we both want to see this program succeed. If I find negative things, you will be the first person to know. Then you will be able to make changes as you see necessary to revise the program's activities to bring them in line with what you hope to achieve."

Box 4.8. An Example of the Need for Evaluation

In a newspaper article titled "Staggering Need, Striking Neglect," Cenziper (2009) reported that the District of Columbia Health Department spent millions of dollars on AIDS services but did not collect data on how the funds were used or whether any sick people actually got services. Washington, D.C., has the highest rate of AIDS in the United States. The article included these quotes (Cenziper, 2009, p. A-1):

- "More than $1 million in AIDS money went to a housing group whose ailing boarders sometimes struggled without electricity, gas or food. A supervisor said she was ordered to create records for ghost employees."

- "About $400,000 was paid to a nonprofit organization, launched by a man who once ran one of the District's largest cocaine rings for a promised job-training center that has never opened."

- "More than $500,000 was earmarked for a housing program whose executive director has a string of convictions for theft, drugs and forgery. After the D.C. Inspector General's Office could find no evidence he was operating an AIDS nonprofit group, the city terminated the grant but never sought repayment."

· · · · · · · · · · · E X T E N D I N G   Y O U R   T H I N K I N G · · · · · · · · · · ·

Utilization–Focused Evaluation

 Use Branch

Sample study	Evaluation approach	List the distinguishing characteristics
Walden and Baxter (2001)	Utilization-focused evaluation (UFE)	"An Evaluation Model to Assess the HIV/AIDS-Related Behavior Change in Developing Countries"

Using the description of the Walden and Baxter (2001) study in Box 4.7, answer the following questions:

1. What are the characteristics that illustrate Walden and Baxter's use of the UFE Model of evaluation?

2. What do you identify as the strengths and weaknesses of this model in terms of the types of data that were collected by the evaluators?

3. What do you identify as the strengths and weaknesses of the strategies used in this study that were intended to increase utilization of the results?

4. What would you suggest modifying in this study to improve the usefulness of the results?

Learning Organization Evaluation

As described earlier in this chapter, Preskill and Torres (1999) have provided a model for evaluation called "learning organization evaluation." They work with businesses and schools to establish these organizations' cultures with regard to evaluation. Are they open to evaluation? What kinds of past experiences have they had with evaluation? How can the organizations build evaluation into their everyday practices and then use that information to adapt to changing contextual variables and/or to achieve their goals? Box 4.9 describes a study using this model of evaluation.

Box 4.9. Sample Learning Organization Evaluation Study: The School Reform Study

Sample study	Evaluation approach	Document title
Sutherland (2004)	Learning organization evaluation	"Creating a Culture of Data Use for Continuous Improvement: A Case Study of an Edison Project School"

The Evaluators

Stephanie Sutherland is employed at the Learning Research and Development Center at the University of Pittsburgh. Her role in the evaluation was as a research associate who provided conceptual input into the data collection protocols, data collection, analysis, and report writing. She does say that research teams of two to three people did the data collection, but she does not identify who these other people were.

The Evaluand and Its Context

The evaluand was a 4-year comprehensive school reform program in 12 Title I schools. The school reform took place under the auspices of the Edison Project, which is a private company that takes over public schools or works with charter schools at the current public school funding levels. The evaluation report focuses on the first 2 years of the project.

Philosophical and Theoretical Lens

This evaluation is situated in the Use Branch, as it focused on the promotion and maintenance of a learning culture in organizations (schools) for continuous improvement.

(cont.)

Box 4.9 (cont.)

The evaluator reviewed the literature on building a framework for what is thought to be related to an organization's inclination to use data for improvement. The model suggests that the upper-level policy makers must mandate the use of such data for improvement. Such a mandate is an external motivational force. Factors related to internal motivation also need to be considered; these include people's self-determined actions because they see the value of the proposed changes. Institutional structures need to be modified as well, to respond to increasing demands for accountability. This means that school processes and structures need to be examined to determine how to facilitate the use of data for continuous improvement. This model also includes an element of teaching the stakeholders about evaluation and giving them opportunities to share their learning with others in the organization. All of these elements combine to address the need for a culture change in the organization.

Method

Evaluation Purposes and Questions

The evaluation purpose was to investigate and evaluate school change efforts as part of an initiative to increase the school's use of data for continuous improvement.

Stakeholders and Participants

The evaluator conducted 46 interviews with principals, teachers, other staff members, parents, and students. In addition, she conducted 12 interviews with state officials, the superintendent, the assistant superintendent, and other high-level administrators.

Data Collection

The schools use data from the Edison Benchmark system to monitor progress of students. This is an online system of 15-question tests in reading, language arts, and math that teachers can use to get immediate feedback on students' learning at an individual or group level. The evaluators also conducted observations in classrooms that corresponded with the site visits used to do the interviews. They created observation logs and field notes, and integrated these with the interview data.

Management and Budget

The article does not include information about management and budget.

Meta-Evaluation

Sutherland says that there was no meta-evaluative component to this study.

Reports and Utilization

The interview data revealed that the districts had responded to the evidence-based mandates by making a commitment to support the schools in their analysis and use of data. The teachers viewed the improvements that they witnessed in students as reinforcing and as engendering more internal motivation to use the data. Other teachers continued to see the emphasis on testing and benchmarks as sources of stress. Sutherland (2004) states: "It is hoped that the findings from this investigation will be used in concert with results from other studies, so that the elements required to create and sustain a culture for continuous improvement using data can be further empirically identified, and that a more robust framework can be developed" (p. 290).

Preskill and Torres (1999) identify three inquiry phases in the learning organization evaluation model:

1. *Focusing the inquiry.* Team members determine what issues and concerns the evaluative effort will address, who the stakeholders are, and what questions will guide the evaluative inquiry.

2. *Carrying out the inquiry.* Organization members determine the most appropriate inquiry design; methods of data collection, analysis, and interpretation; and methods of communicating and reporting strategies.

3. *Applying learning:* Organization members develop strategies that address the evaluative inquiry's outcomes, design and implement action plans based on these strategies, and monitor the progress of actions taken.

During each of these phases, the stakeholders engage in learning processes that include dialogue; reflection; asking questions; and identifying and clarifying values, beliefs, assumptions, and knowledge. In the Sutherland (2004) study, the learning processes were evident in the use of literature reviews, engagement with stakeholders, and examination of policies. Interviews with stakeholders are also points of dialogue that allow multiple points of view to surface and allow exploration of shared meanings. This results in a stronger sense of community and increases the likelihood that the stakeholders will be open to learning.

Reflection is another important learning strategy in the learning organization model of evaluation. This enables stakeholders to think about the innovation, recognize their own feelings about the change, and challenges them to align their values and their behaviors. In the Sutherland (2004) study, teachers wanted to improve their teaching, and for some of them, the continuous use of data was viewed as contributing to that goal.

Organization Evaluation

 Use Branch

Sample study		Evaluation approach	List the distinguishing characteristics
Sutherland (2004)		Learning organization evaluation	

Using the description of the Sutherland (2004) study in Box 4.9, answer the following questions:

1. What are the characteristics that illustrate Sutherland's use of the Learning Organization Model of evaluation?

2. What do you identify as the strengths and weaknesses of this model in terms of the types of data that were collected by the evaluators?

3. What do you identify as the strengths and weaknesses of the strategies used in this study that were intended to increase utilization of the results?

4. What would you suggest modifying in this study to improve the usefulness of the results?

Empowerment Evaluation

As noted earlier, **Dave Fetterman** and **Abe Wandersman** developed the approach to evaluation called empowerment evaluation. Box 4.10 describes an example of such an evaluation, conducted by Fetterman (2009). The basic principle guiding empowerment evaluation is that the program staff is in charge of the direction and execution of the evaluations, while an evaluator serves as a critical friend, coach, advisor, or guide (Fetterman, 2009). Fetterman and Wandersman (2005) provide the following definition of empowerment evaluation: "It is an approach that aims to increase the likelihood that programs will achieve results by increasing the capacity of program stakeholders to plan, implement, and evaluate their own programs" (p. 27).

The role of the evaluator in empowerment evaluation is not as an expert or director. Rather, the evaluator plays the role of a critical friend, which is more akin to being a coach or advisor. The critical friend helps the stakeholders to identify their goals and strategies for changes needed to reach those goals, using data as the basis for their decisions. These result in the stakeholders' empowering themselves to make changes to improve their programs.

Box 4.10. Sample Empowerment Evaluation Study: The Medical Education Study

Sample study	Evaluation approach	Document title
Fetterman (2009)	Empowerment evaluation	"Empowerment Evaluation at the Stanford University School of Medicine: Using a Critical Friend to Improve the Clerkship Experience"

The Evaluator

David Fetterman is the President of Fetterman and Associates. At the time this evaluation was carried out, he was the Director of Evaluation, Division of Evaluation, Stanford University School of Medicine.

Philosophical and Theoretical Lens

Fetterman's study is situated in the Use Branch, because it focused on allowing the project people to decide for themselves what was needed in terms of an evaluation, as well as to plan and implement the evaluation so that they would be in a good position to use the results.

The Evaluand and Its Context

The Stanford University School of Medicine curriculum includes rotations for students through a variety of clerkships. The students rated two of the clerkships very low, and the medical school wanted to evaluate the clerkships to figure out how to respond to these low ratings.

Method

Design

The evaluator scheduled a meeting with the medical school faculty members involved in each problematic clerkship. During the meeting, he presented the student and faculty ratings. The group then discussed possible reasons for the low ratings and decided that there were three time points where evaluation could be useful: orientation, and the middle and end of the clerkship. The group made a list of things that could be done to improve their performance, such as putting orientation information online, as well as reviewing students' performance at midclerkship and providing them with feedback.

Evaluation Purpose and Questions

The evaluation's purpose was to determine whether the new strategies designed by the faculty were working.

(cont.)

Box 4.10 *(cont.)*

Stakeholders and Participants

Students, faculty, and administrators participated in the evaluation.

Data Collection

The School of Medicine administrators, faculty, and students created a statement of the goals for their program and assessed how well they believed they were accomplishing those goals. They then reviewed the low rankings on the two problematic clerkships and agreed that changes were needed. They "created new goals, related to the activities they just rated and discussed, and new strategies to accomplish those goals" (Fetterman, 2009, p. 200). The evaluator helped the groups conduct surveys, focus groups, interviews, and observations.

Management and Budget

The evaluation tools helped determine whether the new strategies were successful. The information gathered midway through the clerkships was given to the group members, who were then able to make any necessary changes in the program. Illustrations of the baseline data compared to the second collection of data showed clearly how curricular changes had been made. No budget information was included.

Meta-Evaluation

Fetterman (2009) judged that the evaluation was effective, because the program changes resulted in higher ratings for both of the clerkships in question.

Report and Utilization

The data were used to make midcourse corrections in the two clerkships. The clerkships both showed significant improvement in student ratings in less than 1 year.

Empowerment evaluation has three steps:

- First, the stakeholders identify the mission of their organization.
- Second, they "take stock" by identifying what needs to be evaluated, and are given "dots" to vote on their priorities for what is most in need of evaluation. They then rate the organization on how well it is doing in each of the priority areas, usually on a scale of 1 (low) to 10 (high).
- The third step is "plan for the future," in which the stakeholders decide what needs to be changed for them to address the weak areas identified in step 2. The stakeholders then decide what evidence is needed to see whether the changes that they identify are working as intended. The evaluator provides guidance at this point in regard to methods of data collection, but the stakeholders conduct the evaluation themselves.

Critique of Empowerment Evaluation

Empowerment evaluation has been the object of criticism, on the grounds that it abdicates the role of the evaluator to program participants who do not have the skills to undertake an evaluation, even with a professional evaluator as a coach (Stufflebeam, 1994; Scriven, 2005; Sechrest, 1997). Two reviews of empowerment evaluation studies indicated that little evidence was available to indicate that the intended outcome of empowering those who participated in the evaluation or the program beneficiaries occurred (Miller & Campbell, 2006; Patton, 2005).

· · · · · · · · · · · E X T E N D I N G　Y O U R　T H I N K I N G · · · · · · · · · · ·

Empowerment Evaluation

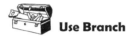 **Use Branch**

Sample study	Evaluation approach	List the distinguishing characteristics
Fetterman (2009)	Empowerment evaluation	

Using the description of the Fetterman (2009) study in Box 4.10, answer the following questions:

1. What are the characteristics that illustrate Fetterman's use of the Empowerment Model of evaluation?

2. What do you identify as the strengths and weaknesses of this model in terms of the types of data that were collected by the evaluator?

3. What do you identify as the strengths and weaknesses of the strategies used in this study that were intended to increase utilization of the results?

4. How would you suggest modifying this study to improve the usefulness of the results?

Practical Participatory Evaluation

Practical participatory evaluation rests on the assumption that stakeholders who are in positions to make decisions about programs need to be involved in the evaluation process in meaningful ways. Box 4.11 describes a study using this approach to evaluation.

Box 4.11. Sample Practical Participatory Evaluation Study: The Disability Rehabilitation Study

Sample study		Evaluation approach	Document title
Sharma and Deepak (2001)	(C B R hòa binh)	Practical participatory evaluation	"A Participatory Evaluation of a Community-Based Rehabilitation Programme in North Central Vietnam"

The Evaluators

Manoj Sharma is a professor in the Health Promotion and Education program in the College of Education, Criminal Justice, and Human Services at the University of Cincinnati. Sunil Deepak is the head of the Medical Support Department of the Associazione Italiana Amici di Raoul Follereau (AIFO) in Bologna, Italy. (Note: The words "hòa binh" in the icon for this study mean "peace" in Vietnamese.)

The Evaluand and Its Context

In 1976, the World Health Organization (WHO) acknowledged that throughout the world, 90% of people with disabilities were neglected and not receiving primary health care or rehabilitative services. In recognition of this marginalization, WHO launched an initiative called "community-based rehabilitation" (CBR), which would bring needed services to persons with disabilities by tapping resources already available in their communities. The five basic principles of CBR are as follows:

- Utilization of available resources in the community.

- Transfer of knowledge about disabilities and skills in rehabilitation to people with disabilities, families, and communities.

- Community involvement in planning, decision making, and evaluation.

- Utilization and strengthening of referral services at district, provincial, and national levels, so that personnel are able to perform skilled assessments with increasing sophistication, make rehabilitation plans, and participate in training and supervision.

- Utilization of a coordinated, multisectoral approach.

Vietnam is one of the world's poorest countries and is typical in its neglect of people with disabilities. At the time of the study, Vietnamese families subsisted on $320 a year; more than one-third of the population was under 14 years of age; average life expectancy was 58 years; one-third of all infants born died within their first year of life; and clean water and appropriate sanitation conditions were out of reach for almost half of the rural population. Only 3.1% of the federal budget was spent on health care for the entire population, and people with disabilities were very likely to benefit from this set-aside.

CBR was introduced to Vietnam in 1987. In 1992, WHO invited an Italian NGO, the AIFO, to establish a 3-year pilot project in a north central province to focus on the medical needs of people with disabilities. The AIFO partnered with a Vietnamese NGO called the Viet Nam Rehabilitation Association (VINAREHA). In 1996, the European Union (EU) supported a VINAREHA 3-year CBR project in five north central provinces whose goals were these (Sharma & Deepak, 2001, p. 353):

- Training of a nucleus of trainers that would train the peripheral level staff as well as volunteers.
- Transfer of knowledge from the rehabilitation workers to the PWD [persons with disabilities] and their families about disabilities and rehabilitation.
- Promotion of a multisectoral approach through the formation of CBR committees in the provinces for the planning and implementation of the programme activities.
- Use of appropriate technology for the production of simple orthopaedic appliances, utilizing the locally available raw materials.
- Improving the referral services for rehabilitation at district and province levels.
- Promoting the integration of children with disabilities in normal schools.
- Enhancing the role of organizations of PWD for promoting activities for protection of their human rights.
- Promoting economic self-sufficiency for PWD through creation of rotating credit funds, professional training, and employment.

Philosophical and Theoretical Lens

Sharma and Deepak (2001) wrote:

> The participatory approach used in this evaluation has its roots based on the principles of liberation theology, social activism, community psychology and rural development. The approach builds on accepting the potential of the people, focusing on the reality of experiences rather than thrusting knowledge [on people], respecting the views of the community rather than pushing outside ideas, and working from a mutually shared terrain rather than imposing theoretical ideas onto the community. The approach utilized in this evaluation is based on the postmodernist paradigm that discards the notion of objective reality and emphasizes value on meaning and interpretation. (p. 353)

The evaluators used a participatory approach because it is a robust approach that works well in a situation like this. It also empowers the local project team members in various aspects of evaluation, and thereby enhances their capacity to independently carry out evaluation tasks in the future. Despite the evaluators' intent to situate their work in social activism, they acknowledge that their evaluation focused more on the views of the service providers than on those of persons with disabilities. Since these findings were used to submit a report, publish an article, and obtain additional funding, and not for social action, it is placed in the use category rather than the social justice category.

The role of the principal evaluator (Manoj Sharma) was that of a facilitator and sympathetic critic. He provided training on various aspects of evaluation to the local

(cont.)

Box 4.11 *(cont.)*

team, and helped to develop a "strengths, weaknesses, opportunities, threats" (SWOT) framework for the project and its impact.

Methods

Design

The evaluation team used a practical participatory approach to evaluation design. The evaluation was facilitated by Manoj Sharma, with support from the local project team in Vietnam. Members of the local team led the focus groups, conducted the interviews, and helped with translations. This was Sharma's first visit to Vietnam. He was not familiar with Vietnam, but he was trained in the participatory approach. The local team that helped with data collection was from Vietnam and was well versed in the local culture. Several constraints (such as time and budget) prevented the interviewing of all stakeholders, so CBR national members randomly selected five districts of three provinces to be included in the evaluation. The district personnel then selected the communes where all people with disabilities and personnel involved in CBR were contacted for interviews. At the commune and village levels, only joint semistructured interviews were given. The facilitator's English was translated into the villagers' primary language, Kinh, and responses were retranslated and transcribed.

Evaluation Purposes and Questions

The purpose of this participatory evaluation was to determine the extent of the success of a 3-year (1996–1999) CBR program based on the WHO model, which ran in five north central provinces in Vietnam. The evaluation examined the findings against the principles of CBR set by the WHO model to discover what was successful in order to develop implications for future CBR programming.

As noted above, SWOT framework was used for collecting data. The primary questions posed for reflection were these:

1. *Strengths:* What are some of the strong aspects that you think the program has been able to accomplish in the past 3 years?

2. *Weaknesses:* What are some of the difficulties that you think the program has encountered in the past 3 years?

3. *Opportunities:* What are some of the areas that you think the program can consolidate and augment over the next 3 years?

4. *Threats:* What are some of the areas that you think the program will face difficulties in over the next 3 years?

Stakeholders and Participants

The stakeholders were categorized at five levels: the central level, provincial level, district level, commune level, and village level. These different levels of services reflect the administrative setup of Vietnam, where certain specialized services (such as reconstructive surgery) are available only at the central level in Hanoi or at the provincial headquarters level. At the time of the study, each provincial hospital had a rehabilitation unit with rehabilitation doctors, for providing referral level support including technical appliances. At district-level health centers, there were only general doctors and nurses. At the village and commune levels (a commune is a group of adjacent villages), there were only health workers and community volunteers, who had received limited training in CBR.

Data Collection

Data collection was carried out over a 2-month period by Sharma. Participatory data collection utilized semistructured interviews and focus group discussions. All six central personnel were members of the national CBR committee and participated in an English-only focus group, followed by individual semistructured interviews. Participatory data at the provincial and district levels were collected jointly, except for two of the six focus groups (one of which consisted only of district-level participants and the other only of the corresponding provincial-level participants). The other focus groups were made up of CBR committee members and two members of each district and province steering committee. The focus groups and semistructured interviews were guided by the SWOT framework, with the addition of probing questions when needed. Participant-generated topics were welcomed and encouraged.

> The data were recorded in the form of notes in a field book. Then the data were collated in three categories: (1) village and commune level; (2) district and province level; and (3) national level in the four identified themes: (1) strengths; (2) weaknesses; (3) opportunities; and (4) threats. Each idea expressed by participants was written down. If the statements supplemented an existing idea, it was added to the already written statement. Efforts were taken to document all the ideas mentioned by the participants. Finally, the data were re-collated across levels along the four themes. The data analysis was done by transcribing the field notes on a computer word processor. The researcher and facilitator involved with data collection and analysis was in no way involved with any aspect of programme administration or management. (Sharma & Deepak, pp. 354–355)

Management and Budget

The project lasted 3 years (June 1996–June 1999), and the data collection was done in June and July 1999. A grant from the EU and the AIFO paid for the facilitator's fee and travel expenses.

Meta-Evaluation

The "evaluation of the evaluation" was done by preparing a manuscript and submitting it for close scrutiny by a panel of peer reviewers at the journal *Disability and Rehabilitation*. The reviewers asked several questions and provided various comments, which helped in clarifying some more aspects of the evaluation. Meta-evaluation was also done by the funders, who expressed satisfaction with this report.

(cont.)

Box 4.11 (cont.)

Reports and Utilization

The findings were shared with those CBR personnel and persons with disabilities involved with the 3-year project, as one purpose of the study was to plan for future programming. The findings were also shared with the EU and AIFO, which provided continued funding for this project.

REFLECTIONS FROM AN EVALUATOR

In terms of some reflections about the process and challenges, since I [Sunil Deepak] didn't participate in the specific field evaluation, my comments should be seen more as cumulative ideas that come with hindsight and looking at different evaluations in many CBR programs. Evaluations in CBR programs sometimes focus more on views and perceptions of personnel and program managers than on persons with disabilities and communities themselves. Even when evaluations take note of views and perceptions of persons with disabilities, certain groups—for example, persons with intellectual disabilities, mental illness, multiple disabilities, hearing loss, and speech disabilities—may not be included or adequately represented. In some countries with strong central control of governments and bodies such as people's committees, people may not be willing to express any critical thoughts, so evaluators need to look for other evidence and maybe use indirect ways to elicit information. Language and cultural barriers, already a problem, become even more important in such contexts.

King (2005) offers many ideas for how to conduct practical participatory evaluation. She recommends the active involvement of stakeholders in ways that helps build their capacity to do evaluation themselves. Because this creates additional time demands in the form of meetings, training sessions, assignments related to data collection, and ongoing interactions with the evaluators, evaluators need to consider whether the culture and climate are supportive of a participatory evaluation. A necessary follow-up to the evaluation training is continual monitoring to see whether the stakeholders' evaluation capacity is improving. Practical participatory evaluation is a responsive process, in that changes may need to be made if interim data suggest that changes are necessary; the method for making such decisions should be a collaborative process. Thus frequent and effective communication between the evaluators and the stakeholders at all levels is crucial. Consideration should be given to both oral and written reports with joint collaboration on the format and content of the reports. King (2005) also recommends creating an advisory group, developing an internal evaluation infrastructure, increasing stakeholders' capacity to use test scores, and instituting action research activities.

Practical Participatory Evaluation

 Use Branch

Sample study		Evaluation approach	List the distinguishing characteristics
Sharma and Deepak (2001)		Practical participatory evaluation	

Using the description of the Sharma and Deepak (2001) study in Box 4.11, answer the following questions:

1. What are the characteristics that illustrate Sharma and Deepak's use of the Practical Participatory Model of evaluation?

2. What do you identify as the strengths and weaknesses of this model in terms of the types of data that were collected by the evaluator?

3. What do you identify as the strengths and weaknesses of the strategies used in this study that were intended to increase utilization of the results?

4. What would you suggest modifying in this study to improve the usefulness of the results?

Critiques of the Use Branch

Brandon and Singh (2009) reviewed evaluation studies that focused on use, and reported that they could not find evidence in the majority of the studies to suggest that the evaluation findings were actually used. The studies were also generally weak in terms of establishing the validity of the data collection instruments. Hence Brandon and Singh concluded that it was probably better that the evaluation findings were not used more, as the data collection was insufficient to support the recommendations that came from the studies. If evaluators want to improve the use of their studies, these authors suggest that they pay more attention to rigor in methods.

········· E X T E N D I N G   Y O U R   T H I N K I N G ·········
Use Branch Evaluations

1   If you were about to conduct a use-based study, what two lessons from Walden and Baxter's (2001) study would you keep in mind in your own study?

2. Ordinarily when individuals learn that their project, work, or program will be evaluated, they react negatively. As mentioned earlier, people can have "evaluation anxiety" and resist cooperating with the evaluators. They may have had a negative experience with a previous evaluation. Imagine that you are meeting with a group of stakeholders who are told they must cooperate with you, the evaluator. What speech could you prepare to convince the group that using a UFE or empowerment evaluation methodology will be beneficial and sustainable, and will work for them and not against them?

3. Deepak reflects in Box 4.11 that it isn't always possible for an evaluator to speak directly to those who are beneficiaries of the program being evaluated—specifically, "persons with intellectual disabilities, mental illness, multiple disabilities, hearing [disabilities,] and speech disabilities." According to *The Program Evaluation Standards* (Joint Committee, 2011, p. 23), "Evaluations should devote attention to the full range of individuals and groups invested in the program and affected by its evaluation." As an evaluator, what kind of effort can or should you make to include people with disabilities in the evaluation process?

Your Evaluation Plan: Your Philosophical Stance

Begin writing your understandings of the pragmatic paradigm and the Use Branch as a way of clarifying your own thinking about your philosophical beliefs and how they might influence the way you conduct an evaluation. This can become part of your evaluation plan later, when you decide which approach you will use.

 ### Moving On to the Next Chapter

Evaluators who were concerned with the meanings ascribed to evaluation findings, and the need to reflect the complexity of the perspectives within those findings, developed the Values Branch of evaluation. They proposed the use (primarily) of qualitative methods in order to capture the diversity of stakeholders' experiences and the implications of different values for determining how to interpret those findings. In Chapter 5, we will examine the Values Branch of evaluation. Evaluators in this branch focus on the intended users as a means to increasing the impact of their evaluations.

*   *   *

Remember the studies below, as we refer to them again in later chapters.

Use Branch

Sample study	Evaluation approach	Topical area
Stufflebeam, Gullickson, and Wingate (2002)	Context, input, process, product (CIPP) evaluation	Housing for poor people in Hawaii
Walden and Baxter (2001)	Utilization-focused evaluation (UFE)	Condom use among sex workers
Sutherland (2004)	Learning organization evaluation	School reform in high-poverty areas in the United States
Fetterman (2009)	Empowerment evaluation	Improving clerkships for medical students
Sharma and Deepak (2001)	Practical participatory evaluation	Community-based rehabilitation (CBR) with disabled persons

Preparing to Read Chapter Five

Branch	Paradigm	Description
Methods	Postpositivist	Focuses primarily on quantitative designs and data
Use	Pragmatic	Focuses primarily on data that are found to be useful by stakeholders; advocates for the use of mixed methods
Values	**Constructivist**	**Focuses primarily on identifying multiple values and perspectives through qualitative methods**
Social justice	Transformative	Focuses primarily on viewpoints of marginalized groups and interrogating systemic power structures through mixed methods to further social justice and human rights

As you prepare to read this chapter, think about these questions:

1. What are the characteristics of the constructivist paradigm?

2. How do those characteristics influence the practice of evaluation?

3. Which major thinkers have contributed to the approaches associated with the Values Branch?

4. How did the ideas grow from the early days to the present in this theoretical context?

CHAPTER FIVE

The Constructivist Paradigm

and the Values Branch

Imagine that you have developed a partnership with the stakeholders of a program designed to lessen the occurrence of cyberbullying. From the beginning of the evaluation until its end, you engage the stakeholders with questions and discussions; you modify your approach on the basis of their responses. You are open to learning and modifying your evaluation process according to what they share with you. You are interested in knowing their lived experiences from how they perceive the world. Imagine that this process puts aside the importance of predetermined outcomes, but focuses on the stakeholders as your evaluation partners, whom you respect and who open up to you. You learn that cyberbullies are less likely to harass classmates after participating in an antibullying campaign, but the stories they have written and shared with you change the direction of questions you could be asking their teachers. Is this evaluation? Yes, it is. Welcome to the Values Branch.

House (1990) has summarized the movement of evaluation thinking in the direction of the Values Branch:

> Philosophically, evaluators ceased to believe their discipline was value-free and realized their practice entailed promoting the values and interests of some groups over others, though they were by no means clear on what to do about this discovery. They struggled with the seemingly conflicting demands of being scientific on the one hand and being useful on the other. Politically, evaluators moved from a position in which they saw themselves as technical experts opposed to the evils of politics to a position in which they admitted evaluation itself was an activity with political effects. These conceptual changes were stimulated by the rapidly evolving social context, as the United States itself changed character.
>
> If diverse groups wanted different things, then collecting the views of people in and around the programs themselves seemed to make sense. Qualitative methodology useful for obtaining the views of participants came into vogue. Qualitative methods had long been employed in anthropology and sociology, but had been judged to be too subjective for use in program evaluation. Led by evaluators like Robert Stake and Barry MacDonald, qualitative methodology developed a following, a practice, and eventually research rationales. (p. 25)

I (Donna M. Mertens) entered the evaluation field at about the time when what came to be known as the "paradigm wars" began. These were heated debates between advocates of quantitative methods and advocates of qualitative methods. Evaluators who believed that priority had to be given to the values inherent in the human interactions that are part of evaluation were proposing the use of qualitative methods. Evaluators who believed in the importance of objectivity and neutrality had long advocated experimental designs as the "gold standard" for evaluators (see Chapter 3). Alkin (2004) included the following evaluators in the branch that focuses on values: Scriven, Eisner, Stake, Guba and Lincoln, House and Howe, myself, and Greene. In the present text, we have added Shaw, Parlett, and Hamilton to the Values Branch, and we have moved House and Howe, myself, and Greene to the Social Justice Branch (described in Chapter 6). The philosophy that guides the Values Branch is briefly explained, followed by commensurate theoretical positions in order to build a composite picture of current views of "values" as a theoretical basis for evaluation. Examples of studies that reflect the Values Branch are used to illustrate how these theoretical perspectives are manifest in practice. Advantages and challenges associated with approaches reflecting this branch are discussed.

The Constructivist Paradigm

The historical philosophical roots of the constructivist paradigm can be found in the late-1700s work of Immanuel Kant, which challenged the empiricists' claim that the only appropriate subject for research is that which we can sense and therefore measure (Ponterotto, 2005). Kant (1781/1966) held that we humans also create knowledge by using processes inside our heads. By experiencing, processing, and making meaning of what we experience, we create reality that goes beyond the experience of interaction with external stimuli. Kant influenced the thinking of Wilhelm Dilthey, who wrote about the different goals for natural sciences and human sciences. The former strives to provide scientific explanation, while the latter's goal is to achieve understanding of the meaning of social phenomena. Dilthey emphasized the importance of lived experience examined within a particular historical context. Schwandt (2000) adds that a constructivist attempts to reach an understanding of meaning from the perspective of the persons who have the experiences. It is possible that the persons themselves do not fully understand the experience. Thus the act of evaluation becomes one of making visible understandings for stakeholders through the use of appropriate methods.

Another important strand of philosophical thought relevant to the constructivist paradigm is that of Edmund Husserl, who was influenced by Dilthey, among others (Wertz, 2005). Husserl contributed to the beginning of the phenomenological movement in philosophy and psychology. He elaborated on concepts related to researching consciousness in order to better understand human experiences and behaviors. This led to a shift in focus for researchers who held the philosophical position that it was important to understand a research problem from the participants' perspective. The connection between Husserl's work and the constructivist paradigm is illustrated in this passage:

> Husserl [1936/1970] sensed a growing disillusionment, beginning around the turn of the [20th] century, with the narrowness of science, with its inability to address the deepest questions of humanity concerning subjectivity, the meaning of existence, and the free shaping of the future in the face of the portentous upheavals and unhappiness in modern times. The exclusion of subjectivity and values from a science directed at purely material bodies prevented even the human sciences from addressing the most pressing and decisive questions for humanity by

putting aside the concepts and methods of natural science and employing a thoroughgoing description of the conscious constitution of what Husserl called the "lifeworld," he attempted to ground the physical sciences and the human sciences as achievements of consciousness as well as to address questions of subjectivity, values and free self-determination to which natural science had been indifferent. The world of science is a creative, humanly constructed one rather than a mirror of an independent reality. In response to this crisis in the philosophy of science, the search for truth criteria has turned away from references to "reality" to moral, socially established, and practical values. (Wertz, 1999, p. 134)

Axiology (Ethics)

Constructivists have called attention to the importance of researchers' awareness of their own values and reflections on how their values influenced the process and outcomes of the research (Ponterotto, 2005). They hold that it is not possible for researchers to eliminate the influence of their values; rather, these should be consciously treated as an integral part of the research process. Guba and Lincoln (1989), in an early work, discussed values in terms of their influence on the research process—from formulating the focus of the research to making decisions about who to include, how to collect data, and what to do with the findings. In a later work, Guba and Lincoln (2005) have moved toward a transformative view of ethics. They align their beliefs with critical theory and present this description of their axiological assumption: "Propositional, transactional knowing is instrumentally valuable as a means to social emancipation, which is an end in itself, [and] is intrinsically valuable" (p. 198). Although all constructivists may not endorse this as their axiological assumption, it is at this point that Guba and Lincoln's axiological assumption approaches an intersection with the transformative paradigm (see Chapter 6).

How can research participants be unaware of their reality until it is revealed through interaction and reflection? During a group discussion with deaf women in a rural Brazilian town, one deaf woman who had just returned with her family from the state capital (20 miles away) related how freely deaf women lived in the city. Several deaf women in the group said they felt as if they lived in a cage compared to "city" deaf girls, who had easy access to deaf men to date and marry, independence to go to movies and clubs, and the freedom to travel on public transportation. When I asked why the women didn't go to the city on their own, they replied, "Deaf women don't go to the city." I asked them, "Why not?" The discussion started slowly, as they thought of all the reasons they couldn't go: Their families let their deaf sons out, but not their deaf daughters; their neighbors might think they were "loose" if they went to the city; all the money they earned was supposed to go to their families and not for their own needs. The women gradually began to see how negative attitudes about being deaf and female kept them "caged," and how generations of deaf women before them had accepted their situations. A lively discussion ensued of plans to save for bus tickets with side jobs, to travel safely as a large group, and to ask two deaf male relatives to accompany them on the first trip. "The second trip we'll go on our own!" This was the beginning of weekly Friday trips to the Deaf Association's meetings in the city. Although it was not easy at first, with time it soon became "what deaf women did" on Friday nights.

Ontology (Reality)

Constructivists hold that there are multiple, socially constructed realities (Guba & Lincoln, 2005). This assumption reflects a relativist view of reality, because reality is constructed by individuals through reflection upon their experiences and in interaction with others. Many qualitative researchers (although certainly not all) tend to be relativists, believing that reality exists in multiple mental constructions that are "socially and experientially based, local and specific, dependent for their form and content on the persons who hold them" (Guba, 1990, p. 27). Reality is constructed by the research participants through interactive dialogue with the researcher, called the **hermeneutic process** (Ponterotto, 2005). As mentioned previously, participants may be unaware of the meaning of their reality until it is revealed through interaction and reflection (Schwandt, 2000).

Epistemology (Knowledge)

The epistemological assumption for constructivists is already reflected in the ontological assumption. The constructivist epistemological assumption is that researchers and the participants interact through meaningful dialogue and reflection to create knowledge (Guba & Lincoln, 2005). Ponterotto (2005) states:

> The epistemology underlying a constructivist position requires close, prolonged interpersonal contact with the participants in order to facilitate their construction and expression of the "lived experience" being studied. Constructivists–interpretivists advocate a transactional and subjectivist stance that maintains that reality is socially constructed and, therefore, the dynamic interaction between researcher and participant is central to capturing and describing the "lived experience." (p. 131)

Methodology (Systematic Inquiry)

In order to be able to construct reality and uncover hidden meanings, researchers need to have prolonged involvement with the participants. Hence the methodologies most commonly associated with the constructivist paradigm come from the qualitative tradition. Researchers' methods include the use of hermeneutical dialogue, interviews, observation, and document/artifact review (Mertens, 2010). A researcher needs to be immersed in a community's everyday activities for a long period of time in order to have sufficient opportunities to engage in reflective dialogue with participants. Lincoln (2010) reminds us that constructivists are not limited to qualitative data collection. She states that from her earliest writings with Guba in the 1980s to this day, she wishes to

> establish firmly, once and for all, that I am not against quantitative methods, nor am I against mixing them when appropriate. What concerns me is mixing paradigms, or metaphysical models, or, worse yet, simply declaring that one's philosophical belief system associated with research and inquiry are meaningless or irrelevant. (p. 7)

Philosophical Assumptions of the Constructivist Paradigm and the Values Branch

Using the table below, answer the following questions:

1. Can you imagine what a constructivist evaluation would look like?

2. How would the evaluator set up the evaluation?

3. Would the evaluator be involved with the stakeholders or not?

4. How would the evaluator's assumptions guide her/his decisions?

The Constructivist Paradigm and the Values Branch

Description	Axiological assumption	Ontological assumption	Epistemological assumption	Methodological assumption
Focuses primarily on identifying multiple values and perspectives through qualitative methods	Evaluator aware of own values and those of others	Multiple, socially constructed realities	Meaningful dialogue and reflection to create knowledge	• Qualitative, but quantitative too • Participatory

Values Branch Theorists

Michael Scriven's academic background is in philosophy, logic, and mathematics (Oral History Project Team, 2005). Because of his recognized expertise in critical thinking, he came to evaluation as a member of a team that was developing a national social science curriculum. As he wondered about how to determine the effectiveness of the curriculum, he came upon the work of Robert Stake (discussed later in this chapter) and Daniel Stufflebeam (discussed in Chapter 4); this conflu- ence supports the metaphor of branches of a river or currents in the ocean that flow into each other, rather than branches of a tree that are separate from each other. However, Scriven dis- agreed with Stufflebeam that the purpose of evaluation is to provide information for decision making. He argued that the

Values Branch Theorists

Michael Scriven
Eliot Eisner
Robert Stake
Ian Shaw
Malcolm Parlett
David Hamilton
Egon Guba
Yvonna Lincoln

purpose of evaluation is to determine the merit and worth of the evaluand. As noted in Chapter 1, "merit" refers to the intrinsic value of something (how good is it?), and "worth" refers to the value of the evaluand in a particular context (how valuable or necessary is the evaluation in this context?). Both these concepts involve a judgment of value against different sets of criteria. Hence we place Scriven in the Values Branch.

Among Scriven's contribution is the idea of **"goal-free evaluation"** (Scriven, 1991). Scriven developed this idea because he was concerned with the bias associated with having an evaluator hired by a program's developers, as well as by the notion that evaluators should limit their activities to examining whether programs have achieved their stated objectives. He describes his thinking about goal-free evaluation as follows:

> I thought of the possibility of a sacrificial intermediary who would take the contract and then would hire staff to do the fieldwork, to whom he would not reveal the goals of the program but tell them where the program could be seen in action and where control groups could also be seen in action, at least comparison groups. (Oral History Project Team, 2005, p. 386)[1]

Scriven (1967a) wrote a chapter entitled "The Logic of Evaluation" for an American Educational Research Association monograph, in which he proposed the terms "formative evaluation" and "summative evaluation." As noted in Chapter 1, formative evaluation is intended to provide feedback as a program is being developed and implemented, in order to make improvements in the program. Summative evaluation is done at the end of a program, in order to make a summative judgment about the extent to which the program has accomplished its goals. These terms are defined and illustrated in Chapter 1. Formative and summative evaluations can be conducted within any of the evaluation branches; their use is not restricted to the Values Branch.

Elliot Eisner (1976a, 1976b, 1977, 1979a, 1979b) also felt that something was missing in the methods and use approaches to evaluation; he felt that they could make important contributions to the field, but that they could not capture a complete picture of what a program was supposed to do or how well it was done. He believed that evaluation was one way of knowing, but he raised these significant epistemological questions: "How is it that an individual knows? What forms are employed in order to know? And how does one represent what one knows to others?" (Eisner, 1979b, p. 12). His answers to these questions form the basis for an approach to evaluation that is more values based than previous approaches. He argues that knowledge is much more than what can be measured or represented by words and numbers. We humans have five senses, which provide us with many different ways of knowing that are not adequately expressed in words or numbers (e.g., visual images, physical movements, smells). Eisner has used the following metaphor to explain how his views of knowledge and evaluation approaches contrast with those of Methods Branch theorists:

> To cast a net into the sea that is unintentionally designed to let most of the fish get away, and then to conclude from those that are caught of what the variety of fish in the sea consists is, at the very least, a sampling error of the first order. Then to describe the fish that are caught in terms of their length and weight is to reduce radically what we can know about the qualitative features of the ones that have been caught, not to mention the features of those that the net failed to catch in the first place. (Eisner, 1979b, p. 14)

Eisner was one of the early evaluators who argued for the use of qualitative approaches to evaluation (along with Stake, Guba, and Lincoln). He developed the concepts of "evaluation connoisseurship" and "evaluation criticism."[2] He has described evaluation connoisseurship as "the art of appreciation. It is the result of having developed a highly differentiated array of anticipatory schemata that enable one to discern qualities and relationships that others, less well differentiated, are less likely to see" (p. 14). He continues: "The critic's task is neither to use the work as a stimulus for psychological projection, nor is it to be the subject of judicial pronouncements. The function of the critic is to illuminate, to enable others to experience what they may have missed" (p. 15). Eisner's (1991) *The Enlightened Eye* provides an intellectually compelling body of work on the philosophy and practice of qualitative, interpretive, and critical inquiry.

As you will see in Chapter 13 on preparing reports, qualitative evaluators are encouraged to write in rich detail, so as to convey the complex pictures that make possible a deeper understanding of programs than is possible with the didactic, expository language commonly used in evaluation reports situated within other branches.

Robert Stake (1975a, 1975b, 1981, 1991, 2004) was another pioneer in the advancement of qualitative approaches to evaluation through the development of the "responsive evaluation" approach.[3] Stake reacted against what he called a "preordinate" approach to evaluation (Methods Branch)—that is, evaluations using stated goals, objective tests, program personnel standards, and research-type reports—as well as evaluations focused on decision making (Use Branch). He proposed evaluation that is *responsive* to the stakeholders. An evaluation is responsive "if it orients more directly to program activities than to program intents, if it responds to audience requirements for information, and if the different value perspectives of the people at hand are referred to in reporting the success and failure of the program" (Stake, 1991, p. 65). Moreover, the responsive evaluator should let the issues that frame the evaluation arise from interaction with the stakeholders. These issues should then lead to decisions about data collection strategies. The important matter for the evaluator is "to get his [*sic*] information in sufficient amount from numerous independent and credible sources so that it effectively represents the perceived status of the program, however complex" (Stake, 1991, p. 69).

Stake has made a clear distinction between responsive evaluation and other approaches that are more commonly associated with the Methods Branch:

> Responsive evaluation is a search for and documentation of program quality. It uses both criterial measurement and interpretation. The essential feature of the approach is responsiveness to key issues or problems, especially those experienced by people at the sites. It is not particularly responsive to program theory or stated goals; it is responsive to stakeholder concerns. The understanding of goodness rather than the creation of goodness is its aim. Users may go on to alleviate or remediate or develop or aspire, but the purpose of this evaluation is mainly to understand. (Stake, 2004, p. 89)

> **Values Branch Theorists**
>
> Michael Scriven
> Elliot Eisner
> Robert Stake
> Ian Shaw
> Malcolm Parlett
> David Hamilton
> Egon Guba
> Yvonna Lincoln

Values Branch theorists in the United Kingdom include **Ian Shaw** (1999) and **Malcolm Parlett** and **David Hamilton** (1972), who wrote about the need to include qualitative approaches in the form of case studies and illuminative evaluation as manifestations of their belief in the constructivist paradigm. Parlett and Hamilton (1972) used the metaphor of evaluator as social anthropologist. They called their approach "illuminative evaluation," because it reflects the depth of understanding that evaluators can achieve when they are immersed in the program context. An evaluator's responsibility is to report day-to-day reality as a means of uncovering hidden meanings and complexities. This requires the evaluator to make use of qualitative methods such as observation, ongoing conversations with participants, and noting use of language as a doorway to understanding assumptions and relationships.

Egon Guba and **Yvonna Lincoln** have made significant philosophical, theoretical, and methodological contributions to the Values Branch of evaluation. As mentioned previously, Guba began his career working with Stufflebeam at Ohio State University, where he went from being an advocate of randomized controlled trials (see Chapter 3) to using the CIPP model of the Use Branch (Chapter 4) to conceptualizing an approach to evaluation that clearly places him in the Values Branch (Stufflebeam, 2008). Guba coined the term "naturalistic approaches to evaluation" in 1978; this concept became the topic of a book he coauthored with Lincoln (Guba & Lincoln, 1981). **Naturalistic evaluation** was seen as an emergent approach allowing an evaluator to observe a program in its natural state without preconceived hypotheses (as opposed to the experimental approach, which is preordinate, in that the independent and dependent variables are carefully defined and controlled before the study begins).

Guba and Lincoln have acknowledged that they were influenced by Stake's (1978) and Eisner's (1978) early work in case studies and connoisseurship evaluation (see Lincoln, 1991). Eisner's work, they say, emphasizes the importance of involvement with stakeholders in a respectful way that will allow the stakeholders to contribute to the evaluation process so as to reveal things to themselves and the evaluators that are unknown at the beginning of the study. Stake's work, they say, emphasizes bringing together science and art in the form of creating narratives that tell the stories of the stakeholders.

In 1989, with the publication of *Fourth Generation Evaluation,* Guba and Lincoln moved away from the label "naturalistic" because it had so many different meanings; it was not possible to establish a clear identity for the approach to evaluation that this label was intended to describe. Hence they changed the label to **fourth-generation evaluation.** Because their early work was situated primarily in the evaluation of educational programs, they viewed evaluation as having moved through three prior generations: use of testing and measurement as the first generation, use of objectives and tests (à la Tyler) as the second, and judgment (the decision-based models) as the third. Their fourth-generation approach is a manifestation of the constructivist paradigm, in that it includes intensive involvement with stakeholders in the design, conduct, and building of meaning based on the evaluation data.

Theory to Practice

Many evaluation approaches have their origins in the constructivist paradigm and build on the work of these theorists. The approaches reviewed here include goal-free evaluation, case study approaches, connoisseurship evaluation, and responsive evaluation. Some other names for constructivist approaches include naturalistic evaluation, interpretive evaluation, hermeneutic evaluation, narrative evaluation, ethnography, autoethnography evaluation, oral history, ethnomethodology, symbolic interaction, and phenomenology.

Goal–Free Evaluation

Scriven (1991) proposed goal-free evaluation as an approach, in order to free the evaluator from the bias associated with evaluating only the objectives that program development personnel think are important. He reasoned that if a program has significant effects, they should be obvious to an observer who has not been informed about the intended effects. Goal-free evaluations are also excellent for identifying unintended side effects of a program, both positive and negative. Goal-free evaluations should be conducted by external evaluators who are not immersed in the implementing organization. A goal-free evaluation was included as one of the approaches in the Stufflebeam et al. (2002) Hawaiian housing study, summarized in Chapter 4 (see Box 4.3). As we have already explained the evaluand and methods in Chapter 4, we only present a summary of the goal-free component of that study in Box 5.1.

Box 5.1. Sample Goal-Free Evaluation Study: The Hawaiian Housing Study

Sample study	Evaluation approach	Document title
Stufflebeam, Gullickson, and Wingate (2002)	Goal-free evaluation	"The Spirit of Consuelo: An Evaluation of Ke Alca Ho'ona"

Method

A goal-free evaluation component was included, in which an evaluator who did not know the goals for the project collected data from participants about the project's accomplishments, in order to ascertain unintended consequences and give additional credibility to the goal-based evaluation.

The goal-free evaluation strategy is an interesting approach that is designed to bolster the credibility of other evaluation findings. Stufflebeam and colleagues hired several evaluators who understood the general context of the project, but they were not told the specific project goals. These evaluators used typical evaluation data collection strategies based on interviews and observations to determine what goals the staff and participants viewed as having been achieved. In this way, the evaluators could not be viewed as biased by the foreknowledge of what they "should" be looking for. This strategy is useful to identify unintended outcomes of the project. They used the following goal-free questions (Stufflebeam et al., 2002, p. 70):

▓ What positive and negative effects flowed from the project?

▓ How are these effects judged regarding criteria of merit, such as quality of construction, quality of communication and collaboration within the community, quality of organization and administration, etc.?

(cont.)

Box 5.1 (*cont.*)

■ How significant were the project's outcomes compared with the needs of the involved families and the needs of the surrounding environment?

REFLECTIONS FROM THE EVALUATORS

The goal-free evaluators obtained and reported assessments of the project from the perspectives of community groups, including other community developers, government officials, and law enforcement personnel. The Consuelo Foundation's president and staff found the goal-free evaluation results to be very interesting and useful, and a good addition to our primary evaluation reports.

· · · · · · · · · · E X T E N D I N G Y O U R T H I N K I N G · · · · · · · · · ·

Goal–Free Evaluation

Suppose an evaluator used a goal-based evaluation for a project that created public gardens in an abandoned lot and taught nearby residents how to grow and cultivate fruits and vegetables. As fresh produce was prohibitively expensive and of poor quality in the local grocery, it was hoped that personal gardens would increase the amount and quality of nutritional foods in the neighborhood. The evaluator learned that the families did use the plots, harvested a variety of vegetables and some fruits, and served them with meals.

1. If you were the evaluator and performed a goal-free evaluation, what would you have done differently?

2. How would you have proceeded in order to ascertain what the goals of the project were in reality?

3. You might have asked the families whether the gardens had been a success, and the responses might confirm that the goal of the project was reached, but that other unintended outcomes resulted. What types of unintended outcomes might you expect to emerge from such a project? Consider such factors as increased income, contact between people in the neighborhood, and making the neighborhood a safer place to live.

4. The residents of this community, especially the children, benefited greatly from this project as they became healthier, learned about gardening and the importance of eating well and cooperating with their neighbors. What if, as the evaluator, you learned that one of the residents had harvested three marijuana plants and had sold it for a profit to some neighbors?

Case Study Approaches

Many Values Branch theorists propose the use of case studies as a mechanism for gaining understanding about the day-to-day activities of a program as a way of uncovering hidden meanings. The Los Angeles Unified School District wanted an evaluation of its Title I Achieving Schools initiative, which was implemented in the K–12 school system to support the use of promising school-level practices in elementary schools in high-poverty areas (Barela, 2008). The evaluator adopted a case study approach, which is summarized in Box 5.2.

Box 5.2. Sample Case Study: The Los Angeles School Achievement Study

Sample study	Evaluation approach	Document title
Barela (2008)	Case study	"Title I Achieving Schools"

The Evaluator

Eric Barela serves as a senior educational research analyst in the Los Angeles Unified School District's Planning, Assessment, and Research Division.

Philosophical and Theoretical Lenses

In order to be responsive to the diversity in and between schools, and to capture the implementation of changes that were locally based, the evaluator chose a case study design. This is in keeping with the assumptions of the constructivist paradigm. Interestingly, Barela places this study in the Use Branch rather than the Values Branch, because he considers use to be a very important part of the evaluation process. This is reflected in his decision to include budget data from the sample schools because such data were important to the decision makers.

The Evaluand and Its Context

The Los Angeles Unified School District is a very large, public, diverse, urban school district. It has a student enrollment of about 700,000 students and employs about 84,000 people. The specific evaluand consisted of the Title I Achieving Schools, which had received funds from the U.S. Department of Education to implement promising practices in high-poverty areas. "These funds are to be used to enact systemic standards-based reform while allowing for adaptability to local conditions" (p. 532).

Method

Design

The evaluator used a case study design to compare two types of schools: schools that met their Adequate Yearly Progress targets for at least 2 years, and those who had not

(cont.)

Box 5.2 (cont.)

done so. Adequate Yearly Progress targets are required by U.S. federal legislation—the No Child Left Behind (NCLB) Act. The NCLB Act specifies that all relevant subgroups of students (based on student ethnicities, socioeconomic disadvantage, English language learner status, and disability status) must show adequate progress in English/language arts and math. Adequate progress is defined in terms of a benchmark year and subsequent measures in the years following for each school. If a school misses even one of these targets, it is placed on a Watch List. Barela, in an interview with Christie (2008, p. 536), described his design choice this way: "To me, when looking at best practices in high achieving schools, the most sensible approach is a case study design. We already know things are working in our AAA schools. It is with case studies that we learn about why and how things are working."

The evaluator chose eight schools that had met their Adequate Yearly Progress goals and four that were on the Watch List. The schools were matched on the basis of the percentage of low-income students, overall number of students, and percentage of English language learners. All Title I schools must have at least 65% of their students living in poverty.

Evaluation Purposes and Questions

The evaluation had two main purposes. The first was to inform school district decision makers about how the high-achieving schools used their funds. The funds are intended to be used to supplement the core curriculum, such as by hiring more teachers, providing professional development, or providing additional enrichment activities beyond the school day. The second purpose was to determine how these schools implemented their core curriculum, with particular attention to English language learners and students with disabilities. This resulted in two questions: "The first question was compliance driven and the second learning driven, focusing on identifying best practices" (Barela, in an interview with Christie, 2008, p. 536).

Stakeholders and Participants

The major stakeholders were considered to be the decision makers in the school district. In this case, the primary stakeholders were the directors of the agency that commissioned the study (the office responsible for monitoring the district's Adequate Yearly Progress). These directors also were responsible to their own supervisor, the Executive Director of Educational Services. Other stakeholders included the local school administrators, teachers, parents, and Title I coordinators.

Data Collection

The evaluator chose the design, selected the sample of cases, and collected the data. The decision makers wanted to decide which schools would be included in the study, but the evaluator insisted on preserving the confidentiality of the schools' names; hence the administrators did not participate in selecting the schools, nor did they know which schools were eventually chosen. Data were collected through 131 days of observations in classrooms and 66 school-related meetings. The evaluator also interviewed 37 administrators and 61 teachers, and conducted a document review of the schools' plans for how they would use the funds to address particular areas of weakness in achievement of the subgroups of students identified in the NCLB Act.

Management and Budget

Barela has described this as a small study, compared to others done in the school district's Planning, Assessment, and Research Division. It had a budget of $150,000. All the data were collected in a 5-month period, from February to June 2006. He described the generation of the budget figure this way:

> There is some background that helps to explain how we decided upon the budget for this study. Our Director is responsible for reviewing all proposals that come through the District for external evaluation work. An external evaluator had proposed a study of high achieving schools (Academic Achievement Award—AAA schools) for $150,000 focusing on just 5 schools and interviewing just a few principals. After reviewing the proposal internally, my Director thought he would give our Division a chance to propose an alternative project. Dr. Hayes and I were asked to develop a competing proposal for the same cost, which turned out to be the study I conducted. (Barela, in an interview with Christie, 2008, p. 535)

Meta-Evaluation

The school district evaluators who conduct internal evaluations do not need to go through an ethics board review. They do have to get permission from the individual school principals when they want to collect data. Barela has concluded that his methodology was sufficiently rigorous, because the primary stakeholders did not criticize his methods when he was meeting with them.

Reports and Utilization

The evaluator shared monthly memos with the primary stakeholders and responded in a timely manner to any questions they had. Barela has indicated that use was very important and was built into the design of the study. He discussed the implications of the politics of working in a large school district as part of the important use-related considerations. Many of his division's reports are included in major newspapers. The evaluator prepared a report that included not only the qualitative data, but quantitative data about the percentage of teachers certified in bilingual cross-cultural languages, the percentage of English language learners in the schools, the students' achievement levels in English, and budget allocations and expenditures. Barela sent the report without recommendations to the primary stakeholders, so that they could work with him to co-construct recommendations. At the time of Barela's interview with Christie (2008), the report had not been made public. Barela explained to Christie that the primary stakeholders received a copy of the report and indicated that they wanted it to be treated as an internal document to be used to create a list of best practices for Title I schools.

(cont.)

Box 5.2 (*cont.*)

REFLECTIONS FROM THE EVALUATOR

[Note: The following reflections are all quoted from the Christie (2008) interview with Barela.]

Something that has become evident to me while at the LAUSD is that there is a big difference between a useful and used evaluation. I can do really good work and produce a useful evaluation and still it won't be used. So, I decided to show [the two key stakeholders] the study findings, minus my analytic take. I wanted to know, based on what we [the evaluation team] observed, what they [the two key stakeholders] thought some of the recommendations should be? I see my role as helping to facilitate and guide that conversation. We met regularly to work on recommendations. At first, it was an exercise in editing, with them reading through the report and asking me to change words. But then we got to the real purpose, making meaning of our findings. (p. 541)

[Barela offered reflections in this interview about the barriers he experienced in this study and how he overcame them:]

The most significant barrier we encountered, and this is typical across all of the studies I have conducted, is resistance from school staff. Often times when school personnel hear the word "evaluation" they think personnel evaluation. This is a constant struggle. I am always explaining how personnel evaluation and program evaluation are two very different activities and that we are in the business of conducting program evaluation. But, there is a general sense of paranoia around evaluation that is very difficult to offset.

One of the main strategies I use is open communication. I am very transparent about our confidentiality policy. I explain that we will maintain confidentiality not only with District administrators, but also with school administrators. If a teacher says something critical about a principal, I need to be clear that I am not going to disclose what was said to the principal, while the same is true if a principal says something critical about the District. Nonetheless, it is still a struggle because some people just don't believe that is how we [his division] work. (p. 539)

[He also reflected upon the limited use made of his report:]

CHRISTIE: *In retrospect, what would you have done differently to make the report more useful?*

BARELA: *Make it a lot shorter. I wanted to include all of the findings with all of the supporting evidence and explanation. I wanted it to be comprehensive. So I ended up with an 84-page report, plus a 10-page executive summary. (p. 541)*

[He explained that the division now recommends that the body of reports not exceed 30 pages. Additional supporting information can be included in appendices.]

········· E X T E N D I N G   Y O U R   T H I N K I N G ·········
Case Study Approaches

Values Branch

Sample study	Evaluation approach	List the distinguishing characteristics
Barela (2008)	Case study	

Using the description of the Barela (2008) study in Box 5.2, answer the following questions:

1. How are case studies in keeping with the assumptions of the constructivist paradigm?

2. What was the purpose of the Barela evaluation in the Los Angeles Unified School District?

3. Why did Barela choose a case study evaluation, and do you agree with his choice? Explain.

4. Barela did not include a list of recommendations with the results of the evaluation. Instead, he worked with the stakeholders to create recommendations. What is your opinion of this practice?

Connoisseurship Evaluation

Connoisseurship evaluation was proposed by Eisner (1979a, 1991) as a methodological application of the "phenomenological philosophical stance." He described an evaluator's role as that of an educational critic who is tasked with writing in a way that will enable the reader to vicariously participate in the events constituting the aspect of classroom life about which the critic speaks. "Such participation makes it possible for readers to know that aspect of classroom life emotionally. Through it they are able to know what only the artistic use of language can provide" (Eisner, 1979b, pp. 15–16).

Eisner has further described the evaluator's task as that of bringing fresh eyes to see what might be disregarded or overlooked by someone who is used to being in the classroom or the particular context in which the evaluation is taking place. He has also emphasized the critical need for trust between the evaluator and the stakeholder, in order to illuminate such things in a way that is helpful to the stakeholder. An example of a connoisseurship evaluation is summarized in Box 5.3.

Now let's discuss what "phenomenological philosophical stance" means. In "phenomeno-logical," you can see the word "phenomenon," which is from Greek and means "that which appears." Phenomenology is the study of the appearance of things according to how they are subjectively experienced. The two of us (Mertens and Wilson) have been teaching for many years at Gallaudet University, where everyone communicates in American Sign Language. We may miss aspects of our classroom that nonsigners who have never been immersed in deaf culture will perceive. Their description of the classroom might include how noisy it is, or how students' signing differs in speed, space, and size of signs, depending on whom they are signing to. "That which appears" and is taken in by each observer differs, depending upon the observers' life experiences.

Box 5.3. Sample Connoisseurship Evaluation Sample Study: The Imagination and Creativity Study

Sample study	Evaluation approach	Document title
Trotman (2006) 🇬🇧	Connoisseurship evaluation	"Interpreting Imaginative Lifeworlds: Phenomenological Approaches in Imagination and the Evaluation of Educational Practice"

The Evaluator

David Trotman conducted this study as part of his EdD degree requirement. At the time of the study, he was Principal Lecturer in Education and Professional Studies at Newman College of Higher Education in Birmingham, England.

Philosophical and Theoretical Lenses

Trotman gives an extensive explanation of phenomenology as the philosophical frame for his evaluation study. The ontological and epistemological assumptions associated with phenomenology guided the study, in that Trotman tried to come to an under-standing of the essential meaning of the experience of imagination and creativity in primary pupils and how that is perceived by their teachers.

The Evaluand and Its Context

In the United Kingdom, educators have expressed increased interest in creativity and emotional intelligence. As part of an effort to increase school self-evaluations, Trotman conducted a study in six primary schools to evaluate students' creative, imaginative, and emotional development.

Method

Trotman has described his methods as including interviews, observations, and discussion of participant diaries. He decided on the focus of the study as "teacher interpretations of pupils' creative, imaginative and emotional experiences in primary phase teaching" (Trotman, 2006, p. 247). He does not provide details about the implementation of the specific methods.

Design

Trotman describes his intended design as a phenomenological study that would not have preordinate methods, but would evolve as he entered the lifeworld of the participants. He would engage in reflective intuition to clarify the experiences that he observed and that the participants consciously shared with him. He describes his methodology as "eidetic phenomenology," also known as "transcendental phenomenology." Moustakas (1994; cited in Trotman, 2006, p. 247) described eidetic phenomenology as the researcher's trying to describe "'things in themselves' and to enable such phenomena to enter consciousness and be understood in relation to its meaning and 'essences' in light of intuition and self-reflection." According to Husserl, the goal is a transformation of the individual or the experience, so that essential insight occurs via a synthesis of what exists in conscious awareness and what exists in the world. In order to do this, evaluators need to set aside their own biases, prejudices, and beliefs regarding the object of study.

Evaluation Purposes and Questions

The purpose of the evaluation was to establish a fuller picture of educational practice related to imagination and emotional intelligence in order to develop better classroom pedagogy. In addition, Trotman wanted to increase teachers' capacity to make use of qualitative data in their decision making. These were the evaluation questions: How do teachers judge student learning in the creative, imaginative, and emotional spheres? What can phenomenological approaches to understanding educational practice in the interpretation of pupils' imaginative and affective experience offer educators for school self-evaluation?

Stakeholders and Participants

Trotman is not specific about the characteristics of the participants or the way they were selected. He wrote: "Drawn from a range of professional roles, the research participants reflected a range of responsibilities and experience" (p. 250). He then lists 12 names of people who participated in pilot discussions with him. These conversations did not explicitly mention the terms "creativity" or "imagination."

Management and Budget

No information is provided about the time or budget for this study.

(cont.)

Box 5.3 (*cont.*)

Meta-Evaluation

Trotman acknowledges that the jargon associated with phenomenological studies is foreign to most teachers. A challenge is to find appropriate language for teachers and evaluators to share in such studies. Another challenge is preventing the evaluator's own personal feelings from coloring those of the participants. As the evaluator attempts to reveal meanings, they journey into the territory of interpretation. According to Eisner (1991), interpretation occurs at the intersection of connoisseurship and criticism. The critic makes clear what is experienced and explains its meaning.

Reports and Utilization

Trotman indicates that different educators had different perceptions of the importance of nurturing creativity and imagination for students. He concludes: "If imaginative life-worlds are to be subject to educational evaluation, then as this research would suggest, alternative strategies need to be sought that have some congruence with the qualities and characteristics espoused by these participants" (p. 259).

· · · · · · · · · · E X T E N D I N G   Y O U R   T H I N K I N G · · · · · · · · · ·
Connoisseurship Evaluation

 Values Branch

Sample study	Evaluation approach	List the distinguishing characteristics
Trotman (2006)	Connoisseurship evaluation	

Using the description of the Trotman (2006) study in Box 5.3, answer the following questions:

1. What are the characteristics that illustrate Trotman's use of the Connoisseurship Model of evaluation?

2. What do you identify as the strengths and weaknesses of this model in terms of the types of data that were collected by the evaluator?

3. What do you identify as the strengths and weaknesses of the strategies used in this study that were intended to reveal the emotional aspects of the educational experiences?

4. What would you suggest modifying in this study to improve the explicit acknowledgment of the evaluator's and stakeholders' values?

Responsive Evaluation

According to Stake (1991), a responsive evaluation includes an agreement to begin the study with observations, the time and place for which are negotiated with stakeholders. The evaluator will use the data from the observations to prepare brief reports that include narrative data, product displays (e.g., student work), and graphs. Stakeholders are then asked to indicate what aspects of the preliminary report are of value to them and what diversity of opinions exists among them in this respect. Stakeholders are further asked to react to the accuracy of the reports, the importance of the various findings, and their relevance. All of this can be done fairly informally; the evaluator does keep a written record of what is presented and of the stakeholders' reactions.

Stake says that the choice of evaluation questions is a reflection of values for what is considered important. Much as Scriven does in describing goal-free evaluation, Stake warns evaluators to avoid heavy reliance on what the program stakeholders put forth as program goals. Evaluators have a responsibility to look at what is happening in the program first, and then to choose value questions and criteria for judging merit and worth. Stake also suggests the avoidance of narrow measures of achievement as indicators of the success of a program. A responsive evaluator can use such measures if they are of interest to the various stakeholders in the program.

> After getting acquainted with a program, partly by talking with students, parents, taxpayers, program sponsors, and program staff, the evaluator acknowledges certain issues or problems or potential problems. These issues are a structure for continuing discussions with clients, staff, and audiences, and for the data-gathering plan. The systematic observations to be made, the interviews and tests to be given, if any, should be those that contribute to understanding or resolving the issues identified. (Stake, 1991, p. 67)

If other issues emerge during the evaluation, the evaluator can be responsive to those issues at that time. A sample responsive evaluation is summarized in Box 5.4. Conducting an evaluation that is responsive to the needs of the program stakeholders, as this one was, will ensure that what the stakeholders have learned through their active participation is meaningful and is more likely to be used for improving and enhancing programs.

················ E X T E N D I N G   Y O U R   T H I N K I N G ···········

Responsive Evaluation

1. What comments might a postpositivist make about using a responsive evaluation?

2. After you have responded to this question, read Box 5.4 and consider other comments a postpositivist might make.

Box 5.4. Sample Responsive Evaluation Study: The Dance Injury Prevention Study

Sample study	Evaluation approach	Document title
Abma (2005)	Responsive evaluation	"Responsive Evaluation: Its Value and Special Contribution to Health Promotion"

The Evaluator

Tineke Abma is an associate professor in the Department of Medical Humanities, Vrije University Medical Center, Amsterdam. She specializes in using qualitative and mixed methods to evaluate health care programs. She "argue[s] that this kind of evidence is important in the context of health promotion, because it enhances the understanding of human behaviour, it promotes holistic thinking, offers contextual information and brings in the perspective of the community or target group" (Abma, 2005, p. 279). A team of three evaluators conducted the study. The junior evaluation team member used the evaluation as part of her master's thesis. She was seen as an asset because she was a student and a musician and could comfortably access and interact with the students who participated in the study. The senior evaluators are university professors, therefore they assumed that they could more easily relate to the teachers at the schools.

Philosophical and Theoretical Lenses

Robert Stake (originally, 1975a; more recently, 2004) developed the theory and methods of responsive evaluation design that Guba and Lincoln (originally, 1989; more recently, 2005) later used as a foundational concept for their development of the constructivist paradigm in research and evaluation. Abma connects Guba and Lincoln's work with notions of narrative, storytelling, and "hermeneutic dialogue." (See "Reflections from the Evaluator," below, for Abma's definition of this type of dialogue.) Responsive evaluation as understood by Abma places priority on the involvement of and dialogue among all stakeholders, with deliberate attention to those whose voices represent those with less power. The evaluation is designed to be responsive to stakeholders' interests; therefore, they are involved in the process of developing questions, selecting participants, and interpretation of findings. The evaluator facilitates identification of issues and arranges opportunities for dialogue for the stakeholders to explore each other's beliefs, values, and perceptions.

The Evaluand and Its Context

Abma (2005) cites literature related to the intensive training and performance schedules for dancers and musicians that make physical and mental demands that lead to serious injuries. A growing awareness of this problem led the Dance Academy of the Higher School for the Arts in Amsterdam to develop an injury prevention program.[1] This program had four components:

1. Physical exams and advice were provided at the times of auditions.

2. Regular consulting hours were provided with a physiotherapist, an orthopedic surgeon, and the coordinator of the program.

3. The students received lessons in anatomy and injury prevention, including healthy eating habits, stress management, warming up, cooling down, and starting back after an injury.

4. The physiotherapist taught the teachers lessons on prevention of injuries and other health problems.

The evaluation team's literature review (which followed the analysis of the first set of data) indicated that acknowledgment and treatment of injuries were taboo subjects for many dancers, because they feared that they would not be allowed to continue their training or be chosen to perform if they revealed their weaknesses.

Methods

Design

The evaluation team used a mixed methods design (Greene, Kreider, & Mayer, 2005; Stake & Abma, 2005). The schools had collected many types of quantitative data (total number of injuries, kinds of injuries, consultations with paramedics, etc.). These data were used as input for discussions with the stakeholders to complement the qualitative data from the interviews, and to clarify and enliven the quantitative data by using the lived experiences expressed in the stories from the students and teachers.

(cont.)

[1]Abma's (2005) evaluation study also examined the injuries of musicians at the Conservatoire in Amsterdam, but for the sake of illustration, this box describes only the evaluation of the injury prevention program at the dance academy.

Box 5.4 (cont.)

Evaluation Purposes and Questions

> The coordinator of the program and the Board of Directors wanted to gain more insight in the value of the injury prevention program for students and teachers. There were questions regarding the effectiveness of the program and information was needed to further optimize the program. The coordinator noticed for example, that despite the program the incidence of injuries remained high and that prevention, in the regular curriculum, was still a largely ignored dimension.... Those who commissioned the project wanted to improve the quality of the injury prevention practice at both schools and [to obtain] information [on] how to modify this practice. The aim of the evaluation was to motivate students, teachers and medical experts on injury prevention to reflect and think about ways to improve the quality of their practice. (Abma, 2005, p. 282)

Stakeholders and Participants

The evaluators selected a project group to help monitor the evaluation, which included the coordinator of the injury prevention program at the academy, a director of the music conservatory program, and a staff member from the School for Higher Education of the Arts. The stakeholder groups identified by the evaluations included the students, teachers, and medical experts. Initially the project group thought that only the medical experts needed to be included as stakeholders; however, the evaluators argued successfully to also include the students and teachers because they would be affected by the results of the evaluation. They felt that inclusion of the three groups was essential to the quality of the findings.

Data Collection

"Over the course of a year, the junior evaluator worked for three to four days a week at the schools attending regular lessons, special body-awareness lessons and consulting hours as well as concerts and student performances" (Abma, 2005, p. 282). In addition, the evaluators conducted initial interviews with two representatives of each of these stakeholder groups: students, teachers, and medical specialists. The evaluators asked the project committee to recommend individuals who represented these stakeholder groups who had also experienced some kind of injury. The participants' responses about the treatment of the topic of injuries at the school were used as a basis for storytelling workshops with students and teachers (separately), in which short segments of the results of the previous interviews were read and discussed by the workshop participants.

The published version of the evaluation did not give details of the indicators or data analysis procedures.

Management Plan and Budget

The project lasted a year (April 1997–April 1998). The salary of the junior evaluator and her travel costs were financed by the Dutch Health Care Foundation for Students. The senior evaluators did their research work for free as community service.

Meta-Evaluation

The team members met every 2 weeks to review the methodology and to examine how the influence of their own positioning and prejudices might influence the project. They also conducted meta-evaluation activities throughout the entire project by involving groups of stakeholders in the project. For example, they met with the project group before the evaluation started, to discuss the evaluation design and who should be included (the stakeholders). They also discussed other issues such as methodology related to data collection strategies and recruitment of participants; ethics related to privacy, anonymity, and confidentiality; and financial aspects (the cost of the evaluation). As a result of this meta-evaluation process, the evaluators modified the focus of their study to emphasize the psychodynamics that prevented students and teachers from attending to health issues in the form of injuries. This group also contributed to decisions about how the results would be disseminated.

Results of the meta-evaluation are partially reflected in a section of the published report entitled "Lessons Learned":

> Stories offer a way of reaching a deeper understanding of lived experiences and are an appropriate vehicle for reflexive conversations because of their openness and ambiguity. [And] engaging key decision-makers appeared to be an important strategy to gain acceptance for the findings.
>
> Finally, we experienced that the conditions for a responsive evaluation were not optimal in the schools. The schools were characterised by asymmetrical relationships between teachers and students, while responsive evaluation requires a certain power balance to give all stakeholders a fair chance in the process. Health and self-care were sensitive topics in the schools and surrounded by many taboos. Furthermore the Conservatoire teachers [the music school teachers; see footnote 1 in this box] were not very interested in joining the evaluation, while responsive evaluation requires the participation of as many stakeholders as possible. As evaluators we took these conditions into account by investing a lot of time in developing conditions of trust and safety. We, for example, respected the wish of one student not to publish her story because she feared sanctions. Furthermore, we decided not to bring students and teachers physically together in the evaluation process, but invited them to respond to each other via written stories. In order to increase stakeholder participation research activities were integrated in regular lessons and meetings, and not too time-consuming. (Abma, 2005, p. 286)

Reports and Utilization

The evaluators wanted to stimulate dialogue based on their findings; therefore, they created four scenarios that reflected educational practices in the school. The scenarios were connected to the school's mission, which included both high standards and individual development, and to the nexus of responsibility (individual/collective). The scenarios were used to portray practical consequences of different emphases along these two dimensions. After presenting the scenarios, the evaluators distributed their report to various stakeholder groups, including members of the school community, the project group, and the board of the directors. These stakeholder groups were responsible for making recommendations for concrete actions that could address the issues that surfaced in the evaluation.

(cont.)

Box 5.4 (cont.)

REFLECTIONS FROM THE EVALUATOR

The way of working sketched here has been further developed and validated in many other evaluation projects. A central idea remains that responsive evaluation fosters practice improvement through ongoing dialogues between various stakeholder groups. From a hermeneutic perspective, dialogue is considered to be a searching process between people; through their interactions, people may redefine their standpoints, and a fusion of horizons may take place. In the project described, dialogues occurred among the students as they were exploring why, for instance, most of them were so unwilling to stop training lessons when they experienced pain. Although a student might initially state, "You should go on," others would begin to ask questions and say, "Well, yes, but isn't anticipating the possible injury in the long run better?" As pointed out, stories proved to be helpful here, because anyone could relate stories to their own experiences.

As we work in places with vulnerable groups (elderly people, psychiatric patients, and so on), we have been concerned with the question of how to engage those marginalized groups in dialogues with other stakeholders. We do not act as advocates of these groups, but try to connect to them and their lifeworld experiences to help them to articulate their intimate voice. We see that people need each other's support and a safe environment to interact with their surroundings and to become stronger and more articulate. Lately we are also working with client research partners and cultural brokers to be better prepared to connect with certain groups.

This idea of support is not restricted to marginalized groups. In our work with professionals, we also increasingly create learning platforms or networks (communities of practice) to enable professionals from various organizations engaged in a certain practice to share and reflect on their learning experiences. So in this case we might have set up a network of creative, engaged teachers from both the Dance Academy and the Conservatoire to express and further elaborate on their experiences with injury prevention. Data from the evaluation study could have been used as input for discussions.

A final reflection concerns the use of mixed methods strategies. This is also a strategy that has been further elaborated on in our later projects. We prefer to bring in quantitative data to evoke discussions among stakeholders, and to understand the world behind the numbers. This often implies that we have to work with experts in those fields (epidemiologists, statisticians) and to engage them in our work, and vice versa. In most cases we now work with mixed, or transdisciplinary, evaluation teams.

To conclude, our work has become more participatory and more emancipatory over the last several years, but the core notions of dialogue, storytelling, emergence, collaboration, and mutual learning remain central to our responsive evaluation approach.

········· **EXTENDING YOUR THINKING** ·········

Responsive Evaluation

 Values Branch

Sample study	Evaluation approach	List the distinguishing characteristics
Abma (2005)	Responsive evaluation	

Using the description of the Abma (2005) study in Box 5.4, answer the following questions:

1. Since Abma's evaluation process was responsive to feedback from the dancers, teachers, and administrators, rather than being an evaluation focusing on predefined outcomes, the stakeholders may have felt that the evaluation results truly reflected their issues and concerns. What, then, do you see would be some of the advantages of using a responsive evaluation?

2. When would you decide to use a responsive evaluation?

3. What are your thoughts about engaging in dialogue with stakeholders in an evaluation? Is this idea comfortable or uncomfortable for you? Explain.

Your Evaluation Plan: Your Philosophical Stance

Begin writing your understandings of the constructivist paradigm and the Values Branch as a way of clarifying your own thinking about your philosophical beliefs and how they might influence the way you conduct an evaluation. This can become part of your evaluation plan later, when you decide which approach you will use.

Moving On to the Next Chapter

As you have no doubt already sensed, the way evaluators actually do their work muddies the lines between the branches. For example, the Abma (2005) study was based on a responsive evaluation stance, which is associated with the Values Branch. However, in her reflections on that study, Abma indicates that she sees overlap between the responsive approach and the Social Justice Branch, and that her more recent work is increasingly reflective of this branch. Denzin and Lincoln (2005) revealed their movement toward a transformative/social justice stance when they wrote: "We want a social science that is committed up front to issues of social justice, equity, nonviolence, peace, and universal human right. We do not want a social science that says it can address these issues if it wants to" (p. 13).

Hood and Hopson (2008) provide a bridge from the Values Branch to the Social Justice Branch when they acknowledge the contributions of Stake, Guba, Lincoln, Parlett, and Hamilton as innovators in the promotion of evaluation approaches that recognize values as a primary consideration. They single out responsive evaluation (Stake, 1976a), naturalistic evaluation (Guba, 1978), and MacDonald's (1976) approach as major influences, because these approaches "are most amenable to the facilitation of the evaluation process so that the perspectives of the least powerful stakeholders in the evaluation are meaningfully included in the evaluation" (p. 414). In Chapter 6, we discuss the transformative paradigm and look at theorists who have contributed to the development of democratic evaluation approaches in the Social Justice Branch.

* * *

Remember the studies below, as we refer to them again in later chapters.

	Values Branch	
Sample study	**Evaluation approach**	**Topical area**
Stufflebeam, Gullickson, and Wingate (2002)	Goal-free evaluation	Housing for poor people in Hawaii
Barela (2008)	Case study	Los Angeles Unified School District case study
Trotman (2006)	Connoisseurship evaluation	Imagination and creativity
Abma (2005)	Responsive evaluation	Injury prevention in a dance academy in the Netherlands

Notes

1. Scriven's (2003) contributions to theory also include his conceptualization of evaluation as a transdiscipline, as described in Chapter 1.

2. Eisner (1979) called these "education connoisseurship" and "educational criticism." We have changed the former term to "evaluation connoisseurship," because his work has applicability to many disciplines besides education.

3. Stake (1991) acknowledges other evaluators who also advanced theories and approaches commensurate with responsive evaluation, including Malcolm Parlett (Scotland), Barry MacDonald and David Hamilton (England), and Lou Smith and Bob Rippey (United States).

Preparing to Read Chapter Six

Branch	Paradigm	Description
Methods	Postpositivist	Focuses primarily on quantitative designs and data
Use	Pragmatic	Focuses primarily on data that are found to be useful by stakeholders; advocates for the use of mixed methods
Values	Constructivist	Focuses primarily on identifying multiple values and perspectives through qualitative methods
Social justice	**Transformative**	**Focuses primarily on viewpoints of marginalized groups and interrogating systemic power structures through mixed methods to further social justice and human rights**

As you prepare to read this chapter, think about these questions:

1. What are the characteristics of the transformative paradigm?

2. How do those characteristics influence the practice of evaluation?

3. Which major thinkers have contributed to the approaches associated with the Social Justice Branch?

4. How did the ideas grow from the early days to the present in this theoretical context?

CHAPTER SIX

The Transformative Paradigm
and the Social Justice Branch

From childhood, I (Donna M. Mertens) had a strong sense of privilege and inequity in the world. I first came to consciousness of this when my family moved from Washington State to Kentucky in the early 1960s. In Washington, I had only seen people who looked like me—white, middle-class, able-bodied, and standard-English-speaking. In Kentucky, I saw that many black people lived in the slums in the inner city. The black people did not live in my neighborhood or go to my school or swimming pool. When I asked a teacher at my school why there were no black people at my school, she patted me on the head and said, "Honey, they just prefer to be with their own kind." When I compared the conditions I lived in and those of the black people I saw, I wondered how they could prefer living in overcrowded, run-down buildings, and sitting on their porches in the sweltering heat and humidity instead of going to the swimming pool. As this was the 1960s in the United States, it coincided with the civil rights era. Even at that young age, I wanted to know: What were the effects of the civil rights movement? Was the War on Poverty improving living conditions for the poor people in our country?

As I matured, I realized that I wanted to align my life work with the pursuit of human rights. I also realized that reading about things in the newspaper was good, but not enough to bring about social change. I hypothesized that if I could respectfully enter a marginalized community as a researcher and evaluator, I could test my evolving hypothesis that, together, we could work for social justice. My many years at Gallaudet University—the only university in the world whose mission is to serve deaf and hard-of-hearing students—have provided me with the opportunity to test that hypothesis and to examine the intersection of the many dimensions of diversity associated with less access to social privileges. That is how I came to situate myself in the transformative paradigm.

Alkin (2004) did not have a Social Justice Branch on his evaluation tree, because he placed four evaluators who explicitly worked for social justice on the Values Branch (House, Howe, myself, and Greene). In this chapter we make the argument that there is a significant difference between the Values Branch, which can be used to support social justice evaluations, and the Social Justice Branch, which holds that social justice is the primary principle guiding evaluators' work. Therefore, we include the previously mentioned theorists in our discussion below, along with many other evaluators who have contributed to the Social Justice Branch.

The Transformative Paradigm

The assumptions constituting the transformative paradigm pull together many strands of philosophy that focus on issues of power and on addressing inequities in the name of furthering human rights and social justice. Kant's (1781/1966) view of the purpose of philosophy as subjecting reality to critical review in order to illuminate the dynamics of subjugation, as well as Hegel's (1812/1929) illumination of the master–slave relationship and emphasis on the importance of dialectics and history, led the way to the development of one of those philosophical strands (Kincheloe & McLaren, 2002). Marxism began in the mid-1800s with a focus on the alienation of the worker and inequities related to economics and social class, with the goal of changing the conditions of the working class[1] (Marx, 1978). Philosophers at the University of Frankfurt am Main (known as the Frankfurt School) rejected a narrow interpretation of Marxism that focused on challenging capitalism. Neo-Marxists such as Max Weber and Georg Simmel expanded on Marxist philosophy and used it as a basis for the development of critical theory, which examined the meaning of societal critique and social change in terms of addressing inequities based on race and class.

Philosophers who extended thinking about the value-laden perspective of inquiry and the acceptance of using social justice as the starting principle for research and evaluation include Marcus (1998), Habermas (1971), and Horkheimer (1972). Notably, Habermas contributed the idea that social discourse can be used as a means for fostering emancipation—a process he called "communicative rationality." These philosophers paved the way for contemporary philosophers such as Sirotnik and Oakes (1990) and House and Howe (1999) to focus on the concepts of deliberation and democracy as bases for social transformation. People living in democracies have the freedom to question laws and public policies, for example, and then to question the social and institutional conditions that support them.

Several subsequent theoretical frameworks are consonant with the philosophical views of scholars such as Habermas, Kincheloe, and McLaren (2005) and provide the following description of any critical theory: "A critical social theory is concerned in particular with issues of power and justice and the ways that the economy; matters of race, class, and gender; ideologies; discourses; education; religion and other social institutions; and cultural dynamics interact to construct a social system" (p. 92). This statement indicates that critical theorists are aware of the dimensions of diversity that are relevant to an understanding of social inequities. However, additional philosophical strands need to be brought into the transformative paradigm's tent to understand the viewpoints of philosophers who are members of marginalized groups. These include feminists such as Irigaray, Kristeva, and Cixous (see Kincheloe & McLaren, 2005). They also include indigenous and postcolonial philosophers such as Asante (1992), Chilisa (2005, 2011), Bewaji (1995), Eze (1998), Gyekye (1995), Mbiti (1970), and Coetzee and Roux (1998), from Africa; Henry and Pene (2001), who are Māori; Freire (1970) from Latin America; and Cajete (2000) and LaFrance and Crazy Bull (2009), who are Native Americans/American Indians. In addition, they include queer theorists such as Plummer (2005); African American philosophers such as Du Bois (1903/1989), Malcolm X (1992), and Bassey (2007); Latino/Latina philosophers such as Solorzano and Delgado Bernal (2001) and Valdes (1996); and disability rights theorists such as Mertens, Holmes, and Harris (2009), Sullivan (2009), and Meekosha and Shuttleworth (2009).

Each of these philosophical and theoretical perspectives contributes to the framework for the transformative paradigm, because they address issues of power inequities, the impact of privilege, and the consequences of these for achieving social justice. A comprehensive review of these philosophies and theories is beyond the scope of this textbook, although it would be a very interesting intellectual journey to pursue. As a compromise, we provide you with references on these philosophical stances and refer to them throughout this text, as they have implications for theory and approaches to evaluation. For example, although African critical theory shares many similarities with Western critical theory, it offers a more nuanced position with regard to "recognizing the situation or lived-context of Africana people's being in the world" as having been influenced by a legacy of slavery, domination, oppression, and diaspora (Gordon, 1997; quoted in Bassey, 2007, p. 915). Its focus is on the critique of black subjugation and dehumanization (Asante, 1992; Bassey, 2007). Bassey provides an important distinction between Western thinking and African critical theory, in that Westerners focus on the liberation of the individual and Africans focus on the liberation of all black people from oppression. "Africana critical theorists are well aware that for the oppressed, individual consciousness is inextricably linked to the collective" (Bassey, 2007, p. 919).

Another important philosophical strand for the transformative paradigm is the one associated with transformative participatory research. As noted in Chapter 4, participatory research has several different philosophical bases. Practical participatory research emanates from pragmatism. Transformative participatory researchers recognize their philosophical and theoretical roots in Marxism (Fals Borda, 2001), feminist theory (Brydon-Miller, Maguire, & McIntyre, 2004), and critical theory (Bradbury & Reason, 2001).

> The transformative paradigm offers a meta-physical umbrella that brings together these various philosophical strands. It is applicable to people who experience discrimination and oppression on whatever basis, including (but not limited to) race/ethnicity, disability, immigrant status, political conflicts, sexual orientation, poverty, gender, age, or the multitude of other characteristics that are associated with less access to social justice. In addition, the transformative paradigm is applicable to the study of the power structures that perpetuate social inequities. Finally, indigenous peoples and scholars from marginalized communities have much to teach us about respect for culture and the generation of knowledge for social change. Hence, there is not a single context of social inquiry in which the transformative paradigm would not have the potential to raise issues of social justice and human rights. (Mertens, 2009, p. 4)

Although Denzin and Lincoln (2005) were writing about critical theory as a paradigm, their succinct summary of it as a paradigmatic framework reflects the assumptions associated with the transformative paradigm: "This paradigm … articulates an ontology based on historical realism, an epistemology that is transactional, and a methodology that is both dialogic and dialectical" (p. 187). Discussion between the evaluator and stakeholders is a key characteristic of the epistemological process for the transformative paradigm.

Axiology (Ethics)

The transformative paradigm's axiological assumption rests on four primary principles (Mertens, 2009):

■ The importance of being culturally respectful

■ The promotion of social justice

■ The furtherance of human rights

■ Addressing inequities

The evaluator needs to be aware that "discrimination and oppression are pervasive, and that evaluators have a moral responsibility to understand the communities in which they work in order to challenge societal processes that allow the status quo to continue" (Mertens, 2009, p. 48). The ethical principles of ethics, respect, beneficence, and justice are relevant for the transformative evaluator, just as they are in the other paradigms. However, these principles are given somewhat different interpretations in the transformative paradigm:

> Respect is critically examined in terms of the cultural norms of interaction in diverse communities and across cultural groups. Beneficence is defined in terms of the promotion of human rights and an increase in social justice. An explicit connection is made between the process and outcomes of evaluation studies and the furtherance of a social justice agenda. (Mertens, 2009, pp. 49–50)

Ponterotto (2005) describes the differences between the constructivist and the transformative paradigms in terms of their specific foci and the imperative for action associated with them. Constructivists are cognizant of their positionality and the influence of their values in the inquiry process. Transformative evaluators take this a step further by deliberately expecting that their values in regard to social justice and human rights will influence the process and outcomes of their work. The transformative evaluator focuses on "unequal distributions of power and the resultant oppression of subjugated groups," and "a preset goal of the research is to empower participants to transform the status quo and emancipate themselves from ongoing oppression" (Ponterotto, 2005, p. 204). Box 6.1 provides a hypothetical example.

The transformative axiological assumptions carry complex implications for attempts to define ethical practice for evaluators. These complexities can be seen in the following discussion of cultural competence and the revision of ethical guidelines for relevant professional associations.

Ethics, Evaluation, and Cultural Competence

Mertens (2009, 2010) and Kirkhart (2005) recognize that concerns about diversity and multiculturalism have pervasive implications for the quality of evaluation work. Kirkhart introduced the term "multicultural validity" in her presidential address at the 1994 AEA conference; she defined this as "the vehicle for organizing concerns about pluralism and diversity in evaluation, and as a way to reflect upon the cultural boundaries of our work" (Kirkhart, 1995, p. 1). She later expanded on this concept by providing five justifications for considering validity from a multicultural perspective (Kirkhart, 2005, p. 23):

1. Interpersonal—The quality of the interactions between and among participants in the evaluation process.

2. Consequential—The social consequences of understandings and judgments and the actions taken based upon them.

Box 6.1. A Hypothetical Example of a Transformative Evaluation

An evaluator visits a school for the deaf. She notes that the power structure is made up of white, hearing administrators and teachers. Deaf people are employed only as teacher aides. The evaluator asks the teacher aides whether there are any deaf full-time teachers. They reply that there are not; it has never been done.

The evaluator then asks the teachers why there are no deaf full-time teachers. They reply that the deaf assistants have never been able to pass the teacher certification exams, even though they have bachelor's degrees in education. When the evaluator asks the school's principal about the lack of deaf full-time teachers, he replies that it has never been done and that his hands are tied: If the deaf assistants cannot pass the certification test, he cannot hire them as teachers. The evaluator notes the power structures that serve as barriers to the employment of the deaf assistants in positions as full-time teachers as part of her report.

After the deaf assistants read the report, they take it to the administrators and explain that they want to be given the opportunity to retake the certification test. They ask for support for test preparation, and they ask whether the school system can advocate for accommodations in testing (which would include providing interpreters and extended testing time). The administrator replies that this would have budget implications, but he reallocates funds to support this service.

3. Experiential—Congruence with the lived experience of participants in the program and in the evaluation process.

4. Theoretical—The cultural congruence of theoretical perspectives underlying the program, the evaluation, and assumptions of validity.

5. Methodological—The cultural appropriateness of measurement tools and cultural congruence of design configurations.

Kirkhart (2005) went on to argue that evaluation theory has been remiss in acknowledging the important influences of cultural diversity and culturally bound biases, resulting in threats to validity (a topic explored further in Part III of this text).

Lee (2009) provides practical advice for evaluators on the topic of cultural competence, suggesting that an *evaluator* is not "culturally competent," but that with appropriate understandings and experiences, an evaluator can conduct a culturally competent *evaluation*. She describes the acquisition of the necessary understandings and experiences as a journey that involves awareness of important cultural dimensions; cognizance of our multiple social identities and group memberships (e.g., gender, income or educational level, race/ethnicity, disability); and transparent discussions of relevant issues of power and privilege.

··········· **EXTENDING YOUR THINKING** ···········

Cultural Competence

1. Who are you?

2. How do you describe yourself?

3. To what groups do you belong?

4. Does your membership in those groups give you power and privilege?

5. Are you open to self-examination of your culturally based assumptions?

Chilisa (2005) reflects upon the meaning of ethics from an African perspective. She suggests that narrowly defining ethics as protection of the individual fails to protect the evaluated in important ways. Referencing ethics in the African context, she highlights the need to consider ethics as respect for and protection of the integrity of the researched communities, ethnicities, societies, and nations. She contrasts the Western concept of ethics as an "I–you" individualistic perspective with the African concept of "I–we" (as in "I am we; I am because we are; we are because I am") (Goduka, 2000, cited in Chilisa, 2009, p. 413). The African value system is known as *Ubuntu*, which means "humanness" or "humanity," and dictates how people interact with each other (Asante, 1987, 1992).

> *Ubuntu* underscores an I/we relationship where there is connectedness with living and nonliving things; there is brotherhood, sisterhood, guesthood, and community togetherness. Consequently, relationships are not linear but involve circular repetitive, back and forth movements. For indigenous African communities, circular, back and forth movements allow us (speaking as an indigenous researcher) to go back into the past and invoke metaphors from our culture that help us build ethics protocols that promote social justice and respect for postcolonial/indigenous communities. (Chilisa, 2009, p. 408)

The revision of the AEA's (2004) *Guiding Principles for Evaluators* provides one example of how using a different lens to view this set of ethical principles yields different issues. The original principles were accompanied by a statement acknowledging that they were part of the profession's evolving process of self-examination and should be revisited on a regular basis. When the review process was completed for the second edition of the *Guiding Principles,* the categories were essentially unchanged (i.e., "systematic inquiry," "competence," "integrity/honesty," "respect for people," and "responsibilities for general and public welfare"). However, changes did appear in the statements that amplify the meaning of each overarching principle. For example, the following statement was added to the 2004 version of the *Guiding Principles* under the "competence" category:

> To ensure recognition, accurate interpretation and respect for diversity, evaluators should ensure that the members of the evaluation team collectively demonstrate cultural competence.

Cultural competence would be reflected in evaluators seeking awareness of their own culturally-based assumptions, their understanding of the worldviews of culturally-different participants and stakeholders in the evaluation, and the use of appropriate evaluation strategies and skills in working with culturally different groups. Diversity may be in terms of race, ethnicity, gender, religion, socio-economics, or other factors pertinent to the evaluation context. (AEA, 2004)

This change in language arose because evaluators who work in a spirit compatible with the transformative paradigm were given access to the process of reviewing the principles. Box 6.2 displays two definitions of cultural competence in evaluation.

Box 6.2. Definitions of Cultural Competence in Evaluation

These two definitions highlight different aspects of cultural competence, but both sets are important.

Many health and evaluation leaders are careful to point out that cultural competence cannot be determined by a simple checklist, but rather it is an attribute that develops over time. The root of cultural competency in evaluation is a genuine respect for communities being studied and openness to seek depth in understanding different cultural contexts, practices, and paradigms of thinking. This includes being creative and flexible to capture different cultural contexts, and a heightened awareness of power differentials that exist in an evaluation context. Important skills include: ability to build rapport across difference, gain the trust of community members, and self-reflect and recognize one's own biases. (Endo, Joh, & Yu, 2003, p. 5)

Cultural competence in evaluation can be broadly defined as a systematic, responsive inquiry that is actively cognizant, understanding, and appreciative of the cultural context in which the evaluation takes place; that frames and articulates the epistemology of the evaluative endeavor; that employs culturally and contextually appropriate methodology; and that uses stakeholder-generated, interpretive means to arrive at the results and further use of the findings. (Sen-Gupta, Hopson, & Thompson-Robinson, 2004, p. 13)

The concept of cultural competence has become more salient through deliberative discussions of ways to work more ethically in communities with less access to societal privilege. However, the concept itself is fraught with tensions. Pon (2009) has written a provocative article entitled "Cultural Competency as New Racism: An Ontology of Forgetting." He argues that cultural competence as a concept has been used to reify whiteness as the norm and to cast people of color as the "other." This allows evaluators to hold racist views that are based on culture, rather than on biology. He suggests that instead of striving for cultural competence, evaluators should focus on reflexivity that is associated with racism, colonialism, and other manifestations of power.

Controversy in Recognizing Privilege

The University of Minnesota established the Race, Culture, Class, and Gender Task Group to develop recommendations for its teacher preparation program (Gupton, Kelley, Lensmire, Ngo, & Goh, 2009; subsequent quotations are from Schmidt, 2009). The panel said that future teachers should "understand the importance of cultural identity" (p. 4) and "be able to discuss their own histories and current thinking drawing on notions of white privilege, hegemonic masculinity, heteronormativity, and internalized oppression" (p. 4). "Prospective teachers should promote social justice and have an understanding of U.S. history that takes into account the myth of meritocracy in the United States" (p. 11).

Kissel (also quoted in Schmidt, 2009) is the director of the Individual Rights Defense Program, a conservative think tank. He wrote a critique of the University of Minnesota's plan, saying that it is "severely unjust and impermissibly intrudes into matters of individual conscience" (p. 1). He characterized the college's plan as a "mandate that teachers' thoughts, attitudes, values, and beliefs conform to the task group's ideas of 'cultural competence' … As these demands for 'cultural competence' stand today, they are a severe affront to liberty and a disservice to the very ideal of a liberating education that appears to be behind the task group's ideas" (p. 1). Schmidt (2009) cited more vitriolic responses to the University of Minnesota on a local talk show, including the assertion that the school was "one step away from advocating gas chambers for conservatives."

The University of Minnesota responded by saying that the tasks group's goal is to prepare teachers to work with diverse students. This note was also added to the task group's report: "These task group reports are not policy, but a set of working ideas brought forward by these groups for discussion. The broader scope of the teacher education curriculum will be much more comprehensive than any one set of ideas and is still under development" (Gupton et al., 2009, p. 1).

1. Discuss the various positions reflected in the task group's report, the conservative responses, and the university's subsequent action.

2. What do you think is the responsibility of evaluators in terms of knowing their own cultural roots, recognizing their privilege, and subsequently interacting with members of marginalized communities?

3. Discuss evaluation scenarios in which you, as the evaluator, could hold power and privilege.

4. As noted above, Pon (2009) in "Cultural Competency as New Racism: An Ontology of Forgetting?" He argues that cultural competency as a concept has been used to reify whiteness as the norm and to cast people of color as the other. Discuss.

The transformative axiological assumption leads to the ontological assumption in transformative terms, in that issues of power related to who determines what is real become central to the discussion.

Ontology (Reality)

Reality from a transformative perspective is multifaceted. Human beings often believe that they know what is real; however, there are many different opinions about what that reality is. Differences in perspectives on what is real are determined by diverse values and life experiences. In turn, these values and life experiences are often associated with differences in access to privilege, based on such characteristics as disability, gender, sexual identity, religion, race/ethnicity, national origins, political party, income level, age, language, and immigration or refugee status. In contrast to the constructivist paradigm's ontological assumption that reality reflects cultural relativity, the transformative paradigm interrogates versions of reality on the basis of power inequities and the consequences of accepting one version of reality over another.

Guba and Lincoln (2005) use the term "historical realism" to describe this assumption of the nature of reality: "virtual reality shaped by social, political, cultural, economic, ethnicity and gender values; crystallized over time" (p. 193). They emphasize that the ontological assumptions derived from critical theorists (and commensurate with the transformative paradigm)

> tend to locate truth and knowledge in specific historical, economic, racial, and social infrastructures of oppression, injustice, and marginalization. Knowers are not portrayed as separate from some objective reality, but may be cast as unaware actors in such historical realities (false consciousness) or as aware of historical forms of oppression, but unable or unwilling, because of conflicts, to act on those historical forms to alter specific conditions in this historical moment (divided consciousness). Thus the foundation for critical theorists is dualist: social critique tied in turn to raised consciousness of the possibility of positive and liberating social change. (p. 204)

Ponterotto (2005) concurs that reality is best understood in terms of power relations and views of reality that are shaped in social, cultural, and historical contexts.

This relates back to Pon's (2009) point that claims of cultural competence should not be allowed to obscure the influence of power in what is determined to be real, what meaning is attached to experiences, or how the oppressive processes of marginalization are investigated. He uses as an example the portrayal of Australian Aboriginal mothers and their culture as deficient, thus justifying the placement of Aboriginal children in residential schools where they could be forced to erase their memories of their native culture.

············ **E X T E N D I N G   Y O U R   T H I N K I N G** ············
Identifying Differences in Paradigms

1. How would evaluators using the transformative and constructivist paradigms see the evaluand differently?

2. What examples can you think of that would illustrate this difference?

Epistemology (Knowledge)

The transformative epistemological assumption holds that knowledge is neither absolute nor relative. Rather, it is constructed within a context of power and privilege with consequences attached to which version of knowledge is given privilege. In order to know a community's realities, the evaluators need to have an interactive link with the community members. "Knowledge is socially and historically located within a complex cultural context" (Mertens, 2010, p. 48).

In order to come to an understanding of knowledge within this context, an evaluator needs to have a close and collaborative relationship with the stakeholders, including community leaders and members. This brings to the surface issues of effective communication and use of language. If there is a language difference between the evaluator and the community, then the language of the community should take precedence. If necessary, the evaluator can make use of an interpreter; however, the challenges associated with using an interpreter need to be critically examined. The evaluation focus, purpose, design, implementation, and utilization should be developed through a cooperative process between the evaluator and community members.

Relationships between evaluators and communities are fraught with tensions and challenges, yet are also ripe with opportunities to enrich the evaluation process and thus the use of its findings. The transformative axiological and ontological assumptions lead to the epistemological assumption that knowledge is constructed within a context of power and privilege, and thus that a trusting, culturally respectful relationship must be developed between the evaluator and the community (see Figure 6.1). When the community welcomes the evaluator and embraces the interrogation of inequities, then the evaluator can work in a close relationship with the community.

What is the evaluator's role when the context of the evaluation is one of overt oppression, such as circumstances in which violence is done to gay men or lesbian women, or a white supremacist group controls the political system in a community? In regard to the latter situation, Kendall (2006) asserts that the evaluator in such circumstances needs to interrogate the notion of privilege and especially unearned privilege associated with the color of a white person's skin. (Although she is referencing the problem of racism, she also acknowledges that oppression occurs on the basis of many other dimensions of diversity, such as classism, sexism, heterosexism, the institutionalized primacy of Christianity, and able-bodiedism.) She writes:

> All of us who are white, receive white privileges.... We can use [these privileges] in such a way as to dismantle the systems that keep the superiority of whiteness in place. One of the primary privileges is having greater influence, power, and resources.... We must be aware of how the

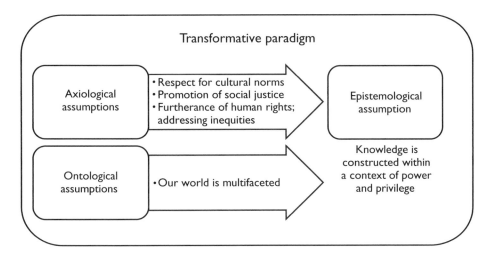

Figure 6.1. The axiological, ontological, and epistemological assumptions underlying the transformative paradigm.

power holders oppressed all people of color to shape the country as they wanted it.... We can dismantle [this system] if we know it well and work together toward that goal. (pp. 62–63)

· · · · · · · · · · E X T E N D I N G   Y O U R   T H I N K I N G · · · · · · · · · ·

Privilege

1. Are you a person of privilege? How do you know if you are or aren't?

2. If you are, how will this affect the work you do?

3. If you are not a person of privilege what will your role be if you work with those who are?

African American, African, and Latino/Latina scholars have written about epistemologies from their respective cultural positions. **Delgado Bernal** (1998) writes about Chicana feminist epistemology. **Mercado-Martinez** et al. (2008) write about an emerging evaluation approach appropriate in the context of Mexico and adjacent areas. **Bewaji** (1995) and **Chilisa** (2005, 2009) write about African epistemologies and philosophies. Wright (2003) cites the work of **Scheurich** and **Young** (1997, 1998) on "coloring epistemologies." **Ladson-Billings** (2000) writes about an "ethnic epistemology," and **Dillard** (2000a, 2000b) about an "endarkened feminist epistemology" (p. 198). For example, Dillard describes the an endarkened feminist epistemology as leading to evaluations in which the inquiry process is a political and utilitarian endeavor associated with an obligation to the black community. Evaluation should serve as a tool to disrupt the hegemonic paradigms associated with oppression of black people. She calls for a "transformation at the epistemological level if education research [evaluation] is to truly change or transform" (Dillard, 2000a, p. 663). The evaluator's role then becomes one of a supportive, reflective activist in the community, who challenges the prevailing research and evaluation establishment.

Guba and Lincoln (2005) describe this epistemological position as "transactional/ subjectivist with value-mediated findings" (p. 193). Morrow (2007) explains that the epistemology is transactional in the sense that evaluators and participants interact with each other in order to come to a shared understanding of what is known. It is subjectivist in that evaluators are cognizant of their and the participants' values, and they expect that their commitment to social justice and human rights will influence the evaluation process and findings.

Methodology (Systematic Inquiry)

The transformative methodological assumption is derived from the three prior assumptions. The methodology employed is not tied to a single approach. Rather, methodological decisions are aimed at determining the approach that will best facilitate use of the process and findings to enhance social justice; identify the systemic forces that support the status quo and those that will allow change to happen; and acknowledge the need for a critical and reflexive relationship between the evaluator and the stakeholders.

In order to plan and conduct a study that is commensurate with these assumptions, the evaluator can use a qualitative data collection strategy as a point of establishing a dialogue between the evaluator and the stakeholders. Guba and Lincoln (2005) describe this methodological stance as "dialogic/dialectical" (p. 193). Mixed methods designs are common in transformative methodologies when they meet the information needs identified. The methodological decisions are made with a conscious awareness of contextual and historical factors, especially as they relate to discrimination and oppression. Thus the methodological assumptions encompass ways to identify who needs to be included and how to include them so that authentic participation is possible.

No single methodology is associated with the transformative paradigm. Rather, evaluators are encouraged to rethink all of their methodological decisions in order to bring them into alignment with the transformative assumptions. For example, sampling needs to be reframed to identify which dimensions of diversity are relevant in the context of the community and what types of communication issues need to be addressed in order to allow for effective communication. Issues of power need to be explicitly acknowledged in terms of the evaluator's and the various community members' roles.

> The transformative paradigm also leads us to (1) reconsider data-collection decisions so we are more inclined to use mixed methods; (2) become consciously aware of the benefits of involving community members in the data-collection decisions and the appropriateness of methods in relation to the cultural issues involved; (3) build trust to obtain valid data; (4) make the modifications that may be necessary to collect valid data from various groups; and (5) tie the data collected to social action. (Mertens, 2009, p. 60)

The next section of this chapter describes the thinking of Social Justice Branch theorists. This is followed by explanations of various transformative approaches and examples of evaluation studies to illustrate these approaches. As a point of contrast, Box 6.3 provides a summary of a study that used only sophisticated quantitative statistical analyses to support the need for diversity in higher education.

Box 6.3. Diversity in Higher Education

A white student sued the University of Michigan because of what he considered to be reverse discrimination. That is, he contended that he was not admitted because the university accepted a less qualified black student. Gurin, Dey, Hurtado, and Gurin (2002) used two large-scale databases that included variables related to the extent of diversity, formal and informal interactions between students of diverse backgrounds and learning outcomes. They conducted a sophisticated statistical analysis that revealed the significant effects of both formal and informal interaction across racial and ethnic groups in terms of student academic and social growth. The U.S. Supreme Court was swayed enough by such research to uphold the consideration of applicants' race by Michigan's law school in its 2003 ruling in *Grutter v. Bollinger*. Gurin et al. argue that their results support the need to continue using affirmative action policy to ensure racially and ethnically diverse student bodies.

- - - - - - - - - - - E X T E N D I N G   Y O U R   T H I N K I N G - - - - - - - - - -

Philosophical Assumptions of the Transformative Paradigm and the Social Justice Branch

Using the table below, answer the following questions:

1. Can you imagine what a transformative evaluation would look like?

2. How would the evaluator set up the evaluation?

3. Would the evaluator be involved with the stakeholders or not?

4. How would the evaluator's assumptions guide her/his decisions?

The Transformative Paradigm and the Social Justice Branch

Description	Axiological assumption	Ontological assumption	Epistemological assumption	Methodological assumption
Focuses primarily on viewpoints of marginalized groups and interrogating systemic power structures through mixed methods to further social justice and human rights	Respect for cultural norms; beneficence is defined in terms of the promotion of human rights and increase in social justice; reciprocity is necessary	Rejects cultural relativism; recognizes that various versions of reality are based on social positioning; conscious recognition of consequences of privileging versions of reality	Interactive link between evaluator and participants (stakeholders); knowledge is socially and historically situated; need to address issues of power and trust	Qualitative (dialogic), but quantitative and mixed methods can be used; contextual, cyclical, consideration of historical factors, especially as they relate to oppression

Social Justice Branch Theorists

Historically, few Social Justice Branch theorists were recognized in the evaluation community; however, many such theorists are now emerging (see Box 6.4). Hopson and Hood (2005) conducted a historical study of the overlooked contributions of African American evaluators in a project called "Nobody Knows My Name." This section includes a description of those now recognized evaluators, as well as the present-day theorists who base their work in democracy and social justice. These include (but are not limited to) theorists whose diverse perspectives reflect feminism, critical race theory (CRT), human rights theory, disability/deaf rights theory, indigenous theories, and queer/LGBTQ theory.

Hopson and Hood (2005) undertook the "Nobody Knows My Name" project in order to bring to light the contributions of African Americans to program evaluation. Hood and Hopson (2008) particularly note the work of African American scholars **Asa Hilliard, Aaron Brown, Leander Boykin,** and **Reid E. Jackson,** who contributed to the theory of evaluation within the context of studying discrimination in schools for black students. This excerpt from Hood and Hopson's discussion of Asa Hilliard's work illustrates the potency of his contribution to evaluation from an Afrocentric perspective:

> In 1989, Hilliard combined his Afrocentric perspective with his observations about evaluation at the annual meeting of the American Evaluation Association in his keynote address entitled "Kemetic (Egyptian) Historical Revision: Implications for Cross-Cultural Evaluation and Research in Education." In particular, he reminded evaluators that they are engaged in the "manipulation of power and therefore politics in its truest sense.... Different approaches to evaluation can result in the painting of very different pictures of reality" (p. 8). (Hood & Hopson, 2008, p. 414)

Hood and Hopson also emphasize the important contribution of Hilliard (1984, p. 120) with regard to connecting evaluation with democracy. Hilliard wrote:

> Educational evaluation in a democratic society must be based on a special view of the person and his or her relationship to others and the environment. The environment includes culture, social class, history, family, and political condition. Each person in an environment actively interacts with it in a way that transforms reality. The natural relationship between people and their environment is a reciprocal. Evaluation in education (which is based on recognizing and understanding active learners within a context in a reciprocal relationship between person and context) is evaluation that fits the real world and makes it possible for evaluation to serve democratic needs. (Quoted in Hood & Hopson, 2008, p. 411)

In the United Kingdom, early theorists who connected their evaluation work with the pursuit of social justice included **Barry MacDonald** and **Saville Kushner.** MacDonald (1976) developed his theory of evaluation from his work at the University of East Anglia's Center for Applied Research in Education. He proposed the idea of democratic evaluation that encompasses the concepts of access, participation, and shared ownership in evaluation. Kushner (2005) has elaborated on this concept by describing how evaluations that use emergent designs can generate democratic capital by including divergent voices in the process and searching for alternative explanations of what is worth knowing. The evaluator's role is to theorize about the shape and process of the evaluation with the

Box 6.4. Social Justice Branch Theorists

Deliberative democratic evaluation	Feminist	LatCrit	Indigenous	African American/ CRT
Barry MacDonald	Kathryn Sielbeck-Bowen	Dolores Delgado Bernal	**African**	Stafford Hood
Saville Kushner	Sharon Brisolera	Francisco Mercado-Martinez	Bagele Chilisa	Rodney Hopson
Ernest House	Cynthia Dillard		John Bewaji	Asa Hilliard
Kenneth Howe	Denise Seigart	Francisco Valdes	**Native American**	Aaron Brown
Jennifer Greene	Elizabeth Tischler	Lilia Fernandez	Marie Battiste	Leander Boykin
Katherine Ryan	Bessa Whitmore	Tara Yosso	Cheryl Crazy Bull	Reid E. Jackson
	Debra Langan	Daniel Solórzano	Joan LaFrance	James Scheurich
Human rights	Mavis Morton	**Disability/ deaf rights**	Doug Brugge	Michelle Young
Thomas Schwandt	Mary Brabeck	Donna Mertens	Mariam Missaghian	Gloria Ladson-Billings
Donna Mertens	Kalina Brabeck	Martin Sullivan	**Māori**	Henry Frierson
Marco Segone	C. Quince Hopkins	Carol Gill	Fiona Cram	Veronica Thomas
Karen Kirkhart	Mary P. Koss	Raychelle Harris	Linda T. Smith	
	LGBTQ	Heidi Holmes		
	Jeffrey Todahl			
	Sarah Dodd			

stakeholders. MacDonald and Kushner have also contributed to the theory of evaluation by suggesting that the evaluator should cede control of the evaluation to the stakeholders.

Ernest House and **Kenneth Howe** (1999) also developed a theory of evaluation related to democracy, which they labeled the "deliberative democratic approach" to evaluation.[2] Kushner (2005) has explained that democratic evaluation is different from deliberative democratic evaluation (DDE)

> in that democratic procedures are built into the action from its earliest stages, in access and design negotiations. [DDE] focuses more on transactions subsequent to evaluation reporting. One radical implication of the approach is that in terms of theory that explains and guides educational practices, the wheel has to be reinvented with each study (not that we cannot learn across studies). This does not deny replicability or a role for formal theory, but it does require us to reconceptualize both in relation to democratic rights in inquiry. Theory, for example, becomes a resource rather than a determinant, subject to the judgment of those (practitioners and citizens) whose lives it purports to explain; methodology becomes a site for the forging of consensus over priorities and meaning rather than merely seeking the "best fit" between a sample of our methods "repertoire" and the characteristics of the evaluand. If this renders unstable our theoretical and methodological sureties, it ought not to disable us as interpreters and observers of change. It merely shifts the basis of our expertise from noun to participle: We should be experts not in theory and methodology but in theorizing and in methodological thinking. (p. 581)

House and Howe's (1999) description of DDE suggests that this theory is not limited to transactions subsequent to evaluation. Rather, they identify three principles of DDE—inclusion, dialogue, and deliberation—that are brought into the evaluation context at the very beginning and serve to inform the evaluator's thinking throughout the process. "Inclusion" means that all relevant interests of stakeholders are taken into consideration. "Dialogue" refers to the process of engaging in conversation between the evaluators and stakeholders in order to determine their interests, opinions, and ideas. "Deliberation" means that the evaluator and stakeholders think reflectively about the issues that surface, in order to identify preferences and values. Through these three principles, the evaluator is able to bring to visibility aspects of the context that might remain hidden without this approach.

Katherine Ryan (2005) expands the idea of DDE by the derivation of a fourth principle: mutual accountability (MacDonald, 1976; Simons, 1987). Social change will come about because all stakeholders, including policy makers, are held accountable. If disparities arise between the original intent of a policy and the outcomes, then a change in direction is warranted. "Democratic accountability aims to redistribute or equalize power relations" (Ryan, 2005, p. 538) through the process of public discourse based on the collection and review of multiple sources of data.

Jennifer Greene (2007) has also contributed substantially to the Social Justice Branch in her theoretical writings, particularly in regard to the role of values and advocacy in evaluation. She has called upon evaluators to be aware of their values and to share those values with stakeholders to allow for a critical examination of how their values influence the evaluation study. In an interview with Tarsilla (2010b), Greene explained the need for pluralistic values and described how previous theorists have contributed to our understandings of linking our values with stakeholder needs. She identified five main genres of evaluation practice that are associated with different values because they serve different stakeholder needs:

> These needs include: (1) the efficiency interests of policymakers (Weiss), (2) the accountability and ameliorative interests of on-site program managers (Patton), (3) the learning, understanding and use (Cronbach); (4) the understanding and development interests of direct service staff and affiliates (Stake); and (5) the democratic and social change interests of program beneficiaries and their allies (democratic evaluation). (Greene, quoted by Tarsilla, 2010b, p. 211)

Greene (2007) acknowledges that it is not possible or even necessary to address all these needs in one evaluation, as the stakeholder's needs vary from study to study. However, evaluators do need to be cognizant of their underlying assumptions and values. Greene has built upon the work of theorists described above, particularly that of Ernie House. She describes evaluation's role as that of "democratizing public conversations," meaning that all persons who have a legitimate stake in the evaluation should have their voices heard. Her commitment to democratic pluralism as a means to bringing the voices of people from marginalized communities into the mix is the reason she is placed in the Social Justice Branch. She emphasizes the importance of engaging in ongoing conversations with stakeholders as a means to creating change for the betterment of society. Her methodological stance is slightly different from that described in the earlier section on transformative methodological assumptions: Her work might better be described as "methodologically dialectical" (i.e., as an avenue to bring about critical conversations across paradigms—a topic discussed in Chapter 9).

Ryan and Schwandt (2002) edited a volume presenting evaluation approaches that seek to advance a role for evaluators oriented toward social criticism and social transformation; this volume included contributions by Hopson (2002) and by **Donna Mertens** (2002; see also Mertens, 2009, 2010). Additional theorists with this orientation include **Marco Segone** (2006) who writes about a human-rights-based approach to evaluation in the international development sector, described as follows:

> Within a human rights approach, evaluation should focus on the most vulnerable populations to determine whether public policies are designed to ensure that all people enjoy their rights as citizens, whether disparities are eliminated and equity enhanced, and whether democratic approaches have been adopted that include everyone in decision-making processes that affect their interests. (Segone, 2006, p. 12)

He notes that a human rights approach should include the democratic principles described previously, as well as the utilization focus discussed in Chapter 4. The United Nations Children's Fund (UNICEF; 2009a, 2009b), with the endorsement of the IOCE and the International Development Association, prepared a report based on a meeting of 85 evaluation organizations that maps future priorities for evaluation situated in a human rights framework.

In addition to these broader calls for theory that addresses discrimination and oppression in evaluation, some theorists write from a particular perspective. For example, several different approaches use race/ethnicity as a theoretical framework. These include culturally responsive evaluation (Hood, Hopson, & **Frierson**, 2005); CRT (**Thomas**, 2009); Latino/Latina CRT or LatCrit (**Valdes**, 1998; **Fernandez**, 2002); and indigenous theories originating from the communities of the Māori (**Cram**, 2009), Africans (**Chilisa**, 2005, 2011), and Native Americans/American Indians (**LaFrance** & **Crazy Bull**, 2009).

Hood et al. (2005a) note the influence of Stake's responsive evaluation in their extension of ideas to the Social Justice Branch. Culturally responsive evaluation requires a full consideration of cultural context in evaluation conducted within communities of color and/or poverty in order for the evaluation to have value. Culturally responsive evaluators are aware of the influence of cultural lenses on their abilities to conduct competent evaluations. They note the value of sharing salient characteristics with the community, such as skin color, while at the same time acknowledging that such characteristics do not in and of themselves qualify an evaluator to conduct a culturally responsive evaluation. The basic premise involved in culturally responsive evaluations asserts that the evaluator use "methods and approaches that are responsive, respectful, ethical, and beneficial to these communities" (Hopson & Hood, 2005b, p. 89).

CRT is an extension of critical theory that is focused on inequities based on race and ethnicity. **Daniel Solórzano** (1997) describes the role of CRT as providing a framework to investigate and make visible those systemic aspects of society that allow the discriminatory and oppressive status quo of racism to continue. Thomas (2009) has described the implications of CRT for evaluators as creating an ethical responsibility for "addressing unequal relations of power, advocating social justice, challenging the dominant hegemonic paradigms, and opening up new spaces for decolonized knowledge production" (p. 57).

LatCrit theory (Valdes, 1998; Fernandez, 2002) is similar to CRT, except that its focus is on inequities associated with the educational, social, and legal positioning of Latinas/Latinos, especially those in the United States. Solórzano and Yosso (2001) describe LatCrit theory as a framework for critically examining the structural racism that affects Latinas/Latinos. LatCrit also includes a directive to work for social change in this community by resisting the deficit view of its members.

Indigenous theorists include those who address the needs of the Māori (Cram, 2009; **Smith**, 1999), African Botswanas (Chilisa, 2005, 2011), Native Americans/American Indians (**Battiste**, 2000; LaFrance & Crazy Bull, 2009; **Brugge** & **Missaghian,** 2006); Canadian First Nations people (Mi'kmaq College Institute, 2006), Australasians (Australasian Evaluation Society, 2006), and indigenous communities in general (**Osborne** & **McPhee,** 2000). Cram (2009) and Smith (2004) theorize about the need to challenge the status quo by foregrounding inequalities and social justice. Indigenous peoples have suffered in many ways from the oppression brought upon them by colonizers. For example, Māori people (like many other indigenous peoples) were robbed of their land by white settlers. The resulting lack of trust between indigenous peoples and white settlers negatively influences current relationships between evaluators and community members when the evaluators are not from that community.

These conditions have led many indigenous groups to develop ways to decolonize research and evaluation involving them, in the form of creating their own "terms of reference" for conducting evaluation studies in their communities. For example, Māori people have put forth terms of reference stating that systematic inquiries will be conducted by Māori, for Māori, and with Māori (Cram et al., 2004). LaFrance and Crazy Bull (2009) provide an excellent description of the way that Native American tribes control access to who conducts research and evaluation studies in their communities. One of the key principles that must be acknowledged is that each tribe is a sovereign nation with its own government and regulation; the second principle is that a tribe must be informed about the potential benefits for individuals and the community as a whole before it decides to participate in an evaluation study.

Scholars such as **Sullivan** (2009; see also Mertens, Sullivan, & Stace, 2011) have developed disability rights theories. Following in the footsteps of other civil rights groups, people with disabilities have demanded to have more control over their lives and over research and evaluation done on them. They have coined the phrase "Nothing about us without us." One major aspect of disability rights theories is the separation of impairment (based on a biological condition) from disability (the oppressive social response to disability). This aspect situates the "problem" in the societal response to a person's impairment, rather than in the person. If society responded appropriately, then there would be no disability. In regard to the conduct of research and evaluation, Sullivan (2009) reminds us of the diversity in the disability community:

> The questions of diversity, especially in terms of impairment, is of ubiquitous concern for disability researchers [evaluators] as different forms of impairment not only necessitate different approaches and methodologies but also generate different subcultures in which disability assumes different meaning and which call for a more nuanced approach to research [and evaluation]. (p. 71)

One clear example of this diversity comes from the perspective of many members of the deaf community, who do not view themselves as disabled (**Harris, Holmes,** & Mertens, 2009). Rather, they see themselves as a linguistic and cultural minority group that needs to fight against oppression by "audists" (people who think that hearing people are superior to deaf people because they can hear). Harris et al. (2009) have adapted the Aboriginal terms of reference (Osborne & McPhee, 2000) to the American Sign Language community. They note the importance of respecting deaf culture and sign language throughout the evaluation process.

Feminists such as **Sielbeck-Bowen, Brisolara, Seigart, Tischler**, and **Whitmore** (2002), **Langan** and **Morton** (2009), **Brabeck** and **Brabeck** (2009), and **Hopkins** and **Koss** (2005) have contributed to the development of feminist theories of evaluation. The essence of such theories is to "expose the individual and institutional practices that have denied access to women and other oppressed groups and have ignored or devalued women" (Brabeck & Brabeck, 2009, p. 39). Feminists are concerned with political and activist agendas and with striving for improved social justice for women.

Hopkins and Koss (2005) note that there are many variations of feminist theories, including "liberal, cultural, radical, Marxist and/or socialist, postmodern (or poststructuralist), and multiracial feminism" (p. 698). Liberal feminists strive for equality of treatment between men and women. Cultural feminists argue that equal treatment of men and women will not redress inequities, because of the legacy of a sexist society that results in substantial differences in resources and opportunities for men and women. Cultural feminists focus on correcting the devaluation of women's experiences and contributions to society by recognizing the importance of human relationships and narrative methods of communication. Radical feminists focus on oppression based on sexism, which is manifested as men's dominance over women. Marxist and socialist feminists include class and economic issues in addition to gender. Thus they tend to focus on such topics as unpaid work in the home, poverty reduction among women, and exploitation of sex workers. Postmodern or poststructuralist feminists question the binary male–female categories and argue for the deconstruction of gender roles to correct the subjugation of women by men. These traditional categories are redefined to recognize the full spectrum of possible gender roles. Multiracial feminists look through both the race and gender lenses to identify inequities that result from this intersection. (Recall the "endarkened feminist epistemology" and similar epistemologies discussed earlier in this chapter.) Multiracial feminists also connect themselves with the indigenous and postcolonial theorists discussed previously.

Queer/LGBTQ theorists such as **Jeffrey Todahl** focus on gender and sexual identity issues in evaluation. **Sarah Dodd** (2009) discusses theories that have arisen in LGBTQ communities. While Dodd acknowledges uniqueness and diversity within and between each of these communities, commonalities exist in the form of recognizing discrimination and oppression on the basis of sexual orientation. Sexual minorities are likely to be present in many evaluation populations; however, evaluators may be unaware of their inclusion because of the stigma attached to "outing" oneself. Queer/LGBTQ theorists question the heterosexist bias that pervades society in terms of power over and discrimination toward sexual orientation minorities. Because of the sensitivity of the issues surrounding LGBTQ status, evaluators need to be aware of safe ways to protect such individuals' identities and ensure that discriminatory practices are brought to light in order to bring about a more just society.

"Listen to me and take seriously the situation that I am in" (Todahl, Linville, Bustin, Wheeler, & Gau, 2009, p. 34). This quotation comes from an evaluation of sexual assault support services for LGBTQ people and the specific needs of their communities in the Pacific northwest. Many studies exist in relation to sexual assault of children and adults in the United States, but rarely has sexual orientation been considered in research. Although empirical evidence concerning sexual assault and persons in LGBTQ communities is minimal, nonempirical literature points to social conditions (discrimination, marginalization, and social oppression) that make access to health care, social services, and criminal justice difficult for poor LGBTQ people. In order to capture these people's lived experience obtaining sexual assault support services, Todahl et al. (2009) were conscientious about preserving the privacy and confidentiality necessary for the stakeholders to feel confident and comfortable enough to voice the opinion that there was low community awareness and support for them in time of need. Given this opportunity to state their concerns and needs, the LGBTQ communities were able to share their belief in the importance of changing attitudes about LGBTQ persons in the community at large, in increasing access to LGBTQ-friendly services, and in developing and implementing LGBTQ sensitivity-training protocols for key social and health service delivery systems.

As noted in Chapter 4, participatory evaluation can be practical or transformative. Cousins and Whitmore (1998) have distinguished between practical participatory evaluation (discussed in Chapter 4) and transformative participatory evaluation. Both approaches involve community members in decision making about the evaluation; however, the latter does so with an explicit recognition of power issues in granting or denying access to resources and opportunities. Community members who are denied access on the basis of dimensions of diversity associated with oppression and discrimination are invited to participate, and appropriate supportive mechanisms are brought to bear to ensure that they can do so authentically. Transformative participatory evaluation consciously brings in the voices of those most oppressed in order to bring about social change.

Theory to Practice

The Social Justice Branch makes use of many different approaches, including DDE, country-led evaluation (CLE), CRT, indigenous evaluation, culturally responsive evaluation, disability- and deaf-rights-based evaluation, feminist evaluation, and transformative participatory evaluation. The criteria for quality in all these types of evaluation are rooted in issues of social justice and human rights. Lather (as a contributor to Moss et al., 2009, p. 506) offered this reflection on "touchstones" that determine quality in the context of educational research/evaluation:

> Given this positioning, my quality touchstones are three. The first one is that regardless of paradigm I look for research that has some sense of the history, sociology, philosophy, ethics of inquiry, and what might be called a rigor of reflective competence. I'm very interested in redefining rigor so that it includes a certain sense of the history and philosophy of research, so that people can situate what they are doing within these more foundational discourses. Second, as opposed to assuming a unified idea of science and homogeneous standards, I'm interested in quality indicators that fit paradigmatic assumptions, across the spectrum from earlier naturalistic and constructivist paradigms to discourse theory, ethnographic authority, critical, feminist, and race-based paradigms and more recent post-structuralisms.
>
> Validity in qualitative research ranges from correspondence models of truth and assumptions of transparent narration to practices that take into account the crisis of representation. Some scholars call for new imaginaries altogether, where validity is as much about the play of difference as the repetition of sameness (Scheurich, 1996). From such a perspective, validity is recognized as part of the power and political dimensions of the demarcation of what is and is not science, what is "good" science, and who gets to say. As such, validity is far more about deep theoretical and political issues than about a technical issue or an issue of allegiance to correct procedure.

Deliberative Democratic Evaluation

The inclusion of a democratic perspective in evaluation is evidenced in several of the theories described in this chapter. One of these, DDE has three methodological requirements: All relevant interests need to be included; the evaluation process is dialogical in order to identify stakeholder interests; and the evaluation results are deliberated upon by the relevant stakeholders. House (2004) conducted a DDE of a bilingual program, and this is summarized in Box 6.5.

House (2004) has noted 10 points about DDE that merit attention:

1. *Cultural acceptability.* DDE can only be applied in settings that are democratic. The political system in the United States is democratic; however, it is controlled to a large extent by the rich and powerful elite. Hence deliberation is important as part of the democratic process, to challenge the influence of the powerful.

2. *Cultural diversity.* Evaluators need to be aware of the diversity within communities. Latinas/Latinos may share a language, but they can differ in many other respects (e.g., economic status, value of education, aspirations for their children, level of education, and citizenship). Cultures are not internally uniform.

Box 6.5. Sample DDE Study: The Denver Bilingual Program Study

Sample study		Evaluation approach	Document title
House (2004)	HOLA!·HI! COLORADO	Deliberative democratic evaluation	"Democracy and Evaluation"

The Evaluator

Ernest House is Professor Emeritus in the School of Education at the University of Colorado at Boulder. He is one of the original members of the AEA and its predecessor organizations.

Philosophical and Theoretical Lenses

House used a DDE approach.

> The three principles are inclusion of all relevant stakeholder views, values, and interests; extensive dialogue between and among evaluators and stakeholders so they understand one another thoroughly; and deliberation with and by all parties to reach conclusions (House and Howe, 1999). The conclusions might be jointly constructed rather than made entirely by the evaluator. (A checklist for DDE is on the website of the Evaluation Center at Western Michigan University: *www.wmich.edu/evalctr/checklists.*) (House, 2004)

Because stakeholders are enlisted at many points, the evaluator's role in DDE is extended beyond the traditional. Since a range of views, values, and interests are considered, the hope is that the conclusions will be sounder, that participants will accept and use the findings more; and that an evaluation becomes a democratic practice that faces up to the political, value-imbued situation evaluators often find themselves in. House attempted to establish complete transparency in order to avoid appearing to be more supportive of one side than the other. House hired two former principals who were Latinos to collect the data in the schools.

The Evaluand and Its Context

Denver, Colorado is located in the Southwest United States and has a large Spanish-speaking community, largely as a result of immigration from Mexico. Its school system was under court order to provide instruction in Spanish for students who did not know English until they reached a sufficient level of English proficiency to participate in regular classes. The school district developed a bilingual program called English Language Acquisition, which was then reviewed and accepted by the Congress of Hispanic Educators and the U.S. Department of Justice. The court appointed House to monitor the implementation of this program. Emotions ran high on both sides of the issue; the school district and the plaintiffs had major trust issues. As the Latino/Latina population increased, animosities arose among these immigrants, the Anglo business establishment, and the African Americans (who viewed the Latinos/Latinas as a threat to affordable housing and entry-level jobs). Some of the newer immigrants followed distinctive cultural traditions, such as taking their children out of school for a month to attend fiestas in Mexico.

Method

Design

The study was not designed to compare ways to teach English in general; therefore, a randomized controlled design would not work in these circumstances. House (2004) describes his approach:

> I met with interested groups in the community, including the most militant, those bitterly opposed to bilingual programs and those who wanted total bilingual schools. I listened, responded to their concerns, and included their ideas in my investigations. I followed up on information they provided using traditional research methods. I thought about holding meetings open to the public but decided against such meetings since I was afraid they would degenerate into shouting matches. The emotions were too raw. I developed quantitative performance indicators of program success based on the school district's data management system. I discussed the indicators with all parties until everyone accepted them as indicators of progress.

Evaluation Purposes and Questions

The purpose of the evaluation was to monitor the implementation of the court-ordered bilingual education program.

Stakeholders and Participants

House distinguished the Latinos/Latinas families had been in the United States for many years from the more recent immigrants (mostly from Mexico). Many teachers and administrators were from "old" Latino/Latinas families; this gave them a shared language with the newer immigrants, but also differentiated them from that group, because many of the new immigrants were poor and uneducated. Of the school district's 70,000 students, 15,000 needed instruction in Spanish. The stakeholders were thus the students and their families, the educators in the school system, and the parties in the court case. House did not interact with these stakeholders directly; rather, he interacted with their representatives in the form of a council that he met with twice a year. The council included the lawyers from both sides of the court case.

Data Collection

> For data I constructed a checklist based on the key elements of the program to assess each school. I submitted the checklist to all parties and used their recommendations to revise it. I hired two retired school principals to visit and assess individual schools with the checklist. Since they were former principals, the school district trusted them. Since they were Latinos and supported bilingual instruction, the plaintiffs trusted them. I encouraged the school district staff to challenge the evaluation of each school where they disagreed. We hashed out disagreements face-to-face. (Eventually, the school district developed its own checklist to anticipate which schools might have problems.) (House, 2004)

(cont.)

Box 6.5 (cont.)

Sampling schools was not an option, because the court ordered monitoring of every individual school.

Management and Budget

House met with the stakeholders from both sides twice a year to share his progress with the evaluation. The evaluation lasted 5 years.

> My written reports went to the presiding judge three times a year. As court documents, the reports were public information the local media seized on. I asked the school district officials and the plaintiffs how I should handle these requests. They preferred that I not talk to the media. It would inflame the situation. So I referred all inquiries to the stakeholders and made no public comments beyond my written reports. (House, 2004)

There is no specific information given about the budget.

Reports and Utilization

House (2004) writes:

> Many different issues arose over a five-year period. For example, the lawyers representing the Latinos[/Latinas] suspected the school district was forcing schools to move students into English classes prematurely. So I paid close attention to the proficiency level of the students when they were transferred to English and to the procedures used to assess them. Lawyers from the US Justice Department were afraid students would be taught with inferior materials. So we assessed the Spanish versus English teaching materials to ensure the quality was similar. Even the lawyers on the same side had different concerns....
>
> The parents themselves disagreed. Some wanted their children immersed in English immediately so the students could get jobs. Most wanted their children in Spanish first, then English. Legally, parents could choose what their children should do. We discovered that many schools did not make these choices clear to parents. So we attended to whether the options were presented to parents at each school in ways they could understand.
>
> The most militant Latino[/Latina] group in the city wanted full cultural maintenance of Spanish rather than transition to English. I met with the leader of this group in the café that served as political headquarters in the Latino[/Latina] part of Denver. I listened to her concerns. There was little I could do about cultural maintenance since I had to work within the court document, which precluded it. However, I could investigate issues that caused her to distrust the schools. For example, some school principals were not identifying Spanish-speaking students because they were afraid their teachers would be replaced by Spanish teachers. We reported this to school district officials, who resolved the problem.

Meta-Evaluation

House (2004) reports that the evaluation was at least partially successful based on the following changes in the school district.

> Now, after five years—preceded by twenty years of militant strife—the program is almost fully implemented. The issue seems to be defused for the school district. The opposing groups can meet in a room without casting insults at each other. I am not saying the groups love each

other, but they can manage their business together rationally. The conflict is nothing like when we started.

REFLECTIONS FROM THE EVALUATOR

In summary, the Denver evaluation dealt with the politics of the program. It dealt with specific issues arising from the views, values, and interests of those most concerned. The face-to-face meetings among the key stakeholders proved critical. In addition, the transparency of my actions as evaluator was also critical. Without stakeholders' understanding what I was doing, I don't believe trust could have evolved. The evaluation became a mode of communication, negotiation, and common understanding. During the study, I employed the usual research methods we use—checklists, tests, and performance indicators. What was different was how the study was framed.

I believe this evaluation incorporated a democratic process that gave voice to stakeholders. Its legitimacy to participants rested on fair, inclusive, and open procedures for deliberation, where those in discussion were not intimidated or manipulated (Stein, 2001). Of course, those involved still do not agree on all issues, and they never will. Some value disagreements are intractable, but that does not mean we cannot handle them.

3. *Faithful representation.* It is not possible to involve all stakeholders in the deliberation process (recall that there were 15,000 Latina/Latino students in the Denver case). Thus the evaluator needs to select representatives from the stakeholder group in such a way that all stakeholders believe their representation to be legitimate.

4. *Authentic processes.* The democratic process must be authentic in the sense that foregone conclusions are not allowed to prevail.

5. *Structured interaction.* The evaluator needs to establish a structure to control the nature of interactions among the stakeholders, in order to prevent domination by one group over another.

6. *A focus on issues.* One way to structure interactions is to keep them focused on specific issues that need attention and discussions of the types of evidence that need to be brought to bear to illuminate those issues.

7. *Rules and principles.* The AEA's (2004) has a set of *Guiding Principles for Evaluators* are specific enough to inform decisions, but flexible enough to be responsive to contextual differences. These apply in DDE as well as in other evaluation approaches.

8. *Collaboration.* "The evaluators' role in deliberative evaluation is one of collaboration, not capitulation" (House, 2004). If the stakeholders make unreasonable requests, the evaluator should not capitulate in the interest of smoothing thing over. Rather, the evaluator needs to reference principles, guidelines, courts, or

other legitimate authorities to substantiate their position to maintain a balanced perspective and focus on the salient issues.

9. *Balance of power.* Power differences are inherent in most evaluation contexts. The evaluator needs to be aware of the sources of power differentials and to arrange circumstances so that those in a position of less power are not intimidated or silenced.

10. *Constraints on self-interest.* Democratic societies are not exempt from corruption; people often seek to satisfy their own selfish interests. Evaluators do not have a magic solution to this challenge, but they can emphasize the need to put the greater good above individual self-interests.

In addition to the challenges associated with self-interest, House has noted several other potential difficulties in attempting to implement a DDE. When an evaluation is emotionally and politically charged, it can be difficult to involve the general public without putting the outcomes of the evaluation at risk or having the evaluation compromised. In addition, evaluations are just one small part of the overall dynamic that swirls around complex societal changes. Hence the influence of the evaluation itself may be limited by larger societal forces.

· · · · · · · · · · **EXTENDING YOUR THINKING** · · · · · · · · · ·
Deliberative Democratic Evaluation

 Social Justice Branch

Sample study	Evaluation approach	List the distinguishing characteristics
House (2004)	Deliberative democratic evaluation (DDE)	

Using the description of the House (2004) study in Box 6.5, answer the following questions:

1. What are the characteristics that illustrate House's use of the Deliberative Democratic Evaluation Model?

2. What do you identify as the strengths and weaknesses of this model in terms of the types of data that were collected by the evaluator?

3. What do you identify as the strengths and weaknesses of the strategies used in this study that were intended to address issues of social justice?

4. What would you suggest modifying in this study to improve the potential for social change based on the process and results of the evaluation?

Country–Led Evaluation

The international development community's desire to approach evaluation from a human rights perspective has led to the development of an approach to evaluation called CLE. CLE arose because evaluations conducted by donor agencies or their consultants did not instill a sense of ownership of the programs in the home country. Segone (2009) suggests that partner countries can lead evaluations and thus feel more ownership for the program and the evaluation findings. The partner country should decide what is to be evaluated and how, as well as how the findings are interpreted and used. The Pennarz et al. (2007) study, summarized in Box 6.6 illustrates CLE.

Box 6.6. CLE Study: The Bosnia-Herzegovina Poverty Reduction Study

Sample study	Evaluation approach	Document title
Pennarz, Holicek, Rasidagic, and Rogers (2007)	Country-led evaluation (CLE)	*Joint Country-Led Evaluation of Child-Focused Policies within the Social Protection Sector in Bosnia and Herzegovina*

The Evaluators

These four evaluators are listed as authors of the final report: Johanna Pennarz, Reima Anna Maglajlic Holicek, Esref Kenan Rasidagic, and Dane Rogers. They work for a private consulting firm called ITAD, which undertakes evaluations in the United Kingdom and around the world.

Philosophical and Theoretical Lenses

A human rights/social justice lens was used as the basis for the evaluation. This is in keeping with the mission of UNICEF and the needs of the region.

The Evaluand and Its Context

The evaluation took place in Bosnia-Herzegovina following the 1992–1995 war. This country is the poorest state of the former Yugoslavia, with 72% of the adults living in poverty. The situation is worse for Roma, refugees, and returnees. Households with more than two children are most likely to be poor. The government developed a Medium-Term Development Strategy in 2004–2007 as a guide to poverty reduction. UNICEF worked in partnership with the Bosnia-Herzegovina government and other donor agencies to implement and evaluate this strategy.

The evaluation was conducted as a team approach, with external consultants and country-level evaluators working in partnership. The consultants provided capacity-building experiences for the local-level evaluators.

(cont.)

Box 6.6 (*cont.*)

Method

The major data collection methods included document reviews, reviews of statistical data, in-depth interviews with key stakeholders, institutional visits, surveys, and case studies.

Design

This evaluation is described as a joint CLE, in that the external consultants provided guidance and support for the local-level evaluators. The basic premise of a CLE is that a participating country will feel more ownership of the evaluation and be able to shape the evaluation in ways that are viewed as useful for decision makers in that country.

Evaluation Purposes and Questions

The "terms of reference" for the evaluation listed two purposes:

1. To represent an ex-ante evaluation for the BiH EPPU [Bosnia and Herzegovina Economic Policy and Planning Unit, later renamed the Directorate for Economic Planning or DEP] to inform and structure the production of the strategic social sector documents in 2007, including a) recommendations to address the weaknesses of the system in reaching its developmental objectives, and b) recommendations on policy development criteria, as well as indicators for monitoring and evaluation of social policy implementation process; and,

2. To inform UNICEF's Mid Term Review and UNDAF [United Nations Development Assistance Framework] Evaluation, assessing UNICEF's contribution to the BiH Social Protection sector, including a) capacity to develop evidence-based policies, and b) develop more structured and coherent approaches to policy development and implementation. (Pennarz et al., 2007, p. 62)

Pennarz et al. (2007) note a later change:

> Following negotiations between the evaluators and the stakeholders, the purpose was changed to a review of evidence-based policy making in relation to Children's Allowances in BiH and UNICEF's contribution to development of evidence-based, child-focused methodologies in the social protection sector. (p. 5)

Sample evaluation questions included the following (Pennarz et al., 2007, p. 71):

3.1.   What are the mechanisms for the implementation of policies that regulate Children's Allowances?

3.1.1. How have they been supported/funded?

3.1.2. Are these mechanisms efficient?

3.1.3. What has been achieved in terms of outputs from these mechanisms (i.e., improved targeting)?

3.2.   What are the mechanisms addressing key gaps/barriers in relation to Children's Allowances?

3.2.1. How have they been supported/funded?

3.2.2. Are these mechanisms efficient?

3.2.3. What has been achieved in terms of outputs from these mechanisms?

Stakeholders and Participants

Key stakeholders included the ministry officials concerned with social policies; national statistical agencies; local governments; NGOs (e.g., lobby groups, universities, and unions); and international donor agencies (e.g., the UNDP, UNICEF, and the World Bank).

Management and Budget

The evaluators present a list of the main steps taken in the joint CLE, which began with the definition of the purpose and scope of the evaluation, identification of stakeholders, and development of an evaluation framework. After presenting the evaluation framework to key stakeholders, the evaluators then developed detailed evaluation questions and a work plan. They identified appropriate cases for in-depth studies and moved on to the data collection and analysis. They held thematic workshops to discuss the preliminary findings and obtain stakeholder input before the final report was prepared and disseminated. There is no mention of the budget, but presumably the evaluation was supported by funds from UNICEF.

Meta-Evaluation

Time constraints prohibited full achievement of the goals of a CLE. This limited the extent to which the process could be participatory. The CLE did help build relationships among key actors, clarified roles and responsibilities, and identified activities that will benefit the process in the future.

Reports and Utilization

The study results highlighted the continued problems with providing protection to children in this context, especially those who are Roma and/or come from families with more than two children. The evaluators recommended legislative and institutional reform, as well as the development of a more efficient social protection system that includes effective partnerships with governmental agencies at all levels, with NGOs, and with donor agencies. The government has made a commitment to human rights and social protection; however, economic conditions are not favorable enough to allow it to follow through on this commitment.

CLE is not without its problems. Tall (2009) points out the need to give serious consideration to the purposes and dynamics of CLE. Countries that receive development aid may feel threatened if they conduct an evaluation that is critical of the donor. A country and a donor agency may have different perspectives on the meaning of evaluation. The capacity to conduct an evaluation that has merit in the eyes of stakeholders may need to be built in the country. This may require a cultural shift in the country's governmental agencies if they have not been accustomed to using evaluation data for decision making.

In addition, this may call for a release of control by the donor agencies—not only from how the evaluation is conducted, but also from what the aid funds are used for. Tall writes:

> Ownership is the key factor to reverse the development trends where poverty remains despite significant economic growth recorded in African countries. What it implies is the need to allow countries to decide, by themselves, how they would like to make use of their financial resources … and how they will manage its use to produce results. In other words, this is about ownership of development and development evaluation. (p. 129)

· · · · · · · · · · · E X T E N D I N G   Y O U R   T H I N K I N G · · · · · · · · · · ·

Country–Led Evaluation

 Social Justice Branch

Sample study	Evaluation approach	List the distinguishing characteristics
Pennarz, Holicek, Rasidagic, and Rogers (2007)	Country-led evaluation (CLE)	

Using the description of the Pennarz et al. (2007) study in Box 6.6, answer the following questions:

1. What are the characteristics that illustrate Pennarz et al.'s use of the Country-Led Evaluation Model?

2. What do you identify as the strengths and weaknesses of this model in terms of the types of data that were collected by the evaluators?

3. What do you identify as the strengths and weaknesses of the strategies used in this study that were intended to address issues of social justice?

4. What would you suggest modifying in this study to improve the potential for social change based on the process and results of the evaluation?

CRT Evaluation

Critical race theorists work through a lens of discrimination based on race or ethnicity to interrogate the effects of racism in the provision of services for communities of color. The CRT evaluation approach provides a means to make visible inequities related to differences in power in social, educational, and political systems. The sample study conducted by Fierro (2006) and described in Box 6.7 provides insights into how to conduct an evaluation positioned in CRT.

Box 6.7. Sample CRT Evaluation Study: The Philadelphia Welfare-to-Work Study

Sample study	Evaluation approach	Document title
Fierro (2006)	Critical race theory (CRT) evaluation	*African American Agency within Welfare Agencies: A Critical Study of African American Mothers with Transitional Custody*

The Evaluators

The evaluation team was composed of three members: a senior social work professor, a social scientist, and a database specialist.

The senior social worker (who holds an MSW degree) was also the founder of the community-based organization that implemented the program. He brought to the evaluation knowledge of the organization, its philosophy, and its internal workings, as well as over 30 years of social work and networking experience with local agencies and service providers.

The social scientist, Rita S. Fierro, had a master's degree in sociology and was working toward a PhD in African American studies. The database specialist also held human resources responsibilities and brought to the evaluation computer expertise and knowledge of staff inner workings.

Philosophical and Theoretical Lenses

This evaluation incorporated two opposing theoretical perspectives.

As a PhD student in African American studies, Fierro was aware of racial oppression, institutional racism, and the unique African American cultural perspective in the U.S. experience. This framework led her to organize and measure the impact of integrating culturally relevant topics into participants' training. Except for database information, which workers collected at intake, Fierro conducted all data collection. As such, the data collection process was never judgmental.

> Aware of how commonly my respondents' lifestyle was judged, I was mindful to not be judgmental. I avoided personal comments until I was certain the respondent was comfortable with me or asked me to do so. I became a little more informal over time. My respondents knew, from the occasional Ebonics expressions I used and my passion for African American Studies that I was often comfortable around Black people. However, I knew, as white, that I was under continual scrutiny; therefore I only spoke of my studies when the respondents asked me to, and was mindful to not sound "preachy." I answered most personal questions with sincerity and was rarely evasive. (Fierro, 2006, p. 90)

The senior social worker had a color-blind, deficit-focused perspective on transitional custody parents. For him, as frequently for the rest of society, the challenges that parents faced were grounded in their own deficiencies and were in no way attributable to social factors. From this perspective, culture-centered perspectives are inadequate. He had no involvement in the data collection, but took the lead on planning the evalua-

(cont.)

Box 6.7 (cont.)

tion. For this reason, results from the cultural empowerment experiment were limited to the expanded study.

These two perspectives clashed often, and kept the evaluation from being one coherent body of research. For the purpose of this discussion, the evaluation and the expanded study are presented. In this internal evaluation, the senior social worker handled the politics of the evaluation by deciding what information would be communicated to the organization and how. Fierro functioned as a manager of the data collection, analysis, and report writing, by revising the database, organizing and analyzing all data, speaking to parents, attending meetings, and working with workers to fill in missing data. As she became more familiar with the parents' stories, she became more and more a passionate advocate for a change in the child welfare system and an adequate representation of parents' experiences. The expanded study was her dissertation work. The database specialist created the program's database and revised data input and output files.

In the expanded study, the social scientist coined the term "transitional custody parents" to correct the erroneous evaluation use of "noncustodial parents" to indicate parents who lost custody to the state. The revised term is used here except in quotations from the original evaluation report.

The Evaluand and Its Context

This study was a program evaluation of a welfare-to-work (WtW) program in Philadelphia. It took place within the first politically charged years after welfare reform. Parents who lose custody of their children face multiple challenges in reuniting with their children. As they struggle to fulfill the requirements of the child welfare system, they confront unsympathetic legal and welfare systems as well. Most parents lose custody because of neglect, not abuse. Poverty is frequently confused with neglect.

This WtW program made an attempt to overcome the conflicting child welfare and welfare systems by enrolling parents who had children in the system and then helping them overcome their barriers to employment by (1) networking on their behalf with local service providers and institutions; (2) providing job training, resume assistance, domestic violence workshops, health resources, child care, and housing vouchers; and (3) providing a friendly environment. The employment advisors assigned to each participant contacted agencies if the participant needed resources or accommodations. Program stakeholders met monthly with representatives of local agency providers, in "infrastructure meetings" where challenges were overcome via networking.

The program was based on two assumptions: that by removing parents' barriers to employment, they would be able to regain custody; and that institutions would be more favorable to institutions advocating for individuals than to individuals alone.

Method

Design

A mixed method process and outcome design was chosen for this evaluation. The quantitative measures (database analysis, surveys, pre–post tests on experiment) favored the measurements of outcomes. Via qualitative methods (ethnographic interviews, observations, and focus groups), Fierro explored the context within which participants lived and operated.

Evaluation Purposes and Questions

The main objectives of the WtW outcome evaluation were as follows:

1. Assess the impact of the WtW program by analyzing the extent of its achieved outcomes (employment, housing, and reunification);

2. Outline the demographics of the most successful population of WtW clients;

3. Compare—among WtW clients—the population of general welfare recipients to the population of noncustodial parents in terms of demographics, employment barriers, attendance and contacts with staff, and program outcomes;

4. Determine the relevance of the WtW infrastructure to WtW clients;

5. Offer suggestions to improve service delivery, program implementation, and policy planning.

The goals of the expanded study (Fierro, 2006, p. 66) were as follows:

1. To outline the experience of African American transitional custody mothers within the welfare, child welfare and legal systems;

2. To explore the mothers' own definitions of success and empowerment;

3. To assess whether infusion of African American cultural content would affect their personal empowerment, sense of control and Afrocentric belief system;

4. To highlight what impact a more culturally and educationally wholistic approach had on the clients' experience throughout their time at the WtW program.

The ethnography's "grand tour" questions were these: "What is the personal background of transitional custody mothers and what has been their experience within the system? What have they learned that they think would be helpful to other mothers? (Fierro, 2006, p. 69).

Stakeholders and Participants

Program workers, local agency and provider representatives, and participants were program stakeholders. In the first 2 years, program participation was open to all parents looking for employment. Beginning in 2002, participation was limited to parents who had lost their children to the state and wanted to regain custody. Most participants were female (88%), single (91%), and African American (89%). Participants in the expanded study were all mothers.

Data Collection

The following data were collected throughout the evaluation, according to the original (December 2004) report:

(cont.)

Box 6.7 (cont.)

■ Data on demographics, employment barriers, education, and program status were collected for 571 clients enrolled (starting in September 1999) in the WtW database.[1]

■ Focus groups (71 in all) were conducted once a week for 6 weeks with clients enrolled in five cycles, starting in September 2003 and ending in April 2004.[2]

■ Two employment advisors conducted phone follow-ups with their clients after the end of the program: a senior employment advisor ($n = 253$ clients) and a second employment advisor ($n = 37$ clients). Out of the 290 clients called, 153 were reached (52.75%).

■ To allow the staff's experience to emerge from the evaluation, staff surveys were handed out. A total of 10 staff surveys were collected.

■ Attendance records were collected for 134 clients enrolled after February 2002 in the first 6–7 weeks of the WtW program.

■ Number, type, and intensity of contacts between clients and staff were collected for 149 clients enrolled from February 2002 to April 2004.

In the expanded study (Fierro, 2006), an ethnography and an experiment were conducted. The ethnography included the following:

■ Ethnographic interviews were conducted with 13 program participants to reflect various issues present in the lives of transitional custody mothers; the sample was stratified on age, number of children, reason for loss of custody, marital status, housing status, and employment status.

■ Ethnographic interviews were conducted with four women working in the welfare, child welfare, and legal systems.

■ Participant observations (12 in all) were conducted with single clients.

■ Observations were made of meetings and workshops.

■ Focus groups (21 in all) were conducted.

The experimental data collection included the following:

■ A posttest was administered to a control group (5 people) that experienced workforce skills training in its traditional job-training form.

■ Two experimental groups (25 people) completed a pretest and posttest, and

---

[1]For evaluation purposes, 100 variables were chosen out of the total 330.

[2]Focus groups were conducted with clients enrolled starting in October 2002. For present purposes, however, only 2003–2004 focus groups are taken into account.

experienced the infusion of African American cultural and historical content in the form of workshops and activities in the first 7 weeks of the WtW program.

▨ Surveys (104 in all) were administered after 15 of the activities.

The program lasted 5 years (October 1999–October 2004). The evaluation began in 2001 and ended in 2004. The extended study was completed in 2006. The program and senior social work professor's compensation were funded by the U.S. Department of Labor. The database manager was a full-time Temple University employee. The social scientist's salary was financed by Temple University and the Department of Labor.

Meta-Evaluation

In the expanded study, Fierro made some critical reflections about the evaluation's process and her own expectations. This was what she had expected:

> a) women to experience stigma in the system, as African Americans; b) to see a white system against Black mothers; c) mothers to tell me that Black social workers were better than white ones; d) to not be able to overcome the differences that separated me from the mothers; among age, race, culture and education I thought race was the hardest. (Fierro, 2006, p. 88)

The senior social worker encouraged Fierro to explore, in the expanded study, whether the program and evaluation assumptions were true. The basic assumption—that participants' barriers to employment and to reunification were the same, and that when the latter were overcome the former would be as well—was false. The expanded study also states that the term "noncustodial parents" was and is inappropriate, as this term indicates parents who lose custody to their partners, not to the state. The breadth and depth of the data collected across the evaluation and the expanded study together brought this understanding. The expanded study made use of a new, more appropriate term, "transitional custody parents," for parents who lost custody of their children to the state.

The ethnography showed the depth of the obstacles that a mother had to overcome, both personally and systemically. Many mothers had childhood traumas that were being repeated over time, and were further blocked by their frustrations of dealing with an ineffective, punitive system that lacked transparency. Many futile attempts to gather data from the Pennsylvania Department of Human Services regarding the official reasons children were taken confirmed this. Years of networking experience with the department yielded no results in accessing data. Furthermore, Fierro's combined experience with the infrastructure's representatives and the mothers' personal lives showed the child welfare and welfare systems in deep contrast, with different requirements, but both equally punitive in outlook. Mothers were often caught in the middle. The extended study included an historical analysis that showed the origins of such systems and described how, over time, the child welfare, welfare, and legal systems had reinforced each other in perpetuating institutional racism.

Mothers reported experiencing a sense of empowerment from participating in the

(cont.)

Box 6.7 (cont.)

evaluation, because they had the unique opportunity to share their experiences with other mothers and learn from each other.

Reports and Utilization

Process evaluation findings were shared with administrators and agency representatives at meetings throughout program implementation. In the last program year, the infrastructure committees were asked to report on major policy and programmatic challenges and suggestions in one of five areas: job training, mental health, education, housing, and child care. At the end of the evaluation, the evaluators and representatives from each committee presented results to members of different agencies across the city.

REFLECTIONS FROM THE EVALUATOR

I have presented at a variety of conferences and meetings during and after the evaluation's completion. The results of the extended study have also been submitted for publication. Since 2006, I have also been participating as a parent advocate in an activist grassroots organization that supports parents in overcoming the challenges of the child welfare system and regaining custody of their children. I am contributing to a dossier (report) and a documentary on the topic.

· · · · · · · · · · · E X T E N D I N G   Y O U R   T H I N K I N G · · · · · · · · · · ·

CRT Evaluation

 Social Justice Branch

Sample study	Evaluation approach	List the distinguishing characteristics
Fierro (2006)	Critical race theory (CRT) evaluation	

Using the description of the Fierro (2006) study in Box 6.7, answer the following questions:

1. What are the characteristics that illustrate Fierro's use of the Critical Race Theory Evaluation Model?

2. What do you identify as the strengths and weaknesses of this model in terms of the types of data that were collected by the evaluator?

3. What do you identify as the strengths and weaknesses of the strategies used in this study that were intended to address issues of social justice?

4. What would you suggest modifying in this study to improve the potential for social change based on the process and results of the evaluation?

Indigenous Evaluation

Indigenous peoples are quite diverse—not only in terms of their tribal/ethnic group affiliations, but in many other respects, such as gender, economic status, and disability. The commonality that drives indigenous evaluation approaches is an experience of colonization and oppression by more powerful outsiders. In many cases, this takes the form of denigrating the cultures and traditions of the indigenous peoples. Many indigenous scholars have contributed to evaluation approaches that reclaim indigenous ways. Moewaka Barnes and Te Ropu Whariki (2009) provide guidance for indigenous evaluations based on their work in the Māori community. These authors describe Māori evaluation in terms of its concerns with values and power. "A Māori evaluation is controlled and owned by Māori, meets the community's needs, reflects the culture of the Māori people, questions dominant culture and norms, and aims to make a positive difference" (p. 9). In Māori evaluations, relationships are critically important; this implies the need for trust and a long-standing relationship, as well as a sense of reciprocity. These characteristics are similar when applied to other indigenous approaches to evaluation, with the caveat that each group has important unique characteristics. By way of comparison, consider Bowman's (2005) description of an indigenous approach to evaluation based on her membership in and evaluation work with American Indian communities:

> An Indigenous Self-Determination Evaluation Model respects, recognizes, and values the inherent worth of Indian culture; is responsive to the communities' needs as voiced by all members of the Tribal community; builds evaluation designs and processes around Indian assets and resources; and literally and figuratively employs Indians in every part of the process (program, policy, implementation, evaluation) to heal, strengthen, and preserve Indigenous societies for the next 7 generations.

An example of an indigenous evaluation study is presented in Box 6.8.

Box. 6.8. Sample Indigenous Evaluation Study: The Study of the Mental Health Services in Indian Country

Sample study	Evaluation approach	Document title
Cross, Earle, Echo-Hawk Solie, and Manness (2000)	Indigenous evaluation	"Cultural Strengths and Challenges in Implementing a System of Care Model in American Indian Communities"

(cont.)

Box. 6.8 (cont.)

The Evaluators

Terry Cross is a member of the Seneca Nation, Holly Echo-Hawk Solie is a member of the Pawnee/Otoc Nation, and Kathryn Manness is a member of the Huron Nation. They and Kathleen Earle work for the National Indian Child Welfare Association.

The Evaluand and Its Context

American Indian children face many stresses in life—poverty, unemployment, accidental deaths, domestic violence, alcoholism, child neglect, and suicide—emanating from a historical legacy of discrimination and oppression. Traditional models of mental health care have not been effective in providing appropriate treatment for these children. The Center for Mental Health Services funded five projects based on a culturally appropriate model for members of the American Indian community. The National Indian Child Welfare Association was contracted to conduct an evaluation of these five projects.

Philosophical and Theoretical Lenses

The evaluators describe their approach as using a relational model based on the American Indian medicine wheel. The medicine wheel is divided into four quadrants that represent the balance among context (culture, community, family, peers, work, school, and social history), mind (cognitive processes such as thoughts, memories, knowledge, and emotions), body (physical aspects such as genetics, gender, fitness, sleep, nutrition, and substance use), and spirit (spiritual practices/teachings, dreams, symbols, positive–negative forces, intuition). Cross et al. used these four quadrants to design an indigenous evaluation strategy.

The evaluators established their credibility by means of their American Indian heritage, as well as by respectfully entering the communities through hosting social events to introduce themselves and the evaluation to the communities. They invited the parents and children to a luncheon and gave an additional $35 honorarium to those who participated in the focus groups.

Method

Design

The relational model involved the use of the medicine wheel quadrants to guide the decisions about data collection.

Evaluation Purposes and Questions

The evaluation questions centered on the balance achieved in the four quadrants as a result of participating in the programs. The context quadrant included questions such as this (all questions are from Cross et al., 2000, p. 104). "How does your program draw upon extended relationships to help parents help their children?" A sample mind question was this: "How has the program helped you develop strategies that use Indian ways for addressing the needs of your child?" The body quadrant contained questions related to the importance of medical wellness as part of mental or emotional wellness, as well as the role of exercise, nutrition, sleep, and avoidance of alcohol, tobacco, or other drugs. A sample context question was this: "Have you or your child participated in any cultural activities to improve physical health, e.g., special tribal celebrations with food served to mark the occasion?" Spirit, the final quadrant, explored the blending of Christianity with American Indian traditions, as well as adaptations of Christian practices and participation in traditional American Indian spiritual revitalization. A sample spirit question was this: "Have you or your family participated in any rituals or ceremonies to help restore balance to your lives?"

Stakeholders and Participants

The stakeholders included parents, children, service providers, community members, and staff from all five programs. The key informants included medicine people, elders, and other important community members.

Data Collection

The data collection was accomplished by the use of focus groups and key informant interviews. The questions were matched to the four medicine wheel quadrants (see above).

Management and Budget

The sites were asked to schedule two or more group meetings that would allow 2–3 hours of time together over a period of 1–3 days. The focus groups and individual interviews included up to six separate interviews, which included a campout with staff, parents, children, and spiritual leaders. All scheduling was done at the convenience of the service providers and families. The evaluators were paid by a grant; however, the budget amount was not mentioned.

Meta-Evaluation

The evaluation identified a number of important themes, such as the importance of responding to the posttraumatic stress that is prevalent in Indian families, due to historical oppression and multigenerational traumas associated with alcoholism or relocation. Tribes also have many strengths that can be brought into the provision of mental health services, such as crafts, ceremonies, sweat lodges, and use of indigenous languages. The evaluators felt affirmation that what they were doing was effective.

Reports and Utilization

The evaluation data were shared with representatives from each site to determine their accuracy and appropriateness. The evaluators compiled a description of each of the five projects. The evaluators were able to identify a number of promising practices for the provision of effective mental health services for Indian children, including involvement of extended family and use of traditional teachings. The results were reported within the framework of the four medicine wheel quadrants. The evaluation report also highlighted the need to identify additional resources to support this approach to mental health services, because it is time-intensive and the need is great.

Indigenous Evaluation

 Social Justice Branch

Sample study	Evaluation approach	List the distinguishing characteristics
Cross, Earle, Echo-Hawk Solie, and Manness (2000)	Indigenous evaluation	

Using the description of the Cross et al. study in Box 6.8, answer the following questions:

1. What are the characteristics that illustrate Cross et al.'s use of the Indigenous Evaluation Model?

2. What do you identify as the strengths and weaknesses of this model in terms of the types of data that were collected by the evaluator?

3. What do you identify as the strengths and weaknesses of the strategies used in this study that were intended to address issues of social justice?

4. What would you suggest modifying in this study to improve the potential for social change based on the process and results of the evaluation?

Culturally Responsive Evaluation

Johnson (2006) has outlined the unique characteristics associated with a culturally responsive evaluation. One of the first steps is to determine the appropriate focus for the evaluation. In culturally responsive evaluation, the focus is determined with a conscious awareness of various dimensions of diversity (such as race/ethnicity, income, and language). Staff and evaluators are selected whose backgrounds and expertise match the relevant dimensions of diversity. The step in the evaluation in which the evaluand is defined is informed by input from the program management, staff, and participants. A specific effort is made to make explicit the assumptions underlying the evaluand. Possible interpretations and ways to establish validity of results are proactively discussed, along with how the interpretations will occur and how they will be shaped to be responsive to the needs of the community. Data collection tools and strategies are adapted to be suitable to the community, making whatever accommodations are necessary (for language, format, etc.). Data analysis involves the following principles: sensitivity to and understanding of the cultural context, use of appropriate disaggregation, discussion of possible interpretations with program management, and again making the assumptions explicit. Reports in culturally responsive evaluations include a description of contextual and cultural factors, methodological accommodations, alternative interpretations along with supportive evidence, and descriptions of how data can be used for continuous program improvement. Box 6.9 (pp. 202–204) summarizes a study using culturally responsive evaluation.

· · · · · · · · · · · **EXTENDING YOUR THINKING** · · · · · · · · · · ·

Culturally Responsive Evaluation

 Social Justice Branch

Sample study	Evaluation approach	List the distinguishing characteristics
Zulli and Frierson (2004)	Culturally responsive evaluation	

Using the description of the Zulli and Frierson (2004) study in Box 6.9, answer the following questions:

1. What are the characteristics that illustrate Zulli and Frierson's use of the Culturally Responsive Evaluation Model?

2. What do you identify as the strengths and weaknesses of this model in terms of the types of data that were collected by the evaluator?

3. What do you identify as the strengths and weaknesses of the strategies used in this study that were intended to address issues of social justice?

4. What would you suggest modifying in this study to improve the potential for social change based on the process and results of the evaluation?

Disability- and Deaf-Rights-Based Evaluation

As noted previously, diversity within disability communities (and the deaf community, which does not view itself as "disabled") is of paramount concern in evaluations that are designed to address issues of social justice. The evaluator needs to be aware not only of those dimensions associated with different types of disability, but also of characteristics such as language use, gender, and others that are contextually relevant. Appropriate accommodations are needed to ensure that stakeholder participation is supported. Mertens, Harris, Holmes, and Brandt (2007) conducted an evaluation of a master's degree program in one university to prepare teachers who are deaf or hard of hearing and/or from ethnic/racial minority groups to teach children who are deaf and who have an additional disability. Box 6.10 (pp. 204–207) describes this study.

Box 6.9. Sample Culturally Responsive Evaluation Study: The Upward Bound Study

Sample study		Evaluation approach	Document title
Zulli and Frierson (2004)		Culturally responsive evaluation	"Evaluating an Upward Bound Program"

The Evaluators

At the time of the study, Rebecca A. Zulli was a senior research associate at the North Carolina Education Research Council, with responsibility for oversight of the development and production of the annual First in America Report Card. Henry T. Frierson was Professor in the Division of Educational Psychology, Measurement, and Evaluation in the School of Education at the University of North Carolina (UNC) at Chapel Hill, and was also Director of the Research Education Support Program. He is now Associate Vice President and Dean of the Graduate School at the University of Florida. Both evaluators are African Americans.

Philosophical and Theoretical Lenses

The evaluators situated their work within the culturally responsive evaluation stance, as it is explicated by Frierson, Hood and Hughes (2002, p. 63): "Culturally responsive evaluators honor the cultural context in which an evaluation takes place by bringing needed, shared life experience, and understandings to the evaluation tasks at hand." The evaluators saw their role as "to actively respond to and investigate the potential impacts of cultural responsiveness and cultural competence on the program" (Frierson et al., 2002, p. 83).

The Evaluand and Its Context

Upward Bound is a federally funded initiative designed to improve participation in postsecondary education for students from economically and educationally deprived backgrounds. The specific focus of this evaluation was the Upward Bound program implemented at UNC Chapel Hill.

Method

Design

A transformative culturally responsive design was used for this study. Decisions about how to proceed and what was important emanated from the theoretical stance of the evaluators in concert with discussions with stakeholders. The evaluators used a cyclical design, which allowed them to modify their procedures based on evidence collected in earlier stages of the project.

Evaluation Purpose and Questions

The purpose of the evaluation was to examine the program's merit and worth (i.e., the value of having the program and the extent to which it was accomplishing the goals for the program). In addition, the evaluators focused on the identification of program characteristics to which its success could be ascribed, including cultural factors. For example, how did shared characteristics for the program staff and participants influence the success of the program?

Stakeholders and Participants

Program staff and program participants were viewed as the primary stakeholders. Program alumni and parents of students in the program were also included.

Data Collection

The evaluators conducted semistructured interviews with program staff members to determine their perceptions of the program, their own life experiences, and similarities between themselves and the program participants. Focus groups were also conducted with program staff, participants, parents, and program alumni; data from these sources were used to design questionnaires that were distributed to larger samples of participants and parents. In addition, 64 individual interviews were conducted with participants over a 3-year period to determine changes over time in their academic success and their perceptions of the program's contribution to that success. Data analysis consisted of searching for patterns in the data that reflected factors related to participants' success, as well as aspects of cultural responsiveness that were part of that process.

Management and Budget

The evaluation occurred over a 3-year period. The budget for the evaluation consisted of funds from the federal government grant that supported the implementation of the Upward Bound program at UNC Chapel Hill.

Reports and Utilization

The evaluators conducted data analysis throughout the period of the evaluation; hence they were able to use preliminary findings to modify the scope of the evaluation as appropriate. For example, their early analysis revealed the important contribution of instilling motivation for success to predicting capacity to succeed in postsecondary education. The evaluators used this finding to justify emphasizing the collection of more in-depth data in later stages of the study about the role of motivation and how cultural responsiveness contributed to increased motivation.

The evaluators made a full effort to capture the essence of the Upward Bound program, so that the value and worth of the program could be determined by the participants, their parents, and the key decision makers, and so that the information from the evaluation could be presented to society in general.

Meta-Evaluation

The evaluators shared their interpretations of the data with the program stakeholders, in order to increase their confidence that they had correctly understood the cultural context of the program and appropriately interpreted the experiences of the staff and participants.

Box 6.9 *(cont.)*

REFLECTIONS FROM THE EVALUATORS

In keeping with a culturally responsive approach, the initial primary challenge was gaining the trust of the key stakeholders, including the participants and their parents, to ensure them that we wanted to gain accurate data and provide information that accurately reflected the program. When we were collecting qualitative data in particular, we constantly communicated with participants in the study to ensure that our interpretations of the data were accurate. The notion was promoted that the evaluation was conducted for the stakeholders, particularly those who had to make decisions regarding the program. Further, those individuals were informed that it was important to provide us with evaluation questions that they actually wanted answered. Communication was critical in this process.

Box 6.10. Sample Disability- and Deaf-Rights-Based Evaluation: The Study of Teacher Preparation in Deaf Education at Gallaudet University

Sample study	Evaluation approach	Document title
Mertens, Harris, Holmes, and Brandt (2007)	Disability- and deaf-rights-based evaluation	*Project SUCCESS Summative Evaluation Report*

The Evaluators

Donna M. Mertens is a hearing professor of research and evaluation, with many years of experience evaluating programs in the deaf community. Heidi Holmes and Raychelle Harris are PhD students who are both deaf; they use American Sign Language and consider themselves to be culturally deaf. Susan Brandt is a deaf PhD student who has a cochlear implant, which allows her to speak and hear in most situations.

Philosophical and Theoretical Lenses

A transformative deaf rights approach was used to inform the development of the evaluation. This meant having an awareness of the relevant dimensions of diversity that are associated with differences in power and access to resources and opportunities in the deaf and hard-of-hearing communities.

The role of the evaluation within this framework was to document the project's accomplishments and raise questions surrounding mechanisms for meaningfully involving diverse groups in the process of constructing an understanding of what happened and possibilities for future options. To this end, the evaluators needed to ensure that the evaluation team was representative of the intended stakeholder groups and that effective communication in the first language of the stakeholders could occur.

The Evaluand and Its Context

Gallaudet University's Department of Education received a 7-year grant from the U.S. Department of Education to develop and implement a teacher preparation program that was designed (1) to increase diversity in the teacher candidate pool and (2) to prepare teachers who had expertise with students who are deaf and have a disability. (Again, recall that culturally deaf people do not consider themselves to be disabled.) The program was to emphasize the active recruitment and mentoring of graduate students who were deaf/hard of hearing and/or were from underrepresented groups. Ten students were to be recruited each year. Technology, collaborative skills, assessment, action research, and parent consultation skills were to be stressed throughout the program. High expectations and standards for future teachers and the children they would teach were to be promoted and modeled through a commitment to excellence and innovation. Mentoring and a summer seminar for graduates of this innovative program were to be provided in the year beyond graduation, to increase the retention of beginning teachers.

Method

Design

The evaluators used a transformative cyclical mixed methods design that allowed for early data collection results to inform each subsequent step in the process.

Evaluation Purposes and Questions

The project director asked for a summative evaluation that would satisfy funding requirements. The evaluation team negotiated to expand this purpose to include informing the university and the broader teacher preparation community on issues of discrimination and oppression that needed to be made explicit to prepare teachers effectively for the target population. Sample evaluation questions included the following:

- How effective were the recruitment strategies?
- How effective were the support services?
- How effective were the course offerings?
- How effective were the field-based experiences?
- How well prepared were the graduates to teach the deaf and hard-of-hearing students with a disability?

Stakeholders and Participants

In addition to the funding agency, the stakeholders included the faculty and administrators at the university who were responsible for teacher preparation programs; staff at cooperating schools where the teacher candidates did their field placements; the teacher candidates over the 7-year period; and the students these teachers taught.

Data Collection

The evaluation team developed a work plan for the evaluation that included a listing of the evaluation questions and data collection strategies associated with each question. Data

(cont.)

Box 6.10 (cont.)

collection began with document review of the request for a proposal, the proposal that was submitted to the U.S. Department of Education, and the 6 years of annual reports that the project filed with the funding agency. An evaluation team was then developed that included the hearing professor, two culturally deaf American Sign Language users, and the deaf cochlear implant user. This team discussed the focus of the evaluation and shared it with the project director and other stakeholders. The methodology was outlined to include a 2-day period of observation during a 3-day reflective seminar held for all program graduates. Based on the observation, the evaluators created interview questions that they used on the third day to investigate relevant points. The hearing evaluator (Mertens) and the cochlear implant user (Brandt) interviewed the hearing and hard-of-hearing graduates; the two culturally deaf evaluators (Holmes and Harris) interviewed the deaf participants who used American Sign Language. The results of these interviews were used for two purposes: to investigate the successes and challenges of the graduates in depth, and to develop an online survey that was sent to all the graduates who were not able to attend the seminar. The results of the observations, interviews, and survey were used as a basis for interviewing the university faculty and the staff from the cooperating schools. The final report reflected all the data collection sources.

Management and Budget

Mertens assembled a team of evaluators. The evaluation team members reviewed the documents and conducted the observations. They met at the end of each day to determine subsequent actions. The interviews of reflective seminar participants were as described above. One of the graduate students took primary responsibility for the Web-based survey. The team worked together to analyze the qualitative and quantitative data. Mertens conducted the interviews with the university faculty and the cooperating school staff members. The team members wrote the report together and made presentations at professional conferences for teacher preparation programs in the United States and Canada. The evaluation budget was $5,000.

Meta-Evaluation

The evaluation was assessed according to the major categories for quality in educational evaluations: utility, feasibility, accuracy, and propriety. The evaluation findings were used throughout the project, as well as at the conclusion of the formal evaluation. The methods for data collection were intertwined with previously scheduled events for program graduates. The accuracy of the findings is supported by the overlap among findings from different sources. The evaluators prepared a proposal that was approved by the Gallaudet University Institutional Review Board at each stage of data collection. In addition, cultural issues for effective communication were addressed by the composition of the evaluation team.

Reports and Utilization

As noted in the "Method" section, this was a cyclical evaluation design, in which each data collection moment was used to inform subsequent steps in the evaluation process. The reading of the documents led to an awareness of the intended purposes of the project and potential areas of challenge. The observations led to the development of the interview questions. The documents, observations, and interviews were used to develop the online survey. The results of these prior data collections and analyses were used to formulate interview questions for the staff and faculty. The findings of the overall study were used to inform the faculty and staff about strengths and ongoing concerns related to the preparation of teachers for students who are deaf or hard of hearing and who have a disability. The university education department recognized that its graduates needed continuing support in order to address the complex challenges that they encountered in their classrooms. The department set up an online mentoring system that originally was accessible only to students in the multiple-disabilities program. However, graduates of other programs in the department asked whether they could be included in the online mentoring system. All these new graduates thus have access to the experiences of other new graduates, early career teachers, and the university faculty.

· · · · · · · · · · · E X T E N D I N G   Y O U R   T H I N K I N G · · · · · · · · · ·

Disability– and Deaf–Rights–Based Evaluation

 Social Justice Branch

Sample study	Evaluation approach	List the distinguishing characteristics
Mertens, Harris, Holmes, and Brandt (2007)	Disability- and deaf-rights-based evaluation	

Using the description of the Mertens (2007) study in Box 6.10, answer the following questions:

1. What are the characteristics that illustrate Mertens et al.'s use of the Disability and Deafness Rights Evaluation Model?

2. What do you identify as the strengths and weaknesses of this model in terms of the types of data that were collected by the evaluator?

3. What do you identify as the strengths and weaknesses of the strategies used in this study that were intended to address issues of social justice?

4. What would you suggest modifying in this study to improve the potential for social change based on the process and results of the evaluation?

Feminist Evaluation

Sielbeck-Bowen et al. (2002; cited in Mertens, 2009, p. 64) have presented the following principles of feminist evaluation as they are derived from Western research literature:

1. The central focus is on gender inequities that lead to social injustice; every evaluation should be conducted with an eye toward reversing gender inequities.

2. Discrimination or inequality based on gender is systemic and structural.

3. Evaluation is a political activity; the contexts in which evaluations operate are politicized, and the personal experiences, perspectives, and characteristics evaluators bring to evaluations lead to a particular political stance.

4. The evaluation process can lead to significant negative or positive effects on the people involved in the evaluation.

5. The evaluator must recognize and explore the unique conditions and characteristics of the issue under study; critical self-reflection is necessary.

6. There are multiple ways of knowing; some ways are privileged over others.

7. Transformative knowledge that emanates from an experiential base is valued.

Box 6.11 describes a study that used feminist evaluation.

Box 6.11. Sample Feminist Evaluation Study: The Study of School-Based Health Issues in Australia, the United States, and Canada

Sample study	Evaluation approach	Document title
Seigart (2007)	Feminist evaluation	"Gender and Healthcare: Why Australian Men Can't Get Vasectomies"

The Evaluator

Denise Seigart is a faculty member in the department of health sciences at Mansfield University in Mansfield, Pennsylvania.

Philosophical and Theoretical Lenses

Seigart identifies herself as a feminist and states that she brings a feminist lens to her evaluation work.

The Evaluand and Its Context

Seigart undertook a multiyear evaluation of school-based health care programs in the United States, Canada, and Australia. (This summary focuses primarily on her work in Australia.) A feminist evaluator is cognizant of inequities on the basis of gender, as well as race, class, religion, economics, and culture.

Method

Design

Seigart used a qualitative case study design to collect information about school-based health care in the United States, Australia, and Canada.

Evaluation Purposes and Questions

The purpose of the evaluation was to provide information about the health care needs of children, barriers to provision of health care through schools, and variables that influence the provision of health care in school settings. Seigart (2007) explained that during the course of the research, gender inequities in access to health care were uncovered, along with the impact of tying health care to employment "on women and children, and the valuing (or devaluing) of women's work with regard to the provision of health care for children in schools" (p. 1).

Stakeholders and Participants

The stakeholders for the Australian portion of the study included the Australian Medical Association, nursing faculty, community/school nurses, teachers, school administrators, community leaders, parents, and family members, as well as health agency and school staff in southeastern Australia.

Data Collection

Seigart used three data collection methods: document review, observation, and interviews. She interviewed representatives of all the stakeholder groups except physicians. She completed a document review revealing that physicians in Australia favored limiting the practice of nurse practitioners and midwives. This position was substantiated through data collected in interviews with midwives. She observed in hospitals, community health agencies, and schools. Her questions focused on the health needs of children, barriers to care, and cultural differences in the approaches to providing care. She also identified issues such as the territorialism of the Australian Medical Association, which denies nurse practitioners and midwives the right to practice in certain areas. In addition, the Catholic Church impinges on the provision of health care services in some areas by limiting the content of sex education in the schools, limiting access to birth control and condoms (particularly for adolescents), and influencing access to abortions or vasectomies by denying these services in its health care facilities (thus effectively denying these services to entire communities in some areas).

Management and Budget

The evaluation took place during the fall semester, in which Seigart lived in a rural community in southeastern Australia and traveled to other areas in this part of the country. The research in Australia was funded by a Visiting Professor Fellowship awarded by Charles Sturt University and a sabbatical award made by Mansfield University.

(cont.)

Box 6.11 (cont.)

Meta-Evaluation

Seigart analyzed her evaluation according to the feminist principles for evaluation, as well as the criteria for credibility for qualitative research. She also shared all data with her Australian and Canadian faculty colleagues, and sought their feedback and reflections.

Reports and Utilization

While in Australia, Seigart analyzed her results by utilizing a grounded theory approach, analytic memos, and the principles of feminist evaluation. She also sought out the reflections of an Australian colleague who likewise utilizes a feminist research approach. In addition, she shared the preliminary results with nursing faculty in Australia during a presentation and sought feedback from the group at that time. She prepared a presentation for the annual meeting of the AEA, following continued research on this topic in Canada.

As noted in Box 6.11, Seigart's (2007) evaluation uncovered inequities on the basis of gender, racism, and classism. The evaluator was sensitive to these systemic inequities because of her feminist identification. For example, she noted that one Australian school principal said there was no need to have a school health program; the reason given was that the Aboriginal people preferred to go to the emergency room for their health issues, because it was air-conditioned and had a television. Other individuals, including health care workers, also expressed this opinion. Classism was noted as well: Those with only public health insurance were often required to wait long periods of time to receive care, particularly for nonemergency services (speech therapy, hip replacements, etc.). Those who could purchase private insurance had no such wait. The politics of the study were palpable, in that several health care agencies and schools denied Seigart access to conduct interviews at their locations without completing a lengthy ethics review at each site where she desired to interview nurses or teachers. She had already completed and passed two ethics reviews at two universities, but these approvals were not necessarily considered adequate by some health care agencies or schools. Seigart addressed this barrier by using informed consent forms with individuals outside their work settings and using the "snowball" method of sampling (see Chapter 11). That is, she asked her respondents to nominate other persons she could approach for an interview. The knowledge created by her evaluation has the potential to stimulate change in the provision of school health care in the Australian setting.

Gender analysis is an approach that is used to uncover inequities based on gender. It is commonly used in international development evaluations; it is discussed further in Chapters 8, 9, and 10.

Feminist Evaluation

 Social Justice Branch

Sample study	Evaluation approach	List the distinguishing characteristics
Seigart (2007)	Feminist evaluation	

Using the description of the Seigart (2007) study in Box 6.11, answer the following questions:

1. What are the characteristics that illustrate Seigart's use of the Feminist Evaluation Model?

2. What do you identify as the strengths and weaknesses of this model in terms of the types of data that were collected by the evaluator?

3. What do you identify as the strengths and weaknesses of the strategies used in this study that were intended to address issues of social justice?

4. What would you suggest modifying in this study to improve the potential for social change based on the process and results of the evaluation?

Transformative Participatory Evaluation

Transformative participatory approaches to evaluation are similar to practical participatory approaches; however, the former are conducted with the intent to stimulate action that is directly related to the furtherance of social justice. In such an evaluation, the evaluator seeks to include people who are marginalized, in order to address the power inequities that serve to block their achieving this goal. The Infant Feeding Research Project (IFRP) used outcome mapping in its second phase as a planning, monitoring, and evaluation tool (see Chapter 7). The purpose of the IFRP was to contribute to the decrease of pediatric HIV/AIDS in southern Africa by enhancing the effectiveness of infant feeding counseling through the design of an alternative counseling format, as described in Box 6.12.

Nurturing the relationships needed to implement transformative participatory evaluation takes additional time and resources. Evaluators need to be able to stay flexible and responsive, so that the desired changes in the program come from the participants. Capacity building in the use of transformative participatory methods (and concept mapping) is needed, so that the stakeholders are able to understand the process and buy into it. This approach can then be used to influence policy changes that may be needed to bring about the desired outcomes. Buskens and Earl (2008) built the capacity of the

Box 6.12. Sample Transformative Study: The African Study of Breast Feeding to Prevent HIV/AIDS

Sample study		Evaluation approach	Document title
Buskens and Earl (2008)		Transformative participatory evaluation	"Research for Change: Outcome Mapping's Contribution to Emancipatory Action Research in Africa"

The Evaluators

Ineke Buskens is a cultural anthropologist who has lived in the Republic of South Africa for over two decades. Sarah Earl is a senior program specialist with the International Development Research Centre in Ottawa, Canada. She specializes in international development that engages social activism with international development. Outcome mapping was used by the IFRP team members who participated in the second phase, in which the counseling format was implemented.

Philosophical and Theoretical Lenses

"In an international development context, action researchers seek to improve the lives of marginalized people both through the process of enquiry as well as through the practical application of the research findings" (Buskens & Earl, 2008, p. 173). Sixteen researchers participated in the first phase of the research, which was an ethnographic exploratory study. Four of these 16 researchers continued in the second phase, which was an action research phase where the intervention (the counseling format) was tested. Outcome mapping was used by the four action researchers and the coordinating team members to keep their action research process "on track." The research process involved the research team members and the counselors on a very deep personal level; change and personal transformation were on the agenda for everybody involved.

The Evaluation and Its Context

The IFRP was designed to reduce the transmission of HIV/AIDS from mother to child though a counseling program with mothers in Namibia, the Republic of South Africa, and Swaziland. The norm in the region is for mothers to combine formula and breast feeding; however, this approach is associated with the highest transmission rates from mother to child. "Evidence suggests that in exclusive breast feeding the virus is digested like all other protein, with minimal risk of transmission" (Buskens & Earl, 2008, p. 177). The evaluation was implemented at 11 sites.

Method

Design

The research was conducted in two phases, as noted above. The first phase was an ethnographic study that lasted for a year and was designed to show how the mothers and infants participated in the program. The results of the first phase indicated that the counseling was not effective, and that the relationship between counselors and mothers was so troubled that mere enhancement of the counseling by sensitizing the counselors to the mothers' perspectives and realities would not have the desired effect either. Hence a counseling format was designed that was grounded in a different counseling technique (brief motivational interviewing instead of Rogerian counseling) and in a perspective of "woman-centeredness" (which would stimulate the counselors to take responsibility for the intragender dynamics that would play a role in their relationship with the mothers). This new training program was provided to the counselors. In this phase of the research project, outcome mapping was used.

Evaluation Purposes and Questions

The research question of the second phase was this: "How can counselors be prepared effectively for their task?" (Buskens & Earl, 2008, p. 179).

Stakeholders and Participants

The stakeholders included the counselors, the researchers (who also acted as trainers of the counselors), the mothers and their children, and the personnel at the clinics in which the counseling took place.

Data Collection

The outcome mapping was conducted constantly throughout the process of the second phase. Outcome mapping is an evaluation tool developed by Canada's International Development and Research Centre. It is used for strategic planning and evaluation to help plan and assess the influence of the evaluative process and its findings by identifying the linkages between interventions and desired changes in behavior. (This strategy is discussed in greater detail in Chapter 7.) Through this process, the counselors were invited to reflect on their own learning process and give their perspectives on the counseling and counseling-training experience. The first phase of the research project was conducted during a 1-year period. The time period for the second phase of the evaluation was not explicitly stated.

Meta-Evaluation

The decision to "scale up" the project to additional locations was accepted as evidence of the quality of the evaluation work.

Reports and Utilization

The findings from the first phase revealed that the counseling program was not effective. These findings were used to revise the training program for the counselors. The constant use of the outcome mapping allowed the evaluation findings to be used to make changes as necessary throughout the second phase. The results were also used as a justification for expanding certain elements of the program to other HIV counseling programs in other countries in southern Africa.

(cont.)

Box 6.12 (*cont.*)

REFLECTIONS FROM THE EVALUATORS

Outcome mapping was a tool that allowed the evaluation team to use their time with stakeholders efficiently and effectively. The project manager's major responsibility was to clearly allocate tasks and to facilitate open communication. Outcome mapping facilitates learning across sites, because the experiences of each site are shared in a similar format. A close partnership between the funder and the evaluators is an important component in enhancing the use of the findings. The evaluators need to make clear that the power to influence the project is shared with the other stakeholders.

counselors and mothers by training them in the use of outcome mapping as a tool for assessing their progress toward achieving their goal of encouraging breast feeding as a means to reduce HIV/AIDS transmission. The results of their study were used to justify a policy change by the World Health Organization (WHO, 2010). The WHO revised its 2006 guidelines for HIV-positive mothers and breast feeding to recommend that these mothers be provided with antiretroviral drugs (AVRs) in their 9 months of pregnancy and 5 months after giving birth. Also, mothers should be encouraged to breast-feed their babies exclusively for the first 12 months of life. The United Nations also reported that use of AVRs at this early stage and exclusive breast feeding are yielding positive results in preventing mother-to-child transmission (Joint United Nations Programme on HIV/AIDS [UNAID], 2009).

· · · · · · · · · · E X T E N D I N G   Y O U R   T H I N K I N G · · · · · · · · · ·
Transformative Participatory Evaluation

 Social Justice Branch

Sample study		Evaluation approach	List the distinguishing characteristics
Buskens and Earl (2008)		Transformative participatory evaluation	

Using the description of the Buskens and Earl (2008) study in Box 6.12, answer the following questions:

1. What are the characteristics that illustrate Buskens and Earl's use of the Transformative Participatory Evaluation Model?

2. What do you identify as the strengths and weaknesses of this model in terms of the types of data that were collected by the evaluators?

3. What do you identify as the strengths and weaknesses of the strategies used in this study that were intended to address issues of social justice?

4. What would you suggest modifying in this study to improve the potential for social change based on the process and results of the evaluation?

- - - - - - - - - - **EXTENDING YOUR THINKING** - - - - - - - - - -
The Social Justice Branch in Evaluation

1. Obtain any of the following resources, read them, and discuss how they illustrate the Social Justice Branch in evaluation.

Cousins, J. B., & Whitmore, E. (1998). Framing participatory evaluation. *New Directions for Evaluation, 80,* 5–23.

Fetterman, D. (2001). *Foundations of empowerment evaluation.* Thousand Oaks, CA: Sage.

Furrobo, J.-E., Rist, R., & Sandahl, R. (Eds.). (2002). *International atlas of evaluation.* New Brunswick, NJ: Transaction.

Hanberger, A. (2001). Policy and program evaluation, civil society, and democracy. *American Journal of Evaluation, 22*(2), 211–228.

House, E. R., & Howe, K. R. (1999) *Values in evaluation and social research.* Thousand Oaks, CA: Sage.

Karlsson, O. (1996). A critical dialogue in evaluation: How can interaction between evaluation and politics be tackled? *Evaluation, 2,* 405–416.

King, J. A. (1998). Making sense of participatory evaluation. *New Directions for Evaluation, 80,* 57–67.

Kushner, S. (2000). *Personalizing evaluation.* London: Sage.

MacDonald, B., & Kushner, S. (2005). Democratic evaluation. In S. Mathison (Ed.), *Encyclopedia of evaluation* (pp. 109–113). Thousand Oaks, CA: Sage.

Mark, M. M., Henry, G. T., & Julnes, G. (2000). *Evaluation.* San Francisco: Jossey-Bass.

Murray, R. (2002). Citizens' control of evaluations. *Evaluation, 8*(1), 81–100.

Patton, M. Q. (2002). A vision of evaluation that strengthens democracy. *Evaluation, 8*(1), 125–139.

Ryan, K. E., & DeStefano, L. (Eds.). (2000). Evaluation as a democratic process: Promoting inclusion, dialogue, and deliberation. *New Directions for Evaluation, 85.*

Simons, H. (1987). *Getting to know schools in a democracy.* London: Falmer.

2. As an evaluator, would you be willing to be a supportive, reflective activist in the community who challenges the prevailing research and evaluation establishment?

Your Evaluation Plan: Your Philosophical Stance

Begin writing your understandings of the transformative paradigm and the Social Justice Branch as a way of clarifying your own thinking about your philosophical beliefs and how they might influence the way you conduct an evaluation. This can become part of your evaluation plan later, when you decide which approach you will use.

*   *   *

Remember the studies below, as we refer to them again in later chapters.

Social Justice Branch

Sample study		Evaluation approach	Topical area
House (2004)	HOLA!·HI! COLORADO	Deliberative democratic evaluation (DDE)	Denver bilingual program
Pennarz, Holicek, Rasidagic, and Rogers (2007)		Country-led evaluation (CLE)	Bosnia-Herzegovina poverty reduction study
Fierro (2006)		Critical race theory (CRT) evaluation	Welfare-to-work program in Philadelphia
Cross, Earle, Echo-Hawk Solie, and Manness (2000)		Indigenous evaluation	Mental health services in Indian country
Zulli and Frierson (2004)		Culturally responsive evaluation	Upward Bound program in North Carolina
Mertens, Harris, Holmes, and Brandt (2007)		Disability- and deaf-rights-based evaluation	Teacher preparation in deaf education at Gallaudet University
Seigart (2007)		Feminist evaluation	School health issues in Australia, the United States, and Canada
Buskens and Earl (2008)		Transformative participatory evaluation	Breast feeding to prevent HIV/AIDS in infants in Africa

In Part III

Social Justice Branch evaluators may place themselves within one particular theoretical perspective, such as feminist or CRT; however, they also need to be cognizant of the many dimensions of diversity that influence the evaluation context. Bledsoe and Graham (2005), using multiple theoretical perspectives and approaches, evaluated an early literacy program for African American families living in poverty. They discuss the use of the inclusive evaluation approach (Mertens, 2003) in order to include traditionally powerful stakeholders such as funders, administrators, and staff, as well as to provide accurate and credible representation to those whose voices have been traditionally excluded from or misrepresented in the evaluation process. In their evaluation, this meant doing a careful demographic study of the full range of diversity in the community; this study allowed them to recognize that in addition to the African American and Latina/Latino populations (which made up roughly 80% of the community), the other 20% were immigrants from various countries in Latin America, the Caribbean, and Eastern Europe. The evaluators brought this information into their discussions with the staff members as a means to keep issues of culture and power differentials at the forefront of the evaluation process. Bledsoe and Graham (2005) also used several evaluation approaches in this study that have been discussed in previous chapters: theory-driven approaches (including logic modeling), empowerment evaluation, and UFE. Acknowledging the permeable borders in the evaluation landscape is a good segue into Part III of this book, "Planning Evaluations."

Notes

1. Recall that Denzin and Lincoln (2005) labeled two separate paradigms "critical theory" and "participatory theory." As explained earlier, we reject this labeling in order to maintain consistency in the levels of abstraction from paradigm to theory to approach.

2. Compatible ideas have been advanced by MacDonald (MacDonald & Kushner, 2005), Simons (1987), and Kushner (2000) (Barry MacDonald was the first to develop a concept of democratic evaluation back in the 1970s); by Karlsson (1996, 2003), Segerholm (2003), and Hanberger (2001); and by Krogstrup (2003) in Denmark. The Scandinavians have carried democratic ideas farther than anyone. In Australia, Savaya, Elsworth, and Rogers (2009) have introduced such ideas into their work.

PLANNING EVALUATIONS

Part III of this book provides details for planning evaluations. It takes into consideration unique aspects of evaluation, as well as those parts of evaluation planning that overlap with applied research methods. It begins with strategies for determining what is being evaluated (the evaluand) and identifying contextual variables of relevance for the study. In order to know what is to be evaluated, the evaluators need to have interactions with a preliminary group of stakeholders, so implicit in this first step is identification of stakeholders who are in a position to contribute to this part of the planning process.

The path for planning an evaluation is not linear; however, there is a logical flow to the steps, even while the steps are revisited as you progress through the planning process. Three examples from evaluation studies illustrate this point.

- *Example 1: Emerging list of stakeholders.* The evaluator needs to identify stakeholders with whom to begin the process of planning. However, the planning process will probably lead to the identification of additional stakeholders who need to be involved in the evaluation.

- *Example 2: Planning for use at the beginning of the evaluation.* A naïve evaluator might think that use is a topic addressed when the evaluation is over. However, Patton's (2008) work on utilization affirms that use needs to be considered from the very beginning of an evaluation. Therefore, the topic of use is included in every chapter, because this is an integral concept throughout the planning and implementation of an evaluation.

- *Example 3: Meta-evaluation.* The study of the quality of the evaluation might also be assumed to occur at the end of the evaluation; however, Hedler and Gibram (2009) suggest that meta-evaluation needs to occur throughout the process of the evaluation, from beginning to end.

In Part III, you will move from understanding what is to be evaluated and its context, to determining the purpose of the evaluation, appropriate questions, further identification of stakeholders, and planning for use and meta-evaluation. You will then be ready to make use of applied social science strategies, such as planning the design of the evaluation, identifying participants and sampling strategies, selecting or developing data collection instruments and procedures, and analyzing the data and disseminating the findings. It should be noted that in Part III, these topics are discussed in the specific context of evaluation. In addition, issues of culture are highlighted throughout, because these have surfaced as critical concerns in terms of validity and ethics in evaluation. Practical guidance is provided that will allow you to plan an evaluation of an evaluand of your choice. Specific web-based resources are also provided to enhance your abilities to plan these aspects of the evaluation.

Part III consists of these chapters:

■ Chapter 7. Working with Stakeholders: Establishing the Context and the Evaluand
  • Identifying Stakeholders
  • Human Relations
  • Interacting with Stakeholders
  • Developing Partnerships/Relationships
  • The Evaluand and Its Context
  • Sources That Inform the Identification of the Evaluand and Context
  • Depicting the Evaluand
  • Planning Your Evaluation: Stakeholders, Context, and Evaluand

■ Chapter 8. Evaluation Purposes, Types, and Questions
  • Purposes and Types of Evaluation
  • Multipurpose Evaluations
  • Purpose: To Gain Insights or to Determine Necessary Inputs
  • Purpose: To Find Areas in Need of Improvement or to Change Practices
  • Purpose: To Assess Program Effectiveness
  • Purpose: To Address Issues of Human Rights and Social Justice
  • Multipurpose Evaluation Strategies
  • Generating Questions
  • Planning Your Evaluation: Purposes and Questions

■ Chapter 9. Evaluation Designs
  • Quantitative Designs
  • Qualitative Designs
  • Mixed Methods Designs
  • Making Choices about Designs
  • Evaluation Checklists
  • Planning Your Evaluation: The Design of the Evaluation Study

Preparing to Read Chapter Seven

As you prepare to read this chapter, think about these questions:

1. What is your role as an evaluator in the identification of the evaluand?

2. How will you identify appropriate stakeholders for the evaluation?

3. How will you work with your stakeholders? Will your relationship be purely academic, or will it also be personal?

4. If your characteristics (race, gender, sexual orientation, etc.) do not match the community's characteristics, how will you deal with the possible emerging issues of power and privilege?

5. Is an evaluation logic model logical to use? Read on and find out!

CHAPTER SEVEN

Working with Stakeholders

Establishing the Context and the Evaluand

You have already read about a wide variety of evaluands that reflect many disciplines and issues, such as programs to provide youth mentoring, address homelessness and unemployment, provide effective mental health services, increase literacy skills, provide safe housing, improve schools, and prevent HIV/AIDS. An evaluand may seem pretty clear in the published version of an evaluation; however, this clarity generally comes from many hours of discussions and revisions during the evaluation planning and implementation phases. The evaluations discussed in earlier chapters have also been conducted in a wide variety of contexts and countries across the globe, with diverse cultural groups who use different languages and live in different socioeconomic conditions. These contextual factors influence what is chosen to be evaluated and how that determination is made.

Evaluation planning can begin in many different ways: a phone call from a person previously unknown to you who says, "I have a program that needs to be evaluated"; an email from someone who is preparing a proposal to develop a new program that needs an evaluation plan; or a request to expand on previous evaluation work with members of a community with whom you have an ongoing relationship. What these beginning points have in common is that you as the evaluator are interacting with another person or persons. Hence issues of human relations are inevitably part of the process of planning an evaluation. A second important thing to note is that evaluands come in all stages of being implemented—from existing only as an idea in a principal investigator's head to a firmly established program or one that is undergoing changes.

Identifying Stakeholders

Once the initial contact has been made between a client and an evaluator, both parties need to consider who needs to be involved in the process of planning the evaluation. As defined in Chapter 1, stakeholders are people who have a stake in the program: They fund, administer, provide services, receive services, or are denied access to services. It is usually wise to spend some time and effort thinking about which stakeholders need to be included at the very beginning; this can help avoid political disasters at the end of evaluations if the proper people were not involved. On a more positive note, the quality of the evaluation will be enhanced with representation of diverse interests, especially by inclusion of traditionally marginalized groups (Prell, Hubacek, & Reed, 2007). Appropriate stakeholders are sometimes identified by default, including only those who have power in positions related to the evaluation. The selection of stakeholders can also be an evolving process, with some stakeholders identified early in the process and others added as the relevant issues become clarified. In relatively small projects, the identification of stakeholders may be fairly straightforward. However, in larger projects, strategies for selection of representatives from stakeholder groups will probably need to be employed.

Identification of stakeholders is context-specific. Two lists of categories of stakeholders are displayed in Box 7.1; these will give you an idea of how many and what types of diverse groups can be considered in identifying stakeholders. The first list is based on a study of projects specifically focused on substance abuse prevention (Center for Substance Abuse Prevention [CSAP], 2008).

Box 7.1. Two Samples of Stakeholders for Evaluations, Listed by Category

Substance abuse prevention (based on CSAP, 2008)	Integration of gender in policy for poverty reduction strategies (based on UNIFEM, 2010)
Law enforcement	Various ministry officials, such as finance, economic planning, and others (health, education, trade, industry, labor, social development, natural resources, and environment)
Education	
Youth	
Criminal justice	Elected officials
Civic organizations	Civil society (e.g., NGOs, community-based organizations, faith-based groups, trade unions, private sector associations), with specific attention given to relevant dimensions of diversity within these groups (e.g., rural–urban, disability groups, women's groups)
Parents	
Faith-based organizations	
Elderly persons	
Businesses	World Bank staff involved in poverty reduction planning, especially those responsible for the World Bank Joint Staff Assessments/Joint Staff Advisory Notes, because they assess the quality of poverty reduction plans and make their recommendations for funding or debt reduction to the World Bank and International Monetary Fund
Human service providers	
Health care providers	
Military	
Colleges and universities	International agencies, such as United Nations agencies and international donor agencies (e.g., CARE, Oxfam, Save the Children, ActionAid)
Ethnic groups	
Government	Representatives from the sectoral groups that represent infrastructure, agriculture, education, health, and employment
Elected officials	
Child care providers	

The second list of stakeholders is based on the United Nations Development Fund for Women's (UNIFEM, 2010) *Guide to Integration of Gender in Policy for Poverty Reduction Strategies*, which provides ideas for how to involve different stakeholders in the development and revision of national poverty reduction policies and how to integrate issues of gender into these policies. UNIFEM suggests that evaluators begin by working with project staff to identify who is responsible for the poverty reduction plan in each country. The World Bank maintains a website with this information (***www.worldbank.org/prsp***), and another website maintained by VENRO, an umbrella organizations of NGOs in Germany, contains similar information (***www.prsp-watch.de***). Once the person responsible for poverty reduction strategies in each country is identified, then the project staff and evaluator need to identify other stakeholder groups to involve, such as those listed in Box 7.1.

Broad categories that are contextually relevant can be helpful in identifying stakeholders for specific evaluation studies. Evaluators can determine which stakeholder groups have relevance by recalling their own experiences in particular contexts, reading literature related to the particular context, conferring with knowledgeable members of the community, and asking for specific recommendations to represent diverse viewpoints. Evaluators should be aware of the need to include stakeholders who represent diverse perspectives and positions of power. They should also be aware of the need to provide support for those stakeholders who require it for authentic participation. This support might take the form of transportation, stipends, a safe meeting environment, interpreters, food, or child care. Evaluators working with stakeholders require careful attention to their interpersonal skills, because human relations are critical in conducting high-quality evaluations, as discussed in the next section.

········· **E X T E N D I N G   Y O U R   T H I N K I N G** ·········

Identifying Stakeholders

Machik is an NGO that is building new opportunities for education and training with Tibetans living in a small, isolated village in a deep valley. With support from donors, they have opened the Ruth Walter Chungba Primary School in this rural community. Imagine that Machik has asked you to evaluate the impact the school has made on the community. You need to decide with the school authorities and the donors who the stakeholders are in this community. Who would you ask to participate in this study, and why? (Read about the school and watch a video at this website: ***www.machik.org/index.php?option=com_content&task=view&id=24&Itemid=50***)

Human Relations

The nature of the relationship between the evaluator and stakeholders is an area of tension in the evaluation community, as exemplified by the different paradigmatic perspectives on this topic:

■ Methods Branch evaluators tend to favor having a *distant relationship,* in the belief that this will protect the evaluator from developing biases toward particular stakeholder groups.

- Use Branch evaluators see the necessity of *forming a relationship* with the stakeholders who are the primary intended users, so the evaluator can be responsive to their needs and thus enhance the possibility of use of the findings.

- Values Branch evaluators believe that the evaluator *needs to be involved with the community sufficiently* to reveal the viewpoints of different stakeholder groups accurately.

- The Social Justice Branch evaluators *directly address differences in power between themselves and various stakeholder groups,* with a conscious awareness of the need to bring those who have traditionally been excluded from decision-making positions into the process.

These differences in the nature of evaluator–stakeholder relationships lead to differences in the processes used to define the evaluand and understand its context.

· · · · · · · · · · E X T E N D I N G Y O U R T H I N K I N G · · · · · · · · · ·
Human Relations Skills for Evaluators

Two eminent scholars in the evaluation community see the importance of human relations very differently. Read the two passages below, and discuss your own thoughts and positioning with regard to this issue. First, Patton (as a contributor to Donaldson, Patton, Fetterman, & Scriven, 2010) writes:

> Human beings are in a relationship to each other and that relationship includes both cognitive and emotional dynamics. The interpersonal relationship between the evaluator and intended users matters and affects use. That interpersonal relationship is not just intellectual. It is also political, psychological, emotional, and affected by status and self-interest on all sides. What the astute evaluator has to be able to do, which includes the essential competencies to do that, is to be able to engage in relationships. (p. 25)

In contrast, Scriven (also as a contributor to Donaldson et al., 2010) writes that interpersonal skills are not necessarily important for evaluators:

> Michael [Patton] finds one of these to be a great strength, namely having lots of interpersonal skills. Forget it, guys! The way that evaluation works, and always will, is that it inhabits ninety niches. One of those niches is to be found in Washington in every agency, e.g., in the office of its inspector-general. Here are to be found the desk evaluators. Most of them don't have to have interpersonal skills any more than anyone in any kind of office job; and they don't need them. All they're doing is analyzing the reports, and they're very important people because they're the first line of advice and back-up to the decision makers. What we need from them is good analytic skills. It's not that I don't think that it's a good thing to have good interpersonal skills; it is that one must not put them in as minimum requirements for every evaluator. (p. 24)

1. What do you think about these two positions?

2. What merits do their arguments have?

3. Do you personally agree more with one than the other?

4. What are your reasons for your own positioning on the topic of human relations skills in evaluation?

Interacting with Stakeholders

Kirkhart (2005) has noted that the validity of an evaluation is influenced by "interpersonal justification" (i.e., the quality of the interactions between and among participants and the evaluator). Evaluators bring their own cultural lenses to the planning process, and these affect their interactions with stakeholders in terms of who is involved in the process and how. Lincoln (1995) has reinforced the importance of the quality of human relations in evaluation by suggesting that an evaluator needs to know the community "well enough" to link the evaluation results to positive action within the community. Evaluators must critically examine the meaning of "well enough"; what does this mean? Indigenous researchers provide insights into the nature of relationships that they would interpret as indicating that an evaluator is appropriately situated to work in their communities.

Lessons from the Māori

Cram (2009) and Smith (1999, 2004, 2005), who work in the indigenous Māori community in New Zealand (Aotearoa), have provided guidance to the meaning of *Kaupapa Māori* (which means "a Māori way"). *Kaupapa Māori* can be applied to many aspects of life; it implies the development of a relationship that is respectful of Māori cultural, social, and economic well-being. Cram (2009) provides a list of cultural values derived from Smith's (1999) work, which she translates into expectations for evaluators' interactions in their community. These include the following:

- *Aroha ki e tangata* (respect for people). Evaluators establish relationships with people via situating themselves within the history of the community (genealogically if possible; through personal connections if no genealogical link is present), with the assistance of the community elders. Another aspect of respect for people is to be knowledgeable about appropriate rituals in terms of entering the community (such as who to contact, how to approach people, bringing of gifts, etc.).

- *He kanohi kitea* (a voice may be heard, but a voice must be seen). Māori people expect that an evaluator will come into their community to allow the community members to see for themselves who this person is. Community meetings, called *hui,* are often used as a forum for evaluators to meet stakeholders, explain the study, and ask permission to proceed.

- *Titro, whakarongo ... korero* (watch, listen ... talk). An evaluator shows respect for Māori people by listening to what they say before he/she talks. This process of first looking and listening conveys the value that the evaluator places on the contributions of the community members.

- *Manaaki kit e tangata* (looking after people). In the context of the evaluation, the essential meaning of this concept is that the evaluator establishes a reciprocal relationship with the stakeholders. The stakeholders are providing access to their community and information in the form of data; the evaluator can offer small gifts or services, capacity-building activities, networking, and access to the evaluation findings.

◾ *Kaua e takahia te mana o te tangata* (do not trample on the *mana* [authority] of the people). Māori people want to know what an evaluator is saying about them before the results are released outside the community. As most communities would, the Māori do not want to be portrayed as having something wrong with them (a deficit view). Rather, they want to be portrayed in a balanced way, with both their strengths and their challenges.

◾ *Kia mahaki* (be humble). An evaluator should share the results with the Māori community in a way that helps the community take action on its own behalf. The community members can be provided with the tools necessary to fight for their own rights and challenge oppressive systems.

· · · · · · · · · · E X T E N D I N G   Y O U R   T H I N K I N G · · · · · · · · · ·
Māori Cultural Values and Evaluation

1. Reciprocity is seen as valuable in evaluations conducted in the Māori community. How would this principle translate to evaluation situations outside the Māori community?

2. What is your opinion with regard to the implications of applying these Māori cultural values in other evaluation contexts?

3. What could evaluators learn about the establishment of relationships with stakeholders from these Māori cultural values?

4. What might some evaluators find objectionable concerning the Māori's expectations of the evaluators' interactions in their community? Why would they object?

5. What do you know about yourself that might enhance or inhibit your ability to work in an evaluation context with regard to cultural values and backgrounds?

6. Symonette (2004) suggests that evaluators need to be aware of who they are themselves, as well as who they are in relation to community:

   Even more important for the viability, vitality, productivity and trust-building capacity of a transaction and relationship cultivation is multilateral self awareness: self in context and self as pivotal instrument. Who do those that one is seeking to communicate with and engage perceive the evaluator as being? … Regardless of the truth value of such perceptions, they still rule until authentically engaged in ways that speak into the listening. (p. 100)

   How would you answer this question: Who do others think that you are? If you are in an evaluator role, who do others think you are?

Power and Privilege

Power and privilege are concepts discussed in prior chapters. Here the emphasis is on strategies for evaluators to use to bring themselves and the communities they work with to consciousness of the dynamics of power and privilege, as well as on meaningful ways to engage those who have traditionally had less power in evaluation contexts. Two action researchers, Heron and Reason (2006), provide the following strategies as ways both to be self-reflective and to monitor the evaluator's engagement with communities in culturally respectful ways:

- *Research cycling.* Evaluators should be prepared to go through the inquiry process several times. This cycling process allows for repeated episodes of action and reflection that can help refine understandings and reduce distortions.

- *Authentic collaboration.* Evaluators and stakeholders need to devise strategies for interactions that allow for the development of an egalitarian relationship. The interaction dynamic needs to be designed so that stakeholders are motivated to have sustained involvement and allow every voice to be expressed.

- *Challenging consensus collusion.* Individuals have the right to challenge the assumptions that underlie the knowledge being created or the process by which it was created.

- *Managing distress.* Group processes typically have moments of stress and tension; a process needs to be in place to handle this distress respectfully.

- *Reflection and action.* A cyclical process that includes phases of action and reflection allows needed changes to occur.

- *Chaos and order.* Reflective action is difficult when a system is in total chaos. Evaluators should encourage divergent thinking and also bring the system back into balance so that the group can move forward toward its goals.

· · · · · · · · · · **EXTENDING YOUR THINKING** · · · · · · · · · ·

Power and Privilege

1. How do we understand the dynamics of power when participatory methods are employed by the powerful?

2. Whose voices are raised, and whose are heard?

3. How are these voices mediated as issues of representation become more complex with the use of participatory methods in larger-scale planning and consultation exercises? (Note: These first three questions are from Mertens, 2009, p. 85.)

4. The culturally responsive approach to evaluation places emphasis on matching the characteristics of the evaluation team with those of the community, particularly in terms of race. Frierson, Hood, and Hughes (2002) suggest that data will not be valid if they are collected by people who are not attuned to the program's cultural context. What if you are a member of the community? How does that

(cont.)

prepare you to work in that community? What if you are not a member of a community? To what extent is it necessary to share salient characteristics of a community?

5. Recall the discussion of cultural competence in Chapter 6. How does cultural competence come into the discussion of interactions in evaluation contexts?

6. When evaluators enter a community, they may find that they hold power in a way they have not before. For example, an elderly female evaluator may be more respected in this community than in her home culture. List situations where you must be cognizant of the increased or decreased power you hold as a result of personal characteristics that may affect your relationship with the stakeholders (age, gender, education, ethnicity, sexual orientation, etc.).

Developing Partnerships/Relationships

A large community of immigrants and refugees settled outside Lowell, Massachusetts, in a relocation effort for people from Laos who had assisted the United States in the years preceding the Vietnam War. When the United States lost the war, the government followed through on its promise to move members of the Laotian community who had been their allies to a safe place. The presence of such a large community in what had previously been a very working-class, white, mainstream American community did not go unnoticed by researchers. Researchers motivated by a desire to create knowledge, to work with an exotic community, or even simply to do good inundated the community with their study teams. Silka (2005) and her colleagues at the Center for Family, Work and Community at the University of Massachusetts, Lowell, noted that the immigrants and refugees were not benefiting from the research. They developed a model for partnership research and evaluation between a consortium of universities and the Laotian community, in order to protect the community from exploitative research that did not directly benefit the community. Silka and her colleagues have developed a set of tip sheets to guide researchers and evaluators who conduct studies in the Laotian community; several of these tip sheets are summarized in Box 7.2. They have wider applicability in the development of partnerships with other communities as well.

Box 7.2. Developing Ethical Partnerships: Tip Sheet Summaries

◼ *Initiating Partnerships: Gathering the Players,* by Darcie Boyer. This is the initial step in the process of acting on a felt need, identifying others who share a concern in the community and in the research or evaluation world, finding appropriate ways to contact and communicate with potential partners, and planning to have a community meeting to discuss the potential partnership.

◼ *Ethical Considerations in Participatory Research: The Researcher's Point of View,* by Mary-jane Costello. Researchers need to be aware of the diversity of perceptions as to what constitutes ethical practice in various communities.

▨ *Partnership-Based Research: How the Community Balances Power within a Research Partnership,* by G. Martin Sirait. Partnerships should be arranged so that both researchers and participants are recognized as having power in that context.

▨ *Everything You Always Wanted to Know about IRBs,* by Sokmeakara Chiev. IRBs, or Institutional Review Boards, are mandated by U.S. federal legislation for any organization that receives federal funds to do research. Communities can institute IRBs of their own with membership from within their cultural group. (Note: IRBs are discussed more extensively in Chapter 11.)

▨ *Overcoming the Roadblocks to Partnership,* by Marie Martinelli. Communities can ensure that they derive benefits from proposed research or evaluation by forming community advisory boards, actively participating in the planning process, and considering successful models of partnerships that might transfer to their own situation.

▨ *Knowledge Creation in Research Partnerships,* by Pascal Garbani. Researchers need to work together to create knowledge in a manner that respects differences between and within groups.

Source: Based on Center for Family, Work and Community at the University of Massachusetts, Lowell (2004). The Center's home page is *www.uml.edu/centers/cfwc.*

Many indigenous peoples prefer to speak of "relationships" rather than "partnerships." For example, Māori, Native Americans, and Africans share an emphasis on connectivity and extend it beyond relationships among human beings to include the wider environment, ancestors, and inanimate objects. For them, "partnership" implies more of a contractual relationship that may still reflect inequities and exploitation. "Relationship" means that there is a deeper connection at multiple levels in terms of where we are from and who our people are. It means that the evaluators understand the culturally appropriate ways of a community and see the evaluation as a journey that they take together with community members, with opportunities for mutual learning, participant control, and evaluator accountability (Cram, Ormond, & Carter, 2006).

Partnerships or relationships are not easy to develop and may not be smooth throughout their existence. Kirkhart (2005) suggests the following considerations that are related to effective partnerships and relationships. First, relationships in evaluation take time and effort to develop. Evaluators often work in compressed time frames with limited budgets that constrain their ability to be responsive to multicultural dimensions. Second, cultural responsiveness requires knowledge, emotions, and skills. These are complex and not easily taught. Third, evaluators need to be able to interact with the stakeholders in the evaluation in ways that are culturally respectful, cognizant of the strength in the community, and facilitates desired change. This means that they need to be flexible with the design and implementation of the evaluation in order to be responsive to these factors. Finally, evaluators, particularly if they are from outside the community, need to avoid cultural arrogance in several forms: imposing their own cultural beliefs on the stakeholders, pre-imposing a design on the evaluation, or mistakenly thinking that they accurately under-stand the culture in which they are working.

Evaluators can also work with community members on capacity building. The capac-ity building can be reciprocal, in that the evaluators will have knowledge and skills to teach from their perspective and the community members have knowledge, skills, and attitudes to teach from theirs. Teams of evaluators can be formed that allow strengths from all sides to be represented in the evaluation planning. Caldwell et al. (2005) describe effective evaluator teams formed with academic and tribal representatives. They do point out that one challenge with this approach arises from concerns about confiden-tiality and anonymity, especially in small communities where identities can readily be recognized.

· · · · · · · · · · · E X T E N D I N G   Y O U R   T H I N K I N G · · · · · · · · · ·
Developing Partnerships

Think about the evaluation you intend to plan.

1. At what point will you involve the community?

2. How will you prepare yourself for meeting the community? (By reading about the culture, etc.?)

3. How will you approach that community?

4. What benefits do you see for the community?

5. How will you demonstrate your respect for its culture and traditions?

The Evaluand and Its Context

The theme of AEA's annual meeting in 2009 was "Context and Evaluation." Debra J. Rog, the 2009 president of AEA, defined context in these terms:

> Context typically refers to the setting (time and place) and broader environment in which the focus of the evaluation (evaluand) is located. Context also can refer to the historical con-text of the problem or phenomenon that the program or policy targets as well as the policy and decision-making context enveloping the evaluation. Context has multiple layers and is dynamic, changing over time. (Rog, 2009, p. 1)

The contrast in terms of how evaluators from different branches view context was captured in the opening plenary session of the 2009 AEA meeting. Bickman (2009), a theorist from the Methods Branch, said that context was always something that he called "extraneous variables"—in other words, variables that were not of central concern but had to be controlled, so that the validity of the intervention could be determined apart from contextual factors. His perspective contrasted sharply with that of Bledsoe (2009), who is situated in the Social Justice Branch. She indicated that understanding the context was critical about the less powerful in the evaluations that she conducted, in order to challenge assumptions by the more powerful. With those two anchor points, we now explore several types of contextual variables and the implications of these contextual variables for the identification of the evaluand and the methods used in the evaluation.

Contextual variables include those associated with the local setting (time and place), as well as with the broader context—the history of the problem and its proposed solutions, as well as politics and legislation that have relevance for the evaluand. The range of stakeholders and their cultural differences are also contextual variables that need to be considered. These contextual variables influence who is involved (stakeholders), how they are involved, the evaluation questions, the type of evaluation undertaken, use of evaluation findings, and decisions about analysis and dissemination of results. The following questions can help stimulate your thinking about contextual variables and their implications:

▨ What dimensions of context influence the type of evaluation questions that can be addressed?

▨ How does the nature of the political context influence utilization? How does it interact with the type of evaluation conducted?

▨ What dimensions of context influence the choice of methods?

▨ How does culture within context affect evaluation practice?

▨ How do our evaluation theories guide us in thinking about context?

▨ How can we learn about context in multisite studies?

▨ What are the implications of a context-sensitive evaluation for analysis and dissemination?

▨ How can we incorporate context into our evaluation inquiries?

Here is an example from the Hawaiian housing study (Stufflebeam et al., 2002; see Chapter 4, Box 4.3) of the identification of contextual variables. The local setting for the housing project was on Oahu's Waianae Coast, one of the most depressed and crime-ridden areas in the state. The project stretched over 7 years. The funding agency placed high value on self-help and sustainability; this value system influenced the design of the program as well as the evaluation. Contextual variables of particular importance centered on the characteristics of the intended beneficiaries—specifically, the extent of their needs and their abilities to follow through on the expectations for helping to build and pay for their houses. These contextual variables influenced who was finally accepted as the target audience and how local people were used in the role of data collectors. As noted in Box 4.3, the original intent of the program was to serve the poorest families. However, these families could not get the mortgages, so the focus of the project was shifted to the working poor.

············ **EXTENDING YOUR THINKING** ············
Questions about Context

Reflect on the excerpt of Rog's (2009) explanation of context and the discussion of contextual variables in this section.

Now return to the sample studies summarized in boxes in Chapters 3–6. Use the questions listed earlier in this section to analyze relevant contextual variables in at least one sample study. Think about how the authors either considered or did not consider these contextual variables.

Sources That Inform the Identification of the Evaluand and Context

Developing a focused identification of the context and the evaluand can be approached through a number of different strategies:

- Funding agencies establish priorities and provide information in requests for proposals (RFPs) about the context and the program that needs to be evaluated. Another version of a funding agency request is a request for a program to be developed with the requirement for an evaluation plan in the proposal.

- Traditional scholarly literature reviews can provide valuable information about the context and the evaluand in terms of what is already known about the setting and the program. This type of resource is generally found through databases of articles available in university and sometimes community libraries, or online for a fee.

- Theoretical frameworks for evaluation approaches can provide guidance to the the variables that are important (e.g., an indigenous evaluation will emphasize specifics of the targeted culture), as well as a basis for decisions about appropriate components of a program. Theoretical frameworks can inform the evaluator and stakeholders about power differences on the basis of race/ethnicity, gender, sexual identities, disabilities/deafness, religion, class/socioeconomic status, and other characteristics associated with discrimination and oppression.

- Web-based resources are now available (sometimes overwhelmingly!). Here, an evaluator can read about past evaluations, recommended evaluation strategies for this type of evaluand, and relevant contextual factors. Web-based resources can also include databases such as those posted by the U.S. Census Bureau.

- "Grey literature" (i.e., that which is not published) can be a valuable resource, especially to gain the perspectives of those who have not been in the privileged scholarly or technological circles that would be represented in the first several strategies. This literature can include program-produced documents such as brochures, project reports, self-studies, past evaluations, conference papers, policy statements, newsletters, newspapers, fact sheets, and more.

▓ Group and individual strategies can be used, such as interviews, surveys, focus groups, concept mapping, and outcome mapping, as well as indigenous methods based on traditional community meeting ceremonies and rituals.

▓ Advisory boards are commonly used to guide evaluators throughout the process of planning and implementing an evaluation.

▓ New technological tools such as satellite imagery and mapping can be used to provide valuable contextual information about the locations of roads, buildings, services, and natural terrain.

We discuss all of these strategies in more detail below.

Funding Agencies

Funding agencies typically include government agencies and foundations. The U.S. government has a website that lists opportunities to apply for more than $400 billion in federal monies from over 1,000 different programs (***www.grants.gov***). In addition, many agencies offer their own funding opportunities at their websites (e.g., the U.S. Department of Education). Obtaining funds from federal agencies usually brings a fairly prescriptives set of requirements for how the funds can be used. On the other hand, foundations also offer many potential funding opportunities through a web portal (***lnps.fdncenter.org***); larger foundations offer such opportunities at their own websites. Foundations tend to have priority interest areas, but they are generally more flexible than government granting agencies. Box 7.3 provides contrasting statements from a federal agency's and a foundation's RFPs.

Box 7.3. Government and Foundation RFPs

The U.S. Department of Justice (2009) offers funding for a tribal youth program that includes the following program requirements:

[The Office of Juvenile Justice and Delinquency Prevention] seeks applicants to establish or expand a mentoring program that offers a mixture of core services and engages youth with activities that enable them to practice healthy behaviors within a positive pro-social peer group. The target population should be youth at risk of gang activity, delinquency, and youth violence.

The goals of this mentoring program are to prevent gang activity, delinquency, and violence by doing the following:

(1) Offering at-risk youth core services that fulfill their adolescent developmental needs within the context of a positive pro-social peer group, including:

▓ A multi-modal mixture of services that may include, but is not limited to, life skills and psycho-educational training, mental health counseling, job placement, community service projects, and structured afterschool recreational, educational, and artistic/culturally enhancing activities.

▓ Emphasizing long-term relationships with mentors and key staff, who are nurturing and supportive adults.

(cont.)

Box 7.3 (cont.)

(2) Developing structured mentoring relationships that include the following:

■ A relationship that lasts 2 or more years with significant contact between the mentor and mentee where the mentee views the mentor as a friend, not an authority figure.

■ Significant training for the mentor.

■ Oversight of the mentoring relationship.

■ Data collection to track the relationship and positive outcomes arising from the mentoring relationship.

■ Structured activities for the mentors and mentees to participate in together.

The Ford Foundation (2010) also supports grantees to develop and implement projects for youth mentoring, but it does not have explicit requirements about the nature of the program. Rather, it has issued this broad statement:

We make grants to develop new ideas and strengthen organizations that reduce poverty and injustice and promote democratic values, international cooperation and human achievement. To achieve these goals, we take varied approaches to our work, including supporting emerging leaders; working with social justice movements and networks; sponsoring research and dialogue; creating new organizations; and supporting innovations that improve lives. These methods of problem-solving reflect our values and the diverse ways in which we support grantees.

The foundation also describes a model of philanthropy that it has pursued for more than 70 years: to be a long-term and flexible partner for innovative leaders of thought and action. Lasting change in difficult areas, such as the reduction of poverty, protection of human rights, and establishment of democratic governance after a dictatorship, requires decades of effort. It involves sustained work with successive generations of innovators, thinkers, and activists as they pursue transformational and ambitious goals.

Cheek (2005; cited in Mertens, 2009, p. 112) offers the following cautionary questions before you accept money from a funding agency:

■ Who owns the data and what can you do with the data?

■ What if the funder wants to suppress results of the study? Or wants to exclude parts of the results?

■ What exactly is the deliverable (e.g., product expected by the funder)?

■ In what time frame?

■ Reporting requirements?

■ What if there is a disagreement about the way the research or evaluation should proceed?

Scholarly Literature

Many funding agencies require a scholarly review of literature on the evaluation topic in order to provide evidence of knowledge in the field, of the need for the proposed project, and directions to inform the proposed scope of work. Searching databases is very easy for evaluators in the developed world, especially those who work in universities. A list of commonly used databases is provided in Box 7.4. These are generally searchable for free at universities and for a modest fee for people in other settings. Most of these databases can be searched by topic, author, or title. Many databases now have full text documents electronically available to users; this eliminates the need to actually visit the library to obtain the documents.

Box 7.4. Scholarly Databases

Psychology

The American Psychological Association (APA) produces the following databases:

- PsycARTICLES. This database contains full text articles from 42 journals published by APA and related organizations. The dates of coverage vary; the earliest articles are from 1988, but APA is developing PsycArchives, which has over 100 years of content coverage.

- PsycINFO. This database indexes and abstracts over 1,300 journals, books, and book chapters in psychology and related disciplines (1887–present).

- PsycBOOKS. Textbooks published by APA and selected classic books from other publishers are found in this database.

Social Science

- Social Science Journals (ProQuest). Social science journal articles published from 1994 to the present.

- Sociological Abstracts. This is an online resource for researchers, professionals, and students in sociology and related disciplines. Sociological Abstracts includes citations and abstracts from over 2,000 journals, plus relevant dissertation listings, abstracts of conference papers and selected books, citations of book reviews and other media, and citations and abstracts from Social Planning/Policy and Development Abstracts.

- Social Work Abstracts. Index to articles from social work and other related journals on topics such as homelessness, AIDS, child and family welfare, aging, substance abuse, legislation, community organization, and more.

Education

- Education Complete (ProQuest). Indexes more than 750 titles on education, including primary-, secondary-, and university-level topics. Almost 500 titles include full text.

(cont.)

Box 7.3 *(cont.)*

░ Educational Resources Information Center (ERIC). A bibliographic database covering the U.S. literature on education; a key source for researchers, teachers, policy makers, librarians, journalists, students, parents, and the general public. Accessible to the public at *www.eric.ed.gov*.

Dissertations and Theses

░ ProQuest Dissertations and Theses. Dissertations and theses published in the United States and internationally.

Lawless and Pellegrino (2007) describe an evaluation they were planning to determine how to prepare teachers to use technology in their classrooms to enhance learning. They began with a very extensive literature review, which focused on "what is known and unknown about professional development to support the integration of technology into teaching and learning. To answer such questions, we have assembled bodies of literature that are relevant to the design of research studies, the evaluation of the quality of the evidence obtained therein, and the possible utility of conclusions" (p. 577). To this end, they examined a multipart literature: what constitutes professional development, how technology is integrated into the classroom, what influences teachers to adopt technology, the multiple roles that technology can play in this context, the quality of previous research on this topic, and the long-term impacts technology has had on teachers and administrators. They used this literature review to "lay out the kinds of questions that should be asked in evaluating how states, districts, and schools have invested their technology integration funds and the nature of the research designs and sources of evidence that might be used to better answer questions about what is effective and why" (p. 578).

In an evaluation of the sustainability of health projects, Scheirer (2005) provides this description of her literature search strategy:

> The search was conducted using the search string "sustainability OR routinization OR institutionalization AND health OR healthcare," in all major relevant bibliographic databases, for the years 1990 to 2003, including PubMed, ProQuest, the Librarians Index to the Internet, and NLM Gateway. The abstracts of potentially relevant citations were examined to determine if the original research included data collected about any aspect of sustainability after the initial funding had ended. Full texts of all relevant articles were then obtained. A few studies were already known to me from prior related work. In addition, reference lists of obtained articles were examined for any additional studies, such as those using different terminology. The systematic review did not include articles or how-to-do-it commentaries about sustainability that did not report empirical data, although these articles were consulted for their conceptual frameworks and approaches. These procedures yielded 19 studies that met the criteria for inclusion: reporting data collected about the status and/or influences on health program sustainability (including case studies). The review included all available studies that met these criteria, not a sample of them. (p. 327)

The use of scholarly literature is a critical part of enhancing our understanding of the context in which the evaluation is taking place. However, it is limited by the fact that various gatekeepers decide what will be published and what will be archived in a database. Therefore, evaluators should be cognizant of this limitation and engage in other types of search strategies to identify important contextual variables.

Theoretical Frameworks

The theorists whose work is described in Chapters 3–6 provide evaluators with a multitude of theoretical frameworks to choose from in their planning work. These theories can range from theories of literacy development to theories of community involvement. Theories provide a framework for thinking, highlight relevant concepts, and suggest dynamic relationships between those concepts. Here are some examples of evaluations that used theoretical concepts:

- Bowman's (2005) evaluation of a tribal education model in a technical college in Wisconsin was based on an indigenous theory from the Native American community. The geographic coverage area of the technical college included members of three tribes. The evaluators sought out each tribe's individual customs, culture, language, and epistemological views based on their tribal traditions.

- Donaldson and Gooler (2002) conducted a theory-based evaluation of a job search training program in California. The underlying theory of the program was based on identifying the skills and psychological factors that were necessary for the participants to find employment and improve their mental health. The theory held that the participants needed to increase their job search confidence, their job search skills, and their problem-solving strategies in order to achieve the intended outcomes.

- Seigart's (2007) study of school-based health services in Australia (see Chapter 6, Box 6.11) used a feminist theoretical framework, which focused on power differentials based on gender (as well as race and class) in the planning, implementation, and use of the evaluation.

- Brady and O'Regan (2009) used Rhodes's model of mentoring as a theoretical framework for their youth mentoring evaluand. This model is presented graphically in Chapter 3, Box 3.2.

Web-Based Resources

The proliferation of web-based resources sometimes makes me (Donna M. Mertens) wonder what we would do if we didn't have the World Wide Web anymore. This is probably unimaginable to many people younger than I am, and I admit that life would be a lot harder for me if it happened. The major search engines of today may not be the major search engines of tomorrow. The two major search engines that I currently use (*www.google.com* and *www.yahoo.com*) provide access to printed documents, pictures, graphics, images, news, videos, discussion groups, maps, and more. Evaluators can locate a great deal of information about contexts of evaluations and experiences with similar evaluands through web searching. Here are two examples:

▓ Bowman (2005) used data from the U.S. Census Bureau for the year 2000 to determine that the technical college serves 4,880 members of three tribal communities: Fairwater Country Pawnee, Lake du Forest, and Moon Lake Sioux. Wisconsin's largest Indian population is in the city of Green Bay. This coincides with the U.S. Census Bureau's finding that 90% of American Indians/Native Americans live off reservations.

▓ Sharma and Deepak (2001) gathered contextual data for their evaluation of CBR in Vietnam (see Chapter 4, Box 4.11) from several websites, including the World Bank, the Central Intelligence Agency (CIA), and UNICEF. They were able to report on the gross national product of Vietnam, the density of its population, its population growth rate, and other demographics such as health indicators, age, life expectancy, infant mortality, literacy rates, access to clean water, and government budgets.

"Grey Literature"

Evaluators should always seek program documents that have been produced before the start of the evaluation process. The quantity and quality of these documents will vary widely, depending on the history of the evaluand. Even if a new program is planned, it is probably going to occur in a context that has some kind of paper trail. When I conducted an evaluation of a residential school for the deaf, I asked to see their self-study report and their accreditation report. In addition, I asked to see the curriculum guides and the student conduct rules. All of these documents gave me an overview of the evaluation context. The APA (*www.apa.org/psycextra*) has listed the following documents as examples of "grey literature": research reports, policy statements, annual reports, curricula materials, standards, videos, conference papers and abstracts, fact sheets, consumer brochures, newsletters, pamphlets, directories, popular magazines, white papers, and grant information. Examples of using "grey literature" in evaluation practice include the following:

▓ Mertens et al. (2007; see Chapter 6, Box 6.10) read over the RFP for the teacher training program that they evaluated, as well as the university's proposal and annual reports for the 6 years prior to the evaluation.

▓ Bowman (2005) located and reviewed the initial needs assessment that was conducted in Wisconsin and was used as the basis for the development of the tribal education model for on- and off-campus activities. She was also able to determine that there had been no electronic, print, or annual data since the time of that report until she undertook her evaluation study in 2004.

▓ Brady and O'Regan (2009; see Chapter 3, Box 3.2) cited the Atlantic Philanthropies annual report for 2007 as a source of historical information that set the context for their evaluation of the youth mentoring program in Ireland. The Atlantic Philanthropies foundation has funded programs to improve people's lives through education and knowledge creation since the 1990s. The foundation reported that early initiatives in this area were not as effective as they had hoped because of lack of coordination, depending on volunteers, and relying on multiple unpredictable funding sources. Within the Foroige agency in Ireland, the foundation funded a pilot project of a BBBS model of youth mentoring.

Group and Individual Strategies

Evaluators can use group and individual strategies such as concept mapping, brainstorming, interviews, surveys, and focus groups, as well as indigenous methods based on traditional community meeting ceremonies and rituals. Steps for conducting group and individual interviews are described in the chapter on data collection. Here we provide examples of the use of these strategies and indigenous methods for the purpose of determining the evaluand and its context.

Bowman (2005) included the use of focus groups and individual interviews in the Native American community in order to determine what their needs were for tribal-related education. She integrated the medicine wheel into the interviews (similar to the Cross et al. [2000] study summarized in Chapter 6, Box 6.8). She structured the questions based on the four quadrants of the medicine wheel. In addition, she provided time for informal interaction following the focus group process to allow people to socialize and share experiences that might not have surfaced during the focus group. The data from the focus groups and individual interviews were used to develop recommendations for changes in the tribal education model, the evaluand of interest in this study.

Africans have traditional tribal gatherings that can be used as a basis for dialogue about context and needs (Chilisa & Preece, 2005). The group gatherings in Botswana are called *kgotla*; these involve the village council in the main village, with the chief or his assistant in charge of the process. Smaller *kgotla* can be held in outlying areas with the head tribesman as the facilitator, or even in extended families with the elders facilitating the process. These gatherings can be used to identify problems and potential solutions. One downside to this process is that it has traditionally excluded women and children. Therefore, evaluators will need to work with the communities to develop appropriate strategies for all stakeholders' views to be represented.

Concept Mapping

Trochim (1989) developed the technique of "concept mapping," which has been applied in many different contexts. The steps in the process involve having participants brainstorm either possible outcomes or specific factors that influence those outcomes. The next step is to edit the statements to reduce repetition. Participants are then asked to rate the outcomes on two dimensions—importance (compared to other factors), and feasibility over the next few years—on 5-point scales where 5 indicates "extremely important" or "extremely feasible." Sophisticated statistical procedures (multidimensional scaling and hierarchical cluster analysis, discussed in Chapter 12) are then applied to the data to produce configurations revealing which of the statements are rated most similarly. Different types of maps can be used to demonstrate how the statements can be organized and used to understand the underlying theory of the project.

Trochim, Milstein, Wood, Jackson, and Pressler (2004) used concept mapping with the Hawaii Department of Health to determine factors of importance that affect individuals' behaviors related to avoidance of tobacco, improvement of nutrition, and increased physical activity. Project participants brainstormed factors that they believed influenced individuals' behaviors, and then rated them according to their importance and feasibility. The concept mapping revealed that factors could be categorized in terms of policies and laws, environment infrastructure, children and schools, coalitions and collaborations, community infrastructure, information and communication, and access. These results were used by the state's governor in the official state plan, approved by the legislature, and used to create sustainable change in Hawaii.

Outcome Mapping

Buskens and Earl (2008; see Chapter 6, Box 6.12) offer a strategy similar to concept mapping called "outcome mapping." These two strategies are similar in many respects; however, Buskens and Earl offer insights into the application of outcome mapping within the context of transformative participatory evaluations in international development. Outcome mapping deliberately involves subgroups of stakeholders in the process of determining how interventions fit into the overall development process. It begins with four questions (Buskens & Earl, 2008, p. 174):

1. What is the program's vision?
2. Who are its boundary partners?
3. What changes in behavior are being sought?
4. How can the program best contribute to these changes?

"Boundary partners" are defined as "the individuals, groups, or organizations with whom the program works directly and with whom the program anticipates opportunities for influence" (p. 190). Boundary partners are similar to stakeholders; however, Buskens and Earl make the distinction that boundary partners are the subgroups interacting most closely with each other. Hence, instead of having big stakeholder meetings with everyone represented, they tend to have team meetings of relevant boundary partners. For example, the core management team for the IFRP had the following boundary partners (Buskens & Earl, 2008, p. 183):

■ Action researchers

■ Training development team

■ IFRP trainers

■ IFRP desk researchers

■ Funders

■ Motivational Interviewing Southern African Network (MISA)

■ Department of Family Medicine at University of Stellenbosch

■ Health researchers in southern Africa

The action researchers had their closest associations with the nurse counselors and the project management team, who constituted their boundary partners. The boundary partners for the mothers who participated in the project were the nurse counselors with whom they worked. These teams deliberated on the program's vision and desired changes in behavior. Buskens and Earl then discuss how the program could provide the conditions necessary for that change to occur. The outcome-mapping process is dynamic and ongoing, allowing the boundary partners to examine their progress and to make adjustments to the intervention as deemed necessary.

Advisory Boards

Evaluators often work with advisory boards as a way to get input from representatives of various stakeholder groups. It would not be possible to work with all stakeholders in a national-level study (or a state-level or community-level study, in many instances). Hence the use of an advisory board can allow for important dimensions of the community to be represented. Mertens (2000) worked with an advisory board in a national evaluation of court access for deaf and hard-of-hearing people. The advisory board included representatives of the deaf and hard-of-hearing communities who were diverse in various respects: their choice of communication mode and language (sign language, reading lips, use of voice); backgrounds with the court (attorneys, judges, judicial educators, police officers, and interpreters); and hearing status (hearing, hard of hearing, and deaf). This group was able to provide guidance in regard to the diversity of experiences that deaf and hard-of-hearing people experience in the courts. The group also emphasized the importance of understanding these diverse experiences in order to develop an intervention that could improve court access.

Technological Tools: Satellite Imagery and Mapping

The use of satellite imagery and mapping is a valuable tool that can be used to display current conditions, as well as to compare past and current conditions. An organization called Information Technology for Humanitarian Assistance, Cooperation and Action (*www.ithaca.polito.it*) provided information to help aid agencies plan how to respond when the island country of Haiti was struck by a massive earthquake on January 12, 2010. This organization used geomapping technology to post before-and-after pictures on its website of the areas hit by the earthquake. The before-earthquake satellite photos showed roads, airports, various types of buildings (public and private), and water and electricity centers. The photos taken after the earthquake showed how extensive the damage was to all these facilities. Electricity was not available; telephone cables were damaged; the airport had no fuel or lights, and the road from there into the city was destroyed; the water supply collapsed, and wells were contaminated; the prisons broke open, and the prisoners who survived the quake escaped. The geomapping tool thus provided information that was invaluable in helping the aid agencies understand what the conditions were on the ground, especially since communication systems were not functioning.

Note that many of these strategies for identification of context and evaluand are revisited in our Chapter 8 discussion of the approach to evaluation known as "needs and assets assessment."

Depicting the Evaluand

The evaluand, as the entity that is being evaluated, needs to be specified early in the evaluation-planning process. As mentioned at the beginning of this chapter, evaluands can range in definition from a gleam in a proposing investigator's eye to a well-established program. It is sometimes easier to describe an evaluand that has a long history and ample extant information, although this is not always the case. Sometimes a program that has been around for a while has developed layers of complexity that were not present in the original plans, requiring evaluators to do a bit of investigative work. Programs that are under development may also exist differently in the minds of different stakeholders. One of the greatest services an evaluator can provide in such circumstances is to facilitate discussions among the various stakeholder groups to identify what the various components of the evaluand are, how they work together, and what resources are needed and available to lead to the desired outcomes. Portrayals of evaluands should be considered as working models that will change over time; however, in order to plan an evaluation, a preliminary portrayal of the evaluand is needed.

Evaluands can be depicted in many ways: descriptively or graphically, as static or dynamic entities. Descriptive portrayals of evaluands are typically given as narratives; the object of the evaluation is described, along with the major players and goals. Graphic portrayals of evaluands have typically taken the form of **logic models** or **logical frameworks** (the latter is sometimes shortened to **log frame,** the terminology used in the international development community for logic models). Evaluators from all branches can use all of these approaches to depicting evaluands; however, they may use them a bit differently.

Logic Models and Log Frames

Logic models are most closely tied to theory-based evaluation approaches (although they are used in many evaluation approaches), because the essence of theory-based evaluation is to reveal the underlying theory of how the program intends to achieve its intended outcomes. For example, if I want youth to refrain from using illegal drugs, what is my theory as to how to accomplish that outcome? The logic model is supposed to make the program's theory of change explicit. A theory of change describes how the activities, resources, and contextual factors work together to achieve the intended outcomes.

The W. K. Kellogg Foundation (WKKF, 2004) has published a logic model development guide that starts with a very simple depiction of a logic model. This includes two main components: what the program people plan to do (resources/inputs and activities) and what their intended results are (output, outcomes, impact). This elementary depiction of a logic model is shown in Figure 7.1. "Resources" or "inputs" are those human, financial, and community resources that are needed for the evaluand, such as funding, partnering organizations, staff, volunteers, time, facilities, equipment, and supplies. They can also include wider contextual factors, such as attitudes, policies, laws, regulations, and geography. "Activities" include the processes, events, technology, and actions that are part of the program implementation. These can include such things as education and training services, counseling, or health screening; products such as curriculum materials, training materials, or brochures; and infrastructure such as new networks, organizations, or relationships. "Outputs" are products of the activities and include the quantity and quality of the services delivered by the program, such as the number of workshops taught or the number of participants served. "Outcomes" are the changes in individual participants in terms of behaviors, knowledge, skills, or attitudes. These can be short-term or long-term. "Impact" is the desired change on a broader level for organizations or communities, such as reduction of poverty or increase in health.

The most basic format for a logic model is the outcomes-based logic model, which starts with stakeholders' identifying those outcomes and impacts that are important to them. Any of the group processes described earlier in this chapter can be used for this

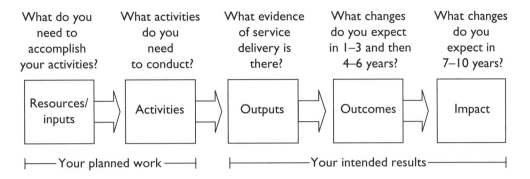

Figure 7.1. Basic logic model template. *Source:* Based on WKKF (2004, pp. 1 and 17).

DD purpose. For example, Fredericks et al. (2008; see Chapter 3, Box 3.4) described a logic model for a project that was supposed to improve services and quality of life for people with developmental disabilities. The stakeholders included a state-level steering committee and a finance team from the state agency in charge of the program. The project had specified goals: "to increase the individualization of service planning and delivery, increase administrative efficiencies, increase person-centered planning, increase consumer choice, increase community integration, and improve the quality of life for consumers—in terms of home, relationships, personal life, work and school, and community" (Center for Policy Research, 2003; cited in Fredericks et al., 2008, p. 254). The evaluators and the steering committee worked together to develop the logic model displayed in Box 7.5.

Box 7.5. Logic Model from the Fredericks et al. (2008) Quality-of-Life Study

Inputs (What is going into the system?)	Process (What is it that we are doing?)	Outputs and short-term outcomes (How will we know when we have done this?)	Long-term outcomes and impacts (Why are we doing this?)
▦ Training for staff to ensure more individualized services	▦ Implementing sites will redesign service delivery efforts based on an individualized service environment	▦ Increases in person-centered planning	▦ Increases in the individualization of service planning and delivery
▦ Resources to train and retain qualified staff		▦ Increases in community integration	▦ Increases in administrative efficiencies
		▦ Increases in consumer choice	

(cont.)

Box 7.5 (cont.)

Inputs (What is going into the system?)	Process (What is it that we are doing?)	Outputs and short-term outcomes (How will we know when we have done this?)	Long-term outcomes and impacts (Why are we doing this?)
▪ Links to community partners that will allow consumers to be more involved in the community, both socially and in a work setting ▪ Increased choices for consumers	▪ Implementing sites will provide services according to the performance contract ▪ Implementing sites will provide services to individuals currently not being served ▪ Implementing sites will serve individuals with a full range of disabilities ▪ Implementing sites will use a new budgeting procedure	▪ Increases in the number of people being served ▪ Financial predictability, as measured by stability in the budgets	▪ Increases in the quality of life for consumers—in terms of home, relationships, personal life, work and school, and community

Source: Fredericks et al. (2008, p. 255). Copyright 2008 by the American Evaluation Association. Reprinted by permission.

The WKKF (2004) logic development guide offers another, more intricate template for a theory-based logic model. Like the simpler logic model just presented, this theory-based logic model explains what the project wants to accomplish and how it will accomplish those intended results, but it does so in greater detail and complexity. The theory-based approach begins by clarifying the assumptions that underlie the decisions to plan and implement the evaluand. A template for this type of logic model appears in Figure 7.2. The development of the theory-based logic model follows these steps:

1. Identify the problem or issue. Why is this evaluand needed? What are the conditions in the community that give rise to the need for this program (e.g., high levels of poverty, increased rate of infection from HIV/AIDS, low literacy levels)?

2. List the community's needs and assets. This means listing both the strengths and challenges in the community. For example, strengths might include networks of health care workers, expressed desire to work for change, or access to funds. Challenges might be poor infrastructure in terms of transportation or school buildings or clean drinking water. Part of the contextual analysis should pay attention to issues of power and influences of discrimination and oppression in the evaluation context.

3. Specify the desired results in terms of outputs, outcomes, and impact. As explained above for the outcomes-based logic model, outputs might be services delivered, workshops provided, or number of participants trained. Outcomes are short-term results in the form of changes in individuals' behaviors, skills, efficiency, literacy levels, or disease prevention or treatment. The impacts are the longer-term goals of the project (e.g., reduction of poverty, violence, economic hardship, or hunger).

4. Identify influential factors—both those that are facilitative and those that are barriers to change. These can include legislation or policies that either mandate or inhibit the changes that are needed; history of political stability or civil unrest; economic upturns or downturns; natural disasters; and political or community leadership.

5. Determine strategies (activities) that are needed to achieve the desired results. These might include development of recruitment or training materials, provision

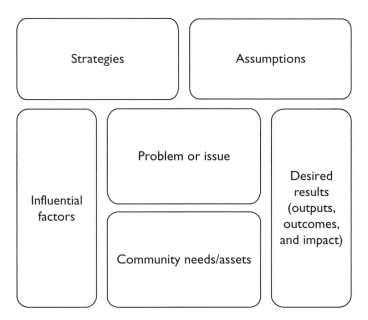

Figure 7.2. Theory–based logic model template. *Source:* Based on WKKF (2004, p. 28).

of services to enhance skills or health, or enhancement of infrastructure or technology.

6. State the assumptions that underlie the project. Why do the stakeholders believe that this course of action in this context will garner the results they desire? What are the principles, beliefs, or ideas that are guiding this project?

An example of a theory-based logic model is displayed in Figure 7.3. This figure is adapted from the work of Kathleen Donnelly-Wijting (2007) for an evaluation of an HIV/AIDS prevention program for deaf youth in South Africa.

In addition to the WKKF (2004) development guide for logic models, a number of other guides are available online:

▭ The Harvard Family Research Project has a guide for developing logic models that is available online (*www.hfrp.org*). The logic model development process is illustrated with an example of a districtwide family engagement program.

▭ The Aspen Institute has developed a tool that includes step-by-step instructions

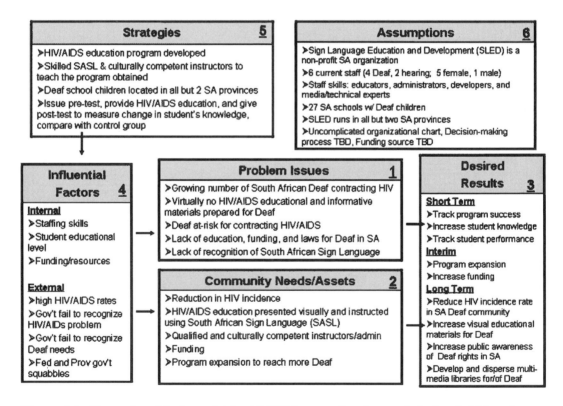

Figure 7.3. Theory-based logic model for HIV/AIDS prevention for youth in South Africa. *Source:* Adapted from Donnelly-Wijting. Used by permission of Kathleen Donnelly-Wijting.

on the development of a logic model within the world of philanthropy. Continuous Progress, a branch of the Aspen Institute's Global Interdependence Initiative, just launched its Advocacy Progress Planner (*planning.continuousprogress.org*). Funded by the California Endowment, this tool illustrates the range of possible outcomes and target audiences that might be relevant to a certain advocacy or policy change strategy. The model helps a user focus on identifying the proper goals of any advocacy effort, which depends on where the issue stands in the policy process.

■ CSAP presents a planning framework for interventions for prevention programs (*captus.samhsa.gov/prevention-practice/strategic-prevention-framework*). Many of the steps fit into the logic model system. Step 1 is to assess the community's needs and readiness for an intervention. Step 2 is to mobilize the community and build capacity as necessary. Step 3 is called "planning" and includes a description of the program, activities, and strategies. The website gives many examples of best practices from the National Institute on Drug Abuse, CSAP, the National Center for the Advancement of Prevention, the Office of Juvenile Justice and Delinquency Prevention, the Department of Education, and the Centers for Disease Control and Prevention (CDC). Step 4 is to implement the program, and Step 5 is to evaluate the program's results and sustainability.

In the field of international development, logical frameworks (log frames) are used instead of logic models. Baker (2000) describes log frames as a statement of objectives that lead to the identification of outputs and impact indicators.

> The use of a logical (log) framework approach provides a good and commonly used tool for identifying the goals of the project and the information needs around which the evaluation can be constructed. The log frame, increasingly used at the World Bank, is based on a simple four-by-four matrix that matches information on project objectives with how performance will be tracked using milestones and work schedules, what impact project outputs will have on a beneficiary institution or system and how that will be measured, and how inputs are used to deliver outputs.... In other words, it is assumed that the project's intended impact is a function of the project's outputs as well as a series of other factors. The outputs, in turn, are a function of the project's inputs and factors outside the project. Quantifiable measures should then be identified for each link in the project cycle. This approach does not preclude the evaluator from also looking at the unintended impacts of a project but serves to keep the objectives of the evaluation clear and focused. Qualitative techniques are also useful in eliciting participation in clarifying the objectives of the evaluation and resulting impact indicators. (p. 19)

Davies (2005) also describes a logical framework as a 4 × 4 planning matrix:

> The four columns are the Narrative—a description of expected changes, Objectively Verifiable Indicators—of those changes, Means of Verification—of those indicators, and Assumptions about external influences on the expected changes, both positive and negative. The four rows are the Activities, which lead via Assumptions on that row to the Output, which leads via Assumptions on that row to the Purpose, which leads via Assumptions on that row to the Goal. (p. 147)

· · · · · · · · · · **E X T E N D I N G   Y O U R   T H I N K I N G** · · · · · · · · · ·

Using a Logic Model

Logic model: Stopping teens from texting while driving

Situation: A high school in Montgomery County is mourning the death of one senior who died in a car accident as he was texting while driving. The problem seems to be complex: Many teens text while they drive; their parents text while driving; teens see other drivers texting while driving; the local police department does not seem to be ticketing or consistently ticketing drivers, despite the law prohibiting driving and texting; and there are limited consequences for the few teens who have been caught texting.

The Montgomery County Teen Unit (MCTU) is planning a campaign to begin a program to teach the teens and the community at large about the dangers of texting while driving. Below are the inputs and processes. What would be some other outputs and short-term outcomes, and some other long-term outcomes and impacts?

Inputs	Process (activities)
Montgomery County grants	MCTU will:
Private funding (telephone companies)	Develop teaching units with driving schools
Parents	Create literature with teens
Montgomery High School	Create public service announcements at high school's TV lab
Equipment	
Volunteers (parents, police, community members, teens)	Engage youth and build relationships
	Write grants for funding
Community partners	Collaborate with county judges for consistent punishments and education
Existing resources	
MCTU Staff	Conduct training for cell phone providers
Materials	Work with police on vigilant and consistent enforcement
Time	
	Discuss initiative at county hall meetings
	Deliver prevention education programs

Outputs and short-term outcomes	Long-term outcomes and impacts
Increased knowledge about the danger of texting while driving	Decrease in the number of teens who text while driving after first probation
Name others:	Name others:

In the international development context, evaluators focus on the United Nations MDGs (these are listed in Chapter 1, Box 1.3). These give evaluators direction in terms of their goals and targets, as well as the indicators they can use to determine whether those goals and targets are being achieved. The World Bank and the United Nations have developed electronic databases that provide helpful information in planning an evaluation for an international development project.

The United Nations developed DevInfo, which contains information about progress toward the achievement of the MDGs by geographic areas (Pron, Oswalt, Segone, & Sakvarelidze, 2009). DevInfo allows planners to target disparities associated with the most vulnerable groups, thus enhancing the possibility of designing interventions that are appropriate within each country's context. The software allows the user to create tables, graphs, and maps that depict the extent of progress toward meeting the MDGs. DevInfo works in concert with three databases developed by the UNICEF Regional Office for Eastern and Central Europe and the Commonwealth of Independent States:

1. The Regional MDGInfo database (*www.regionalmdg.org*) contains the MDGs and locally determined indicators for this region.

2. The MICSInfo database (*www.micsinfo.org*) contains results of Multiple Indicators Clusters Surveys (household surveys to collect data about women and children) from 12 countries and disaggregates the data by region, urban–rural status, ethnicities, wealth, mother's education, and age of children.

3. The MoneeInfo database (*www.moneeinfo.org*) is specific to data on women and children in 27 countries, especially with regard to child protection issues such as institutionalization, living arrangements, and juvenile justice.

Evaluators can use these databases to provide context for their evaluation planning, as well as to inform stakeholders about the extent of needs within various populations.

The World Bank (n.d.) describes its modeling methodologies for monitoring the MDGs as follows:

> The new modeling methodologies being mobilized by the Bank to help understand the challenges of achieving the MDGs at the country as well as global level use powerful new software, including programs to deliver computable general equilibrium (CGE) models.
>
> These are used to analyze macroeconomic data, along with microdata gathered in detailed household surveys.
>
> Policymakers using these tools can analyze various policy scenarios, while also comparing the outcomes of actual policies and programs, with the counterfactuals. These computerized models can explain not only what happened as a result of a given policy, program or project, but what would have happened had it not been implemented.
>
> Such modeling exercises aim to overcome the difficulties encountered in establishing linkages between non-income aspects of the MDGs, such as, for example, the links between public health service provision and child mortality. In its initial phase, the effort will focus on one or two pilot countries, so as to develop a standardized and easily adapted methodology for wider use.
>
> The Bank's Development Data Platform (DDP) is a web-based data tool that provides access to statistics from more than 75 key databases. Users can also access record-level data

and documentation from over three thousand household surveys. The DDP Microdata incorporates both innovative IT design and development and a substantial effort to locate and format household survey data. More information on this tool is available online through the International Household Survey Network.

Descriptive Depictions of the Evaluand

Evaluators always have a descriptive depiction of the evaluand; this can stand alone or can support the graphic depiction of the evaluand in a logic model. All the examples of evaluations presented in this and earlier chapters have either a descriptive depiction of the evaluand or a descriptive and graphic depiction. One framework that is useful for conceptualizing a description of the evaluand is the CIPP model developed by Stufflebeam (see Chapter 4). Box 7.6 contains examples of the types of variables that might be considered for each aspect of the model, as well as applications of these to the evaluand description of a self-help program for women adjusting to breast cancer and its treatment (Sidani & Sechrest, 1999). It provided information about the course of treatment, belief in self, and improving problem-solving and cognitive reframing skills. The course had three components: (1) The cognitive component provided the knowledge needed to understand the condition, treatment, and self-care strategies; (2) the behavioral component addressed women's skills necessary for active participation in their own care, problem solving, and stress management; and (3) the psychological component helped women deal with their feelings. The course used three teaching modes (interactive, didactic, and hands-on experience).

Box 7.6. Evaluand Descriptions Based on the CIPP Model

Component	Variables	Example from Sidani and Sechrest (1999)
Context	Presenting problem; characteristics of the setting (physical and psychosocial features of the environment; social, political, and economic context of the program).	Women with breast cancer receiving therapy.... Physical side effects; need for management to minimize effect on daily functioning.
	Setting: accessibility, material resources needed to deliver the services; the physical layout and attractiveness of the setting; organizational culture; composition of and working relationships among the staff; norms and policies.	Setting: classroom in a quiet setting; written materials; seating arrangements to facilitate discussion; audiovisual materials; space and equipment for demonstrations and hands-on learning.

Component	Variables	*Example from Sidani and Sechrest (1999)*
Input	Critical inputs needed to produce the desired results, including: Client characteristics (e.g., demographics, personality traits, personal beliefs, employment status, level of anxiety, stage of the disease). Resources available to clients (internal and external support factors); access to treatment. Characteristics of the staff: Personal and professional attributes; competency; gender.	Clients: Age, gender, educational level, traits such as sense of control, cultural values, and beliefs. Staff: Communication abilities, demeanor, education background, level of competence or expertise in provided services, preferences for types of treatment, beliefs and attitudes toward target population. Staff members (women) delivering the courses: knowledge about breast cancer and self-help strategies; sensitivity to clients; good communication and teaching skills. Teaching protocol: objectives, content, learning activities, logistical instructions, training for instructors.
Process	Mediating processes, targeted activities, quality of implementation; quantity of process delivered (dosage/strength); frequency, duration; which clients received which components of the project at which dosage; sequence of change expected....	The self-help program had three components: cognitive, behavioral, and psychological. The course was given over six sessions (90 minutes each, once a week). The theoretical process involved this chain of events: attending course, increasing knowledge, engaging in self-care, decreasing uncertainty, improving affect, improving quality of life.
Product	The expected outcomes; reasons why the program was implemented; criteria to judge the effectiveness of the program; nature, timing, and pattern of change expected. (Nature of outcomes included particular changes in the clients' lives or condition; timing refers to when the change was expected to occur—immediately, short-term, or long-term.)	The self-help program expected positive changes in the quality of life about 6 months after the training; it should continue into the future. Improved quality of life was contingent upon the women's improvement in self-care and affect and the reduction of uncertainties.

Mixing Things Up

As most people know, life is rarely a linear pathway. Hence the use of linear models to depict evaluands is limited, because they do not portray deviations from what was planned or iterative changes that occur during the life of a program. A logic model is linear and suggests that action flows in one direction. However, the intended outcomes can focus on changes in participants, as well as changes in staff members as they progress through the project as well. These could lead to additional changes in the program that are not depicted in the logic model. Davies (2004) asserts that linear models are inadequate to depict the complexity of evaluands throughout the life of a project. He suggests that evaluators consider using more complex modeling strategies based on network analysis.

This chapter ends with an example of an evaluand that was depicted in both narrative and graphic form (Box 7.7). It is from an evaluation of a program to promote gender and ethnic/racial equality in Brazil. This is a funding initiative undertaken by the UNDP (2007). (Note: Don't be confused by the format of the chart in Box 7.7. Whereas the previous examples have had the inputs in the first column and the outcomes in the fourth column of the logic model, this UNDP chart is flipped horizontally, so that the inputs are in the fourth column and the outcomes are in the first column.)

Planning Your Evaluation: Stakeholders, Context, and Evaluand

Choose an evaluand for which you can develop an evaluation plan. This may be a program that you experienced at some time in your past, something related to your current position, or even a new idea that you would like to develop. Using one of the models for a logic model presented in this chapter, develop a logic model for your evaluand, at least as you presently understand it. Your understanding is expected to change throughout the planning process; therefore, be prepared to be flexible with this part of the process. Identify potential stakeholders for this evaluand; to the extent feasible, involve the stakeholders in the process of developing the evaluand. After you develop the logic model, write a narrative that explains the context of the evaluand and also provides additional details of what is depicted in the logic model. Share this narrative with a peer; obtain feedback as to the clarity and completeness of your depiction of the context and evaluand. Make revisions as necessary. If possible, obtain feedback from the stakeholders about your logic model and narrative.

Moving On to the Next Chapter

This chapter rests on the assumption that evaluators and stakeholders know what the evaluand should be or is. That is not necessarily the case, however. In Chapter 8, we look at strategies evaluators can use to provide information to stakeholders who are in the process of designing a new intervention or making substantial changes in an existing evaluand. This approach to evaluation is called "needs and assets assessment." We also look at other evaluation purposes and questions that might be used to guide the evaluation; we focus on how answers to those questions might be used to make changes in the organization.

Box 7.7. Inter-Agency Programme for the Promotion of Gender and Ethnic–Racial Equality in Public Policies in Brazil

Descriptive Portrayal of the Evaluand

III. Joint programme outputs

Expected outputs

This joint programme aims to support the implementation of the above-mentioned National Plans, with the following expected outputs:

1. Increased access to public services of excluded and vulnerable population groups.
2. Gender-based violence against women reduced.
3. Gender and ethnic–racial mainstreaming strengthened in public policy formulation, implementation, and monitoring.

Outcomes related to the expected outputs

1.1. Increased access of women, especially black and indigenous women, to reproductive health services (UNFPA, UNIFEM).
1.2. Production of local methodologies for the prevention and reduction of ethnic–racial vulnerabilities to HIV/AIDS among women, adolescents, and youth (UNICEF, UNFPA, UNIFEM).
1.3. Integrated actions aimed to strengthen gender and ethnic–racial institutionality in social control actions so as to ensure the appropriate monitoring and evaluation of direct cooperation among cities, and leveraging the access of women—especially blacks and indigenous—to housing ownership, safety, and keeping (UN-Habitat, UNIFEM, UNDP).

2.1 Support to the Maria da Penha Law[1] Implementation Watch, as a contribution to combating gender-based violence against women (UNFPA, UNIFEM, ILO, UNICEF, UN-Habitat, and UNDP).
2.2. Health, social service, and public security personnel trained to provide humanized nondiscriminatory attention to women and girls in situations of sexual violence and/or exploitation (UNICEF, UNIFEM, and UNFPA).
2.3. Methodological guide for attention to families in situations of violence, with a focus on gender and ethnic–racial vulnerabilities (UNFPA, UNIFEM, ILO, UNICEF, UN-Habitat, and UNDP).
3.1. Public sector managers and social actors trained to mainstream gender and ethnic–racial dimensions in the formulation, implementation, monitoring, and evaluation of policies and actions, as well as in the access to basic services (UNFPA, UNIFEM, ILO, UNICEF, UN-Habitat, and UNDP).
3.2. Public sector managers and social actors trained to mainstream gender and ethnic–racial dimensions in electoral processes, with a view to the increase

(cont.)

---

[1] A law on violence against women sanctioned by the President of Brazil in August 2006, named after the first Brazilian woman to sue (and win) the Brazilian state at the Inter-American Justice Court on gender-based violence.

Box 7.7 (cont.)

in the access of women—especially blacks and indigenous—to elective posts (UNFPA, UNIFEM, ILO, UNICEF, UN-Habitat, and UNDP).

3.3. Tools and indicators for the monitoring and evaluation of [the National Plan of Policies for Women] and [the National Policy to Promote Racist Equality] developed (UNFPA, UNIFEM, ILO, UNICEF, UN-Habitat, and UNDP).

National and local capacities to be strengthened through the programme

▓ Creation, strengthening, and increase of specific bodies for policies for women and for the promotion of racial equality at the top level of the federal, state, and municipal governments.

▓ Implementation of integrated public policies for the building up and promotion of gender and ethnic–racial equality.

▓ Public sector managers trained to mainstream the gender and ethnic–racial approaches, so as to guarantee the implementation of equalitarian public policies.

▓ Fulfillment of international treaties, agreements, and conventions signed and ratified by the Brazilian state in the areas of women's human rights, and combat[ing of] racism, racial discrimination, xenophobia, and related intolerances.

▓ Significant advancements towards the achievement of the MDGs.

▓ Implementation of affirmative action policies as tools for the full enjoyment of fundamental rights and liberties by different groups of women, especially blacks and indigenous.

▓ Promotion of a power balance between women and men, with a focus on black women, in the areas of economic resources, legal rights, political participation, and interpersonal relations.

▓ Progress in combating different forms of violence against women, including sexual exploitation and trafficking, with a focus on black women.

▓ Social participation and control in the formulation, implementation, monitoring, and evaluation of public policies, including the availability of data and indicators to the public and guaranteeing transparency.

Graphic Portrayal of the Evaluand: Excerpts from the Joint Programme Results Framework[2]

Expected outcome

2. Gender and racial–ethnic inequalities are reduced, taking into account territorial heterogeneities.

---

[2]This type of results framework should be done at a sufficiently strategic level that it does not exceed two pages.

Joint programme outcomes[3]	Outputs (by agency)	Indicative activities (by agency)	National and local partners
▨ Increased access to public services of excluded and vulnerable population groups.	1.1. Increased access of women, especially black and indigenous women, to reproductive health services (UNFPA, UNIFEM).	1.1.1. Support to networking of civil society organizations, mainly women's organizations, and especially black and indigenous women's organizations (UNFPA, UNIFEM).	Special Secretariat for Policies for Women (SPM) and the Special Secretariat for Policies for the Promotion of Racial Equality (SEPPIR).
		1.1.2. Support to the continued training and education of public health personnel, aimed to develop reproductive health capacities (UNFPA, UNIFEM).	
	1.2. Production of local methodologies for the prevention and reduction of ethnic–racial vulnerabilities to HIV/AIDS among women, adolescents, and youth (UNICEF, UNFPA, UNIFEM).	1.2.1. Design of methodological material on the prevention and reduction of ethnic–racial vulnerabilities to HIV/AIDS among women, adolescents, and youth (UNICEF, UNFPA, and UNIFEM).	
▨ Gender-based violence against women reduced.	2.1. Support to the Maria da Penha Law Implementation Watch, as a contribution to combating gender-based violence against women (UNFPA, UNIFEM, ILO, UNICEF, UN-Habitat, and UNDP).	2.1.1. Support to the networking of civil society organizations to combat gender-based violence against women, especially blacks and indigenous (UNFPA, UNICEF, UNIFEM, UNDP).	2.1.2. Support to the incorporation of combat to trafficking in persons for sexual exploitation into the scope of the Maria da Penha Law Implementation Watch (ILO, UNIFEM).

[3]Please note that outcomes do not have to be broken up by agency.

(cont.)

Box 7.7 *(cont.)*

Joint programme outcomes[3]	Outputs (by agency)	Indicative activities (by agency)	National and local partners
	2.2. Health, social service, and public security personnel trained to provide humanized nondiscriminatory attention to women and girls in situations of sexual violence and/ or exploitation (UNICEF, UNIFEM, and UNFPA).		
▪ Gender and ethnic–racial mainstreaming strengthened in public policy formulation, implementation, and monitoring.	3.1. Public sector managers and social actors trained to mainstream gender and ethnic–racial dimensions in the formulation, implementation, monitoring, and evaluation of policies and actions, as well as in the access to basic services (UNFPA, UNIFEM, ILO, UNICEF, UN-Habitat, and UNDP).	3.1.1. Seminar for the dissemination of poverty reduction and development promotion strategies for public managers at the federal, state, and municipal levels (UNFPA, UNIFEM, ILO, UNICEF, UN-Habitat, and UNDP). 3.1.2. Production and dissemination of communication material on actions to reduce poverty and promote development (UNFPA, UNIFEM, ILO, UNICEF, UN-Habitat, UNDP).	Special Secretariat for Policies for Women (SPM) and the Special Secretariat for Policies for the Promotion of Racial Equality (SEPPIR).

Joint programme outcomes[3]	Outputs (by agency)	Indicative activities (by agency)	National and local partners
	3.2. Public sector managers and social actors trained to mainstream gender and ethnic–racial dimensions in electoral processes, with a view to the increase in the access of women —especially blacks and indigenous—to elective posts (UNFPA, UNIFEM, ILO, UNICEF, UN-Habitat, and UNDP).	3.2.1. Preparation of reference contents for gender and ethnic–racial mainstreaming in the formulation, implementation, monitoring, and evaluation of policies and actions, and access to public services (UNFPA, UNIFEM, ILO, UNICEF, UN-Habitat, and UNDP).	
		3.2.2. Sensitization and training of public managers in the use of municipal reproductive health indicators (UNFPA, UNIFEM).	
	3.3. Tools and indicators for the monitoring and evaluation of PNPM and PNPIR developed (UNFPA, UNIFEM, ILO, UNICEF, UN-Habitat, and UNDP).	3.2.3. Training of trainers according to outputs 3.1 and 3.2 (UNFPA, UNICEF, UNIFEM, ILO, and UNDP).	

Source: UNDP (2007). Reprinted by permission of UNDP.

Preparing to Read Chapter Eight

As you are halfway through the book, you now have a good understanding of the landscape of the evaluation field, its history, its currently used paradigms, and the different theories and approaches in evaluation. In Chapter 7, you have learned how to identify the stakeholders and establish the context of the evaluand. Do you think by now you can list why evaluations are done?

1. Imagine that your school wants to establish a no-texting policy during classes or meetings. Try to list as many purposes for an evaluation of this type of initiative as you can.

2. Consider the following purposes for an evaluation of the no-texting policy:

   a. Is this a good policy?

   b. How well was it implemented?

   c. What were the results of implementing the policy?

3. What kind of data would you collect in order to address these purposes for the evaluation?

CHAPTER EIGHT

Evaluation Purposes,
Types, and Questions

This chapter moves the discussion from what is being evaluated to why the evaluation is needed, who needs to be involved in the process, and what evaluation questions need to be answered. Evaluation purposes and types are explored that focus on gaining insights into the needs and assets of a community, refining the implementation of a program, assessing program effects, and determining social transformation as a result of the evaluation process and outcomes. At this stage of the planning process, a general statement of how the evaluation findings are expected to be used can be derived from the statement of purpose. More specific plans for the use of data will surface when an evaluator is ready to make the data collection and reporting plans (see Chapters 10 and 13).

This chapter examines numerous evaluation types, organized into four main categories. We also want to add the caveat that most evaluations have multiple purposes. Examples of evaluations are used to illustrate different purposes. As usual, evaluators find themselves in a dynamic state: They need to identify people with whom to work in the initial planning stages (as discussed in Chapter 7), but the members of the stakeholder group may well expand and change as the purposes and questions are developed for the evaluation. This chapter therefore includes additional examples of ways to identify and engage with stakeholders.

Purposes and Types of Evaluation

The theme of the purposes and types of evaluation is one that surfaces at different levels of complexity throughout this text. In this chapter, examples of evaluations are introduced to provide a practice-grounded understanding of various evaluation purposes and types. These examples reflect not only multiple disciplines, but also various levels of evaluation work (e.g., large-scale vs. small-scale, local vs. national vs. international). The purposes and types of evaluation are broadly outlined in Box 8.1. The development of evaluation questions is integrally connected with the evaluation purposes and types; hence this chapter explores sample questions for different evaluation purposes and types.

The broadest purposes for evaluation can be characterized as legitimate or illegitimate. If evaluations are conducted to support foregone conclusions or as public relations pieces, then these are illegitimate purposes for evaluation. Evaluators should use their investigative skills to determine the sincerity of the stakeholders' purposes for requesting an evaluation. Legitimate purposes of evaluation include those listed in Box 8.1 when they are undertaken with an honest desire to gather information that is well balanced and adheres to the *The Program Standards Evaluation* (Joint Committee on Standards for Educational Evaluation, 2011) and relevant ethical principles.

Multipurpose Evaluations

The good news and bad news is that the majority of evaluations are conducted for multiple purposes. The good news is that you are relieved of the burden of deciding on only one purpose; the bad news is that you need to be able to sort through all of these purposes and decide which are appropriate in your context. (That is not really such bad news for those of us who enjoy the challenge.) An evaluation might start with needs and assets assessment, context evaluation, or capacity building; move to process evaluation, monitoring, or formative evaluation; and conclude with some kind of outcome or impact evaluation. Sometimes it will include evaluation for the purpose of replication or sustainability. Any of these purposes can be pursued for the purpose of social justice. Although all of these purposes can be pursued in any of the major evaluation branches, some of the branches put greater emphasis on specific purposes. For example, the Methods Branch puts great emphasis on impact evaluation. The Social Justice Branch puts greater emphasis on the purpose of achieving social transformation. If you look at the examples of evaluations throughout this book, you will see that most reflect one value system more clearly than others, and that most address more than one purpose.

Given the integral relationship between evaluation purposes and types on the one hand and evaluation and questions on the other, most of the rest of this chapter is organized by evaluation purposes and types. Hence you can use Box 8.1 as a guide throughout this chapter. Each type of evaluation is explained and illustrated with a sample evaluation study.

Purpose: To Gain Insights or to Determine Necessary Inputs

Evaluations that serve the purpose of gaining insights or determining necessary inputs are aligned with such evaluation types as context evaluation, capacity building, needs and assets assessment, and relevance evaluation (see Figure 8.1). In this section, each of those types is explained, along with examples of studies that illustrate the purpose, type, and evaluation questions.

Context Evaluation

Recall Stufflebeam et al.'s (2002) context analysis in their evaluation of the Hawaiian housing project (see Chapter 4, Box 4.3), in which they assessed the extent to which the project addressed the needs of the community and the adequacy and appropriateness of resources that were brought to bear in the project. They gathered environmental data about the demographics, economic conditions, available projects and services, and needs of the community members. They also conducted interviews with stakeholders who had contact with members of the targeted community, such as teachers and social workers. They were able to conduct this environmental scan for the first 4 years of the

Box 8.1. Evaluation Purposes and Types

Purposes	*Types of evaluation*
To gain insights or to determine necessary inputs. For example:	▪ Context evaluation
	▪ Capacity building
▪ To assess and build capacity in the community.	▪ Needs and assets assessment
▪ To assess needs, desires, and assets of community members.	▪ Organizational assessment
▪ To identify needed inputs, barriers, and facilitators to program development or implementation.	▪ Relevance evaluation
▪ To determine feasibility of methods to describe and measure program activities and effects.	
To find areas in need of improvement or to change practices. For example:	▪ Implementation evaluation
	▪ Responsive evaluation
▪ To refine plans for introducing a new service.	▪ Participatory evaluation
▪ To characterize the extent to which intervention plans were implemented.	▪ Process evaluation
▪ To improve the content of educational materials.	▪ Monitoring
▪ To enhance the program's cultural competence.	▪ Formative evaluation
▪ To verify that participants' rights are protected.	▪ Developmental evaluation
▪ To set priorities for staff training.	
▪ To make midcourse adjustments to improve participant logistics.	
▪ To improve the clarity of communication messages.	
▪ To determine whether customer satisfaction rates can be improved.	
▪ To mobilize community support for the program.	

(cont.)

Box 8.1 (*cont.*)

Purposes	*Types of evaluation*
To assess program effectiveness. For example:	▨ Outcome/impact evaluation
	▨ Summative evaluation
▨ To assess skills development, knowledge gain, and/or attitude and behavior changes by program participants.	▨ Policy evaluation
	▨ Replicability/exportability/transferability evaluation
▨ To compare changes in provider behavior over time.	▨ Sustainability evaluation
▨ To compare costs with benefits.	▨ Cost analysis
▨ To find out which participants do well in the program.	
▨ To decide where to allocate new resources.	
▨ To document the level of success in accomplishing objectives.	
▨ To demonstrate that accountability requirements are fulfilled.	
▨ To aggregate information from several evaluations to estimate outcome effects for similar kinds of programs.	
▨ To gather success stories.	
To address issues of human rights and social justice. For example:	▨ DDE
	▨ CLE
▨ To broaden consensus among coalition members regarding program goals.	▨ CRT evaluation
	▨ Indigenous evaluation
▨ To support organizational change and development.	▨ Culturally responsive evaluation
▨ To determine inequities on the basis of gender, race, ethnicity, disability, and other relevant dimensions of diversity.	▨ Disability- and deaf-rights-based evaluation
	▨ Feminist evaluation
	▨ Gender analysis
	▨ Transformative participatory evaluation

Source: Based on CDC (1999, p. 12).

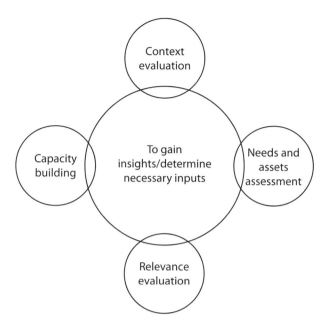

Figure 8.1. Purposes of evaluations related to gaining insights or determining necessary inputs.

project, which is a bit unusual for evaluation studies. Revisit Chapters 4 and 7 to review evaluation questions and methods that are associated with context evaluation.

Capacity Building

When considering who needs to be involved in the evaluation planning, evaluators need to consider the capacities and cultures of the stakeholders with whom they are working.

Preskill and Torres (1999) contributed greatly to strategies to determine the readiness of an organization to participate in and benefit from evaluation studies. Recall from Chapter 4 Preskill and Torres's model for evaluation called learning organization evaluation, in which they argue for the importance of determining the organization's expertise in, experience with, and culture of evaluation. They recognize four main factors that needed to be addressed in a capacity-building initiative: leadership, organizational structures, culture, and communication. This might mean that evaluators start with a group of highly motivated staff members to carry out an evaluation that includes capacity building, on the assumption that success breeds success.

Sutherland's (2004) study (see Chapter 4, Box 4.9) focused on school reform and building evaluation capacity in a school system where poverty runs high. The evaluator needed to be aware of different levels of expertise, attitudes toward evaluation, and willingness to be involved with evaluation at different levels in the organization. In any group or organization, these may be quite different in the top level of management, the lower-level administrators, the service providers, and the participants. Sutherland argued that in her study, the upper levels of administration needed to mandate the use of data for improvement as external motivation to the rest of the organization. Evaluators in other branches might view this approach as appropriate, unnecessary, or too top-down to achieve real change.

Nevertheless, evaluators can benefit from knowing about an organization's past experiences with evaluations, as well as its expertise in and willingness to use evaluation as a way of ongoing improvement. If the expertise is absent or insufficient, then evaluators may need to undertake capacity building within the organization by instituting training programs, workshops, or community meetings to this end. Two contrasting examples of capacity building provide insights into this process—one at an international development agency (Taut, 2007), and the other at a large government research center (Milstein, Chapel, Wetterhall, & Cotton, 2002).

Taut (2007) was engaged to conduct an action research study centered on capacity building in evaluation at an international development agency. She identified the key factors in this process as focusing on a specific organizational need; provision of training through multiple methods that were interactive and directly applicable on the job; and long-term efforts backed up by organizational structures. She began with a needs assessment (discussed below) in order to determine the level of knowledge about evaluation, its current uses, and attitudes toward evaluation. She found that expertise varied considerably within the organization; that the use of evaluation findings was considered to be insufficient; and that many people did not see the usefulness of engaging in more evaluation activities.

This cultural context presented many challenges to capacity building in evaluation, some of which were not overcome in Taut's (2007) study. Capacity building interventions included the following:

1. An expert facilitator provided three 1-day workshops that were attended by 47 staff members. The workshops were designed to provide the staffers with a rationale for increasing their expertise in evaluation and their skills in the conduct of evaluations, as well as an opportunity to plan an evaluation of a project of their own. The goal of having the 47 staff members conduct evaluations was greatly scaled back to the two participants who were willing to do so.

2. The evaluator mentored the participants in the conduct of these two evaluation projects. The staff members who resisted conducting evaluations justified their position on the basis that the organization's management did not provide incentives or support for this kind of work.

3. The organization supported the development and dissemination of additional resources via a website and email discussion groups on evaluation.

4. The organization's evaluation unit staff also attended the workshop and was trained to facilitate future workshops.

Milstein et al. (2002) described a large-scale overhaul of the capacity for the conduct of evaluations in the CDC. The CDC's budget of $2.8 billion is used to control and prevent diseases worldwide. However, agency officials raised concerns about the quality of evaluations conducted under the CDC's auspices, as well as the capability of their staff and many partners to conduct effective evaluations. To address this challenge, the CDC set up a working group with two charges: to produce a framework for evaluation at the

CDC, and to promote program evaluation practice there. The working group convened a larger workshop group to begin the development of the framework, which was then developed and field-tested. They also undertook "listening sessions" over a 5-month period to determine current attitudes toward evaluation and strategies for institutional change. The listening sessions took many forms: individual and group interviews, focus groups, "brown-bag" discussions, and workshops. The evaluators engaged with over 250 CDC staff members and representatives from other related organizations. These sessions revealed the need for a clearly understood definition of evaluation; increased use of logic models or other graphic models to communicate about programs and their evaluations; and the use of multiple methods for evaluation design, methods, data collection, and analysis.

In terms of evaluation capacity building, Milstein et al. (2002) identified the need for support and direction from organizational leadership; increased funding; recruitment of staff with evaluation expertise; organization-wide training; technical assistance for those undertaking evaluations; and sharing of information about strategies for evaluations and use of their findings. These are similar to the elements that were identified in the Taut (2007) study. In addition, CDC contributors recognized the importance of involving community members in the evaluation planning; the need for integration of health information systems to prevent duplication of effort; and the importance of accountability to funders (in the CDC's case, the funding source is the U.S. Congress). The development of training materials was informed by a literature review based on published and unpublished materials, websites, conference proceedings, and the AEA listserv (EvalTalk). The framework was developed on the basis of the data collected from the listening sessions and the literature review.

· · · · · · · · · · EXTENDING YOUR THINKING · · · · · · · · · ·
Evaluation Capacity Building

In a recent post on Patricia Rogers and Jane Davidson's Genuine Evaluation blog (*genuineevaluation.com/how-much-is-enough-evaluation-capacity-building*), one blogger asks, "So my question is, what is that we seek to achieve through [community-]based [evaluation capacity building]—a world full of do-it-yourself evaluators, heaven forbid? What are the potential downsides of taking people away from their work and asking them to contribute to and better understand what we do?" Before you go to the blog to read how other evaluators responded to this question, what would your response be?

Needs and Assets Assessment

"Needs assessment" is a commonly used term when evaluators are at the beginning of the planning process and in a position to provide information to program planners about what the evaluand should entail. This is fine, except that evaluators often focus on needs to the exclusion of assets. This can lead to an overemphasis on needs and to a focus on deficits; the strengths of an organization or community are thus overlooked. When an organization is developing a new program, or when there is a desire to make substantial changes in an existing program, needs and assets assessments can contribute to that process. These assessments can fulfill a number of specific purposes: providing a picture of the community (context); identifying demographic groups and geographic areas in need; providing guidance in the prioritization and use of resources such as funding to address important needs; and convincing policy makers that they should support initiatives in this community (CSAP, 2008). CSAP recommends examining both risk factors (needs) and protective factors (assets). Such conditions are common in evaluation contexts; therefore, this purpose for evaluation is explored further here.

We begin with two quotations from Altschuld and Kumar (2010):

> Needs assessment is the process of identifying needs, prioritizing them, making needs-based decisions, allocating resources, and implementing actions in organizations to resolve problems underlying important needs. (p. 20)

> Formally, need is the measurable gap between two conditions—"what is" (the current status or state) and "what should be" (the desired status or state). (p. 2)

Altschuld and Kumar (2010) thus provide us with a definition of needs assessment and raise the important point that it involves identifying a discrepancy between what is and what should be. (Simply asking people about what they think they need is not considered needs assessment; Altschuld and Kumar call this "needs sensing.") Altschuld and Kumar primarily discuss needs assessment; however, they acknowledge the importance of identifying a community's assets as well. In this section, we integrate the discussion of needs and assets assessments as tools to gain insights into an organization's or communities' needs, strengths, and resources.

For a needs assessment, Altschuld and Kumar present a model that involves three phases of assessment (see Figure 8.2) and three levels of needs (see Figure 8.3). Information for the primary level in Figure 8.3 may be available from organizational databases, although nonparticipants who are eligible for services would probably not be included. Because these stakeholders may be more difficult to reach, evaluators sometimes assume that working with the secondary-level stakeholders can accurately identify the needs at the primary level.

Preassessment methods typically include archival data review (i.e., review of extant reports and databases), as well as data generated by individual and group meetings and interviews. In the preassessment phase, evaluators can ask such questions as these (based on Altschuld & Kumar, 2010, pp. 36–37):

- What issue or problem is concerning you?
- What knowledge do you have about it right now? What resources are available that are relevant to understanding this issue?
- Which groups of people are most affected by the discrepancy between what is and what should be? Are there differences of opinion about this?
- What has the organization done in the past to address this discrepancy? What are the challenges that still remain?

These additional questions (based on *WKKF Evaluation Handbook*, 1998, p. 23) also have relevance for needs and organizational assessments:

Preassessment

■ Ascertaining the status of the organization in terms of what is already known or available about its needs and assets. If sufficient information is available, the evaluator might skip assessment and move on.

Assessment

■ Collecting new information about the organization's needs and assets.

Postassessment

■ Using the information from the first two phases to design appropriate interventions.

Figure 8.2. Three phases of assessment. *Source:* Based on Altschuld and Kumar (2010).

Primary level

■ Includes recipients of services, such as students, parents, clients, patients, homeless people, people with disabilities, or mothers with HIV/AIDS.

Secondary level

■ Includes individuals and groups who deliver the services, such as staff, teachers, administrators, social workers, medical personnel, trainers, and so on.

Tertiary level

■ Includes the systems of support found in organizations, resources, and structures for those who provide the services (e.g., buildings, facilities, classrooms, transportation systems, salaries, benefits).

Figure 8.3. Three levels of needs. *Source:* Based on Altschuld and Kumar (2010).

■ What are the values that underlie this project and how do those map onto the values of the parent organization?

■ What is the nature of the relationship between the project and the parent organization in terms of finances, physical space, and administrative structures?

■ How does the leadership and organizational structure support or impede the success of the project?

■ What are the characteristics of the staff and the leadership?

■ What is the organizational culture with regard to the project and evaluation?

■ What resources are available in terms of funding, staffing, organizational support, expertise, and educational opportunities?

CSAP (2008) provides a sample list of needs (risk factors) and assets (protective factors) in substance abuse prevention contexts (see Box 8.2). Some factors can be either risk or protective factors, depending on what is happening in the community. For example, if drugs are easily available, then this is a risk factor; if not, this is a protective factor.

Box 8.2. Sample Risk and Protective Factors in Substance Abuse Prevention

Community:

■ Availability of drugs

■ Community laws/norms

■ Transitions and mobility

■ Low neighborhood attachment/ community disorganization

■ Extreme economic and social deprivation

Family:

■ Family history of substance abuse

■ Family management problems

■ Family conflict

■ Favorable parental attitudes/ involvement

School:

■ Lack of commitment to school

■ Early and persistent antisocial behavior

■ Academic failure beginning in late elementary school

Individual/peer:

■ Alienation/rebelliousness

■ Friends who engage in the problem behavior

■ Favorable attitudes toward the problem behavior

■ Early initiation of the problem behavior

Source: CSAP (2008).

In Taut's (2007) assessment of the training needs for capacity building in an international development agency, she described her preassessment and assessment activities as document analysis, staff surveys, participant observation, and interviews. The documents were evaluation reports, work plans, strategic plans, and others relevant to the evaluation activities in the organization. The survey was adapted from Preskill and Torres (2001) Readiness for Organizational Learning and Evaluation instrument and from a similar instrument developed by Cousins, Goh, and Lee (2003). The items on the survey asked about the participants' perceptions of evaluation, leadership, structures, communication, and culture; their experiences with and attitudes toward evaluation, monitoring, and reporting activities; and their background and training in evaluation. Her participant observation was conducted over a 3-year period and included everyday activities as well as those specific to evaluation and strategic planning. She interviewed current and past employees to ascertain additional information about the organization's needs and assets. She used this information to move on to the postassessment phase (i.e., using her data to design the intervention described earlier).

Grigg-Saito, Och, Liang, Toof, and Silka (2008) provide an excellent example of assessing both needs and assets in their work related to health services for a Cambodian refugee community in Massachusetts. Recall that Silka's work (see Chapter 7) reflects a social justice orientation through protection of overresearched groups and a cyclical approach to determining needs and developing and testing interventions. Grigg-Saito et al. (2008) began their work in health promotion and outreach by identifying and building on the strengths in the Cambodian community: "strong community input for planning, an influential self-initiated Cambodian Elders' Council, ties to local Buddhist temples, the presence of numerous Cambodian businesses, cultural respect for elders, strong family relationships, and enjoyment of social events" (p. 415). The Elder Council in particular was instrumental in advising the evaluators and program developers about their networks of social support, providing access to Khmer-language radio and TV stations, guiding the development of meaningful cultural events, effective messages about strengthening healthy behaviors (e.g., decreased smoking rates and increased fruit and vegetable consumption). The data collection and program development were bolstered by having bilingual, bicultural staff members who assisted in developing training for the entire staff.

As the Grigg-Saito et al. (2008) example illustrates, the process of mapping community needs and assets can help you do many things:

- Identify existing community action groups and understand the history of their efforts.
- Identify existing formal, informal, and potential leaders.
- Identify community needs and gaps in services.
- Identify community strengths and opportunities.
- Understand your target population (both needs and assets) in order to improve, build, and secure project credibility within the community.
- Create a momentum for project activities by getting community input.

Mapping community needs and assets can also help you determine the appropriateness of project goals and provide baseline data for later outcome evaluations.

Organizational assessment can be a valuable part of needs and assets assessment.

Through an organizational assessment, project staff can examine the internal dynamics of a project to see how these dynamics may be hindering or supporting project success. Questions to be addressed might include the following (WKKF, 1998, p. 23):

- What are the values or environment of the project (internal) and its larger institutional context (umbrella organization)? How are they the same? How do differences in values impede project activities?

- What are the fiduciary, physical space, and other collaborative and administrative relationships between the project and its umbrella institution? How do they relate to project accomplishments or failures? For a proposed activity, are these arrangements adequate?

- What [are] the structure and size of the project in relation to [those] of the umbrella organization?

- How [do] the leadership and organizational structure of the project influence its effectiveness? What is the complexity of the organizational chart? Do organizational decision-making bodies impede or strengthen ongoing or proposed activities?

- What are the characteristics of project staff and leadership? How are project members recruited? What is the organizational culture?

- What resources (e.g., funding, staffing, organizational and/or institutional support, expertise, and educational opportunities) are available to the project and to the evaluation?

- To what extent are opportunities to participate in the evaluation process available for people who have a stake in the project's outcome?

If an organizational assessment does not fully explain the project's strengths and weaknesses in serving its target population, another contextual area to examine might be whether changes in federal and state climates may be having an impact on the community and project.

Furthermore, examining the external and internal contextual environments of a project provides the groundwork for implementation and outcome evaluation. It helps to explain why a project has been implemented the way it has, and why certain outcomes have been achieved and others have not. Evaluating the multiple contexts of a project may also point to situations that limit a project's ability to achieve anticipated outcomes, or lead to the realization that specific interventions and their intended outcomes may be difficult to measure or to attribute to the project itself (WKKF, 1998).

External–internal factors in international development may be political and may influence needs assessments and/or implementation and outcome evaluations. An example is in southern Somalia, where poor governance, years of war, soaring food prices, and drought have been causing a deteriorating humanitarian situation for 2.3 million people, despite interventions by foreign donor agencies. Bradbury, Hofmann, Maxwell, Venekamp, and Montani (2003) reviewed the assessment practices of 36 international aid agencies and 10 donor representatives and reports. They found that humanitarian agencies' needs assessments proved difficult to carry out, and that they used varying conceptual models: Some focused on immediate needs such as food and shelter, while others attempted to measure vulnerability or risk to overall security. They concluded that there were inadequacies and a lack of internal capacity in assessing needs and in monitoring the development assistance; therefore, the humanitarian assistance given was not truly needs-driven, despite the fact that people were in acute life-threatening situations. Instead, slower long-term processes were put into place for disaster mitigation, peace building, and programs for supporting livelihoods. Saving lives was no longer the sole objective, or even the highest-priority objective, of humanitarian interventions. "[The finding that] needs assessments ultimately have little influence on resource allocation, among donors and of many aid agencies, suggests that this is fundamentally a political rather than a technical issue" (Bradbury et al., 2003, p. 57).

· · · · · · · · · EXTENDING YOUR THINKING · · · · · · · · · ·
Needs and Assets Assessment

1. Kretzmann and McKnight (2005) have created the Capacity Inventory, which they use at their Asset-Based Community Development Institute (ABCDI; *www.abcdinstitute.org*). The Capacity Inventory is used with community groups to identify the strengths, skills, and knowledge of their members and other local organizations to build sustainable, strong communities. The inventory is purposefully created to be easy to read by all community members, as they are participants in the process of finding out the needs of the community by first learning what their strengths are. Look at these three tools on the ABCDI website (click on "Resources" and then scroll down to "Mapping tools"):

   a. Introduction to Capacity Inventories

   b. The Capacity Inventory

   c. How to Use the Capacity Inventory

   ABCDI shares several stories of community projects using the asset-based approach (go to the website and click on "Community Stories"). Select one of the stories listed below, and note the assets the evaluators and community members found. Discuss how they used the assets for building and strengthening their programs.

   ▪ KaBOOM!—Building community one playground at a time, Washington, DC.

   ▪ Mercado Central—Community entrepreneurship in St. Paul, Minnesota.

   ▪ Greater Rochester Health Foundation—Neighborhood Health Status Improvement Projects, Rochester, New York.

   ▪ Fig Tree Community Garden—New South Wales, Australia.

   ▪ The Denver Foundation—Strengthening Neighborhoods Program, Denver, Colorado.

   ▪ Seattle's Columbia City—Columbia City Revitalization, Seattle, Washington.

   ▪ Southeast Raleigh Community Garden—Project FACT, Raleigh, North Carolina.

   (cont.)

2. Read the following imaginary scenario:

"Soaring Eagles" is a nonprofit organization that promotes positive development for youth who have incarcerated parent(s) and provides them with counseling and with adult mentors in the community. High school teachers are concerned that increasing numbers of these youth are truant from school; the teachers are especially worried about the effect on graduation rates. A team of school administrators has decided to investigate the situation, and possibly to add services and mentors during the school day in the school.

    a. What can the team do to respond to this question: "What are the underlying needs and conditions that must be addressed?"

    b. Who should be on the committee or work group to collect the data? Which key stakeholders need to be included?

    c. Imagine what data may be available for assessing needs (risk factors) and assets (protective factors).

    d. Determine what data still need to be collected by the team that may not be available.

    e. Determine the best methods to gather the data, and develop a data collection plan. How will the team gather that data? Surveys? Interviews? Collecting documents? Who? What? How?

Relevance Evaluation

In international development evaluation, the "gaining insight" purpose of evaluation is typically labeled "relevance," or the extent to which the aid activity is responsive to the project's priorities as viewed by the donors and government agencies. The OECD DAC (2006a) suggests that questions such as these are helpful in relevance evaluation:

    ■ To what extent are objectives of the program still valid?

    ■ To what extent are the activities and outputs of the current program consistent with the overall aims of the program and the intended outcomes?

    ■ How do these activities contribute to the attainment of the objectives?

Chianca (2008) has criticized the OECD DAC's conceptualization of relevance as being too narrowly focused on the goals and priorities of the donor agencies or the country-level governments, instead of on the needs of the targeted population (primary-level needs, according to Altschuld & Kumar, 2010). This narrow focus on goals may eclipse the true value of the program for the recipients of the services. Chianca suggests that international development evaluation would benefit from a more expansive view of relevance that includes the recipients' views of needs, rather than only the perspectives of the donors and/or government agencies.

Purpose: To Find Areas in Need of Improvement or to Change Practices

The second major category of evaluation purposes is to figure out areas in need of improvement or to change practices; hence the focus is on the implementation of a program, including the processes, materials, staffing, and other aspects of the program in process. This category of purposes includes the following evaluation types (see Figure 8.4): implementation evaluation, monitoring (in international development), process evaluation, formative evaluation, developmental evaluation, responsive evaluation, and participatory evaluation (these last two can also be used for other purposes). These evaluation types are focused on determining why or why not desired outcomes are achieved, and what needs to be changed if the outcomes are not being successfully achieved.

Implementation Evaluation

Implementation evaluation may be needed if a new program is being implemented or if data indicate that goals of an existing program are not being satisfactorily achieved. Implementation evaluations can be focused on identifying strengths and challenges in the implementation of a program; reassessing the appropriateness of the program under changing conditions; assessing the extent to which the appropriate resources were available; measuring perceptions of the program by the community, staff, and participants; determining the quality of the services provided; and monitoring stakeholders' experiences.

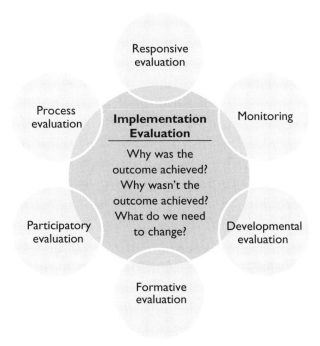

Figure 8.4. Types of evaluation associated with improvement and change purposes.

The WKKF evaluation handbook (WKKF, 1998, p. 24) lists these questions as part of an implementation evaluation:

- What are the critical components/activities of this project (both explicit and implicit)?

- How do these components connect to the goals and intended outcomes for this project?

- What aspects of the implementation process are facilitating success or acting as stumbling blocks for the project?

- How is the program being implemented and how does that compare to the initial plan for implementation?

- What changes might be necessary in organizational structure, recruitment materials, support for participants, resources, facilities, scheduling, location, transportation, strategies, or activities?

- To what extent is the program serving the intended participants? Who is being excluded and why?

Fixsen, Naoom, Blasé, Friedman, and Wallace (2005) divide implementation evaluation into three components:

1. Were the required resources available (e.g., staff qualifications and numbers, ratio of service providers to recipients, supervisor–practitioner relations, locations of service provision, access to and effectiveness of training)?

2. To what extent was the program implemented according to the core components described in the plan?

3. How competent were the service providers, with specific reference to the program's core components?

Fixsen, Panzano, Naoom, and Blasé (2008) describe measures they have used to measure implementation of programs in the area of therapy and child development. These can also be accessed at the National Implementation Research Network website (*nirn.fpg.unc.edu*).

Responsive Evaluation

Stake (1991) raises issues relevant to process evaluation in his discussions of responsive evaluation. He asks about the match between what was planned and what was delivered, the strength of the treatment (sometimes called dosage, i.e., how much of the intervention was actually delivered), effects of providing ongoing feedback to the stakeholders, and changes in the program from its initial stages throughout to its conclusion. Reread the section of Chapter 5 that explains Stake's responsive evaluation, along with the Los Angeles school achievement study (Barela, 2008; see Chapter 5, Box 5.2) and the dance injury prevention study (Abma, 2005; see Chapter 5, Box 5.4). Barela (2008) used responsive evaluation as part of the framework for his case study. His evaluation purpose and question most closely illustrating responsive evaluation were as follows: "The second purpose was to determine how these schools implemented their core curriculum, with particular attention to English Language Learners and students with disabilities. The associated evaluation question is learning driven, focusing on identifying best practices" (Barela in interview with Christie, 2008, p. 536).

In the Abma (2005) study, the stakeholders wanted to know what they could do to decrease the number of injuries for the dancers; they were looking for data to support a change in practices.

Process Evaluation

Process evaluation has been introduced in Chapter 4 as part of the discussion of Stuffle-beam's CIPP model of evaluation theory and practice. This is a good time to review the meaning of process evaluation as it is explained in Chapter 4, along with the summary and discussion of the Hawaiian housing study (Stufflebeam et al., 2002; see Chapter 4, Box 4.3). Chapter 4 includes a rubric for developing and assessing quality of a process evaluation. The process evaluation question that guided Stufflebeam and colleagues in their evaluation was "To what extent were the project's operations consistent with plans responsibly conducted, and effective in addressing beneficiaries' needs?"

King (2007) provides us with strategies for using process evaluation as a means to build evaluation capacity. She includes the context evaluation as a first step (i.e., examining the organization's culture and expertise in evaluation, as well as mandates and accountability demands such as policy, legislation, and funding requirements). The context assessment may reveal people with a passionate interest in evaluation; King calls these passionate people "evaluation champions." She suggests establishing an advisory group headed by an evaluation champion and made up of staff members who have competence, motivation, and a sense of humor. The advisory group will be charged with the responsibility of shepherding the capacity-building process. The evaluator's responsibility is to communicate clearly the intent to build the organization's capacity to conduct evaluations, and to describe the strategies that will be used during the process evaluation to do that. This sets the stage for a synergistic relationship to develop between the evaluator and the advisory group. The evaluator needs to be aware of teachable moments during the planning and implementation of the evaluation, noting when additional instruction might be useful for the group. This might entail providing instruction on data collection methods, validity, reliability, statistical terms, or data interpretation. It also requires interpersonal skills related to conflict resolution, team building, negotiations, and cultural competence. King (2007) also recommends keeping a "paper trail" of the capacity-building activities that can form the basis of a framework for evaluation, just as Milstein et al. (2002) did for the CDC. Reflecting on the process of planning and conducting an evaluation provides opportunities to learn from this experience and build better practices into the next evaluation.

King (2007) also describes several examples of process evaluations that were used to build capacity. In a large school district, she trained staff members in how to write survey items, conduct focus groups, and analyze data. She also worked with a social service agency in which all staffers are required to attend a half-day workshop as an introduction to evaluation, every program has a logic model, and the staff members work together with the evaluation advisory group to improve their skills in evaluation. Another important facet that supports the link between process evaluation and capacity building is access to databases, so that information is accessible and can be shared.

Shen, Yang, Cao, and Warfield (2008) conducted a process evaluation for the purpose of determining the "fidelity of treatment." In other words, to what extent was the program that was implemented reflective of the program as planned? They also raised this question: To what extent were changes made that were necessary once the implementation had begun? Was the program modified in order to be more responsive to the target population or other contextual factors? This set of questions relates to tensions that exist between the various evaluation branches. Evaluators in the Methods Branch would argue that a program has to be implemented as planned, or its effectiveness cannot be validly tested. Evaluators in other branches might argue that adjustments in the program are appropriate in order to increase the value of the program to the participants, enhance use of evaluation findings, and/or further the goals of social justice and human rights.

Monitoring in International Development

Monitoring in international development has been defined in Chapter 1; it involves an ongoing assessment of a project's progress. In this sense, it is a process evaluation. The World Bank (Baker, 2000) distinguishes monitoring and process evaluation as follows: "Monitoring will help to assess whether a program is being implemented as was planned. A program monitoring system enables continuous feedback on the status of program implementation, identifying specific problems as they arise. Process evaluation is concerned with how the program operates and focuses on problems in service delivery" (p. 1).

In international development evaluation, monitoring can focus more on the progress toward outcomes than on the actual processes that are implemented. Chianca (2008) notes that international development evaluators tend to limit their focus to outcomes and impact, and do not give sufficient attention to the quality of the process. He suggests that process evaluation in international development would be improved if it addressed these criteria for quality (based on Chianca, 2008, pp. 46–47):

- Ethicality (e.g., are any ethical norms not observed in the delivery of services to recipients or in the treatment of staff?)

- Environmental responsibility (e.g., are the intervention's activities producing current or future damage to the environment?)

- Scientific soundness (e.g., does the program follow sound scientific knowledge or accepted best-practice guidance of the relevant sector, based on research and evaluations of similar interventions?)

- Adoption of alleged specifications (e.g., is the intervention delivering what was promised?)

- Coverage (e.g., are the targeted people being covered; do men and women, boys and girls have equal access to benefits; and is the intervention covering an appropriate number of recipients?)

- Responsiveness (e.g., is the intervention adequately responding to the changing environment?)

- Stakeholder participation (e.g., do men and women, boys and girls, and/or relevant subgroups in the society have equal opportunities to participate in program decisions and activities?)

- Cultural appropriateness (e.g., are the services and activities being delivered in accordance to local cultural norms?)

Sample evaluation questions for monitoring studies in international development include these from the USAID (2009):

Monitoring Questions

■ Is the program achieving its objectives?

■ Is the program measuring up against performance standards?

Evaluation Questions

■ Which aspects of operations have had an impact on the intended beneficiaries?

■ Which factors in the environment have impeded or contributed to the program's success?

■ How is the relationship between the program's inputs, activities, outputs, and outcomes most accurately explained?

■ What impacts has the program had beyond its intended objectives?

■ What would have occurred if the program had not been implemented?

■ How has the program performed in comparison to similar programs?

. . . . E X T E N D I N G   Y O U R   T H I N K I N G . . . .

Monitoring and Evaluation

In February 2010, USAID opened a new Department of Evaluation, Policy Analysis and Learning. Ruth Levine, the new department's director, spoke at the InterAction Forum in Washington, D.C. (June 2, 2010), stating that the office will be supporting initiatives that apply the best available evidence to make development assistance decisions throughout the world. Levine said that USAID will now use varying evaluation designs in order to ascertain where USAID is making the most impact. USAID Administrator Dr. Rajiv Shah (2010) supported Levine's statement and stated that instead of continuing the practice of generating 800-page evaluations that go unread and unused, that USAID will focus on evidence-based development research.

At the website for Demographic and Health Surveys (*www.measuredhs.com/aboutsurveys/start.cfm*), you can see an illustration of how USAID's monitoring has focused more on the progress toward outcomes than on the actual processes that were implemented in its monitoring of programs. This website states that Demographic and Health Surveys "supports a range of data collection options that can be tailored to fit specific monitoring and evaluation needs of host countries." Enjoy opening the many surveys posted on the site, and consider the questions that are asked of the participants. On the sidebar, there is a link to qualitative data collection tools for monitoring and evaluation. Click on this link and explore what is there. What information might be missing about "process" from these surveys that could be important for the monitoring of these programs? What would you add that might be missing?

Developmental Evaluation

Based on his work in UFE (see Chapter 4), Patton (2010; Donaldson et al., 2010) has expanded on developmental evaluation as a purpose for evaluations that is distinctly different from formative evaluation. He states that developmental evaluation

> is an *additional distinct purpose* that would in *no* way replace formative and summative, but is an additional distinct purpose. I'm arguing that there are kinds of interventions that involve ongoing development, and that the development of something is different from improving it.... *developmental evaluation* ... is a purpose[ful] distinction—to develop through ongoing adaptation, especially under conditions of complexity. (Patton, as a contributor to Donaldson et al., 2010, p. 25; emphasis in original)

When organizations see themselves in a constantly responsive mode based on new developments in the field or reaching new populations, they do not want to stop changing their programs. Hence the notion of formative evaluation's leading to program improvement, followed by a static period in which the program does not change in order to facilitate measurement of outcomes in a summative manner, and does not fit with the organization's needs. This gap between formative and summative evaluations is what Patton uses as a rationale for developmental evaluation. Developmental evaluation focuses on "ongoing adaptation to a changing environment and changing dynamics under the presumption that there will never be a fixed model" (Patton as a contributor to Donaldson et al., 2010, p. 28).

Purpose: To Assess Program Effectiveness

The third major category of evaluation purposes is to assess a program's effectiveness. This category incudes the following evaluation types (see Figure 8.5): summative evaluation, outcome/impact evaluation, policy evaluation, replicability/exportability/transferability evaluation, sustainability evaluation, and cost analysis.

Outcome/Impact Evaluation

Recall from Chapter 7 that evaluation planning typically involves the identification of short- and long-term results for a project. Outcome evaluation focuses on short-term results; impact evaluation focuses on long-term results (see Figure 8.6).

A focus on outcomes or impacts is most similar to the concept of summative evaluation. We have examined the identification of short- and long-term goals and impact in the section of Chapter 7 about logic models.

Evaluators can start outcome/impact evaluations with these questions (WKKF, 1998, p. 28).

■ What are the critical outcomes you are trying to achieve?

■ What impact is the project having on its clients, its staff, its umbrella organization, and its community?

■ What unexpected impact has the project had?

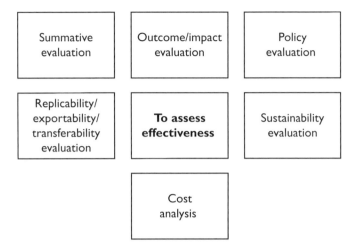

Figure 8.5. Types of evaluation associated with assessing effectiveness.

Outcome/impact evaluations can be useful for demonstrating that a project is or is not achieving its goals; making a case for additional funding, revisions, expansions, or replications; and answering questions about differential effectiveness with subgroups in the community.

Outcomes can be thought of at different levels. For example, at the individual level, evaluators can ask: What difference did this program make in the lives of the individuals who participated in it? An individual difference might be for these individuals to obtain job skills and employment sufficient to support themselves and their families; to obtain medical insurance and child care; or to have improved health status. Contrast such a statement of outcomes with such ideas as that a certain number of people will attend a workshop (this is not specific about the outcome for the individuals). Evaluators should also be aware that interim outcomes may need to be accomplished before the primary

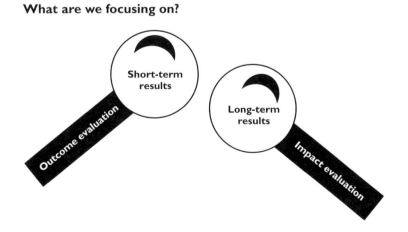

Figure 8.6. Outcome versus impact evaluation.

intended outcomes can materialize. For example, individuals may have to leave an abusive relationship, get secure housing, or stop using illegal drugs before they can fully engage in an employment program.

Often programs are designed to serve individuals and their families; hence outcomes need to be thought about at this broader level. Examples might include improved communication, safety for children, and parent–child interactions. At the even broader community level, outcomes can be thought of as "increased civic engagement and participation, decreased violence, shifts in authority and responsibility from traditional institutions to community-based agencies and community resident groups, or more intensive collaboration among community agencies and institutions" (WKKF, 1998, p. 31).

The Early Childhood Outcomes Center developed a set of outcomes appropriate for infants, toddlers, and preschoolers with disabilities (Bailey et al., 2006). From stakeholders' input, they identified five outcomes that could be used to assess the effectiveness of services for these families:

1. Families understand their children's strengths, abilities, and special needs.

2. Families know their rights and advocate effectively for their children.

3. Families help their children develop and learn.

4. Families have support systems.

5. Families are able to gain access to desired services and activities in their community.

These outcomes provided a framework within which states and the federal government could document whether early intervention and preschool programs were providing demonstrable benefits for families. They also provided the basis for developing measurement systems to determine the extent to which such benefits were attained.

In order to achieve individual-, family-, or community-level outcomes, evaluators need to think of program- or system-level outcomes that might be necessary to support those goals. These might include provision of staff training; development of community–agency partnerships; provision of enrichment activities; modification of incentives; development of information systems; increase in financial support or scholarships; and expanded coverage and improved accessibility to services. Other changes, such as improving program management or organizational effectiveness, might be necessary at organizational levels.

Evaluators can use the following questions (based on WKKF, 1998, p. 32) to begin planning for an outcome/impact evaluation:

- Who is the target population (e.g., women in prison)? What subgroups are important (e.g., women in prison with children)?

- What outcomes (e.g., knowledge, behaviors, attitudes, skills) are you trying to achieve for the various subgroups in the target population?

- What types of measures (e.g., teacher assessments, standardized tests, personality inventories) might be used to measure the achievement of these outcomes?

- What logistical factors (e.g., time, money, expertise, access) need to be considered in making measurement decisions?

How will you use the results? (e.g., if the results reveal one thing, what will you do? If they reveal a different thing, what will you do?)

What are your performance targets (e.g., indicators that you will accept as evidence that you have successfully achieved the desired results)?

Four of the five evaluation criteria for international development interventions that emerged from the OECD DAC (2006a) guidelines relate to impact evaluation: effectiveness, impact, sustainability, and efficiency (Chianca, 2008). According to the OECD DAC, "effectiveness" is defined as the measure of the extent to which an aid activity obtains its objectives. Useful questions to determine effectiveness include these:

To what extent were the objectives achieved or likely to be achieved?

What were the major factors influencing the achievement or nonachievement of the objectives?

Chianca (2008) criticizes this narrowness of the concept of effectiveness, as it focuses on meeting the project's objectives and not the broader concept of meeting the stakeholders' needs. He also suggests that this criterion could be subsumed under the impact criterion.

"Impact" is defined by the OECD DAC (2006a) as both the positive and negative changes produced by a development intervention; these changes may be direct or indirect, intended or unintended. They include the main impacts and effects resulting from the intervention on local socioeconomic, environmental, and other development indicators. Useful questions to determine impact include these:

What has happened as a result of the project or program?

What real difference has the activity made to the beneficiaries?

How many people were affected?

Impact evaluation is usually interpreted as longer-term effects of the intervention.

The World Bank describes impact evaluation as "intended to determine more broadly whether the program had the desired effects on individuals, households, and institutions and whether those effects are attributable to the program intervention" (Baker, 2000, p.1). Although impact evaluations focus on intended effects, they can also reveal unintended effects of a program. The World Bank emphasizes the importance of examining the impact of a program while contrasting this with what would happen if the program had not been implemented (this is called a "counterfactual"). This places the World Bank's view of impact evaluation directly in the Methods Branch, and it is operationalized by the use of experimental and quasi-experimental designs. These have been discussed in Chapter 3 and are elaborated upon in Chapter 9.

Coady, Wang, and Dai (2001) described an example of an impact evaluation conducted in China that was focused on reducing women's fertility rates by educating them about career and cultural opportunities. The program involved 57 poor villages that were randomly assigned either to receive or not to receive the intervention over a 3-year period. Women in the experimental group were employed in such areas as apple processing, tobacco processing, and making handicrafts. They also established a reading room and an entertainment hall in their communities for cultural enrichment. When compared with the control group, the participants in the experimental group had higher incomes, spent more money on their children's education, expressed less desire to have a large family, and reduced the bias toward valuing male children more than female children.

At the World Bank's website (*www.worldbank.org*), you can find examples of impact evaluations in many sectors and in many countries. Many of the examples are from education (school-based management, teacher contracting, enhancing school performance), health (HIV/AIDS prevention and treatment, malaria control), social protection (cash transfer systems, school-to-work transition), and human development (preschools, nutrition). The World Bank uses community-level surveys as data collection methods. It wants to expand impact evaluation to other areas such as water projects, road construction, and governance reforms.

Policy Evaluation

Evaluations can be undertaken for the purpose of evaluating policy or changing policies. Evaluations that are conducted for this purpose need to start by building capacity in the community and evaluation team in regard to the relevant policies and the processes that may be useful to evaluate or change those policies. These policies can range from the organizational level to larger systems (e.g., departments of government) to national legislation. These questions (based on WKKF, 1998, p. 44) can be used to guide a policy-related evaluation:

- What types and levels of policy need to be changed?

- Which persons, agencies, and so on do we need to contact and influence?

- What do they need to hear?

In policy evaluations, stakeholders may be people with power who have their own agendas and ways of doing business. Evaluators need to do their homework as to what these processes are and what types of information would be likely to persuade the policy makers. Clarity and relevance to their constituencies are important criteria for evaluators to consider in their communications with policy makers. Policy makers are responsive to their constituencies; therefore, it is important for evaluators to involve the general public in the evaluation process, so that they can communicate with the policy makers themselves. This might include having meetings with these community members to share the evaluation findings with them in a way that enables the members to communicate effectively with the policy makers.

Jacob (2008) argues that policy evaluation is so complex that it requires having an interdisciplinary team of evaluators. Tensions can run high, and diverse stakeholder groups can be quite vocal about policies related to such topics as abortion, euthanasia, and stem cell research. Some domains require wide-ranging bases of knowledge that are more easily tapped by including people from different disciplines, such as environmental and health sciences. Of course, there will be challenges associated with bringing people from different disciplines together, including questions of resources, communication, and power. Yet many policy evaluations require input from various disciplinary perspectives; therefore, this strategy should be considered.

Gysen, Bruyninckx, and Bachus (2006) have developed an approach to policy evaluation that is designed to measure both intended main effects and unintended side effects of environmental policies (policies related to air pollution, water treatment, etc.). Gysen et al. recognize that main effects can be categorized in the ways we have discussed before: output, outcome, and impact. An example of an output effect might be the number of permits issued or the number of field inspectors in place after a policy has been implemented. The issuing of permits and addition of inspectors do not indicate that environmental changes have happened, but they are necessary steps before stakeholders can take action in that regard. Outcomes are the desired short-term and midterm effects, such as reduced emissions, increase in citations for violators, or increases in recycling. Impact outcomes are those long-term intended outcomes such as improved air or water quality. Side effects can be anticipated or unanticipated and positive or negative; they can also be direct, indirect, or derived. A direct, anticipated side effect might be the establishment of an oversight committee; an indirect side effect of this action might be the development of training materials for the committee. The derived side effect might be an increase in revenue in a community in which the committee, its staff, and consultants reside. An example of a negative side effect can be seen in a policy for mountaintop mining that results in filling valleys with what remains of the mountaintop after the coal has been extracted. The policy states that the mining company is bound to restore the mountain to its original state minus the coal. However, this does not happen in many instances, and the indirect side effect is poisoning the water in the creeks and rivers that drain the valleys. The derived side effects include mudslides that destroy the schools, homes, and livelihoods of the people living in the valley.

Policy evaluations are fraught with complexity, because many variables influence the desired effects (Gysen et al., 2006). For example, air quality may be influenced by a policy that limits industrial emissions, but there are many other sources of contaminants in the air (e.g., vehicular traffic and household consumption). Also, air crosses administrative and governmental boundaries, so changes in policy in one place may be negated or otherwise affected by air that travels from another place. Policies aimed at ameliorating major environmental conditions (e.g., global warming) draw on multiple disciplines, such as physical, social, and biological sciences; therefore, it is necessary to have persons with expertise in these areas as part of the evaluation team. Data collection tools might involve expensive and complex scientific instrumentation. Another concept of relevance to environmental policies is the reversibility or irreversibility of changes (e.g., species' becoming extinct) or the threshold at which dramatic changes will occur (e.g., water temperature and the death of coral reefs). With all of this complexity, it is challenging to provide causal proof of a policy's effectiveness. However, evaluators can work with stakeholders to develop a chain of evidence that links the policy to outputs, outcomes, and impacts, bolstered by scientific measurements from baseline over an appropriate time frame.

Opfer (2006) provides another example of a policy evaluation. This example involved the effectiveness of policies that created charter schools in the southern part of the United States. Opfer was tasked with evaluating the overall effectiveness of the schools in one state as an indication of the effectiveness of the policies. The state department of education agreed that her evaluation questions should be the following (Opfer, 2006, p. 275):

1. How did charter schools compare with traditional public schools in the state with regard to student achievement and stakeholder satisfaction?

2. How was the charter school concept being implemented in the state? Descriptively, how were they being organized, structured, managed, and so on? And what curricular and pedagogical strategies were being used?

3. Finally, what implementation issues were arising in charter schools, and what were the impetuses for these issues?

To answer these questions, Opfer interviewed principals, parents, and teachers; conducted site visits and observed at a sample of the schools; reviewed documents; and surveyed teachers and parents. In addition, she collected archival data on student demographics and achievement. The demographic data and interviews with parents revealed that white parents in one county with a black majority population had used the charter school system to set up schools segregated by race. When Opfer included this result in the evaluation report, the state department of education officials asked her to remove it because it was based on the results of only one school and was not reflective of the overall effectiveness of the charter school policy in the state. She went back to the data and discovered that 18 of the 28 charter schools were at least 20% more white than their districts; she also noted that this state did not have racial balance guidelines in the policy. The state department of education removed this from the revised report, and no changes were made in the policy.

Replication/Exportability/Transferability Evaluation

The WKKF (1998) acknowledges that one purpose of evaluations may be to determine whether a particular project can be transferred to another setting. For instance, this purpose arises when a pilot or demonstration project is implemented with the intent to apply it elsewhere if it is successful. In evaluations of this type, evaluators need to consider the critical contextual factors that would serve to inhibit or facilitate replication. Evaluators also need to examine the contextual conditions in the communities being considered to receive the program and compare them to the original conditions. Important questions would include these (based on WKKF, 1998, p. 27):

- What is unique about this project?
- Can the project be effectively replicated?
- What are the critical implementation elements?
- How might contextual factors affect replication?

Davidson (2005) uses the term "exportability" to indicate that a project may not be transported in its entirety. Rather, the intent may be to export parts of the project, such as its design, approach, or product. Chianca (2008) suggests that the accomplishment of this evaluation purpose requires broader knowledge outside the project being evaluated in order to assess the similarity of the other situations, as well as creative thinking to figure out what modifications might be needed to adapt to new circumstances.

Gueron (2007) offers an example of how replicability of treatments was ascertained through multiple evaluation studies of the effectiveness of various U.S. welfare initiatives. Gueron's position is that use of randomized controlled trials (RCT) (associated with the

Methods Branch) provides the strongest evidence of the replicability of a intervention. She bases her rationale on the presumed control of extraneous variables that an RCT design provides. (This is explained in more depth in Chapter 9.) She lists the following evaluation questions (Gueron, 2007, p. 135):

- Do the programs have any effect, positive or negative? If yes, and the answer is positive, what is the magnitude of the impacts?

- Do these programs offer a solution or an improvement?

- Do impacts vary for different groups of people and types of programs?

- Is there a trade-off between different program goals, for example, between reducing dependency and reducing poverty?

- Is the story all about variation, or are impacts replicable across contexts?

- Can you answer such questions in a way that will be widely believed? In particular, can you use random assignment?

- Are such research tools feasible in the real world of large-scale operating programs?

- Will high-quality information make a difference to policy makers and practitioners?

The program to be tested for its replicability was one that the Ford Foundation had supported in New York City called Supported Work. This program was designed to provide a structured 12-month work experience for people who had been on welfare for a long time, as well as for ex-addicts, ex-offenders, and school dropouts. The outcomes included employment, along with reduction of criminal activities, drug use, and receipt of public welfare funds. In the replication study, the program was expanded to 10 other communities. Individuals could apply to be in the program, and their names would be entered into a lottery; names of those who would participate were randomly drawn. The results indicated replicability of outcomes for women who were previously receiving welfare, but not for the mostly male participants who made up the ex-addicts and ex-offenders.

Qualitative researchers also emphasize the necessity of understanding how a program brings about the desired results as an important element of understanding replicability. Ginsburg and Rhett (2003) base their argument for the importance of qualitative approaches for replicability on the need for a sufficient description of how a program was implemented before it can be implemented in another context. Guba and Lincoln (2005) write about "transferability" rather than "replicability," contending that a researcher has an obligation to provide a sufficient description for the readers to make a judgment about the transferability of results from one situation to another. Erickson and Gutierrez (2002, p. 21) argue that qualitative methods are essential and should be combined with causal methods, because before asking, "Did it work?", readers will ask, "What was the 'it'?" That is, what was the "treatment" as actually delivered? Mixed methods researchers suggest that the combination of quantitative and qualitative methods strengthens an evaluator's ability to draw conclusions about replicability (Mertens, 2009, 2010).

Replicability also bears a relationship to the next evaluation purpose, sustainability, in that similar factors affect whether a project can be replicated or sustained. The Sustainable Agriculture and Rural Development initiative (Powell, 2007, p. 62) suggests that for effective technology transfer or replication in the context of rural development, technologies should have the following characteristics (based on IFAD, 2003; Neely, 2001; Scherr, 1999):

▨ Built on existing local and indigenous technologies or approaches

▨ Based on a widely shared need or problem of the rural poor

▨ Simple to understand and implement

▨ Able to be adopted incrementally

▨ Able to be adapted to local conditions, including adverse climatic conditions

▨ Culturally and socially acceptable

▨ Environmentally sound

▨ Economically viable, enhancing total farm productivity and stability

▨ Affordable to the rural poor in terms of financial and time constraints (e.g., have a rapid return on investment)

▨ Support the diversification of production

▨ Relatively independent on the use of purchased inputs (especially for subsistence production, for farmers distant from road networks or where input markets function poorly)

▨ Low risk and or able to protect the basic survival of the poor, including their food security

▨ Able to be reversed

Sustainability Evaluation

"Sustainability" is defined by the OECD DAC (2006a) as the benefits that continue to accrue after a donor's funding is withdrawn. The idea of international development is to build capacity in communities so they can continue to receive needed services after the donor leaves. The OECD DAC criteria specifically mention the importance of financial and environment factors that support or inhibit sustainability. Useful questions to assess sustainability include these:

▨ To what extent did the benefits of a program or project continue after donor funding ceased?

▨ What were the major factors which influence the achievement or non-achievement of sustainability of the program or project?

Chianca (2008) suggests that additional factors need to be considered, such as political support, cultural appropriateness, adequacy of technology, and institutional capacity.

A major outcome of importance to most funding agencies and communities is sustainability. If a donor provides funds for a specified period of time, it will expect the community to find alternative funding sources to sustain the project, such as state or federal monies, other foundations, private donors, or adoption by larger organizations. In other words, projects need to be able to find a way to obtain long-term support once short-term funding disappears. A growing body of evidence suggests that a program's success over the long term is associated with the ability of key stakeholders to change the conditions within which programs operate, thereby creating an environment where programs can flourish. Important questions in sustainability evaluation include the following (the first two are based on WKKF, 1998, p. 44, and the last three on Scheirer, 2005, p. 320):

- What are the social, political, cultural, and economic conditions that support or hinder a program's growth and sustainability?

- What are effective strategies for creating supportive conditions and changing difficult or hostile environments?

- What happens after the initial funding for a new program expires?

- Do the programs continue or end their activities, or even expand to new sites or new beneficiaries?

- Does the concept of "seed funding" have validity in encouraging the startup of new programs that are then continued by other means?

Sustainability is often a source of tension in the evaluation and program development world, because many evaluations end when the funding period ends. Hence it is difficult actually to collect data about sustainability under those conditions. Sustainability also brings up questions related to realistic expectations:

- If a funder provides monies for 3–5 years to address a problem that has existed for decades, maybe even centuries, what is the likelihood that the community can sustain the effort once the funding is gone?

- What are the power dynamics in the community that either support or inhibit sustainability?

- What conditions need to be in place for sustainability to be a feasible goal?

- How realistic is it to expect that short-term funding can lead to long-term change?

- How is the funded intervention structured to build the necessary capacity and arrange the necessary conditions to allow for sustainable change?

Scheirer's (2005) suggestions for important variables in a sustainability study echo some of the elements listed above for replicability. For example, evaluators can examine the extent to which local community members are involved and their degree of commitment to the program; whether there is a champion for the program who is willing to exert the effort needed to sustain it; and broader socioeconomic and political factors in the community, such as an economic downturn or legislative mandates. If the program has been integrated into the organization so that it is now routine practice, this will also influence sustainability. This routinization will be evident if the program is included in regular budgets, staff members are hired to provide the services, equipment is in place, training is provided, and the organization includes it in its policies and procedures. The actual methods of sustainability evaluation may include mail or telephone surveys, site visits, case studies, and archival data reviews. Most sustainability evaluations are undertaken about 2 years after the funding is stopped. Evaluators use quantitative, qualitative, or mixed methods in these studies.

Savaya, Spiro, and Elran-Barak (2008), using a mixed methods approach, conducted a sustainability evaluation of six projects that operated in Israel between 1980 and 2000. They purposefully selected three programs that survived and three that did not; the programs included interventions for alcoholism, parenting skills, domestic violence victimization, and art therapy for children. Then they conducted interviews with representatives of the programs, as well as document reviews of project proposals, correspondence, evaluation reports, and websites. Interestingly, Savaya et al. reported that the following factors did not guarantee sustainability: meeting an expressed need, positive evaluation outcomes, using a theory of change, stability of the host organization, and adequacy of the original funding. Sustainability was negatively influenced by these factors: lack of innovation in the program, high costs, nonuse of volunteers with professional staff, unwillingness to take risks, and sympathy expressed for the intended beneficiaries. Surviving programs typically had multiple sources of funding and a fund-raising strategy. Savaya et al.'s (2008) findings confirmed Scheirer's (2005), in that surviving programs' host organizations had placed a priority on the services provided by these programs, had champions within these organizations who fought for the programs' survival, and developed networks of support for the programs in the broader community.

Cost Analysis

Cost analysis is an important part of determining the effectiveness of a program. "Cost–benefit or cost-effectiveness evaluations assess program costs (monetary or non-monetary), in particular their relation to alternative uses of the same resources and to the benefits being produced by the program" (Baker, 2000, p. 1). In social programs, it is difficult to put a monetary value on such concepts as learning or health. Therefore, evaluators sometimes focus on cost-effectiveness when the outcomes are not monetarily defined. The main steps in this type of analysis are to identify all the project costs and benefits (easier said than done) and to compute a cost-effectiveness ratio. In order to calculate this ratio, all the costs and benefits have to be quantified. The cost effectiveness ratio is then calculated as the costs divided by the benefits. This allows for comparison of cost-effectiveness across different interventions.

Duwe and Kerschner (2008, see Chapter 3, Box 3.3) provide an example of a cost analysis study of a "boot camp" program to reduce criminal offenders' likelihood of returning to prison. The evaluand was a correctional boot camp modeled after military training that was very regimented, strict, and strenuous. If the offenders successfully completed the program, they were eligible for early release, thus saving the state money and reducing overcrowding in the prisons. If the program did not reduce recidivism, then these cost savings would be wiped out because the offenders would be right back in the system. More details of this study are included in Chapter 9 on the design of cost analysis studies.

· · · · · · · · · · E X T E N D I N G   Y O U R   T H I N K I N G · · · · · · · · · ·

Cost Analysis

An example of these two methods of analysis, using a hypothetical dropout prevention program, is presented below (Kee, 1999).

Hypothetical Cost–Effectiveness and Cost–Benefit Results for Dropout Prevention Strategies

Cost-Effectiveness

The cost-effectiveness of each dropout prevention strategy is determined by dividing the cost for each strategy by its effectiveness (e.g., the percentage increase in the number of students graduating). The result is the cost for each percent increase in the number of students graduating.

Strategy	Costs	Effectiveness	C-E ratio
Mentoring	$80,000	10	$ 8,000
After-school sports	$65,000	5	$13,000

Cost–Benefit Ratio

The cost–benefit ratio for each dropout prevention strategy is determined by calculating each strategy's benefits (e.g., estimates of future earnings increases of participants who stayed in school) and costs (e.g., personnel, materials, equipment) and then subtracting the benefits from the costs to get the net benefit for each strategy. The cost–benefit ratio can also be computed by dividing the dollar value of benefits by the costs (the higher the ratio, the more efficient the program in economic terms).

Strategy	Costs	Benefits	Net benefits	C-B ratio
Mentoring	$80,000	$95,000	$15,000	1.188
After-school sports	$65,000	$75,000	$10,000	1.154

1. In reading the example above, what do you think about placing a monetary value on the benefits of the programs?

2. What do you think about this kind of an evaluation?

3. What intangible benefits are missing from this cost analysis? Should they be included? If so, how can you include them?

"Efficiency" is an economic term for using the least costly inputs to achieve the desired results. Efficiency evaluations usually include comparisons of alternatives to see whether the least costly alternative was used. Important questions include these:

▓ Were activities cost-efficient?

▓ Were objectives achieved on time?

▓ Was the program or project implemented in the most efficient way, compared to the alternatives?

Cost could be expanded to include both monetary and nonmonetary terms (Chianca, 2008). Concerns might also be raised about fixating on the least costly approach. (Anyone who has accepted the lowest bid for a roof repair, only to wake up with water pouring into the living room at the first rainstorm, knows that least costly is not always best!) Efficiency is discussed further in the section of this chapter on cost analysis as a purpose for evaluation.

Purpose: To Address Issues of Human Rights and Social Justice

When an evaluation has an explicit purpose of addressing issues of human rights and social justice, then it is most closely aligned with the transformative paradigm. Such evaluations focus primarily on viewpoints from marginalized groups and the examination of power structures that either impede or enhance the furtherance of human rights. The sample studies in Chapter 6 provide a broad overview of evaluation purposes for studies that address issues of human rights and social justice. We begin here by discussing the evaluation purposes of two Chapter 6 sample studies: the Denver bilingual program study and the Bosnia-Herzegovina poverty reduction study. Then we ask you to extend your thinking about this purpose of evaluation by choosing a Chapter 6 sample study and discussing how it reflects purposes related to human rights and social justice. Next, we provide information about another type of evaluation associated with this purpose (gender analysis). We conclude the section with further comments on transformative evaluation in general.

Deliberative Democratic Evaluation

Recall the Denver bilingual program study (House, 2004; see Chapter 6, Box 6.5), in which the stated purpose was to monitor the implementation of a court-ordered bilingual program. That court order arose from concerns about the right to education and about discrimination based on country of origin, length of time in the United States, and socioeconomic status. House (2004) chose an approach to the evaluation that allowed him to explicitly address these sensitive and critical issues.

Country-Led Evaluation

The purposes of the Bosnia-Herzegovina poverty reduction study (Pennarz et al., 2007; see Chapter 6, Box 6.6) reflect purposes that have already been discussed (i.e., to find areas in need of improvement or to change practices and to assess program effectiveness). However, the evaluators conducted this evaluation with an explicit human rights and social justice purpose. They were conscious of the different levels of power associated with access to social protection for children of different ethnicities and from families of different sizes. In particular, they noted that children from Roma families and those from families with more than two children needed additional resources in order to avail themselves of the right to a safe living environment.

Human Rights and Social Justice Purposes in Evaluation

Select a sample study from Chapter 6 that illustrates one of these types of evaluation:

- DDE
- CLE
- CRT evaluation
- Indigenous evaluation
- Culturally responsive evaluation
- Disability- and deaf-rights-based evaluation
- Feminist evaluation
- Gender analysis
- Transformative participatory evaluation

Explain how the evaluators in the study you have chosen addressed the purposes associated with human rights and social justice.

Now, using the following chart, explain how the human rights and social justice evaluation encompassed other purposes in their studies:

To gain insights or to determine necessary inputs	To find areas in need of improvement or to change practices	To assess program effectiveness
• Context evaluation • Capacity building • Needs and assets assessment • Organizational assessment • Relevance evaluation	• Implementation evaluation • Responsive evaluation • Participatory evaluation • Process evaluation • Monitoring • Formative evaluation • Developmental evaluation	• Outcome/impact evaluation • Summative evaluation • Policy evaluation • Replicability/ exportability/ transferability evaluation • Sustainability evaluation • Cost analysis

Gender Analysis

Many of the approaches used for other evaluation purposes can also be used as methodologies for gender analysis. The difference is that a gender lens is brought to the process, and the purpose is to reveal differential access, participation, and impact by gender. For example, participatory approaches can be used; however, the evaluator needs to be aware of cultural practices that may inhibit full participation of women and to figure out ways to challenge those practices (Theobald, Simwaka, & Klugman, 2006). Also, the evaluator needs to be aware of how his/her own gender may affect access to and openness of stakeholders. Diversity within groups of women and men also needs to be considered in terms of potential stakeholders' exclusion from the process or the project.

The Canadian International Development Agency (1999) offers guidelines on gender analysis and suggests evaluation questions such as these:

- Who will benefit and who will lose from this project in terms of gender, over both the short term and the long term?

- To what extent have women been involved in the development of the program?

- Which organizations from government and civil society have been included?

- How does this project challenge existing gender divisions in regard to labor, tasks, responsibilities, opportunities, access to resources, and control over resources? What are the risks of backlash if changes are made?

- How can government agencies be brought into the process to pursue gender equity?

- What barriers need to be overcome to ensure equity in terms of participation and impact? How are these barriers overcome?

- What data are available that can provide baselines in sex-disaggregated form?

Gender analysis grew out of concerns in the international development world that initiatives were not taking into consideration inequities on the basis of gender. Therefore, many international organizations have developed guidelines for program development and evaluation that focus on such inequities and means to address them. The WHO (2002) has identified 13 different international organizations that have gender analysis handbooks and tools. It defines gender analysis as

> an examination of the relationships and role differences between women and men.... Gender analysis identifies, analyzes and informs action to address inequalities that arise from the different roles of women and men, or the unequal power relationships between them and the consequences of these inequalities on their lives, their health and well-being. The way power is distributed in most societies means that women have less access to and control over resources to protect their health and are less likely to be involved in decision-making. Gender analysis in health therefore often highlights how inequalities disadvantage women's health, the constraints women face to attain health and ways to address and overcome these constraints. Gender analysis also reveals health risks and problems which men face as a result of the social construction of their roles. (WHO, 2002, p. 2)

The WHO (2003) also provides suggestions for conducting a gender analysis:

- Assess the impact on men and women; ensure that women's positions are not worsened by the project, and that the project is not placed at risk by women's positions.

- Make gender equity an important goal of the project, and use it as a lens for the evaluation.

- Be sure that stakeholders participate in the process, and that men and women participate equally in the process.

- ▦ Specifically examine how the program takes into account differences between men and women in terms of roles and responsibilities, norms and values, access to/control of resources, and decision-making power.

- ▦ Develop indicators (addressed in this book in Chapter 10 on data collection) that reflect gender-specific resources, and outcomes that reveal the extent of equity between men and women.

A gender analysis conducted in Kenya as part of that country's National HIV/AIDS Strategic Plan revealed numerous examples of inequities in the initial plan (National AIDS Control Council, 2002). For example, insufficient attention was given to the use of female condoms in terms of affordability and accessibility; to transmission of AIDS through gender-based forms of violence, such as rape and incest; or to lack of sensitivity to women's perspectives in the training materials. In its strategies for intervention, the plan did not include centers for women who experienced rape or incest for counseling and treatment; nor did it address the nutritional needs of men and women who had HIV/AIDS, or the extra responsibilities of women who were taking care of persons with the disease. In addition, the plan did not provide for the collection of sex-disaggregated data on the economic impact of HIV/AIDS. The Gender and HIV/AIDS subcommittee used these evaluation data to revise the plan and its implementation.

The Joint United Nations Programme on HIV/AIDS (UNAIDS) Inter-Agency Task Team on Gender and HIV/AIDS (2005, p. 14) provides a useful set of questions for gender analysis that parallel and extend the questions presented above. These questions are set within the context of evaluations of HIV/AIDS programs; however, we have modified some of them for application to other areas of concern. Here is a sample:

- ▦ Is provision made for the involvement of women and girls and their representative organizations in the design of programmatic interventions?

- ▦ Does the program consciously challenge and transform gender stereotypes and power imbalances between men and women, boys and girls?

- ▦ Does the program encourage a discussion about sociocultural norms and dominant interpretations of masculinity–femininity and related gender roles?

- ▦ Is the program informed by an assessment of the specific factors enhancing the vulnerability of women/girls and men/boys (and/or of specific groups of women, girls, men, and boys) to the problem addressed by the program, rather than focusing exclusively on individual behavior?

- ▦ Does the program pay careful attention to local sociocultural realities in the context of which gender rights will be implemented, and does it use culturally sensitive approaches?

- ▦ Does the program contribute to the empowerment of women and girls?

- ▦ Are opportunities created for men and boys who want to resist and transform gender-related norms and roles?

- ▦ Are men encouraged to be involved in the program?

- ▦ Does the program address gender-based violence, including gender-based violence in the home?

■ Does the program actively and directly contribute to the protection and realization of human rights for all, particularly of marginalized groups and other groups with enhanced vulnerability?

■ Are clear and gender-specific indicators adopted to ensure that the process and outcome of the program can be monitored and reviewed in accordance with human rights standards and principles?

■ Is adequate provision made to ensure that people affected by the problem under study, particularly women and girls and their representative organizations, are involved in the design, implementation, and monitoring of the program?

■ Does the program challenge and transform stereotypes and stigma, particularly those that (unconsciously or deliberately) place blame for the problem on women/girls in general or on specific groups of women/girls (or specific groups of men/boys)?

■ Does the program contribute to equitable access to and use of appropriate care and treatment options for both women and men, girls and boys?

■ Is the program informed by an assessment (conducted with people affected by the problem) of the specific treatment, care, and support needs of women/girls and men/boys?

The UNAIDS book that lists the original questions also includes examples of instruments that can be used to collect data to obtain answers to the questions. These instruments are covered in Chapter 10 on data collection.

· · · · · · · · · · EXTENDING YOUR THINKING · · · · · · · · · ·
Gender Analysis

The United Nations Inter-Agency Standing Committee has created an e-learning course you can take online, and an accompanying book (which you can download) entitled *Different Needs–Equal Opportunities: Increasing Effectiveness of Humanitarian Action for Women, Girls, Boys and Men*. There is also a 2-minute video that is quite captivating (*oneresponse.info/crosscutting/gender/Pages/Training.aspx*). In the second part of the e-learning course, checklists are provided in several areas, including health, nutrition, shelter, water, sanitation, and hygiene. The committee also provides directions for collecting, analyzing, and reporting program-monitoring data.

Go to the course website *www.interaction.org/iasc-gender-elearning*. Scroll down to the bottom of the page and open a couple of the checklists. (Take the course, too, if you are interested!)

■ List the quantitative strategies used to collect data.

■ List the qualitative strategies used to collect data.

■ The suggested strategies will just be one part of a much larger evaluation. What do you think an evaluation without a focus on gender analysis would miss that would be important for professionals working in disaster relief to know?

Further Comments about Transformative Evaluation in General

When the evaluation purpose is social transformation, it is possible to have other purposes that fit within this. Social transformation as a purpose can encompass the purposes
of context, input, process and product evaluations as they have been described in this
chapter. However, like gender analysis, social transformation as a purpose of evaluation
brings with it a lens to reveal inequities on the basis of dimensions of diversity associated
with discrimination and oppression.

Again, recall the various examples of evaluations summarized in Chapter 6. House
(2004) evaluated a court-ordered English language program in Colorado for Spanish-
speaking students. He was careful to obtain viewpoints from diverse groups and to make
the evaluation process as transparent as possible. When issues arose that suggested that
discriminatory practices were being used, such as inferior educational materials in Spanish
or failure to identify Spanish-speaking students, House made sure the evaluation focused
on these issues. He consciously brought a lens of democratic practice to the evaluation as a
way to ensure that social justice issues were addressed. Other sample transformative studies described in Chapter 6 revealed inequities related to race and indigenous status.

The Mertens et al. (2007; see Chapter 6, Box 6.10) evaluation of a preparation program for teachers of deaf students who have a disability provides a model for the way a
transformative purpose leads to a cyclical approach to evaluation. In such studies, evaluators begin with a realization that they need to have sufficient knowledge about the cultural
groups and context to identify who should be involved in the initial evaluation planning.
In the case of the Mertens et al. (2007) study, this meant that the evaluation planning team
should represent the various salient dimensions within the deaf community, including use
of American Sign Language and use of assistive listening devices (e.g., cochlear implants).
Because the evaluation team included deaf, hard-of-hearing, and hearing members, as
well as members using sign language and voice as expressive communication systems, the
evaluators were able to support the needs of the stakeholders in culturally appropriate
ways. Some of the program graduates were hearing, and some were deaf. All graduates
knew American Sign Language; however, not all were native signers.

The identification of the focus and methods of the evaluation began with team meetings and was informed by the reading of program documents and the personal experiences
of the team members. The focus and methods were further shaped by conducting observations of a gathering of program graduates to determine the issues that were most salient for
them, rather than imposing specific questions from the program director's or evaluators'
point of view. The cycle involved the formation of the team, team meetings, observations,
interviews with reflective seminar participants, online survey of graduates, interviews with
faculty and staff from coordinating schools, dissemination of findings to the internal stakeholders and external professional groups, and follow-up to determine changes as a result
of the evaluation findings. At each step of the process, the data were used to determine the
next steps and the specific focus of data to be collected subsequently.

The transformative lens revealed issues of inequities that needed to be addressed,
such as provision of support for hearing graduate students to learn American Sign Language, but lack of support for deaf graduate students to prepare them for certification
tests. In addition, the new teachers explained that they felt inadequately prepared to help
children representing several dimensions of diversity: children who came from homes
where English was not used; children who came to school with no language at all; chil-

dren who had different types of disabilities in addition to deafness (e.g., autism, learning disabilities); and children who came to school using communication systems such as cued speech. The new teachers also expressed surprise at the low expectations that the school held for its students and at how the deaf students were marginalized from the main school community. They wanted to know more about how to challenge these inequities constructively. Following up with faculty and cooperating school staff allowed the evaluation team to use the evaluation findings as a catalyst for change in the curriculum, placement sites, and support for new teachers. Sharing the results with the broader teacher preparation programs for deaf students allowed change to be stimulated more broadly.

Box 8.3. Getting to Outcomes

Accountability questions	*Relevant literatures*
1. What are the underlying needs and conditions that must be addressed? (NEEDS/RESOURCES)	1. Needs/resource assessment
2. What are the goals, target population, and objectives (i.e., desired outcomes)? (GOALS)	2. Goal setting
3. What science-based (evidence-based) models and best-practice programs can be used in reaching the goals? (Best Practice)	3. Science-based and best-practice programs
4. What actions need to be taken so the selected program "fits" the community context? (FIT)	4. Feedback on comprehensiveness and fit of program
5. What organizational capacities are needed to implement the program? (CAPACITIES)	5. Assessment of organizational capacities
6. What is the plan for this program? (PLAN)	6. Planning
7. Is the program being implemented with quality? (PROCESS)	7. Process evaluation
8. How well is the program working? (OUTCOME EVALUATION)	8. Outcome and impact evaluation
9. How will continuous quality improvement strategies be included? (IMPROVE)	9. Total quality management: Continuous quality improvement
10. If the program is successful, how will it be sustained? (SUSTAIN)	10. Sustainability and institutionalization

Source: Adapted from Chinman, Imm, and Wandersman (2004).

Multipurpose Evaluation Strategies

Chinman, Imm, and Wandersman (2004; see Box 8.3) have created a system called "Getting to Outcomes," which includes 10 empowerment evaluation and accountability questions used for successful programming. The first question they ask deals with needs assessment and available resources: "What are the underlying needs and conditions that must be addressed?" They then offer eight steps for conducting a needs and resource assessment (Chinman et al., 2004, p. 17):

1) Set up an assessment committee or work group of members from your group to collect the data. Be sure to include key stakeholders.

2) Examine what data are currently available to assess the risk and protective factors.

3) Determine what data still need to be collected by your group.

4) Determine the best methods to gather the data and develop a data collection plan.

5) Implement the data collection plan.

6) Analyze and interpret the data.

7) Select the priority risk and protective factors to be addressed.

8) Use those priority factors to develop goals and objectives and to select programs/strategies to implement.

Wandersman (2009) gives an example of how a needs assessment for an organization may be addressed. The Fayetteville Youth Network promotes positive youth development and provides substance abuse services. Staff members noticed that a growing number of program participants were getting pregnant; they were concerned about the effect of these early pregnancies. They decided to investigate this more closely, and possibly add a teen pregnancy prevention component. A working group of staff members was formed to take a look at the problem and plan a way to address it.

1. The group members collected information from the state health department:

   ▪ Data on the number of pregnancies in each zip code within Fayetteville. The group then identified one zip code where the majority of teen pregnancies were concentrated.

   ▪ Information about the sexual behaviors of youth across the state, from the state's Youth Risk Behavior Survey.

2. The group surveyed high school students to assess different determinants of sexual behaviors—specifically, their knowledge and attitudes about sexuality, STDs, and contraception.

3. Finally, the group conducted a focus group of staff members at one school, to get their perspectives on the risk factors facing youth in that school.

Generating Questions

Patton (2008) suggests that evaluators facilitate the generation of evaluation questions by the intended users, rather than providing such questions for their consideration. He describes a process that looks somewhat simplistic, yet is highly effective. The process begins with asking the stakeholders to think of something about their program that they would like to know and that would really make a difference. Stakeholders can be asked to make a list of 10 things they really want to know that they could envision using to make their program better. With a large group of stakeholders, small groups can be used to discuss the list and prioritize those about which they feel most strongly. Once the group members reach agreement on the evaluation questions, they can proceed with discussions of which types of data are needed to answer the questions and how they could use that resulting information.

- - - - - - - - - - E X T E N D I N G   Y O U R   T H I N K I N G - - - - - - - - - -
Generating Questions

Try Patton's suggestion for generating evaluation questions with others in your class or in your work setting. Imagine that you are evaluating your program evaluation course, a project you are doing at work, or another program you may be involved in. Jot down 10 evaluation questions that you think would be appropriate for evaluating the program, and put them aside. Now ask the stakeholders (your class members, coworkers, friends) to think of something that they would like to know that would improve the program. Perhaps they will ask questions such as these: "Does the library have the electronic resources we will need to write our papers for this course?" or "Will we be allotted enough time during the work day to practice the skills we are learning in the online tutorial?" After questions are created, prioritize those they feel most strongly about.

1. Was the process of eliciting questions from the group difficult? Were people interested in participating?

2. How did you prioritize the questions? Was this process challenging? Explain.

3. Did the questions that the group developed differ from the original 10 questions you created before this process? Explain why they did or did not differ.

4. What do you think of Patton's suggestion to generate questions in this manner?

Planning Your Evaluation: Purposes and Questions

Based on your choice of an evaluand and identification of appropriate stakeholders, write a narrative about the purpose or purposes of the evaluation, and develop a list of evaluation questions. If it is feasible to do so, complete this part of the planning process in collaboration with the identified stakeholders.

 Moving On to the Next Chapter

After deciding on the purpose and evaluation questions, it is time to begin considering the specific design that will frame the evaluation. This is the topic of Chapter 9.

Preparing to Read Chapter Nine

As you prepare to read this chapter, think about these questions:

1. What does the term "design" mean in evaluation planning?

2. How does an evaluator decide which evaluation design to use?

3. How does an evaluator know that it is the intervention that caused the desired change, and not some other variables?

4. How does the evaluator know whether the results found in one sample will generalize to another sample from the same population? Is this important?

5. Why would anyone believe that using both qualitative and quantitative methods in an evaluation is a step in the right direction for evaluators?

6. Although using a case study or a narrative may sound too narrow and focused for an evaluation, doing so can actually be very effective. Why do you think this might be a good way to approach evaluation?

CHAPTER NINE

Evaluation Designs

"**D**esign" in evaluation is a complex concept. Some statements can be made about design that reflect fairly typical options for evaluators situated in different evaluation branches:

▪ Design in methods-based evaluations is simplistically considered as determining who gets what treatment when and when the effects of that treatment are measured.

▪ Design in the Values Branch usually takes the form of a qualitative approach.

▪ Design in the Use Branch usually involves stakeholders in decisions about the design.

▪ Design in the Social Justice Branch is usually cyclical, in the sense of feeding information back to the stakeholders so that they can make decisions about next steps.

Yet, even in making these statements, we are immediately struck by the need to acknowledge that the design options frequently blur the lines between the different branches. For purposes of providing an explanation of design options, we begin with a description of quantitative designs, followed by qualitative designs, mixed methods designs, and special applications of designs for specific evaluation purposes. Box 9.1 displays design options typically associated with the different evaluation branches and types of evaluation. Note that in this box, the types of evaluation are not aligned with particular designs, because different designs can be used for different types of applications. For example, a needs and assets assessment can use both survey and case study designs; it thus becomes a mixed methods design. Garbarino and Holland (2009) argue for the use of both quantitative and qualitative methods in impact evaluations.

This chapter is organized as follows. First, general quantitative, qualitative, and mixed methods designs are described and illustrated. Then specific applications of designs in evaluation are presented, because they often make use of the basic evaluation designs within a specific context (such as cost analysis, needs and assets assessment, or gender analysis).

Box 9.1. Evaluation Branches, Associated Design Options, and Types of Evaluations

Branches and designs	Types of evaluation
Methods Branch: Quantitative	Context evaluation, capacity building, needs and assets assessment, relevance evaluation
▪ Experimental designs	
▪ Quasi-experimental designs	Participatory evaluation, empowerment evaluation, organizational assessment, implementation evaluation, responsive evaluation, process evaluation, monitoring, developmental evaluation, formative evaluation, UFE
▪ Single-group designs	
▪ Surveys	
▪ Cost analysis	
Values Branch: Qualitative	Outcome/product/impact evaluation, replicability/exportability/transferability evaluation, summative evaluation, training evaluation, cost analysis, policy evaluation
▪ Case studies	
▪ Ethnographic designs	
▪ Narrative designs	DDE, CLE, CRT, indigenous evaluation, culturally responsive evaluation, disability- and deaf-rights-based evaluation, gender analysis, transformative participatory evaluation, feminist evaluation
▪ Phenomenological studies	
▪ Participatory action designs	
Use and Social Justice Branches: Mixed methods	
▪ Concurrent mixed methods designs	
▪ Dialectical (or embedded) mixed methods designs	
▪ Sequential mixed methods designs	
▪ Transformative mixed methods designs	
▪ Impact evaluations and mixed methods designs	

Quantitative Designs

Quantitative designs can be divided into two rough categories (see Figure 9.1): those that are used to determine the effectiveness of an intervention, and those that are more descriptive in nature, such as surveys. Designs to determine the effectiveness of an intervention can involve experimental, quasi-experimental, single-group, and cost analysis designs. The primary purpose of using experimental, quasi-experimental or single group quantitative designs to determine an intervention's effectiveness is to be able to say with confidence that whatever changes that occur in the participants' behavior, knowledge, skills, or attitudes (the dependent variable) are the result of the intervention (the independent variable). The extent to which researchers can make this statement with confidence reflects the **"internal validity"** of the study. Researchers have identified a number of variables that potentially threaten their ability to say that changes are indeed a result of the intervention. These variables are called "extraneous variables," "lurking variables," or "threats to validity."

Experimental and quasi-experimental designs serve the purpose of controlling for the effects of extraneous variables while allowing for the testing of the effects of the intervention. We start this section with a discussion of the extraneous variables that threaten internal validity. We then examine a second type of validity: "external validity," or the ability to generalize the results of a study to the population from which the population was drawn. These discussions are followed by explanations of various types of experimental and quasi-experimental designs and how they are used to control the threats to internal and external validity.

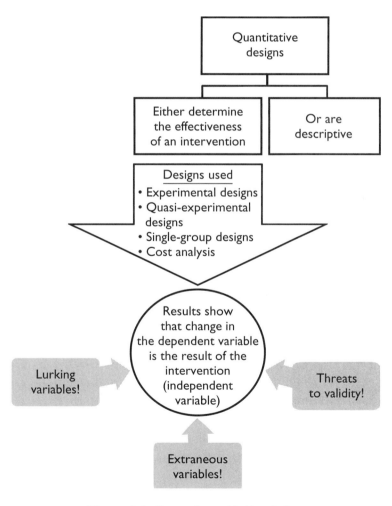

Figure 9.1. Types of quantitative designs.

Internal and External Validity

How does an evaluator know that an intervention, rather than some other variables, has caused a change in the dependent variables? And how does the evaluator know whether the results found in one sample will generalize to the same population from which the population was drawn? These two questions are the essence of two important concepts that Campbell and his associates (Campbell & Stanley, 1963) developed within the post-positivist paradigm: internal and external validity. Internal validity means that an evaluator has controlled the effects of variables other than the treatment, in order to say with confidence that the results are reflective of the treatment. External validity means that the sample is representative of the population, and therefore that if the treatment is applied with another group of people from that population under similar circumstances, it should be effective there as well.

We are sure that you, as an evaluator, can see the benefits of being able to make claims of internal and external validity. We are also sure that you can see the challenges involved in trying to control the variables that might influence outcomes and in trying to establish that a sample is reflective of the population, because of the heterogeneity of groups and because it is difficult to imagine being able to establish similar circumstances in dynamic human systems. Campbell and Stanley (1963) identified a number of threats to validity, also known as extraneous variables, lurking variables, alternative explanations, or rival hypotheses. A list of the threats to validity that we discuss below is given in Box 9.2; this box can serve as your map through the first part of this chapter.

Box 9.2. Threats to Validity

Threats to internal validity

History

Maturation

Testing

Instrumentation

Statistical regression

Differential selection

Experimental mortality

Statistical regression

Experimental treatment diffusion

Compensatory rivalry by the control group

Compensatory equalization of treatments

Resentful demoralization of the control group

Threats to external validity

Lack of an explicit description of the independent variable

Multiple-treatment interference

The Hawthorne effect

Novelty and disruption effects

Experimenter effects

Pretest or posttest sensitization

Different types of measurement for dependent variables

Different times of measurement of dependent variables

Other threats to validity

Lack of treatment fidelity

Poor strength of treatment

Threats to Internal Validity

Box 9.3 gives definitions and examples of some potential threats to internal validity, together with ways of controlling them.

STATISTICAL REGRESSION

One of the more complex concepts internal threats to validity is statistical regression; therefore, we provide the reader with a more detailed explanation of this concept here. Statistical regression is a threat to validity when the research involves use of extreme groups (i.e., participants who are at either the high or low end of the scores on the dependent measure prior to the intervention). It is based in the nature of statistics as a science of probability. If a group is already at the highest point in a continuum, it can either go down or stay the same, hence increasing the probability that a decline in scores may appear as a function of measurement error. For instance, if all members of a group are already scoring at the highest levels and their scores can't go any higher, chances are that any decline in their scores indicates mistakes in the measurement and not in the intervention (e.g., tutoring). The same is true for a group at the lowest point of the continuum; their scores can go up or stay the same. The "improvement" is not the result of the intervention, but the result of the probability basis for measurement and statistics.

EXPERIMENTAL MORTALITY

An example of how evaluators handled attrition comes from the Brady and O'Regan (2009) Irish youth mentoring study. There were 161 youth surveys (98%), 145 parent surveys (88%), and 94 teacher surveys (57%) completed at baseline. (Mentors were not surveyed at Time 1.) At Time 2, a response rate of 83.5% was recorded for the youth survey, 79% for the parent survey, 17% for the teacher survey, and 91% for the mentor survey. At Time 3, return rates were 86% for youth, 80% for parents, 18% for teachers, and 97% for mentors. At Time 4, return rates were 82% for youth, 79% for parents, 6% for teachers, and 96% for mentors. The low response rate from teachers is attributable to the fact that many of the study participants transferred from primary to secondary school during this period and thus the teacher initially nominated was no longer relevant. In addition, teachers proved reluctant to return surveys. The response rate for intervention group youth and parents was slightly higher than for control group youth and parents.

ADDITIONAL THREATS TO INTERNAL VALIDITY

Cook and Campbell (1979) have described further potential threats to internal validity (these are listed in Box 9.2 but not included in Box 9.3):

1. *Experimental treatment diffusion.* People will talk, especially if they really like or dislike something. If members of the experimental group are in close proximity with members of the control group, it is possible that the experimental group might share some information about the intervention. The control group might think that those ideas are worth trying. When the control group implements any part of the intervention, then experimental treatment diffusion becomes operational as a threat to inter-

Box 9.3. Threats to Internal Validity, with Definitions, Examples, and Suggestions for Controlling Them

Threat	Definition	Example	Suggestions for controlling threat
History	Events occurring during a study (other than the experimental treatment) that can influence results.	If, during the Brady and O'Regan (2009) Irish youth mentoring study that measured risky behaviors, the schools had started a drug prevention program, this would have been a "history" threat.	Having two (or more) groups all of which experience the "history" event, but not all of which experience the experimental treatment, can control this threat.
Maturation	Naturally occurring physical or psychological changes in study participants during the study (e.g., participants become tired, older, more coordinated, or better readers just through the passage of time).	Brady and O'Regan had two groups: one that received mentoring, and one that did not. Individuals were randomly assigned to groups. Therefore, any effects of maturation should have been manifested equally within the two groups, leaving only the intervention effects to explain changes.	Having two (or more) groups all of which experience the maturation, but not all of which experience the experimental treatment, can control this threat.
Testing	Administration of a pretest that affects participants' performance on a posttest (i.e., participants become "testwise").	This threat is usually more of a concern when the dependent variable is cognitive or skill development, because participants might become more sensitive to what they are learning than they would have if they had not taken the pretest.	Having two groups, both of which take both the pretest and the posttest, balances out this effect. Also, it can be controlled by not having a pretest.

Threat	Definition	Example	Suggestions for controlling threat
Instrumentation	Having pretests and posttests that differ in terms of difficulty; this can lead to seeming changes that are really due to the difference in the tests.	Brady and O'Regan surveyed their participants three times during the study; however, it was the same survey each time.	Using the same test for both pre- and posttesting is one way to control this threat.
Statistical regression (see the text for more details about this concept)	Having extreme groups in a study (i.e., people very high or very low on a particular characteristic); it is possible that changes will be seen on the dependent variable because of this threat.	The participants in the Brady and O'Regan study were not chosen because they were particularly high or low on any of the dependent measures; hence this threat would not have been a problem in that study.	Having an experimental and a control group will control statistical regression if it is a problem, because it should be reflected in both groups, and then its effects would be the same in both groups. Not using extreme groups also controls this threat.
Differential selection	Differences between the experimental and control groups on important characteristics, other than receipt of the intervention.	One group might have better readers or participants who are older than the other group. Brady and O'Regan randomly assigned participants to treatment or control groups.	Random assignment to experimental and control conditions controls this threat, because characteristics should be randomly distributed in both groups, thus balancing out their effects.
Experimental mortality	Differential dropouts of participants from either the experimental or control groups.	If weaker participants in the experimental group dropped out, then it might give a false impression of positive change. (See text for a more detailed example.)	Random assignment should control for this threat, because theoretically participants would drop out at the same rates. However, evaluators should check to see if this is true.

nal validity. Given the pervasive sharing of information that is possible with electronic means of communication, physical proximity of the two groups is not really necessary for this diffusion to happen. Hence evaluators need a strategy for observing both the experimental and control groups to determine whether the control group is implementing aspects of the intervention. This can be done by making observations in both settings, interviewing participants, or asking participants to keep diaries or logs of their activities.

2. *Compensatory rivalry by the control group.* Stories about resistance to change are easy to come by; change is not always smoothly implemented. Think about times when you are required to change email systems or change your passwords when you are comfortable with (and loyal to) the old way of doing things. This threat is also known as the "John Henry effect," in homage to the legendary railroad builder who wanted to prove that men could build the railroad better than machines. John Henry took on a contest with the new machine (read: experimental intervention). He worked very hard and won the contest, but then died from overexertion. Hence, in some respects, he proved that the old way was better, but only by overcompensating. Compensatory rivalry by the control group occurs when the control condition represents the old way of doing things, and people really believe that it is better than the new way that the experimental intervention represents. The threat of a change can lead members of the control group to try even harder to prove that the old way of doing things is better.

3. *Compensatory equalization of treatments.* If one group receives something and the other group receives nothing, then any effects on the first group may be due to the fact that this group received something, and not to the specifics of what it received. For example, if students participate in a program after school, they spend more time at school and less time out on the streets. Therefore, they may get in less trouble just by virtue of being in school longer and not necessarily because of the nature of the program. Hence evaluators will try to provide something to the control group that will compensate for the extra time at school without giving the control group the actual experimental treatment.

4. *Resentful demoralization of the control group.* If the members of the control group know that the experimental group is getting something, they may become demoralized because they are not getting whatever that is. Brady and O'Regan (2009) directly addressed this threat to validity by offering all youth an opportunity to receive services. The only difference was that the experimental group had mentors as an add-on intervention. Hence their study was not studying the effect of mentoring alone; rather, it was studying the effect of mentoring when it was added to a youth intervention program. They framed this challenge as follows: "The design had to include strategies to avoid 'resentful demoralization' on the part of the control group and ensure that control group participants were sufficiently motivated to continue with the study over the proposed 1.5-year timeframe" (p. 271). They decided that "both intervention and control groups would be offered a basic youth service and mentoring would represent an 'add-on' service for the intervention group. Thus, all research participants would be offered a service. This meant that mentoring would be evaluated as an additional element of youth service provision rather than as a stand-alone program" (p. 272). This strategy also allowed Brady and O'Regan to address one of the ethical issues associated with the use of experimental studies (i.e., denying people who need services access to them).

·········· **EXTENDING YOUR THINKING** ··········
Threats to Internal Validity

1. What threat to internal validity do you spot in the following scenario?

   The name of each student in a classroom was written on a separate piece of paper. All the papers were put in a hat and mixed. Students were assigned to the experimental group and to the control group alternately as their names were pulled out of the hat one at a time. One day at school, the students in the control group were told to go the library and read, and students in the experimental group went to the library to watch videos about the ocean. Asiah and Khadijat, who were in the experimental group, were bored by the ocean video, became disruptive, and were removed from the library. The mean score for students in the control group was 2.0, and the mean score for the experimental group was 3.4. It was concluded that the whale video improved the students' understanding of the threat of the BP oil spill.

2. Create scenarios for two other threats to validity and share with a classmate. Discuss which threats each of you were illustrating in your scenarios.

Threats to External Validity (Generalizability of Treatments)

External validity in terms of a sample's representativeness of the population is addressed in Chapter 11 on sampling strategies. However, several aspects of design influence the evaluators' abilities to claim generalizability of the treatments. These include the following:

1. *Lack of an explicit description of the independent variable.* In order to apply an experimental treatment in another setting after the initial study, it seems obvious that you would have to know precisely what the independent variable was in the first place. In many evaluation studies, however, somewhat generic labels are used to describe the intervention, such as "youth services," "integration of technology," "social skills training," or "innovative reading instructional strategies." Evaluators need to include an appropriate level of detail describing the intervention, so that others can know what needs to be included if they are going to try to implement the same intervention in another setting. The intervention in the Brady and O'Regan (2009) program was the BBBS program, which was described in great detail in a manual for program staff.

2. *Multiple treatment interference.* Interventions typically are multidimensional, meaning that participants experience several things as part of the treatment. The BBBS program was highly structured, with screening, training, and monitoring of the volunteer mentors by a paid case manager (Brady & O'Regan, 2009). The focus of BBBS was on establishment of relationships between the mentors and the youth. However, there is no description of exactly what the mentors did with the youth. One might wonder: Was it sufficient for the mentors to sit and talk with the youth? What if the mentors played sports with their charges? What if they took them out to eat? Were any of these elements that could be viewed as part of the treatment essential for success?

3. *The Hawthorne effect.* This threat to external validity is based on a very old study conducted at the Hawthorne electrical plant on the effects of light levels on productivity (Roethlisberger & Dickson, 1939). The experimenters manipulated the light levels, gradually increasing the light, and then measured the effect on worker productivity. They were not surprised to see that productivity increased with increasing light levels. They then tried the intervention in reverse, gradually lowering the light levels. They were surprised to see that productivity levels continued to increase even as the light levels decreased. They decided that the level of light was not actually the independent variable that was influencing the dependent variable. Rather, the workers increased their productivity simply because someone (the experimenter) was paying attention to them. They felt special, and hence they increased their productivity. (Or they felt threatened, and hence increased their productivity.) Whatever their feelings, the independent variable that was influencing the workers' productivity was not level of light; rather, it was having someone watch them while they worked.

4. *Novelty and disruption effects.* When people are asked to do something new and different, they may embrace it and increase the desired behavior just because it is something new or different. Or they may view it as a disruption of things they are used to and resist the change just because they do not want to change. If either of these dynamics surfaces in an experimental study, changes may be due to the novelty or the disruptive effect, rather than to the inherent quality of the intervention.

5. *Experimenter effects.* This threat to external validity rests on a question: Are the results of the intervention due to the uniqueness of the person who conducted the experiment or who implemented the treatment? If so, then it might be hard for another person to obtain similar results. For example, a very charismatic teacher might be able to reach disaffected youth and teach them algebra by taking them out into the community. Could that treatment be generalized to a similar context, but with a different teacher who was not so charismatic or who did not know the community so well?

6. *Pretest or posttest sensitization.* If you take a pretest, how does that influence your performance on the posttest? If you know you are going to take a posttest, do you engage differently during the program than if you do not have to take such a test? Evaluators want to be sure that the effects they measure are the result of the intervention, and not just the result of participants' being sensitized to certain issues because of a pretest or because they know they will be tested on something at the end of the program.

7. *Different types of measurement for dependent variables.* What is the influence of the type of measurement that is used for the dependent variables? Assume that one evaluator uses a multiple-choice test and another uses an open-ended essay test. If they find different results, is that because they used a different type of dependent measure or because the intervention worked in one context but not in another?

8. *Different times of measurement of dependent variables.* If an evaluator measures the effect of an instructional intervention immediately after the instruction, does that mean that the program is effective? What if the evaluator waits a couple of days, weeks, or months to collect the data? What is the influence of the amount of time between the intervention and measurement of the dependent variable? How long do the effects of the intervention have to last in order to claim that it is effective?

· · · · · · · · · · · **EXTENDING YOUR THINKING** · · · · · · · · · · ·

Threats to External Validity

1. What threat to external validity do you spot in the following scenario?

   Ward was disappointed with the results of his experimental study. He had read Egan's study of "relaxation techniques" used with people who had been searching for employment for over 6 months. Ward used yoga and meditation with 24 Chicago adults who had been unemployed for 6 months, but his results did not show less anxiety in his participants, unlike the results of Egan's study.

2. Create scenarios for two other external threats to validity and share with a classmate. Discuss which threats each of you were illustrating in your scenarios.

Other Threats to Validity

Two other threats to validity are very important to consider when evaluators are testing effects of an experimental treatment. The first is lack of *treatment fidelity*, meaning that the treatment was not implemented as intended. The second is poor *strength of treatment*, meaning that the treatment was not given at a strong enough dosage to justify the expectation of seeing a change. "Dosage" here can mean the length of time that a treatment was implemented (e.g., a few hours, a few days, several weeks, a year) or the amount of time during a set period that the treatment was implemented (e.g., 5 minutes every week over a 6-month time period).

Treatment fidelity is one of the most critical aspects in evaluation studies, because evaluators need to know whether the treatment was implemented according to the specifications. If the evaluators implement the treatment themselves (not usually the case), then they can be sure that it was implemented as planned. However, it is more likely that the treatment will be implemented by teachers, counselors, administrators, staff members, community members, or psychologists, and perhaps it will be implemented in several different venues. Evaluators can recommend strategies for increasing the likelihood that the intervention will be implemented appropriately, such as training the implementers and collecting data on the implementation process as part of the evaluation.

Brady and O'Regan (2009) included a process component in their evaluation that included "a review of the case files of mentored youth ... to establish whether the program was implemented according to the manual. Focus groups with the program staff were also included in the design to collect data regarding their experience of implementing the program" (p. 275).

The strength of treatment also needs to be carefully considered. Is exposure to a new teaching strategy for 30 minutes sufficient to justify the expectation of a significant change in students' abilities to solve math problems? If the innovative math program is implemented over a 6-week period, is that long enough? Or does the implementation need to start in first grade and be implemented over a 5-year period in order for significant changes to be seen? These are all questions of strength of treatment. In the Brady and O'Regan (2009) study, they followed the youth for 18 months. Based on the theory of mentoring that guided the program, this was deemed a sufficient amount of time to see relationships form and to see effects of those relationships in terms of the dependent measures.

Symbols Used in Experimental and Quasi–Experimental Designs

Experimental designs are used in evaluation to test for program effectiveness; the Brady and O'Regan (2009) study is just one example. Experimental designs for evaluation studies have three major characteristics:

- An independent variable that an evaluator can manipulate.
- Use of at least two groups: experimental and control.
- Random assignment of individuals to experimental or control groups.

Experimental and quasi-experimental designs can be depicted with the following symbols, which we use in the discussions of these design types below:

- R stands for random assignment to groups in experimental designs. This means that everyone has an equal chance of being in either the control or experimental groups. Randomization can be achieved by such simple means as putting all the names of possible participants into a hat and randomly drawing out names, or by much more technologically sophisticated means (e.g., using a computer program that does the random assignment).
- O stands for observation (of the dependent variable). The dependent variable is what the evaluator hopes will change after exposure to the experimental treatment; it can be a change in behaviors, attitudes, skills, knowledge, or abilities.
- X stands for the independent variable if there is one independent variable (usually the experimental variable). In evaluation, this is usually the evaluand.

These symbols allow evaluators to succinctly explain the design of their study.

Experimental Designs

The Basic Design: Pretest–Posttest Control Group Design

If an evaluator has two groups (one that gets the experimental treatment and one that does not), administers both a pretest and a posttest to both groups, and randomly assigns participants to each group, then the design will look like this:

$$R \; O \; X \; O$$

$$R \; O \quad \; O$$

Here is what this means: There are two groups (each line represents one group); participants are randomly assigned (R) to each group; both groups take a pretest (O); one group gets the experimental treatment (X); and both groups take the posttest.

The experimental part of the Brady and O'Regan (2009) study used a similar design. Their independent variable was mentoring of youth. It had two levels: One group had mentors; the other group did not. They administered their dependent measure three times—before the experiment began, and at 12 months and 18 months. Therefore, their design could be depicted as follows:

R O X O O

R O   O O

Here, R indicates random assignment to either the control or experimental group; O represents each administration of the dependent measure; and X indicates the experimental treatment (i.e., having a mentor). Notice that the space for a treatment is left blank for the control group because they did not have mentors.

This type of design controls for a number of the threats to validity. First, threats such as history, maturation, and testing are controlled for, because the members of both control and experimental groups are comparable. In the Brady and O'Regan (2009) study, if local schools had instituted a drug prevention program, both the experimental and control groups would have experienced this "event"; therefore, its effect would be canceled out. Instrumentation (a change in the dependent measure) was not a threat, because the evaluators used the same pretests and posttests. Statistical regression is only a problem if participants are selected because they represent extreme groups on the dependent measure. This was not the case in the Brady and O'Regan study.

A potentially serious concern in experimental research is differential selection (i.e., differences between the two groups differ on relevant dimensions beyond reception of the experimental treatment). This threat is controlled by random assignment of participants to experimental and control groups. The reason why random selection is important relates to its theoretical power to balance the characteristics of the different groups, thereby strengthening the argument that the intervention caused the change in the dependent variable, and eliminating other possible causes of changes between groups. For example, random assignment also controls for experimental mortality because, hypothetically, it balances out systematic differences associated with dropping out of the study. In addition, the use of a pretest allows evaluators to compare those who drop out on variables from the pretest, to see whether there are differential characteristics associated with those who complete the study and those who do not.

· · · · · · · · · · · · EXTENDING YOUR THINKING · · · · · · · · · · ·

Using Symbols

Ward randomly assigned 12 people who had been unemployed for 6 months to the control group and 12 people who had been unemployed for 6 months to the experimental group. All workers had been laid off from the Perrara Candy factory, but visited the factory once a week as the Perrara administrators attempted to place them in other work sites. The control group spent 2 hours a week in the employment office waiting room as usual. The experimental group met in the factory's gym and practiced meditation with a Kundalini yoga teacher.

How would you describe this study, using symbols?

Box 9.4. Variations of Experimental Designs

Design	Symbolic description or other information
Posttest-only design	R X O
	R O
Single-factor multiple-treatment design	R O X_1 O O O
	R O X_2 O O O
	R O O O O
Solomon four-group design	R O X O
	R O O
	R X O
	R O
Factorial designs	$A_1 \times B_1$ $A_2 \times B_1$ $A_1 \times B_2$ $A_2 \times B_2$
Cluster randomization designs	No random assignment of individuals; groups rather than individuals are evaluated.

Variations of Experimental Designs

Using the same R, O, X symbols (plus A, B, etc., for factorial designs), evaluators can create several variations of experimental designs. These are summarized in Box 9.4 and described below.

POSTTEST-ONLY DESIGN

In the posttest-only design, no pretest is given, but participants are randomly assigned to groups and a posttest is given. The threats to validity are controlled in this design in much the same way as for the pretest–posttest control group design. One exception is that with no pretest, the threats of instrumentation and testing are not of concern. However, if there are differential completion rates between the experimental and control groups, the evaluator does not have the pretest scores to compare the two groups; this can be a problem in some circumstances. The design for this type of study looks like this:

$$R \quad X O$$
$$R \quad\ \ O$$

SINGLE-FACTOR MULTIPLE-TREATMENT DESIGN

The single-factor multiple-treatment design involves more than two groups. Suppose the Irish mentoring study (Brady & O'Regan, 2009) had included another comparison group that received neither the youth services program nor a mentor. The design for such a study would look like this:

R O X₁ O O O   (Randomly assigned, pretest, mentor posttest, posttest, posttest)

R O X₂ O O O   (Randomly assigned, pretest, service program, posttest, posttest, posttest)

R O   O O O   (Randomly assigned to no-treatment control [neither the youth services program nor a mentor], posttest, posttest, posttest

Each line represents one group. Members of each group were randomly assigned to their group. A pretest was administered, and then posttests were administered at three later times. The X's in this example stand for the two different treatments (X_1, youth services and a mentor; X_2, youth services alone), and the blank space on the third line represents the no-treatment control group (which received neither the youth services nor a mentor).

SOLOMON FOUR-GROUP DESIGN

The Solomon four-group design was developed in order to test the effect of pretest sensitization on the dependent variable. It looks like this:

R O X O

R O   O

R   X O

R   O

That is, four groups are compared on the dependent measure. One of those groups receives a pretest and the experimental treatment; one group receives both a pretest and a posttest, but no treatment. The other two groups do not receive the pretest; one of those receives the treatment, and the other does not. Hence the evaluator is able to test for the effect of taking the pretest on the dependent measure. However, the disadvantage of this design is that it requires having four groups, which necessitates having larger samples and is more costly.

FACTORIAL DESIGNS

A factorial design involves more than one independent variable. In such designs, other alphabetic symbols are more commonly used than X's: A stands for the first independent variable, B stands for the second independent variable, and so on.

Evaluators can also use numbered subscripts to indicate the level of each independent variable. For example, suppose you are evaluating a program that offers job training to individuals who either have or have not graduated from high school. Your study will have two independent variables (high school graduation and job training, with two levels of each variable). The two variables can be indicated as follows:

> A—high school graduation
>
> > A_1—has a high school diploma
> >
> > A_2—does not have a high school diploma
>
> B—job training
>
> > B_1—participates in job training
> >
> > B_2—does not participate in job training

A factorial design provides an opportunity to test for main effects of each independent variable, as well as for interactions between those variables. This can be represented as follows:

$$A$$

$$B$$

$$A \times B$$

$A \times B$ stands for the interaction of the two variables. In the example of high school diplomas and job training, let us assume that the dependent measure is income level. You can test to see whether people who have diplomas have higher incomes than those who do not have such diplomas. You can also test to see whether those who participate in job training benefit more from such training than those who do not participate in the training. In terms of interactions, the comparisons can be made for those who have a high school diploma and job training ($A_1 \times B_1$), those with a high school diploma and no job training ($A_1 \times B_2$), those with no high school diploma and job training ($A_2 \times B_1$), and those with no high school diploma and no job training ($A_2 \times B_2$). This is illustrated in the following matrix:

	Job training (B_1)	No job training (B_2)
Has high school diploma (A_1)	$A_1 \times B_1$	$A_1 \times B_2$
No high school diploma (A_2)	$A_2 \times B_1$	$A_2 \times B_2$

This design will allow conclusions about the effectiveness of the job training program for people with diplomas and those without them.

CLUSTER RANDOMIZATION DESIGNS

Sometimes evaluators cannot randomly assign individuals to conditions, but they can randomly assign groups (e.g., schools or classrooms) to conditions. This resolves some problems and creates others. If data are collected at the individual level (i.e., scores for each student), but randomization is done at the classroom level, then the data for each student need to be transformed to a classroom level in order to be consistent with the design. Such constraints require larger samples and/or the use of sophisticated statistical analyses, discussed further in Chapters 10 and 12.

············ **EXTENDING YOUR THINKING** ············

Variations of Experimental Designs

Both Asiah's and Khadijat's families (see "Extending Your Thinking: Threats to Internal Validity," earlier in this chapter) had moved to the United States from other countries. Both students had lived beside the ocean in their early childhood and had learned much about its beauty and importance from their parents. Two other students in the class were raised in southern Illinois and had never seen the ocean, and two other students had seen the ocean on vacations. The class was just beginning a unit on marine biology, and the teacher wanted them to understand how the BP oil spill had affected the southern U.S. shoreline. She thought that showing the PBS special describing the spill would greatly increase their sense of responsibility of being good stewards of the earth.

1. Imagine how you would create a study with the scenario above, using a factorial design. Describe what the variables are, and write it out symbolically.

2. How would you set up a Solomon four-group design?

3. Now that you know a bit more about Asiah and Khadijat, do you think that there may have been a reason, other than boredom, why they became restless while watching the video?

Ethical Issues in Random Assignment

Random assignment to conditions means that individuals have an equal chance of being in either the experimental or the control group. Brady and O'Regan (2009) used a computer-generated random allocation process to assign youth either to the group with mentors or to the one without mentors.

Ethical questions are associated with random assignment, because it means that some people get a service and others do not, based on the luck of the draw. The research and evaluation communities have devised a number of responses to this dilemma. The World Medical Association (2008) has developed a code of ethics for medical researchers around the globe and recommends that researchers in other domains follow these principles. The Declaration of Helsinki was issued in 1964 and has been revised several times; the most recent version of the declaration was approved in 2008. This declaration states that it is unethical to give no treatment when some treatment is available. However, an experimental treatment can be given to one group, with the caveat that whenever possible the next best treatment be given to the comparison group. The World Medical Association (2008) also writes:

> The benefits, risks, burdens and effectiveness of a new intervention must be tested against those of the best current proven intervention, except in the following circumstances:

> ■ The use of placebo, or no treatment, is acceptable in studies where no current proven intervention exists; or

> ■ Where for compelling and scientifically sound methodological reasons the use of placebo

is necessary to determine the efficacy or safety of an intervention and the patients who receive placebo or no treatment will not be subject to any risk of serious or irreversible harm. Extreme care must be taken to avoid abuse of this option.

As an ethical precaution, Brady and O'Regan (2009) told staff members that there was a limited number of "free passes" they could use if they felt that a particular youth was in circumstances that really required having a mentor. In such cases, they could issue a free pass, and that individual would be placed in the experimental group.

Mark and Gamble (2009) expand on conditions under which denial of treatment might be considered ethical. For example, the control group participants can be offered the service after the study concludes. This is the strategy that Brady and O'Regan (2009) used in their study of the youth mentoring program. The program was designed to serve youth ages 10–18; therefore, they used youth ages 10–14 in their study, meaning that when a youth turned 15 years of age, he/she could be offered a mentor.

Mark and Gamble (2009) say that it is not necessary to provide the control group members with the treatment once the study is completed, as long as they are better off than they would have been without participating in the study. Hence control group participants who are paid for their involvement benefit from the study and therefore are better off. They use an evaluation of the federal early childhood intervention called Head Start as an example. Young children were assigned at random to either Head Start or a control condition, in which their parents were given a list of community agencies serving young children and could pursue referrals to these agencies on their own. The assumption is that children living in poverty would not have access to this specially designed intervention if the government had not made it available to them for this experimental study. If we accept the condition that the United States does not have the resources to provide early childhood services to all of its poor children, then it is acceptable to say that assigning children randomly to have access to those services is ethical.[1]

Another response to concerns about random assignment consists of the use of "stop rules" (Mark & Gamble, 2009). A stop rule is a specific protocol that allows the evaluators to stop the study if significant benefits of a specified size are evident earlier than planned in the study. For example, in a study of the effect of aspirin on the prevention of heart attacks (Hennekens & Buring, 1989), the researchers found that a significant number of men in the control group were having heart attacks, compared to the experimental group. They decided to end the study early in view of these findings and their serious consequences. Stop rules can also be used if the experimental treatment is found to be significantly worse than the control condition, or if harmful unintended consequences are evident.

Quasi–Experimental Designs

Quasi-experimental designs follow the same logic as experimental designs. The big difference between the two approaches is that quasi-experimental designs are used *when random assignment to conditions is not possible*. In studies where the evaluators cannot assign participants randomly to groups, then differential selection is a threat to validity that needs to be given serious attention. For example, if researchers want to know whether having been robbed affects people's views on sentencing of thieves, they are likely to use people who have already been robbed. Evaluators can address this by identifying and measuring background characteristics in each of the groups and comparing to see whether there are important differences between or among them. They can also use statistical processes to control for differences in background characteristics (e.g., multiple linear regression, discussed in Chapter 12), or they can make subgroup comparisons (such as comparing older participants or younger participants from each group).

Box 9.5. Three Quasi-Experimental Designs with Controls for Threats to Validity

Design	Symbolic description
Static group comparison design	$X \quad O$ -------- O Or: $X \quad O_1 \quad O_2 \quad O_3 \quad O_4$ -------------------------- $\quad\quad O_1 \quad O_2 \quad O_3 \quad O_4$
Nonequivalent control group design	$O \quad X \quad O$ ------------- $O \quad\quad O$
Regression discontinuity design	$O \quad C \quad X \quad O$ ------------------ $O \quad C \quad\quad O$

Although participants cannot be randomly assigned to various groups in quasi-experimental designs, evaluators can still choose from a number of quasi-experimental designs similar to those presented in the section on experimental designs. These designs have already been explained in detail; therefore, we choose to provide you with detailed explanations of only three possible quasi-experimental designs. These are summarized in Box 9.5. We assume that you understand that you can use the same designs described previously in circumstances in which you cannot randomly assign participants, with the caveat that you will not have an R at the beginning of these designs (see Box 9.4). The dashed lines between rows in Box 9.5 symbolize the nonrandom assignment to groups.

Static Group Comparison Design

If an evaluator can divide the participants into two (or more) groups, one of which does not get the treatment, then this is the static group comparison design when only a posttest (no pretest) is given. "Static" means that the groups are accepted as they are already; the evaluator does not randomly assign participants to groups. It can be symbolically depicted this way:

$$X \quad O$$
$$\text{--------}$$
$$O$$

In this case, the X stands for the treatment that is administered to the experimental group, and the O stands for the posttest that is administered to both groups.

Another quasi-experimental design of this type is illustrated in the evaluation of a "boot camp" program to prevent return to prison (Duwe & Kerschner, 2008; see Chapter 3, Box 3.3). The design of this study can be depicted as follows:

$$X \quad O_1 \quad O_2 \quad O_3 \quad O_4$$
$$\text{--------------------------}$$
$$O_1 \quad O_2 \quad O_3 \quad O_4$$

In this case, X stands for the experimental treatment (boot camp), and each O stands for one of the dependent measures. The O's that appear below the line are preceded by a blank space, indicating that the control group did not receive this experimental treatment. And the O's are the same dependent measures that were used with the experimental group.

Using the same logic that applies to experimental designs, this quasi-experimental design controlled for the history and maturation threats to validity by virtue of having a comparison group. The testing, instrumentation, and statistical regression threats were not problems, because there was no pretest. However, differential selection and experimental mortality could have been problems because the individuals were not randomly assigned to the groups. In order to address the threat of differential selection, Duwe and Kerschner (2008) used a multistage sampling strategy for selection of control group members. They first screened the control group to eliminate anyone who would not have been eligible for the experimental treatment. They then randomly selected the members of the control group from that eligible group. Finally, they compared the experimental and control groups on 15 variables that were relevant in this study (e.g., sex, age, race, type of offense) to demonstrate the similarities of the two groups. They addressed concerns about experimental mortality by subdividing the experimental group into those who completed the program and those who failed to complete it. This enabled them to compare the effects of dropping out of the program on the same variables for those who completed the program, those who started and dropped out, and those who never entered the experimental program.

One other notable feature of Duwe and Kerschner's (2008) boot camp study was their attention to the strength of treatment. The program was designed to last 18 months and included intensive physical conditioning, drug treatment, and supervision. They noted that these are critical elements influencing the success of such programs.

Nonequivalent Control Group Design

The nonequivalent control group design is similar to the static group comparison design, except that evaluators use a pretest for both the experimental and control groups. This pretest is often referred to as a "baseline" and allows the evaluators to compare the similarities of the two groups before the program begins. It also can be used to control for the experimental mortality threat to validity, because the evaluators can measure to see whether those who dropped out of the program were similar to those who completed it, as well as to those who dropped out of the control group. This design can be depicted as follows:

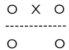

Regression Discontinuity Design

Quasi-experimental designs can also look very different from the standard experimental designs. One of these options is the regression discontinuity design. This type of design is used in evaluation studies in which the intervention and control groups are selected on the basis of scoring above or below a certain cutoff point on a test (Schochet, 2009). In other words, it is used when scores on a continuous measurement are used "to assign the intervention to study units (e.g., school districts, schools, classrooms, or students). Units with scores below a preset cutoff value are assigned to the treatment group, and units with scores above the cutoff value are assigned to comparison group, or vice versa" (Schochet, 2009, p. 238). The rationale for the regression discontinuity design is based on the assumption that the two groups will not show changes from pre- to posttesting unless the intervention is having an effect. The evaluator examines the trend of change between the two groups. If the intervention group shows the same trend of change as the control group, then the evaluator reaches the conclusion that the intervention is having the desired effect.

In regression discontinuity studies, the unit of analysis might be the individual client or student, classroom, clinic or school, or service region or district. For example, Moss and Yeaton (2006) evaluated a developmental English program at the college level. Students come to college with differing levels of ability to write and read English. Some students' skills are considered to be adequate for enrollment in a standard college-level English course. Students who do not enter college with this level of skill are often required to take a developmental English course before they can take the standard course. Moss and Yeaton (2006) used students scoring above and below the cutoff on an English screening test at one college as their two groups in their regression discontinuity study. Here is how Moss and Yeaton describe their design:

> Of the 1,782 students who scored at the developmental level, 1,133 (64%) completed developmental English, and 649 never enrolled in a developmental English course. Of those who completed the developmental English course, 649 (57%) also completed college-level English. It was this group, combined with the 824 nondevelopmental students that constituted our final sample of 1,473. (p. 219)

Using widely accepted notation, the [regression discontinuity] design is illustrated as follows:

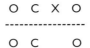

Here, each row references a different group. The O signifies measurement of the pre- and post-tests for each group, and X represents the program that was administered. The C denotes that the groups were assigned by a conditional factor (i.e., participants falling below or at or above a cut[off] score). The top row indicates the group that received the developmental intervention, and the bottom row shows the group that served as a control. (p. 221)

The authors recognized that selection bias (or differential selection) might be a threat to the validity of their study, because the groups differed in their English abilities at the start of the study. This was inherent in the design. However, such a design assumes that "in the absence of the program, the pre–post relationship would be equivalent for the two groups" (Trochim, 1990, p. 122). Regression discontinuity uses the projected trajectory of scores for each group; that is, if the groups did not receive any interventions, what would we expect to see in terms of their performance? The group that is low-performing at the beginning of the study is tracked to see whether the trajectory of its performance is significantly better than would have been predicted without the intervention. And a researcher can determine whether the performance of this actually reflects a performance level similar to that of the group performing at a higher level at the beginning of the study. If the pattern of the originally low-performing group reflects this change, then this is called a "discontinuity in regression analysis" and is accepted as evidence of the program's effectiveness.

Moss and Yeaton (2006) did find this discrepant relationship in their study of the effects of the English development program. Thus they were able to conclude that "students' participation in the program increases English academic achievement to levels similar to those of students not needing developmental coursework" (p. 215). Thus the design allowed the researchers to compare the expected outcomes without the program with the actual outcomes from the program.

It should be noted that Schochet (2009) argues that regression discontinuity requires larger sample sizes than a random assignment design, so that sample sizes will be sufficient for the complex statistics associated with this design. Thus a regression discontinuity design may not be feasible because of the need for a larger sample and associated higher financial costs.

· · · · · · · · · · E X T E N D I N G   Y O U R   T H I N K I N G · · · · · · · · · ·

Quasi-Experimental Designs

1. Think of some circumstances where random selection is not an option and one must use a quasi-experimental design in the evaluation.

2. Give an example of when evaluators might want to use a nonequivalent control group design (first group, O X O; second group, O O).

3. Give an example of when evaluators might want to use a regression discontinuity design (first group, O C X O; second group, O C O).

Single-Group Designs

Sometimes evaluators do not have access to a control group; therefore, they use a single-group design. One such design involves having a pretest and a posttest to be able to demonstrate changes following exposure to the treatment (program). However, an evaluator in such a case is challenged to provide sufficient evidence that the observed changes are the result of the program and not of some other events or circumstances that happened to coincide with the implementation of the program (i.e., the threats to validity are very hard to control). Another possible design is the time series design, which can be used with one group or several groups.

Time Series Design

A time series design includes an intervention and then multiple measures of the dependent variable at various time intervals. Measurements can be made before the intervention to show stability of the behavior without intervention. Then multiple measures are made during and after the intervention to indicate a trajectory of change. The continuity of measures and the pattern of responses on the dependent variable control for many of the threats to validity.

Coryn et al. (2009) integrated a time series design into a success case method (Brinkerhoff, 2003; see explanation of this approach in Chapter 3) study of homelessness and unemployment. Three dependent measures were combined to define success: employment, housing, and reduction of need for government support (e.g., food stamps). The sample was then divided into three groups: high if they met all three criteria, medium if they met one or two of the criteria, and low if they failed to meet any of the criteria. Baseline data on employment, housing, and public assistance were collected before the program began. Then these same measurements were obtained again 6 months, 12 months, and 18 months after program completion. This design allowed the researchers to track any movements from one group into another group (e.g., from low to medium, from medium to high). Movement from a higher to a lower category was associated with variations in strength of treatment; that is, those who did not regularly attend workshops or meetings with case managers tended to move down in levels. The reverse was also true: People who ended up in the high group tended to have high levels of participation in meetings and services. These patterns across time added credibility for claims of the effectiveness of the program.

Surveys

Surveys can be looked at from a design perspective, as well as from a data collection perspective. In this section, we discuss the design options for surveys. Surveys can be used as data collection tools within other evaluation designs; we discuss surveys as data collection tools in Chapter 10.

Survey designs include simple descriptive designs, which occur at a single point in time with the purpose of gaining a descriptive picture of a group on targeted characteristics. Evaluators of a suicide prevention program for women who had experienced abuse at the hands of their partners (intimate partner violence, or IPV) used a descriptive survey to assess the effectiveness of the program (Davis et al., 2009). Davis et al. described their survey as follows:

> Data from an Intervention Satisfaction Survey reveal that the women who participated in the Grady Nia Project are extremely pleased with the services that they receive. Specifically, more than 80% of the women in the project reported that participation facilitated their capacity to talk about IPV and suicidal feelings, to cope more effectively with IPV, and to reduce their suicidality. Over 70% of the women found the Resource Room to be valuable. Overall, close to 90% of the women reported extremely high or high levels of intervention satisfaction. (p. 141)

Cross-sectional designs also occur at a single point in time, but they are administered to several groups at the same time in order to make cross-group comparisons (e.g., a school survey administered to all students in the first, third, and fifth grades can be used to make comparisons across grade levels). Hall, Sedlacek, Berenback, and Dieckman (2007) used a cross-sectional survey design to measure the effectiveness of therapy interventions for women in the military who experienced sexual trauma. They were able to collect data from five facilities and four regions across the United States, and to use the data for comparative purposes.

Longitudinal designs collect data from the same group or cohort over an extended period of time. For example, the Brady and O'Regan (2009) study conducted surveys over the course of the project with the same people to be able to compare changes over time. The U.S. government's National Center for Education Statistics (see, e.g., Planty et al., 2009) undertakes large-scale longitudinal surveys of school systems around the country to measure changes in educational variables such as enrollment, learning outcomes, and educational progress.

Cross-sectional designs have the advantage of requiring less time than longitudinal designs. However, evaluators need to be aware that the threats of maturation, history, and differential selection cannot be controlled in cross-sectional designs. Longitudinal designs have the advantage that the same people provide data over a period of time, so this controls for other sources of variation. However, by the time first graders are in fifth grade (e.g., it is probably not safe to assume that everything is the same in the first grade as it was when they were at that level. So, again, comparisons over time come with their own challenges. Survey researchers have a myriad of other choices to make regarding the means of distribution, doing surveys individually or in groups, methods to enhance returns of the surveys, and strategies for designing the instrument. These are all discussed in Chapter 10.

· · · · · · · · · · EXTENDING YOUR THINKING · · · · · · · · · ·
Surveys

Design	When would you use this design and why?
Simple descriptive designs	
Cross-sectional designs	
Longitudinal designs	

Cost Analysis

As noted briefly in Chapter 8, cost analysis centers on this question: How much does this treatment cost, and is it worth it? This approach looks at effectiveness and efficiency—achieving the most benefit while costing the least for the most people (Fals-Stewart, Yates, & Klostermann, 2005). The terms used in this somewhat simplistic explanation of cost analysis become more problematic and complex with further analysis.

Cost analysis designs can include other types of designs, as well as the unique factors associated with the study of costs. For example, cost analysis assumes that the evaluator can provide an acceptable definition of a program's benefits that can be used to compare benefits across programs. In experimental design terms, this would be the dependent variable. If a cost analysis design is based on a comparison of benefits across programs, then part of the design will include some type of experimental or quasi-experimental component. This strategy then raises many of the challenges associated with these approaches. For example, the evaluator needs to give careful thought to the program chosen for comparison to the evaluand. Should the evaluand be compared to existing practice, to a placebo, or to another variation of the innovative program? Another complication with the term "benefits" is that evaluators need to be aware of the possibility that participants are not receiving benefits from a program; it is possible that they are being harmed. Benefits and harm can also be considered at the individual or societal levels, and can include unintended benefits or harm.

Another layer of complexity is represented in trying to measure costs. Fals-Stewart et al. (2005) provide these definitions and examples of costs:

> *Costs* are defined as the monetary value of resources consumed or otherwise lost as a consequence of an illness or disorder. Costs are often further subdivided into direct costs and indirect costs.
>
> *Direct costs* are those incurred to provide a treatment or service. Direct costs to deliver an intervention may include (a) time (e.g., hours used to deliver the marital or family treatment, time needed to participate by the client and family members); (b) transportation to and from appointments (i.e., mileage costs); (c) materials used in the course of the intervention (e.g., paper-and-pencil measures completed by clients); (d) equipment (e.g., urine assay system in a drug abuse treatment program); (e) rental for space where the treatment is delivered; and (f) overhead costs for operation of the program where the service is provided (e.g., wages of support staff and administrators).
>
> *Indirect costs* are the resources lost due to the disorder. This may include the value of time that could have been used in other activities in the absence of the disorder, such as the cost of lost employment by clients and their family members. (p. 29)

Scriven (2007) recommends that evaluators consider the following:

> (i) money and nonmoney costs, (ii) direct and indirect costs, and (iii) both actual and opportunity costs. They should be itemized by developmental stage—i.e., (a) start-up, (b) maintenance, (c) upgrade, (d) shutdown costs—and/or by calendar time period; by cost elements (rent, equipment, personnel, etc.), and by payee—all of these whenever relevant and possible. Include use of expended but never realized value, if any, e.g., social capital, (e.g., decline in workforce morale). The most common nonmoney costs are space, time, expertise, and common labor (when these are not available for purchase in the open market—if they are so available, they just represent money costs); PLUS the less measurable ones—stress, political and personal capital

(e.g., reputation and goodwill), and immediate environmental impact, which are rarely fully coverable by money. (p. 13)

Hummel-Rossi and Ashdown (2002) expand on the meaning of cost analysis within the educational evaluation domain. Costs should include not just monetary costs, but also both obvious and hidden costs for the entire intervention (e.g., child care or travel costs). They cite an example in special education: Costs could be calculated according to how much additional expense is needed to serve a child with a disability compared to one who is not so identified; or the costs could be calculated by estimating the actual cost of the special education services replacing the regular education services. Hummel-Rossi and Ashdown assert that the latter approach is in line with the "ingredients costs" approach that they favor. Ingredients costs (Levin, 1983) are comprehensive costs; they include *all* costs, even those that do not appear in the budget. Hummel-Rossi and Ashdown's (2002) protocol for cost-effectiveness studies is presented in Box 9.6.

Box 9.6. Cost-Effectiveness Protocol

Component	Recommendation
Perspective	Clearly articulate the goals of the evaluation.
Cost analysis	Use an ingredients approach.
Comparators	Follow existing practice or reasonable alternatives.
Estimation of program effects	Use a rigorous experimental or quasi-experimental design, with attention to identifying hidden and/or qualitative outcomes, and positive as well as negative outcomes.
Outcome measures	Use standardized achievement measures or effect size, if different achievement tests are used. Attempt to measure qualitative residual.
Distributional consequences	Assign all types of costs and effects to appropriate parties.
Analysis of time effects	Annualize costs, take into account inflation, and discount costs over time.
Sensitivity analysis	Explore variations in significant assumptions/parameters and identify their impact on cost-effectiveness ratio.
Decision rule	Remember: Cost analysis is an important source of information in decision making, but not the sole criterion.
Reporting of findings	Write a technical report that includes a reference case and that is available upon request. Results can also be reported in a professional journal.

Source: Adapted from Hummel-Rossi and Ashdown (2002, p. 20), who based it on Barnett (1993) and U.S. Department of Health and Human Services (1996). Copyright 2002 by the American Educational Research Association. Adapted by permission.

Duwe and Kerschner's (2008) evaluation of the boot camp program to reduce return to prison also includes an example of a cost analysis design. They compared the effectiveness of this program (the Challenge Incarceration Program or CIP) with that of the regular incarceration program, using a quasi-experimental design (see earlier discussion in this chapter, as well as Chapter 3, Box 3.3). They also studied whether early release and the reduction in recidivism were associated with cost reductions. For the latter study, they included the costs of the participants' time in the program and the cost of supervision when they were released. They made a distinction between "fixed costs" and "marginal costs." Fixed costs include the expenses of constructing a building and staffing. Marginal costs are those associated with incremental expenses that vary with the number of inmates (e.g., food, clothing, medical services). In their study, Duwe and Kerschner used the marginal costs, because the number of people in the boot camp program was only 1% of the inmates in the system. Since the number was so small, they reasoned that the district would have to have the buildings and staff anyway, so the better choice of cost comparisons was in marginal costs. Here are two excerpts from their article:

> The early release savings were calculated by first segregating CIP participants into 10 separate cohorts by the fiscal year in which they entered Phase I (FY 1993 to FY 2002). Next, program operating costs were determined by counting the total number of days each cohort spent in CIP and then multiplying by the full per diem associated with each phase for that fiscal year. (pp. 632–633)

> The results reported here indicate that CIP significantly reduced the rate at which offenders commit a new crime. But because of the fact that CIP offenders were more likely to come back as supervised release violators, they returned to prison at roughly the same rate as the control group. CIP still produced a recidivism savings, however, because offenders spent, on average, 40 fewer days in prison because of the shorter lengths of stay associated with supervised release violations. Although the total savings were relatively modest at $6.2 million over the 10-year period, the size of the savings, particularly those resulting from the early-release provision, increased nearly every year after FY 1998. (p. 638)

· · · · · · · · · · E X T E N D I N G   Y O U R   T H I N K I N G · · · · · · · · · · ·

Cost Benefits

1. Critics of cost analysis would like to know the answers to such questions as these: How do you put a value on an education? How do you put a value on information? How do you balance the costs and benefits of a seed-planting cooperative that fails economically but has given women a new sense of self, as they have had to learn skills that they believed only men could possess? Can a cost analysis measure these intangible "benefits"? Should it?

2. French et al. (2000) conducted a cost evaluation of a program for substance abuse treatment. Specifically, they compared a full continuum of care (including residential stays) with a partial continuum of care (outpatient care). Imagine that this is your project. What types of costs might you anticipate including in the study?

(cont.)

What sources of information do you think you should use to obtain information about costs? Payment for services is an obvious cost variable, but it might be based on what individuals pay, what insurance companies pay, or agency records. What other types of costs might you consider? Furthermore, what outcomes of the full versus the partial continuum of care might you consider to be important in the French et al. example? Length of drug-free time and reduction of psychiatric symptoms might be two outcome measures. What do you think about placing a monetary value on these outcomes?

Qualitative Designs

Although qualitative designs are typically associated with process evaluations, they do have a place in other evaluation approaches as well. Maxwell (2004) argues that qualitative methods are needed in evaluations that attempt to identify cause-and-effect relationships. Specific criteria for judging the quality of qualitative research—criteria that parallel the concepts of internal and external validity for quantitative evaluations—are presented in Chapter 10 on data collection. However, Erickson (in Moss, Phillips, Erickson, Floden, Lather, & Schneider, 2009)[2] gives us a glimpse into what he considers to be a basis for judging quality in qualitative work:

> For qualitative research, well done means the study involved a substantial amount of time in fieldwork; careful, repeated sifting through information sources that were collected to identify "data" from them; careful, repeated analysis of data to identify patterns in them (using what some call analytic induction); and clear reporting on how the study was done and how conclusions followed from evidence. For qualitative work, reporting means narrative reporting that shows not only things that happened in the setting and the meanings of those happenings to participants, but the relative frequency of occurrence of those happenings—so that the reader gets to see rich details and also the broad patterns within which the details fit. The reader comes away both tree-wise and forest-wise—not tree-wise and forest-foolish, or vice versa.
>
> When I say a study has an educational imagination, I mean it addresses issues of curriculum, pedagogy, and school organization in ways that shed light on—not prove but rather illuminate, make us smarter about—the limits and possibilities for what practicing educators might do in making school happen on a daily basis. Such a study also sheds light on which aims of schooling are worth trying to achieve in the first place—it has a critical vision of ends as well as of means toward ends. Educational imagination involves asking research questions that go beyond utilitarian matters of efficiency and effectiveness, as in the discourse of new public management ... , especially going beyond matters of short-term "effects" that are easily and cheaply measured. (p. 504)

Qualitative designs include case studies, ethnographies, phenomenological studies, grounded theory, discourse analysis, narrative approaches, focus groups, and some forms of participatory action research (other participatory designs use mixed methods). This section includes explanations and examples of case studies, ethnographies, narrative designs, phenomenological studies, and participatory action designs. The topics of grounded theory and discourse analysis are included in Chapter 12; the topic of focus groups is covered in Chapter 10. As with quantitative designs, it is not possible to present all possible qualitative designs in this chapter. Interested readers are referred to these additional sources:

Corbin, J., & Strauss, A. (2008). *Basics of qualitative research: Techniques and procedures for developing grounded theory* (3rd ed.). Thousand Oaks, CA: Sage.

Hesse-Biber, S. N., & Leavy, P. (2011). *The practice of qualitative research* (2nd ed.). Thousand Oaks, CA: Sage.

Marshall, C., & Rossman, G. B. (2011). *Designing qualitative research* (5th ed.). Thousand Oaks, CA: Sage.

Maxwell, J. (2005). *Qualitative research design: An interactive approach* (2nd ed.). Thousand Oaks, CA: Sage.

Rossman, G. B., & Rallis, S. F. (2012). *Learning in the field: An introduction to qualitative research* (3rd ed.). Thousand Oaks, CA: Sage.

Case Studies

Case studies involve in-depth exploration of a single case, such as an individual, a group of individuals, a classroom, a school, a clinic, or even an event (McDuffie & Scruggs, 2008). Case studies are probably the most generic of qualitative designs. They can be combined with other qualitative designs, as in an ethnographic case study or a grounded theory case study. Stake (2004) has addressed the challenge of viewing a case study as a design, a specific method, or a unique form of research. If the evaluation focuses on a specific,

> **Qualitative Designs**
>
> **Case studies**
> Ethnographic designs
> Narrative designs
> Phenomenological studies
> Participatory action designs

unique, bounded system, the likelihood becomes greater that the evaluator is using a case study design. Case studies focus on a complex context and try to understand a particular object or case. Recall the Barela (2008) case study (see Chapter 5, Box 5.2), which studied the case of high-achieving and low-achieving schools that serve children in high-poverty areas in the Los Angeles Unified School District.

Merriam (2001) notes that a case study is (1) particularistic (i.e., it focuses on a particular case); (2) descriptive (i.e., it provides a rich picture of the case under study); and (3) heuristic (i.e., it provides an understanding of this phenomenon). Stake's (2004) responsive evaluation is one type of case study design. Abma's (2005) study of the prevention of dance-related injuries (see Chapter 5, Box 5.4) illustrates the responsive evaluation approach to a case study. In general terms, Stake (2004) recommends that case study designs include the following elements:

- The nature of the case

- Its historical background

- The physical setting

- Other contextual factors, such as economic, political, legal, and aesthetic variables

- Other cases that can be used to inform the understanding of the case itself

- Informants through whom the case can be known

And Yin (2009) makes these suggestions for case study designs:

1. Identify evaluation questions. Usually "how" or "why" questions are good for case studies.

2. Identify propositions, if any. Propositions are like hypotheses that you formulate to begin thinking about why variables might be related.

3. Specify the unit of analysis. This is the bounded system or case that you plan to study.

4. Establish a logical connection between the data and the propositions. Examine evidence to see whether the propositions are supported or not.

5. Develop criteria for interpreting the results.

6. Develop theory based on the data (if this is part of the aims of the study).

Kummerer and Lopez-Reyna (2009) used a case study design to explore the effectiveness of a language and literacy intervention for Mexican immigrant families. The specific bounded system that they investigated was composed of three families with children who were identified as having communication disabilities. The families came from Mexico and were currently living in the United States. They received center-based early childhood intervention services, and the children received speech and language therapy. "The case studies provide a descriptive account of the Mexican immigrant mothers' perceptions about language and literacy learning, their participation in their children's therapy, and implications for service providers in supporting different levels of parental involvement" (p. 332).

Ethnographic Designs

Studies that use ethnographic designs ask questions about the social and cultural practices of groups of people (Mertens, 2010). Ethnographies focus on the lived experiences, daily activities, and social context of everyday life from the perspective of the participants. The purpose is to understand patterns in life associated with systematic connections, such as patterns established through religion or kinship. Ethnographies can vary in scope from a very specific individual experience to a broader level of community experience. In the Use Branch, ethnographies can be conducted in consultation with "intended users" in the communities, who provide their views about what to study, how to study it, and whose voices should be represented. In the Social Justice Branch, ethnographies are more commonly conducted through a theoretical lens; examples include critical ethnography, feminist ethnography, indigenous ethnography, performance ethnography, CRT ethnography, autoethnography, netnography (online ethnography), and photoethnography. Ethnographers sometimes work with these broad theories (called "grand theories"), or they use more personal theories that are more contextually specific.

> **Qualitative Designs**
>
> Case studies
> **Ethnographic designs**
> Narrative designs
> Phenomenological studies
> Participatory action designs

The primary characteristics of an ethnographic design include the following:

- An introductory phase for getting acquainted and figuring out the landscape.
- Drawing boundaries around the study (i.e., setting the boundaries of what will be included in the study and what will be excluded).
- Sustained involvement: 6 months to 2 years, or whatever the circumstances will allow (e.g., 2 weeks).
- Field work: Observations.
- Informal interviews.
- Analysis: Significant themes, verbal descriptions, hypotheses.
- Ethnographic designs can use theories such as feminist, indigenous, disability rights, critical race, sociolinguistics, and other theories.

Frohmann (2005) provides an example of a program evaluation that used ethnography as one of the primary design elements. She was examining the Framing Safety Project, which was designed to allow Mexican and South Asian immigrant women to explore their experiences of violence and develop approaches to create safer spaces. The components included photographs taken by the women (a technique known as "photo-voice," discussed in Chapter 13), community exhibitions of the photographs, and ethnographic interviews and observations. Thus the design of the study was ethnographic participatory action research with a feminist lens. The women in the study were supported in their efforts to take action to improve their own safety, as well as to educate the community about this problem and strategies to overcome it.

Frohmann's (2005) study illustrates the major characteristics of an ethnographic design in evaluation. She began with an exploratory phase to get to know women who were already in an existing support group. She facilitated discussions about the meaning of safety to the participants and about their feelings and experiences with violence. Subsequently she introduced the idea of taking photographs as a means to capture their feelings and experiences by facilitating a discussion about when they had taken photographs in the past and what that meant to them. The women revealed visual images that they associated with the experience of violence; for example, a picture of a clock represented the woman who was waiting at home for her husband, who she knew would return drunk late at night and beat her. When the group members felt ready, they began to take pictures. The boundaries were set in terms of membership in the group and safety concerns, such as being careful not to include themselves or other family members in the pictures for safety reasons. Over a period of several weeks, the women took the pictures and shared them with their fellow participants and the evaluator at the support group meetings. The study continued over an extended period of months, because the second phase of the project involved a community exhibition of their photographs, and the final phase involved in-depth life history interviews of the women and use of the documents from the project (photographs, transcripts of support group discussions, and observational data from the community exhibit and viewers' responses to the exhibit). Frohmann used a grounded theory approach to data analysis (discussed further in Chapter 12) to develop themes that emerged from the data.

Frohmann (2005) describes her work as feminist, because she focused on the importance of the women's own experiences and the need to challenge societal power hierarchies. Here is her description of the feminist ethnographic, action research:

> First, my commitment to empowering the participants meant I chose a method that had the participants, not the researcher or other professionals, identify and photograph significant experiences in their lives. The project is designed to provide participants with a range of private spaces and public settings (support groups, photography exhibits, research interviews, and dispersal of information) in which experiences can be heard. The project participation framework gives women choices of how and when to participate. Second, the knowledge gained from the project can be used for further research and for individual and social action. Third, the project is structured as a collaboration between the participants and me. Fourth, I take a reflexive approach to the research process and I contextualize myself within the project and my writing. (p. 1399)

As discussed elsewhere in this text, feminist theory leads to an examination of power inequities in relationships between men and women. It brings to visibility consequences of those inequities (such as spousal battering), with an eye to social change.

Sociolinguistic Theory and Ethnography

Sociolinguistics is a theory of language use within a social context. For example, Kummerer and Lopez-Reyna (2009) used a sociolinguistic theory as part of their case study, to examine how the children used language to make requests in their environments. The data were gathered in detailed journals kept by the mothers, which revealed the growth in the children's communication abilities from nonverbal communication, gestures, early use of words, and improved articulation.

Hopson, Lucas, and Peterson (2000) provide an example of an evaluation that combined an experimental design (to determine the effectiveness of an HIV/AIDS prevention program) with an ethnographic portion, which was

> implemented to provide rich contextual data derived from interviews, and help encode views of drug-using participants. Social Affiliates in Injectors' Lives (SAIL) goals were twofold: to identify the role of families and support resources in maintaining and adopting HIV risk reduction strategies for high risk individuals, and to assess the association between the HIV-infected person's drug relapse and processes of coping. (p. 35)

The evaluators used ethnographic interviews, which they then analyzed via sociolinguistic strategies to determine the meaning of HIV/AIDS to the people the program was intended to serve.

Real-Time Constraints on Ethnographic Designs

Although evaluators might like to have the luxury of taking 6 months to 2 years to conduct an ethnographic study, logistical constraints (such as time and money) might limit the amount of time they can spend in the field, or information might be needed in a short time frame (such as in evaluations of responses to natural disasters). Rapid assessment is based on both ethnography and action research; it allows for the quick generation of information, with a goal of developing culturally appropriate interventions (McNall & Foster-Fishman, 2007). The United Nations High Commissioner for Refugees (UNHCR; Balde, Crisp, Macleod, &

Tennat, 2011) built on rapid ethnographic strategies to develop real-time evaluation designs that allowed it to be responsive in the early stages of a humanitarian crisis. Specific data collection tools that can be used with these designs are explained in Chapter 10.

· · · · · · · · · · EXTENDING YOUR THINKING · · · · · · · · · ·

Ethnographies

1. Get a taste of ethnography:

   a. View a photoethnography of Mexico's Low Riders (photoethnography) (*www.americanethnography.com/gallery.php?id=102*).

   b. Rent and watch the film *Born into Brothels: Calcutta's Red Light Kids* (2004).

   c. See a slideshow about the iPod nano (netnography, gathering data from online communities) (*www.slideshare.net/Wikonsumer/netnography-ipod-example*).

2. Cook, Murphy, and Hunt (2000) conducted a large-scale evaluation of 19 inner-city schools in Chicago that combined an experimental design with an ethnographic design. The ethnographic part of the evaluation was conducted by Payne (1998) and his colleagues, and included observations at all the schools over the full four years of the study. At the beginning of the evaluation, visits to schools occurred about twice a week, although they became less frequent as the years went by. In addition to these observations, the ethnographers interviewed the staff members who were implementing the program, the local school councils, principals, teachers, and parents. They also reviewed documents related to the team meetings; plans from the youth guidance office, the principals, and selected teachers; and topics covered in retreats and inservice training that were part of the project. "The ethnographic component did not include systematic collection of data on student behavior or in classrooms or in control schools" (Cook et al., 2000, p. 558). Thus the ethnography focused on interactions among adults in the implementation of the program. The ethnography was considered to be a valuable component of the evaluation, because it focused on the degree of implementation of the program. The conclusion based on the ethnographic data revealed that the ethnographers were not willing to classify any school as faithfully following all the program guidelines, although some were listed as close.

   a. Analyze the summary of this study to determine those aspects that identify it as an ethnographic evaluation.

   b. What strengths do you see in the ethnographic design?

   c. What are the implications of these strengths?

   d. What weaknesses do you see in the ethnographic design?

   e. What are the implications of these weaknesses?

Narrative Designs

Narrative designs for evaluation are based on the belief that we can understand the meaning of events by engaging in reflection about the way we talk about them.

> A narrative can be defined as an organized interpretation of a sequence of events. This involves attributing agency to the characters in the narrative and inferring causal links between the events. In the classic formulation, a narrative is an account with three components: a beginning, middle and an end. (Murray, 2008, p. 114)

Qualitative Designs

Case studies
Ethnographic designs
Narrative designs
Phenomenological studies
Participatory action designs

Narrative allows us to restore order to our lives when we encounter disruption (i.e., we try to explain to ourselves why something happened to make sense of it). This act of meaning making is indicative of an active agent role: If we cannot place ourselves in that active agent role, then we experience frustration. Narrative can be considered at the individual level as well as the communal level in terms of how members of a community talk about themselves.

Costantino and Greene (2003) provide an interesting example of a narrative-based design in their evaluation of a storytelling project in the rural Midwestern United States. The idea was for elderly people to tell stories from their own lives to school children, addressing active involvement of seniors, intergenerational communication, and children's knowledge of local history. They started with an interpretive responsive case study design (see the discussion of case studies above). As they encountered the richness of the stories, they realized that adding a narrative framing of the study would be useful. Using the narrative-based design, they "(a) generated important understandings of the interwoven character of the program with its context, and (b) provided windows of unique insight into participants' lived experiences of important program effects and thus unique contributions to assessment of the program's merit and worth" (p. 36). As they evaluated the intergenerational storytelling project, they found that using a narrative approach gave them a clear and significant picture of the quality of the program. They came to this realization after listening to the stories of how the project got started and how it had progressed in the county. They had entered the evaluation thinking that they could devise a chronological timeline and set boundaries around the project. However, the way the people talked about storytelling suggested that such linearity of thinking was not adequate for an understanding of what the project meant to them. Therefore, the evaluators decided to shift their focus to the narratives; they captured "these stories by transcribing them verbatim in order to preserve the participant's voice, not only for its evocative power, but also for the information a speaker's oral performance might provide about the program. We realized that much of what is meaningful to participants in this storytelling program was indeed embedded in the stories they told" (p. 41). Analysis strategies for this type of data are described in Chapter 12.

·········· E X T E N D I N G Y O U R T H I N K I N G ··········

Narrative Designs

"Photostories" (sometimes called "photovoice") are a type of narrative where individuals or community members can share a story visually with photographs. Read one photostory set in Indonesia, where an environmental disaster changed the lives of traditional fishermen and their families (***insightshare.org/resources/photostory/poisonous-stream***).

1. What do you think is effective about this technique?

2. Do you think taking photographs and writing in bubble captions is realistic in an evaluation? Explain.

3. What do you think some of the challenges would be in using this technique?

Phenomenological Studies

Wertz (2005) states that phenomenological inquiry requires the evaluator to set aside prior assumptions

> **Qualitative Designs**
>
> Case studies
> Ethnographic designs
> Narrative designs
> **Phenomenological studies**
> Participatory action designs

in order to gain access, in Husserl's famous phrase, "to the things themselves" … This return to phenomena as they are lived, in contrast to beginning with scientific preconceptions, is a methodological procedure and does not imply that such knowledge is false; it simply suspends received science, puts it out of play, and makes no use of it for the sake of fresh research access to the matters to be investigated. (p. 168)

The purpose of phenomenological inquiry is to shift from a superficial understanding of lived experience to an understanding at a deeper level, as it is experienced in conscious and unconscious ways by the participants. The process of coming to this deeper understanding involves accepting the concrete example of a phenomenon (an experience as described by a participant) and imaginatively varying it in every possible way to reveal its essential features—that is, what is absolutely necessary for this phenomenon to be understood to its fullest.

> Husserl established another important but much misunderstood scientific procedure, one that is fundamental to qualitative research because it enables the researcher to grasp what something is: the *intuition of essence* or the *eidetic reduction*. This method is neither inductive nor deductive; it descriptively delineates the invariant characteristic(s) and clarifies the meaning and structure/organization of a subject matter. (Wertz, 2005, p. 168)

Intentional analysis is an important part of phenomenology, in that humans attach meanings to their experiences based on their understandings of intentions (Wertz, 2005). Individuals have experiences, but they interpret meanings in broader social contexts, called "lifeworlds." These lifeworlds include features of time, space, culture, physical bodies, history, language, religion, and other social phenomena. Phenomenology attempts to understand the meaning of people's experience within this complex context, thus revealing aspects of the experience that the persons may not be aware of themselves.

The Trotman (2006) study was a phenomenological study (see Chapter 5, Box 5.3). Trotman evaluated a program to enhance students' creativity, imagination, and emotional development in six primary schools in the United Kingdom. The phenomenological design is evidenced in his decision to focus on the meaning teachers ascribed to children's creative, imaginative, and emotional experiences. Randall, Cox, and Griffiths (2007) provide another example of a phenomenological design; in this instance, it was used in an evaluation of a program to help nurses in the United Kingdom manage their on-the-job stress. The goal of the evaluation was to determine how the nurses experienced the intervention and how they experienced attempts to implement the intervention in their life spaces. The evaluators explored differences among the participants, which revealed that certain conditions led to changes that were either viewed as positive or negative. For example, one of the outcomes of the intervention was supposed to be planning for more uninterrupted managerial and administrative tasks. When this occurred, the staff reported positive effects in terms of fewer errors, more time for relationship building among staff members, and better paperwork flow. In some contexts, the nurses reported being too busy to sit down and plan how to have that uninterrupted time. Therefore, the results suggested that additional attention needed to be paid to the nurses who found themselves in this situation. Focusing on the meaning of the intervention at a complex and contextual level led to more nuanced conclusions about the effectiveness of the program and recommendations for next steps.

Participatory Action Designs

Participatory evaluation designs can take many forms; they can be pragmatic or transformative (see Chapters 4 and 6). They can be used for a variety of purposes (see Chapters 7 and 8). They can use qualitative or mixed methods designs (mixed methods are discussed later in this chapter). Participatory evaluation designs are used quite pervasively in evaluation, both domestically and internationally. Sharma and Deepak (2001) used a participatory design in their evaluation of a rehabilitation program in Vietnam (see Chapter 4, Box 4.11). Horn et al. (2008) used such a design to evaluate a smoking cessation program for American Indians (see Chapter 1).

As a basic guide to participatory action designs, Heron and Reason (2006) provide this general format:

> **Qualitative Designs**
>
> Case studies
> Ethnographic designs
> Narrative designs
> Phenomenological studies
> **Participatory action designs**

1. Decide on who should be involved, and assemble the group(s). A group size between 6 and 10 people has been suggested as allowing for effective sharing.

2. The group decides on the focus and questions for the research.

3. Researchers and participants observe, engage in action, observe, and record.

4. Researchers and participants immerse themselves in action, and elaborate and deepen their understandings.

5. Group members reassemble and share their knowledge, using this iteration as an opportunity to revise their plans for the next cycle of research.

6. This cycle may be repeated between 6 and 10 times, depending on the complexity of the research context.

Kemmis and McTaggart (2009b), Reason and Bradbury (2008), Whitmore (1998), and Brydon-Miller (2009) have written extensively about participatory action research designs. The essential elements include these:

▓ Community members are involved in a variety of roles.

▓ Involvement of the community can occur through a variety of means: community meetings (see Chapter 7), focus groups, photoethnography, or other methods (discussed more thoroughly in Chapter 10).

▓ The evaluator's role includes working with the community as a change agent.

▓ The focus is on the community's identifying the focus of the research; contributing to decisions about data collection; perhaps working as co-evaluators in data collection; and participating in data analysis, interpretation, and use.

▓ Participatory designs tend to be cyclical, using information gathered in earlier stages to inform the next steps in the process.

Tikare, Youssef, Donnelly-Roark, and Shah (2001) at the World Bank suggest these guiding principles for the use of participatory designs in poverty reduction evaluations. We combine Tikare et al.'s suggestions with ideas from Mertens (2009) to present this list of principles:

▓ *Country ownership.* Governments need to be involved in the participatory process to demonstrate their commitment to the program and its evaluation.

▓ *Outcome orientation.* Evaluators should be clear about the purpose for engaging in the participatory process (e.g., engaging previously excluded groups, addressing gaps in available information).

▓ *Capacity building.* Evaluators should provide capacity-building experiences for community members who have not had opportunities for training in research processes.

▓ *Inclusion.* Participatory designs can be used to include the voices of those who have historically been marginalized, such as women and poor people.

▓ *Use of culturally appropriate data collection.* Use of data collection methods should be based on an understanding of the culture of the community. For visual or illiterate communities, these might include visual methods of data collection. Culturally appropriate ways for participants to contribute their knowledge should be devised.

■ *Transparency.* If the process is transparent, then this will increase the trust and support among the various stakeholders.

■ *Sustainability.* Participatory processes should be grounded in existing policy and programs, so that the probability of action based on the results is increased.

■ *Continuous improvement.* Solutions to poverty will not occur overnight; incremental change is to be expected and tracked.

Box 9.7, which is adapted from Tikare et al. (2001), outlines the steps needed for a participatory design in an international development context. Some of the concepts explained in Box 9.7 are common across other types of participatory designs (e.g., focus groups); some are more specific to international development (e.g., citizen report cards). In addition, Whitmore et al. (2006), Rick Davies (2009b), and Dart and Davies (2003) explain the use of a qualitative strategy commonly used when time is a constraint, called the "most significant change" method. These tools for evaluators are included in Chapter 10.

········· **EXTENDING YOUR THINKING** ·········

Participatory Action Research

A participatory method that has recently emerged is teaching stakeholders how to use video in their gathering of data. "Participatory video" is about getting people to unite and plan together to make change in their community. Go to the InsightShare website to learn about how it is done and watch one of the videos that were made by a community (*insightshare.org/watch/video/what-is-pv*).

1. What do you think is effective about this technique?

2. What would be the advantages of using this participatory strategy to draw out information from stakeholders, as compared to nonparticipatory approaches?

3. What do you think some of the challenges would be in using this technique?

Mixed Methods Designs

As you have probably already realized, evaluators often use mixed methods. House's (2004) study of the court-ordered Denver bilingual program (see Chapter 6, Box 6.5) provides us with an example of how he began with carefully planned meetings with diverse groups of stakeholders to determine how to proceed. These could be looked at as qualitative data collection moments. He then developed a checklist that observers could use to collect quantitative data. He reflected upon the value of the process and data and made necessary modifications. He met with stakeholders twice a year to share the

Box 9.7. Designing a Participatory Process in International Development

Final impact

▦ Effective development and poverty reduction strategies and actions

Key outcomes

▦ Accountable, transparent, and efficient processes for economic decision making, resource allocation, expenditures and service delivery

▦ Increased equity in development policies, goals, and outcomes

▦ Shared long-term vision among all stakeholders for development

Key outputs

▦ Ongoing institutional arrangements for participation and consensus building in government decision-making processes for macroeconomic policy formulation and implementation

▦ Institutional capacity to demystify macroeconomic policies and budgets, analyze data, and promote information exchange and public debates in parliaments, the media, and civil society

▦ Development of mechanisms for negotiation and rules of engagement between key stakeholder groups

▦ Citizen report cards that monitor, for example, the Medium-Term Expenditure Framework and the Poverty Reduction Strategy Program

▦ Development of feedback mechanisms and participatory monitoring systems that enable citizens and key stakeholders within the government to monitor key poverty reduction initiatives, public actions, and outcomes as a part of poverty reduction strategy formulation and implementation

▦ Choice of poverty reduction actions based on a better understanding of the multidimensional aspects of poverty and its causes, including vulnerability, insecurity, and governance

Inputs: Mechanisms and methods

▦ Public information strategy (written and broadcast media, websites, etc.)

▦ Participatory poverty assessments, integrating qualitative and quantitative indicators

▦ Stakeholder analysis

▦ Participatory choice of antipoverty actions to address vulnerability, insecurity, and governance

(cont.)

Box 9.7 (cont.)

▓ National workshops

▓ Regional or local workshops

▓ Focus groups and interviews

▓ Building networks or coalitions of NGOs

▓ Participatory budget formulation and expenditure tracking

▓ Setting up a poverty-monitoring or coordination unit

▓ Citizen surveys and report cards

▓ Preparation of alternative poverty reduction strategy papers or policy proposals

▓ Demystification of budgets through simple summaries and presentations

▓ Sector working groups with multiple-stakeholder representation

Source: Adapted from Tikare, Youssef, Donnelly-Roark, and Shah (2001, p. 239). Copyright 2001 by the World Bank. Adapted by permission.

findings and determine next steps. In House's reflections on the study in Box 6.5, he provides principles he feels are necessary for a deliberative democratic evaluation; he does not specifically address issues of mixed methods design.

Fierro (2006) also used a mixed methods design in the evaluation of a welfare-to-work program (see Chapter 6, Box 6.7). She combined the use of qualitative designs (ethnography and focus groups) with quantitative designs (database analysis, surveys, pre- and posttests). She found that this mixed methods design gave her the outcome data that she needed, as well as in-depth understanding of the participants' experiences.

Chatterji (2005) argues that we evaluators have a moral imperative to conduct mixed methods evaluations because of the complexity of the contexts in which we work. A study that was limited to a randomized controlled trial would not take into consideration the cultural and contextual variables that would be captured by a qualitative study. Yet the use of mixed methods designs has not been as explicitly discussed in the evaluation literature as the use of other designs has been. However, several scholars working in applied research contexts offer examples of explicitly mixed methods designs. Creswell (2009), Teddlie and Tashakkori (2009), Greene (2007), and Mertens (2009, 2010) provide examples of such designs.

Concurrent, Dialectical (or Embedded), and Sequential Mixed Methods Designs

Creswell (2009) describes mixed methods designs as those that include both qualitative and quantitative design elements. The specific designs are based on the temporal relation of the two designs in the study: They can occur concurrently or sequentially. They can also

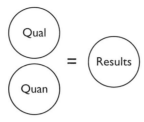

Figure 9.2. Concurrent mixed methods design.

be distinguished as either pragmatic or transformative. If the qualitative and quantitative designs are implemented at the same time in a study, Creswell calls this a **concurrent mixed methods design.** It would look like Figure 9.2. (In this and subsequent figures, Qual is short for qualitative and Quan is short for quantitative.)

Concurrent mixed methods designs can take a dialectical form, as described by Greene (2007).[3] In this design, the quantitative and qualitative designs are implemented fairly independently, perhaps by two teams of evaluators. Then at various points during the study, but especially when the data are analyzed, a dialogue between the qualitative and quantitative evaluators occurs to reveal the similarities and differences of findings from the two methodologies. The opportunity for dialogue across worldviews contributes to the value of this design. This design could look like Figure 9.3.

Creswell (2009) and Teddlie and Tashakkori (2009) refer to a particular type of **dialectical mixed methods design** as an **embedded mixed methods design.** This is a design in which one data set (such as qualitative data) is collected to support the larger data set in a study (such as quantitative data), although dialogue occurs between the two sets of data as just described.

A dialectical (or embedded) mixed methods design was used in the Brady and O'Regan (2009) study of youth mentoring in Ireland (see Chapter 3, Box 3.2). Brady and O'Regan's design is illustrated in Figure 9.4.

If the mixed methods are used sequentially in the study, then this is called a **sequential mixed methods design** (Creswell, 2009). This might look like Figure 9.5 if the quantitative design is implemented first and is used to inform the qualitative design portion of the study, or like Figure 9.6, if the qualitative design is implemented first and its results are used to inform the quantitative portion of the study.

Nastasi et al. (2007) suggest a variation of these designs when the purpose of the evaluation is to provide formative and summative data during the development and implementation of a program. They describe this as a "recurring sequence of qualitative and

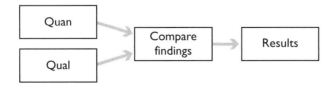

Figure 9.3. Dialectical concurrent mixed methods design.

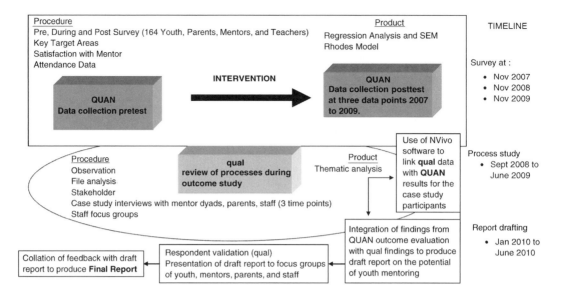

Figure 9.4. Evaluation of Big Brothers Big Sisters Ireland: An embedded mixed methods model. *Source:* Brady and O'Regan (2009, p. 277). Copyright 2009 by Sage Publications, Inc. Reprinted by permission.

quantitative data collection culminating in a recursive qualitative–quantitative process" (p. 165). The design would look like Figure 9.7. The number of iterations would be flexible, depending on the demands of the context:

> Qualitative methods (Qual) are used to generate formative data to guide program development, followed by quantitative evaluation (Quan) to test program effectiveness. Application in another setting can be facilitated by subsequent qualitative data collection (Qual) leading to program design adapted to the new context and participants, which is then followed by quantitative data collection (Quan) to test program outcomes. This sequence can occur across multiple settings and participant groups. Following initial adaptations to local context, program implementation and evaluation can be characterized by a recursive process (Qual ↔ Quan) in which collection of both qualitative and quantitative data inform ongoing modifications

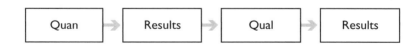

Figure 9.5. Sequential mixed methods design (with quantitative followed by qualitative).

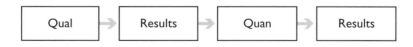

Figure 9.6. Sequential mixed methods design (with qualitative followed by quantitative).

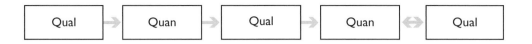

Figure 9.7. A recursive variation of the sequential mixed methods design.

as well as implications for future program development and application. (Nastasi et al., 2007, p. 165)

Transformative Mixed Methods Designs

Transformative mixed methods designs can be concurrent or sequential; however, they most commonly take on a cyclical design. Transformative evaluators start with the community, and they involve the community throughout the evaluation process (see Figure 9.8). A transformative mixed methods design might include these steps:

1. Identify your theoretical lens/worldview (paradigm) as transformative.

2. Identify community members to involve.

3. Develop mechanisms for working together to identify research focus and research questions.

4. Develop a rationale and write a mixed methods purpose statement.

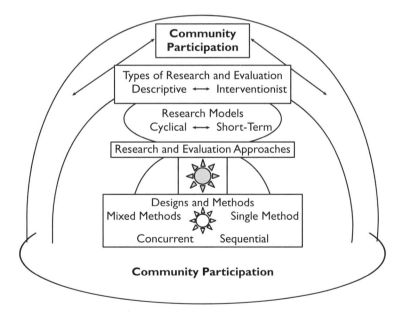

Figure 9.8. Transformative methodologies: The various possibilities. Note the importance of community participation throughout. *Source:* Mertens (2009, p. 138). Copyright 2009 by The Guilford Press. Reprinted by permission.

5. Develop a design for mixed methods.

6. List your qualitative and quantitative data to be collected.

7. Review your qualitative and quantitative data analysis.

8. Draw a diagram of procedures in the design.

The Mertens et al. (2007) study (see Chapter 6, Box 6.10) provides an example of a transformative cyclical mixed methods design (see Figure 9.9). The evaluation began with a request from the project director to Mertens. She asked to review documents and then discussed ideas for the evaluation with the director. He agreed to let the evaluation proceed. The next step in the plan was to hire a team of evaluators who reflected salient dimensions of diversity; in this case, that meant people who were deaf and used either American Sign Language or a cochlear implant that allowed them to hear and speak. This team was assembled, and a series of meetings began in which the team members introduced themselves to each other and to the documents that the project had produced over its lifetime. These meetings and the review of documents were viewed as qualitative data collection moments. The team decided that a transformative cyclical mixed methods design would be useful, starting with observations of the graduates at a reflective seminar, then interviews with seminar participants, followed by a quantitative online survey. Each of the data collection moments informed the next step in the process (e.g., interview questions were developed based on the observations, and online survey questions were based on the interview and observation notes). The results of this phase of the study were analyzed by the team and used to develop questions for interviewing the university faculty and the staff at cooperating schools. The actual words of the new teachers and results of the survey were shared with the faculty and staff, and they were asked to comment on how the program addressed their concerns or what kind of changes might be needed. In this way, the responses of the faculty and staff became the basis for action that could be taken to improve the way the program addressed issues of diversity and marginalization that the new teachers had raised.

Impact Evaluations and Mixed Methods Designs

Impact evaluation has long been associated with strictly quantitative designs, and in particular with the use of experimental or quasi-experimental designs. The prevailing demand

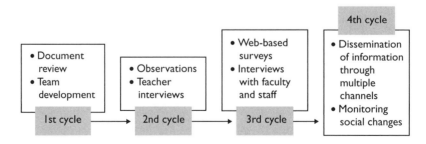

Figure 9.9. Transformative cyclical mixed methods design. Based on Mertens, Harris, Holmes, and Brandt (2007).

was that evaluators do comparative studies, using a group that received a program and comparing this group with what would happen if the program was not provided. This would entail the use of an experimental and a control group, and is known as a "counter-factual approach" in international development. However, the international development community is beginning to voice concerns about the limitations that this imposes on their ability to know what works, who it works for under what conditions, and why it works. Garbarino and Holland (2009), under the auspices of the U.K. Department for International Development, developed a position paper arguing for the combination of quantitative and qualitative designs in impact evaluations. They suggest that evaluations need to look not only at the effects of programs, but also at the effects of programs on different types of people (which might be accomplished by having different groups who represent different characteristics, or by disaggregation of data on one heterogeneous group). They also call for consideration of variables that are difficult to quantify, such as dignity, respect, security, and power.

Impact evaluators can make use of both quantitative and qualitative designs by making use of experimental designs together with participatory and ethnographic designs. (It should be noted that participatory designs can also be mixed methods designs; examples of quantitative and qualitative data collection methods are described in Chapter 10.) Garbarino and Holland (2009) describe mixed methods designs similar to those explained above; they suggest that evaluators can integrate methodologies (e.g., a survey can be used to select a qualitative sample, or qualitative analysis can reveal important topics for a quantitative baseline survey), sequence information (e.g., a qualitative study can inform hypothesis generation for a quantitative study, or qualitative data can be used to inform interpretations of survey results), and merge findings (e.g., results of both quantitative and qualitative parts of the study can be used to make policy recommendations).

Carter (2009) provides an interesting example of a mixed methods impact evaluation of a poverty reduction program in South Africa. He indicated that the quantitative part of the impact evaluation was not sufficient to explain the dynamics of the program's failure to reduce poverty. He combined the quantitative impact study with a qualitative, ethnographic approach called "anecdote circles" (explained further in Chapter 10). Through this mixed methods design, he was able to pinpoint issues that prevented the program from achieving the desired goals. For example, the community suffered from high rates of drug and alcohol abuse, so some of the money was used to support these habits; because cash transfers were sometimes used to pay rent, much of the poverty reduction impact was funneled to landlords rather than residents; and women reported that the police were unresponsive to rape and other crimes of violence against them. Carter suggests that this level of qualitative analysis provides a better understanding of how poverty reduction strategies need to be framed to address specific contextual variables.

Making Choices about Designs

Evaluation purposes commonly drive design decisions. The designs described so far in this chapter provide general guidance for evaluators in deciding what is appropriate for a specific study. However, because of the myriad possible evaluation purposes, design options have developed in the evaluation community that are generally associated with specific purposes. In Box 9.8 we present design options that are typically associated with different evaluation purposes, along with criteria for making decisions about which design option to choose. We urge the reader to use caution when making such decisions, to avoid a rigid interpretation of what is found in Box 9.8. For example, case studies are most typically used to gain insights or to find areas of improvement; however they can be used to document program effectiveness or how it addresses issues of human rights.

Box 9.8. Evaluation Purposes, Designs, and Criteria for Choices

Purpose: *To gain insights or to determine necessary inputs*

Design and choice criteria

▪ Case studies

Use when the evaluation focuses on a small number of sites, and rich detail is needed; caution is advised in attempting to generalize from a small number of cases.

▪ Ethnographies

Use in circumstances similar to case studies when the focus is on an investigation of cultural variables; awareness of diversity within cultural groups is necessary, and caution is advised as in case studies.

▪ Phenomenological studies

Use in circumstances similar to case studies when the focus is on the experience of individuals; awareness of differences between you and these individuals is necessary, and caution is advised as in case studies.

▪ Surveys

Use mail, email, and web-based surveys when information is needed from a large number of participants; data need to be interpreted cautiously because of the lack of personal connection with participants. Personal interviews can be used when more detailed information is required from a smaller number of participants.

▪ Any mixed methods design

Use when both quantitative and qualitative data are needed; be cognizant of the limitations of quantitative and qualitative approaches.

Purpose: *To find areas in need of improvement or to change practices*

Design and choice criteria

▪ Case studies, surveys, any mixed methods design

Use in similar circumstances and with appropriate cautions as mentioned above, when the focus is on understanding the processes that are occurring in an evaluation context.

Purpose: *To assess program effectiveness*

Design and choice criteria

■ Experimental designs

Use when control of extraneous variables is paramount, and in circumstances that permit random assignment to conditions; address the ethical concerns discussed in this chapter.

■ Quasi-experimental designs

Use when control of extraneous variables is paramount, but circumstances do not permit random assignment to conditions; be aware of threats to internal validity, especially differential selection; address the ethical concerns discussed in this chapter.

■ Single-group designs

Use when only one group is available; be aware of threats to validity.

■ Surveys

Use as explained above; be aware of biases due to self-reporting.

■ Cost analysis

Use when the focus is on the expenditure of funds; be aware of assumptions that underlie the numbers.

■ Any mixed methods design

Use as explained above when the focus of the evaluation is on process and effectiveness.

Purpose: *To address issues of human rights and social justice*

Design and choice criteria

■ Transformative (concurrent, sequential, or cyclical) mixed methods designs

Use to gain insights, determine necessary inputs, find areas in need of improvement, change practices, or assess program effectiveness when the focus is on marginalized groups; be aware of cultural differences, diversity within groups, and power inequities.

Evaluation Checklists

The Evaluation Center at Western Michigan University posts checklists on its website that can be helpful for designing various types of evaluations. Box 9.9 provides a list of these.

Box 9.9. Evaluation Checklists

Topic	Author
CIPP Model	Daniel Stufflebeam
Constructivist (a.k.a. Fourth Generation) Evaluation	Egon Guba and Yvonna Lincoln
Deliberative Democratic Evaluation (DDE)	Ernest R. House and Kenneth R. Howe
Key Evaluation Checklist	Michael Scriven
Qualitative Evaluation	Michael Quinn Patton
Utilization-Focused Evaluation (UFE)	Michael Quinn Patton

Source: These checklists are all available at the website of Western Michigan University's Evaluation Center (*www. wmich.edu/evalctr/checklists*).

Planning Your Evaluation: The Design of the Evaluation Study

In light of the evaluand, stakeholders, purpose, and questions, develop a statement of the design that you will use for your evaluation. Use the ideas presented in this chapter to choose a design, or to create one that combines elements of different designs discussed in this chapter. Be sure to be as specific as possible about the components that you will include in the design, and your rationale for choosing this particular design.

 Moving On to the Next Chapter

At this point, you should have a good idea of the philosophical assumptions that guide your work. You should also have developed a plan that describes the evaluand, the purposes of the evaluation, evaluation questions, and the evaluation design. You are now ready to take the next step in evaluation planning: selecting a sample from which to collect data.

Notes

1. Such a condition constitutes a statement in itself about the values that are operating in the United States.

2. This article is based on a panel discussion that occurred at AERA's annual meeting. The printed

version lists the authors in this order; however, the text within the article is attributed to the individuals who made the remarks. We have therefore kept the identity of the speaker that is associated with these remarks, rather than citing them all as Moss et al. (2009).

3. Erickson (Moss et al., 2009, p. 509) eschews the terminology "mixed methods" and opts instead for "multiple methods." His stance with regard to multiple methods is quite similar to the dialogical concurrent mixed methods design discussed by Greene. Erickson states:

> By temperament, I like affirming both sides of a chasm, taking advantage of contradictory truths without trying to erase the contradictions. It seems to me that education research, like social research more broadly, needs to get smarter about which aspects of social life can be appropriately studied as if people were atoms or quarks, or antimatter, and which need to be studied in ways that are radically different from attempts at a social physics because what must be understood and illuminated through narrative description is the life world of their daily practice. To say, "Is this topic appropriate for study from a natural science approach or a human science approach?" is different from saying "Should we use inferential statistics and a randomized field trial or ethnography?" Focusing on the reality of the chasm foregrounds the questions of ontology that I see as fundamental and prior to choices of methods: What is this piece of the world like that we want to study, and for what uses do we want the knowledge that our study might produce?

4. The Network of Networks on Impact Evaluation (NONIE) is chaired by DFID. This network includes representatives from donor agencies, the OECD DAC, the United Nations, and multilateral banks and evaluation associations from developing countries. They are sharing information about impact evaluations. The International Initiative for Impact Evaluation (3ie) is a funding initiative for high-quality impact evaluations (Garbarino & Holland, 2009).

Preparing to Read Chapter Ten

Imagine an NGO established a community-based health program that trains village health workers to teach rural mothers how to prevent the spread of diseases. You will be traveling to this resource-poor country to gather data as part of your evaluation. Before you arrive scenarios like the following have been taking place (Werner & Bower, 1995; copyright 1995 by the Hesperian Foundation; reprinted by permission):

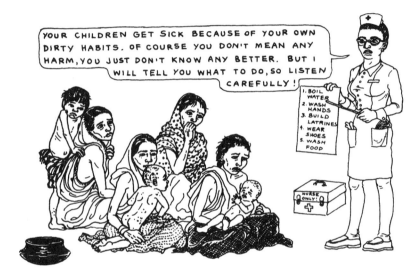

1. What would be some of the challenges you would face in gathering data in this scenario?

2. Would you use quantitative or qualitative strategies or both to collect data from the stakeholders? Explain.

3. What strategies for collecting data might you use in this situation that might be different if you were collecting data on a health program in a U.S. school, and why?

4. How do you think you will be able to earn the trust of the various stakeholders?

CHAPTER TEN

Data Collection Strategies

and Indicators

Data collection is an integral part of evaluation work. This is evident in the sample studies summarized in Part II of this text, as well as in the planning phase of evaluation, which involves establishing the context and describing the evaluand (see Chapter 7). The planning phase of data collection provides yet another example of the nonlinearity of planning evaluations. Data collection strategies are chosen so that they are appropriate for a particular group of people. In systematic inquiry, the selection of people for data collection purposes is called "sampling." An evaluator does need to have a sample in mind in order to plan for data collection. We assume, however, that the identification of stakeholders has given the evaluator a general idea of the people who will make up the sample. Therefore, we have chosen to present this chapter on data collection strategies before the chapter on sampling. The evaluator will be in a better position to select a specific, appropriate sample once the data collection strategies have been identified. Box 10.1 provides two preliminary examples of quantitative and qualitative data collection strategies.

Box 10.1. Examples of Quantitative and Qualitative Data Collection

Quantitative Data Collection

Quantitative data collection is illustrated by the evaluation of final reading outcomes in the national randomized field trial of the Success for All program (Borman et al., 2007, p. 716):

> *Pretests.* All children were individually assessed in fall 2001 (first phase) or fall 2002 (second phase) on the PPVT III [Peabody Picture Vocabulary Test—Third Edition]. This assessment served as the pretest measure for all of the reported analyses.
>
> *Posttests.* During the spring of 2002, 2003, and 2004 (first phase) and the spring of 2003, 2004, and 2005 (second phase), students in the kindergarten longitudinal cohort were individually assessed with the WMTR [Woodcock Reading Mastery Test—Revised].
>
> During Year 1 and Year 2, four subtests of the WMTR were administered: Letter Identification, Word Identification, Word Attack, and Passage Comprehension. During this final year of data collection though, the Letter Identification subtest was not administered because it does not test content that is typically taught in second grade classrooms.

(cont.)

Box 10.1 (*cont.*)

Qualitative Data Collection

Qualitative data collection methods are illustrated by the evaluation of an injury prevention program for dancers described in Chapter 5, Box 5.4 (Abma, 2005, pp. 282–283):

> Over the course of a year, the junior evaluator worked for three to four days a week at the schools attending regular lessons, special body-awareness lessons and consulting hours as well as concerts and student performances. After some time, students spontaneously approached her to talk about their experiences. This "prolonged engagement" (Lincoln & Guba, 1985) enabled her to build up a relationship with the communities. In order to enhance our knowledge of the field, we read several (auto)biographies and interviews with dancers and musicians. Once every two weeks we met as a research team to discuss methodological considerations and to reflect on how our particular position, research agenda, prejudices and main filters influenced the project. We started the evaluation with conversational interviews … with two students (jazz and modern dance), two teachers and two (para-)medical specialists.

Recall that the depiction of an evaluand, whether as a logic model or descriptively, includes specification of outputs (quantity and quality of services delivered), outcomes (short- and long-term changes at the individual level in terms of behaviors, knowledge, skills, or dispositions), and impacts (change at a broader organizational or community level). (See Figure 10.1.) Outcomes and impacts are determined during the process of developing the evaluand, and then they are revisited during the planning of data collection.

During the early stages of planning, an evaluator might ask, "What difference will this program/initiative make in the lives of those served?" During the data collection planning phase, the evaluator asks, "How will we collect data to provide evidence of how we changed the lives of those we served? And what level of performance will we accept as indicating that the program succeeded or failed?" It is not possible for an evaluator to know precisely what outputs, outcomes, and impacts a program will have before it is

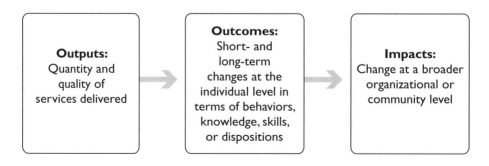

Figure 10.1. Outputs, outcomes, and impacts.

implemented; therefore, the evaluator needs to be in a position to gather data about both intended and unintended consequences of a program.

Outcomes and impacts need to be measured at different levels, such as the individual client level (e.g., better health), the program or system level (e.g., improved partnerships), the broader community level (e.g., increased civic engagement), and the organizational level (e.g., improved management systems) (WKKF, 2004).

At the organizational level, data can be collected for outcomes from the persons employed by that organization, as well as from partnering organizations. Evaluators also need to consider measuring short-term, interim, and long-term outcomes. For example, reduction of violence in a community may require the achievement of short-term outcomes, such as number of children in school; interim outcomes, such as provision of drug treatment centers, employment opportunities, and after-school activities; and finally violence reduction as a long-term outcome. See Figure 7.3 in Chapter 7 (the logic model associated with reduction of HIV/AIDS infection in deaf youth in South Africa) for an example of short-term, interim, and long-term outcomes (Donnelly-Wijting, 2007).

The Fredericks et al. (2008) study (see Chapter 3, Box 3.4) provides an example of **D**Ⓓ different levels of data collection, reasons why they are necessary, and the logical connections between the levels. Recall that their evaluand was a program intended to improve services for people with developmental disabilities. The evaluators identified the individual-level outcomes and impacts as increases in consumer choices and community integration, as well as improvement of the quality of life, for consumers at home and in their relationships, their personal lives, work, school, and the community. To achieve these effects at the individual level, they needed to address organizational outcomes and impacts, including increasing person-centered planning and individualization of service planning, as well as the efficiency of program delivery. This led to the need to collect data at the individual and organizational levels in order to provide a comprehensive picture of program effectiveness.

This chapter is divided into four major sections:

1. A brief introduction to data collection, including how data collection is perceived by the four branches of evaluation.

2. Information to help you make decisions about how you will collect your data:
   a. A description of criteria for quality in data collection.
   b. A generic guide to planning data collection.
   c. Options for data collection (quantitative, qualitative, participatory).
   d. Methods for identifying or developing appropriate data collection instruments and methods.

3. A brief mention of strategies and challenges in mixed methods data collection.

4. A discussion of performance indicators and data collection.

Throughout this chapter, concerns about language and culture are integrated into the discussion of data collection instruments and methods. Evaluators add the concept of indicators to the topic of data collection (i.e., how do the stakeholders know if the evidence presented to them from data collection indicates the extent to which a program succeeded or failed). This topic is illustrated from evaluation studies from multiple sectors. Additional resources for those who want to pursue testing and assessment in more depth are listed below.

Coaley, K. (2010). *An introduction to psychological assessment and psychometrics*. Thousand Oaks, CA: Sage.

Furr, R. M. (2007). *Psychometrics*. Thousand Oaks, CA: Sage.

McIntire, S. A. (2006). *Foundations of psychological testing* (2nd ed.). Thousand Oaks, CA: Sage.

Robinson Kurpius, S. E. (2005). *Testing and measurement*. Thousand Oaks, CA: Sage.

Salkind, N. J. (2005). *Tests and measurement for people who (think they) hate tests and measurement*. Thousand Oaks, CA: Sage.

Wright, R. J. (2007). *Educational assessment*. Thousand Oaks, CA: Sage.

· · · · · · · · · E X T E N D I N G   Y O U R   T H I N K I N G · · · · · · · · ·
Measuring All Levels

Let us imagine that a rural county won a state grant aimed at curbing obesity and encouraging healthier lifestyles for its elderly citizens. Because many young people have left the county for urban living, it has high numbers of elderly citizens, many of whom are inactive and isolated. The county began a program in which seniors were picked up at their homes and had a "Biggest Loser" contest at the senior center. Seniors also met with health care practitioners to develop individual workout plans that allowed them to win a certain number of points for improvements, such as ounces of fat lost or blood pressure points dropped. They could then exchange their points for prizes. In measuring all levels of the program, the evaluators found outcomes and an impact they had not expected, and were able to draw a more comprehensive description of the successes of the program.

Levels at Which to Measure the "Biggest Loser" Program for Seniors			
Outcome	Outcome	Outcome	Impact
Individual client level	*Program or system level*	*Broader community level*	*Organizations*
Seniors stronger and more active	Increased revenue from new gym memberships	Healthier seniors participating in county activities	Organizations adapting programs to accommodate seniors

1. In this imaginary scenario, why would it have been important for the county to have this information? What difference could this data make to the stakeholders?

2. Imagine that the evaluators had only focused on the individual/client level. What would have been lost?

3. Explain in your own words the importance of collecting data and measuring all levels in an evaluation.

Data Collection: An Overview

Data collection is conducted for a variety of purposes, with a variety of strategies and instruments. Although evaluators from each of the four evaluation branches can use any of the data collection methods described in this chapter, evaluators from each branch tend to use particular types of data collection strategies. Evaluators from the Methods Branch tend to use quantitative measures, preferably standardized instruments; their assumptions are that these measures will allow questions to be presented exactly the same way to every participant, reduce evaluator bias, and permit numerical analysis of the data with a determinant standard of error. Evaluators from the Use Branch determine which data collection methods and instruments meet the purpose of the study; they can use methods that are quantitative, qualitative, or both. Evaluators from the Values Branch speak of themselves as instruments and tend to use qualitative data collection methods; their aim is to establish rapport with the participants through sustained contact that allows them to reveal multiple constructions of reality by different constituencies. Evaluators in the Social Justice Branch acknowledge power differences between themselves and the participants, and work to address the implications of these power differences for obtaining accurate information. This entails building trust with the community, being responsive to differences within the community that might require modification of the data collection strategies during the study, and linking data collection to social action.

When making decisions about data collection strategies, evaluators have a conceptual idea and an operational definition of their data collection methods. The conceptual idea is the statement of the attributes of interest; the operational definition is how the data will be collected about those attributes. Often, the work you complete in developing the context and evaluand will lead to ideas of what data are needed and how such data have been collected in the past. For example, in the Borman et al. (2007) study (see Box 10.1), the evaluators were interested in collecting data about children's reading levels (the conceptual idea). They operationalized this idea by selecting two standardized tests: the Peabody Picture Vocabulary Test–Third Edition and the Woodcock Reading Mastery Test–Revised.

Language as an Overarching Issue in Data Collection

Language is a critical issue that permeates decisions about data collection. Myriad issues arise in the discussion of language related to data collection. Sometimes the issues seem obvious: The evaluators and the participants use different languages. Sometimes the issues are less obvious: Participants may have different levels of literacy and thus have different abilities to engage with text, or a different form of the same language may be used in different places (e.g., American English vs. British English, or Spanish in Spain vs. Puerto Rico). Other complications arise when evaluators reflect upon the diversity of the communities in terms of language. For example, Botswana has 25 major languages; South African has 8 official languages (CIA Factbook, 2010). Some languages are only spoken and have no written form (e.g., Hmong); some languages are visual and do not have a spoken or written form (e.g., American Sign Language). Often the dominant or colonizers' language is used by the evaluators, and this sets up power differences in the choice of language for written, oral, or signed data collection.

A seemingly obvious solution to language differences is to translate the data collection instrument (or interview questions) into the appropriate language, and then to do a back-translation into the original language. This makes sense at one level; however, it is not unproblematic. Mukoma et al. (2009, p. 9) conducted an evaluation in Africa that involved the translation of an instrument into four languages. This is how they described the process of translation and back-translation:

> The resulting questionnaire with 188 items in English was translated into Kiswahili, Xhosa, Afrikaans and Sepedi. The translations were done by professional contractors that were not part of the project. To check for accuracy of translation and to ensure that the original meaning was preserved, the translated versions were then translated back into English by individuals who had not been previously involved in the questionnaire development and translation process. The research team checked the back translations to ensure that each question, instructions and response options were accurate. The ordering of items was consistent in all the languages.

Language is much more than a system of symbols we use for communication. Language is part of a full set of cultural baggage, and researchers/evaluators need to be cognizant of the wider cultural implications of the use of language. Guzman (2003; cited in Mertens, 2009, pp. 238–239) notes:

> While translating a measurement tool or having someone who speaks the language of the target population is a step in the direction of cultural sensitivity, these two steps do not constitute cultural competency. As evaluators, we must realize that there is much more to how language functions in a culture, and that a mere translation of certain concepts or measures will not fully capture the experience of the participants.... If an evaluator is not fully aware of a particular culture and how their linguistic patterns shape the behavioral patterns of the individuals from that culture, then the evaluator cannot make logical assessments about the impact of a certain intervention.

Wilson (2007) wrote an interview protocol with administrators, teachers, and parents, to be used for questioning parents about their satisfaction with services they received from an NGO for their deaf/blind children in the Philippines. The questions were translated into Tagalog and then back-translated into English. Although the translations appeared to be correct, the group realized that the content, not the language, would be difficult for uneducated rural parents to understand. The same questions were rewritten to be more comprehensible to parents whose understanding of education was not as sophisticated as that of educated parents. Partnering with members of the language minority group in respectful ways, and building capacities within that group to participate in data collection, are alternatives to consider.

Data Collection Quality in Evaluation Studies

I (Donna M. Mertens) suspect that evaluation's focus on provision of information within the context of a particular project, as well as time and budget constraints, lead to less attention being given to the quality of data collection instruments than in the research world. If evaluators want to know about participant satisfaction or behavior change within a specific project, it is likely that they will develop a brief survey or interview guide focused on that specific context, rather than using or developing a standardized instrument. Brandon and Singh (2009) conducted a literature review of evaluation studies for the purpose of determining the quality of the data produced in those studies. The evaluations collected data about the use of evaluation findings from stakeholder groups in diverse domains. They reported:

> A flaw of nearly all the 52 studies is that insufficient detail is provided about the development of the data collection instruments. This detail is necessary to know the technical quality of the instruments and the procedures for administering them—a key component of content-related validity (Messick, 1989), including narrative reflection methods. Without this detail, we do not know, for example, (a) the extent to which instruments addressed the full conceptual or theoretical domain under study; (b) how well the items capture the aspects of the domain; (c) the degree of reliability of instrument scales; (d) whether the items were carefully written, reviewed, and pilot tested; (e) how carefully data were collected and measurement error was avoided; (f) the manner in which the narrative reflection data were collected and summarized; and (g) the many other aspects of good data collection that affect content-related validity (including reliability) and, ultimately, construct validity. (pp. 131–132)

Although Brandon and Singh's (2009) review focused primarily on the quality of quantitative data collection instruments, their findings should alert evaluators to be mindful of the quality of their data collection instruments and procedures, no matter what data collection methods are used. In the following section, we examine indicators of data collection quality for quantitative and qualitative methods.

Criteria for Quality in Data Collection

The quality of data collected is of utmost importance for evaluators to reach accurate conclusions about a program's functioning and effectiveness. In Chapter 11, we explore the implications of sampling for establishing the quality of data; if the sample is biased or ambiguous, then the best data collection instruments will not provide good data. Criteria for determining the quality of data collection efforts exist for quantitative and qualitative data collection. We discuss these criteria here and extend thinking about quality by examining implications for data collection from the various branches of evaluation.

"Reliability" and "validity" are the most common terms related to the quality of quantitative data collection. Validity essentially means: Does the instrument really measure what it is supposed to measure? Reliability essentially means: Does it do so consistently? Evaluators in the Values Branch (Lincoln & Guba, 2000) have developed parallel criteria for the quality of qualitative evaluations: "dependability" instead of "reliability," and "credibility" instead of "validity." Evaluators in the Social Justice Branch add criteria related to the appropriate inclusiveness of types of data collected, responsiveness to diversity within communities of interest, and facilitation of the furtherance of human rights and social justice.

Reliability and Dependability

Box 10.2 describes different types of reliability and dependability. You should keep in mind that the majority of the scholarship underlying the establishment of reliability and validity has occurred in the realm of educational and psychological test development (AERA, APA, & National Council on Measurement in Education, 1999). Hence evaluators need to be flexible in how they apply these strategies to other types of data collection (e.g., needs and assets assessments, surveys, course evaluations).

Reliability

Reliability calculations need to be done with awareness of the nature of the instrument, how the instrument is administered, and the meaning of the resulting statistics. For example, internal-consistency reliability is based on the assumption that the instrument measures a unitary concept—for example, quality of life. Is quality of life a unitary concept? (This is really a validity question, but it has implications for reliability.) If internal-consistency calculations are high, does this mean that the instrument reliably measures quality of life? If an instrument contains a mix of different types of questions (e.g., demographic, behavioral, attitudinal, and ratings of quality), what types of reliability make sense? Psychometricians and statisticians have developed procedures for establishing reliability for instruments that measure multidimensional characteristics. They recommend the use of item response theory to determine the goodness of fit for each item on a test with the model, yielding an alpha level that indicates divergence from the model at a specified significance level.

Reliability is influenced by how the instrument is administered; this is why Methods Branch evaluators put so much stock in standardization of procedures for administering instruments. If more than one individual is going to administer the instruments, it is important that they receive training to minimize variations that would have a negative impact on reliability.

Reports of reliability are generally included in the "Methods" section of evaluation reports. Here are two examples. Borman et al. (2007, p. 717) described the reliability of their measure of reading as follows:

> The WMTR is nationally normed and has internal reliability coefficients for the Word Identification, Word Attack, and Passage Comprehension subtests of .97, .87, and .92, respectively. The tests were administered by trained graduate students who had experience working with children and administration of tests. (p. 717)

Mukoma et al. (2009) reported on the development and psychometric properties of an instrument to evaluate school-based HIV/AIDS interventions aimed at adolescents in three African sites:

> Methods: The instrument was developed in a series of steps that involved a review of existing instruments; use of empirical data and secondary literature supporting an association between the variables of interest and sexual intercourse or condom use; operationalizing the constructs of the theoretical model employed; and using the objectives of the intervention. Test–retest reliability studies were conducted at each site. Results: The questionnaire demonstrated good internal consistency and adequate test–retest reliability. Cronbach's alpha was higher than 0.50 for all the 10 psychosocial scales, while Cohen's kappa showed poor to substantial test–retest reliability on the sexual behaviour items (k = 0.14 to 0.69). Conclusions: We conclude that the instrument had sufficient test–retest reliability and internal consistency. (p. 37)

Box 10.2. Reliability/Dependability in Data Collection

Reliability: Quantitative data collection

Repeated measures reliability	Coefficient of stability: Evaluator administers the same instrument twice; separated by a short period of time. Results are compared, using a statistic such as a correlation coefficient (see Chapter 12). This is also called test–retest reliability.
	Alternate-form coefficient: Evaluator administers two equivalent versions of the same instrument (parallel forms) to the same group of people. Results are compared, using a coefficient of stability.
Internal-consistency reliability	Participants take one instrument; their scores are subjected to an analysis to reveal their consistency of responses within the instrument, using statistics such as Cronbach's alpha or Kuder–Richardson formula. If respondents answer the questions consistently, then the instrument is considered to be reliable.

Reliability: Quantitative observational data

Interrater reliability	Two observers' data are compared to see whether they are consistently recording the same behaviors when they view the same events. Statistical procedures such as correlation or percentage of agreement can be used to establish this type of reliability.
Intrarater reliability	Intrarater reliability is used to determine whether a single observer is consistently recording data over a period of time. Statistical techniques similar to those used for interrater reliability can be used here.

Dependability: Qualitative data collection

Dependability	Changes in qualitative studies are to be expected, because the evaluator needs to remain in a responsive posture, making adjustments to data collection as new findings emerge. Therefore, the evaluator's responsibility is to maintain a case study protocol that documents changes in understandings and how they have influenced changes in data collection.

Source: Based on Mertens (2009, p. 234).

· · · · · · · · · · E X T E N D I N G   Y O U R   T H I N K I N G · · · · · · · · · ·

Reliability in Coding Qualitative Data

Hruschka et al. (2004, p. 16) present an example of interrater reliability in a study that involved the development of codes and coding of transcripts from open-ended interviews:

> Analysis of text from open-ended interviews has become an important research tool in numerous fields, including business, education, and health research. Coding is an essential part of such analysis, but questions of quality control in the coding process have generally received little attention. This article examines the text coding process

(cont.)

applied to three HIV-related studies conducted with the Centers for Disease Control and Prevention considering populations in the United States and Zimbabwe. Based on experience coding data from these studies, we conclude that (1) a team of coders will initially produce very different codings, but (2) it is possible, through a process of code-book revision and recoding, to establish strong levels of intercoder reliability (e.g., most codes with kappa 0.8). Furthermore, steps can be taken to improve initially poor inter-coder reliability and to reduce the number of iterations required to generate stronger intercoder reliability.

Use this example of coding observation data to identify types of reliability and the process for achieving them.

Dependability

In qualitative studies, the idea of consistency of measurement is less relevant than in quantitative studies, because evaluators have an expectation that the data collection strategies will evolve along with emerging issues in the study. The evaluators' responsibility is to develop a system for documenting what changes occur at what points during the study for what reasons. This can be done by keeping a protocol log (Yin, 2003) that presents publicly inspectable data about the changes. This will enable the conduct of a dependability audit, which involves reviewing project records to determine the extent to which project procedures and changes are documented. McNall and Foster-Fishman (2007) used rapid ethnographic techniques in an evaluation of response to a humanitarian crisis. Here is how they describe their use of a dependability audit:

> Data collection and analyses happened simultaneously during a 4-week period. Phone interviews that lasted between 1 and 2 hrs were conducted with 32 stakeholders. Extensive notes were taken, and digital recordings were done as backup. On the completion of each interview, a case summary sheet was immediately produced in the same manner as described above. Throughout the process, extensive peer debriefing occurred to increase the credibility of the results. The two staff who were conducting the interviews met almost daily to debrief about the themes they were identifying and issues that were emerging. The whole team met weekly to discuss issues and modify the protocol as needed. A detailed audit trail that explained our evaluation processes and changes (dependability audit) was recorded. (pp. 163–164)

Validity and Credibility

In Chapter 9, we have discussed internal validity (did the treatment cause the change in the dependent variable?) and external validity (is the sample representative of the population?) as they are established through design options. In this section, the main focus is on validity in quantitative data collection, which refers to the extent that an instrument measures what it is supposed to measure. For example, if you give a written geography test to a first-grade student that has the item "What does the color blue mean on a map?", and the student (let's call him Jared) does not answer the question, what does that mean? Does it mean that Jared does not know what the color blue on a map means? Or does it mean that he cannot read the test? Or that he is a stubborn, willful child who will not do his work? If this is to be a valid test of geography, the evaluator needs to know the answer to these questions. Several strategies can be used to determine whether the test is valid for determining geographic knowledge or if it is a test of reading ability. For example, the evaluators could read the test to Jared and see whether he can answer the question, or show him a map and ask him to tell them what the color blue on the map means.

Psychologists view validity as a unitary concept that measures the degree to which all the accumulated evidence supports the intended interpretation of test scores for the proposed purpose (AERA et al., 1999; Messick, 1989, 1996). Although validity is recognized as a unitary concept, psychologists recommend the use of different types of evidence to support validity claims (Sireci, 2007). Box 10.3 provides an explanation of different forms of evidence to support validity claims in quantitative data collection, as well as strategies to enhance the credibility of qualitative data.

Box 10.3. Validity/Credibility in Data Collection

Forms of evidence to support validity: Quantitative data collection

Construct validity	This is considered the unitary concept of validity: To what degree does all accumulated evidence support the intended interpretation of scores for the proposed purpose? This unified construct includes content-related, criterion-related, and consequential evidence (Messick, 1989; AERA et al., 1999).
Content-related evidence	Items on the test represent content covered in the program (e.g., did the teacher teach the children that blue on the map means water?). Evaluators can work with content specialists to list the content that is part of the program, and can compare the test items to see whether they correspond.
Criterion-related evidence	Instruments can be used to measure dispositions or behaviors, instead of actually asking the participant to demonstrate those dispositions or behaviors. For example, a scale that is a valid measure of depression can be used instead of observing lengthy therapy sessions. Criterion-related evidence can be used to reveal current characteristics, as well as to predict behavior or dispositions in the future (e.g., reading readiness tests, admissions tests, or having good job skills before being hired). Criterion-related evidence indicates that the measure actually reflects current or future behaviors or dispositions.
Consequential evidence	Evaluators need to be aware of the consequences of using data, especially with regard to the potential to worsen inequities. For example, a test may be used to determine whether deaf people are mentally challenged and overlooks that they lack access to English as a spoken language or opportunities to learn content, and thus could be denied access to appropriate educational opportunities.

(cont.)

Box 10.3 (*cont.*)

Strategies to enhance credibility: Qualitative data collection

Prolonged and substantial engagement	Evaluators need to stay on site for sufficient time to "get the story right." If a study is conducted over too short a time or interviews are conducted with too few people, it is possible that an evaluator will reach "premature closure" (i.e., reach wrong conclusions that would not be reached if additional time were spent in the inquiry context).
Persistent observations	Observations need to be conducted at a variety of times of the day, week, and year (if the study goes on for that long). For example, educators are familiar with the changes in students' behaviors throughout the day, as well as when major holidays are approaching.
Peer debriefing	An evaluator should find a peer with whom to discuss the study at different stages (e.g., beginning, middle, and end). The characteristics of the peer need to be specified, such as being knowledgeable about the topic area but not being directly involved in the study. Or two peers can be found, one of whom shares the evaluator's viewpoints and another who will challenge those viewpoints. The process of working with the peer reviewer needs to be explained (e.g., sharing the evaluation plan or the preliminary results to see whether another pair of eyes would see something differently).
Progressive subjectivity	Evaluators need to be aware of their assumptions, hypotheses, and understandings, and of how these change over the period of the study. Qualitative researchers recommend keeping a reflective journal from the start to the end of a study, in order to document changes in assumptions, hypotheses, and understandings during the course of the study. Such documentation can be used as data to support conclusions.
Member checks	Evaluators can share their data with participants (and, more broadly, stakeholders) to obtain feedback on the perceived accuracy and quality of their work. They can also share preliminary interpretations and draft reports while being vigilant about confidentiality.
Multiple data sources	Qualitative evaluators recommend the use of multiple data sources (different people in different positions) and different data collection strategies: observations, interviews, document reviews to strengthen the credibility of their findings. This was formerly known as **triangulation.**

Source: Based on Guba and Lincoln (1989) and Lincoln (2009).

Validity

Here are some examples of the use of evidence to support the validity of quantitative data. Mukoma et al. (2009, p. 9) provided this description of how they established face and content validity of their instrument to measure the effects of HIV/AIDS prevention programs in Africa:

> To establish face and content validity, the instrument was discussed at a project team workshop and with the advisory boards and expert panels at each site. The advisory boards and expert panels consisted of representatives from nongovernmental organizations, education departments, teachers and students. The questions and response options were checked for vocabulary, culture, language, and age appropriateness. We ensured that the items were consistent with the constructs of the theoretical framework. We also checked that the items reflected the specific objectives of the interventions. For each scale, items that fulfilled these criteria of relevance and appropriateness were retained. Furthermore, correlation matrix analyses were conducted to investigate the construct validity of the scales. It was decided through this process that separate versions of the questionnaire should be administered for males and females as items that were gender specific were cumbersome and some required skip instructions.

Anderson-Butcher, Iachini, and Amorose (2008, p. 49) established the construct validity of a short scale to measure social competence for children and youth. Here is how they described their procedures:

> Our approach to establishing initial reliability and validity evidence for the PSCS [Perceived Social Competence Scale] was to first conduct exploratory and confirmatory factor analyses (CFAs) on the six items with data from a large sample of children and youth. After establishing evidence of factorial validity in this calibration sample, we sought to test whether the factor structure of the scale was robust. We did this by conducting a series of multi-group CFAs designed to test for factorial invariance. Specifically, we tested for gender invariance in the calibration sample, and then tested whether the results from the calibration sample as a whole could be reproduced in independent samples of children (i.e., the cross-validation sample).

Anderson-Butcher et al. (2008, p. 51) then reported the criterion-related validity of the PSCS:

> The final step in our testing of the PSCS was to establish initial evidence of predictive validity. Using the average sum scores from the four items on the PSCS (M = 16.40, SD = 3.57, range = 5–20), we correlated social competence with perceived belongingness (α = .80, M = 17.55, SD = 2.95, range = 5–20) in the cross-validation sample. As expected, social competence was positively and significantly ($p < .01$) associated with perceived belonging among participants (r = .41).

Credibility

Just as Methods Branch evaluators want to assure their stakeholders that they have measured what they say they are measuring, evaluators from the Values Branch want to provide evidence of the believability of their findings. Guba and Lincoln (1989) frame the credibility question as follows: Is there a correspondence between the way the respondents actually perceive social constructs and the way the evaluator portrays the respondents' viewpoints? The strategies to enhance credibility listed in Box 10.3 provide evaluators with alternatives to demonstrate the believability of their findings.

Abma (2005, p. 283) describes the interviews that she and her coworkers conducted in the injury prevention evaluation (Chapter 5, Box 5.4) and the credibility-enhancing strategies they used:

> The interviews were not guided by our topics but by the issues brought to the fore by respondents. We started with broad opening questions, such as "What happened when you were injured and had to stop (temporarily)?" The interviews were all tape-recorded and transcribed. Our interpretations were presented to every respondent in order to give them the chance to comment on our findings ("member checks"). The personal interviews were used as an input for further dialogue via a series of storytelling workshops among groups of students and groups of teachers in both schools. In the workshops, participants were invited to respond to story fragments from the intermediary report. The presented stories were selected because they were like life and critical about the way self-care was approached in the schools. They were edited so that they could be read within a short time period. We decided to give students the stories of their teachers, and vice versa.

Nichols (2004) provides this detailed description of how she ensured the credibility of her data in a study of an early infant program for Cherokee mothers:

> The investigator used multiple techniques such as persistent observation, prolonged engagement, member checks, peer debriefing, negative case analysis, and audit trails to establish trustworthiness and credibility of the findings (Lincoln & Guba, 1985). The researcher moved to the area where the informants live while she collected the data—approximately for 4 months. Trust between the informants and the investigator was increased by her presence and availability in the area. The researcher was able to observe the Cherokee mothers as they provided care to their babies in their homes and in the community. Member checks were made by sharing the data—including emerging definitions, concepts, categories, and theory—with the informants. The researcher shared her analysis of the data with outsiders, other researchers, to get an etic perspective of the data analysis. The researcher interviewed 1 non-Cherokee mother (but of Indian blood) to provide the researcher with a contrasting perspective of Cherokee care. Finally, the researcher maintained records that included (a) the raw data, the tape-recorded interviews and written field notes; (b) data reduction and analysis such as computer printouts from the ethnograph program and memos; (c) data reconstruction and synthesis products; (d) the final report with connections to existing literature and an integration of concepts, relationships, and interpretations; and (e) process notes such as methodological notes, trustworthiness notes, and audit trail notes. (pp. 234–244)

Validity/Credibility in Data Collection for Mixed Methods Evaluations

Concerns about the quality of data collected in mixed methods evaluations overlap with those already discussed for separate quantitative and qualitative studies. However, the use of mixed methods raises additional issues. Leech, Dellinger, Brannagan, and Tanaka (2010) provide food for thought on this topic in the validation framework that they developed specifically to address issues of validity in mixed methods research. They discuss the establishment of construct validity in mixed methods in terms of demonstrating the legitimacy of all sources of data, whether quantitative or qualitative, as providing support for inferences about the phenomenon under study.

················ E X T E N D I N G   Y O U R   T H I N K I N G ············

Mixed Methods and Data Collection

If a mixture of methods is used to obtain data about the same construct, then evaluators need to be cognizant of the sources of evidence to support validity already described for quantitative and qualitative data collection. They also need to give consideration to implications for validity, using a combination of those criteria.

- If the quantitative and qualitative data suggest different outcomes, how can you explain why that happened?
- Is there reason to believe that the quantitative or qualitative data more accurately represents the outcomes of the program?
- If so, how do you support that argument?
- How do you, as the evaluator, support your choice of using both the quantitative and qualitative data collection methods?

Validity/Credibility in Data Collection within the Social Justice Branch

As mentioned at the beginning of this chapter, evaluators from the Social Justice Branch begin data collection by acknowledging power differences between themselves and study participants, as well as the need to establish a trusting relationship with community members. Decisions about data collection are made in consultation with the community, to ensure that these are culturally appropriate and that modifications are made to accommodate important dimensions of diversity within the community. Data collection methods in the Social Justice Branch sport labels similar to those in the other evaluation branches; however, the difference is "in the choice, development, and implementation of the data-collection strategies so that they are grounded in the community and the furtherance of human rights" (Mertens, 2009, p. 234). These considerations therefore become part of the criteria for validity and credibility within this branch. Other implications from the Social Justice Branch for data collection are integrated into subsequent parts of this chapter that describe specific data collection methods.

Planning for Data Collection

You can use this set of steps as a generic guide to planning data collection. In the following sections, specific options for data collection are explored.

- *Step 1.* It is usually best to involve stakeholders in the early planning stages for data collection. They can provide input with regard to appropriate types of data collection methods and instruments, as well as help you decide on any accommodations that may be necessary (e.g., interpreters, visual depiction of language, use of a scribe to record answers).

- *Step 2.* Pilot-testing the data collection instruments and methods is a good idea.

This may involve having a small group of people similar to those who are targeted by the program complete the data collection and share their reflections with you.

■ *Step 3.* Collection of data from human beings (and animals) needs to be approved by ethical review boards. These boards normally ask for the full instrument or list of interview questions, as well as a description of the procedures to be used in collecting and storing the data. This can be a bit of a challenge with qualitative data collection, because of the need to be responsive to each individual's emerging stories and the development of new insights that may need to be pursued, thus necessitating a change in data collection procedures.

■ *Step 4.* Estimate the number of times you will collect data from the participants; you may not know this for sure at the beginning of the study, but you can make an educated guess. Consider the time frame for multiple contacts (e.g., at the beginning, 3 months later, and at the end of the project).

■ *Step 5.* Plan what you will say to the participants when you first meet them (to establish rapport and introduce the study), and at the beginning of the data collection (to obtain informed consent).

■ *Step 6.* Plan how you will record the data. Will participants write their answers on a paper, submit them via computer, audio-record them, or video-record them? Or will you or the support staff take notes?

■ *Step 7.* Reflect on the process of data collection; how can it be improved? What questions have arisen that need additional exploration? How are different stakeholder groups responding differently?

■ *Step 8.* Ensure the quality of the data. If you are taking notes during observations or interviews, review your notes as soon as possible after the session to fill in gaps, correct omissions, and add your own reflections (clearly noted as such). If taping was involved, check the tapes for clarity. If transcripts are created, send them to the participants for member checks. If the data are entered into a database, establish quality checks to be sure that legal values are used throughout; check a sample of responses by more than one person to be sure they are correctly entered.

■ *Step 9.* Plan how to complete data collection. Were additional issues raised for which more data are needed? What strategies will you use to review the data with the participants? Will you provide preliminary reports before final analysis to the stakeholders?

A caveat is in order here. Evaluations are done in education and training, social programs, environmental areas, medical and health settings, business and marketing, transportation, international development, governments and policies, disaster response, agriculture, housing, and gender equity, to name a few settings. Given the diversity and the inherent contextual demands of evaluation, it is not possible to provide detailed instructions for data collection methods for all possible settings. Therefore, the following sections of this chapter provide descriptions of data collection options and resources for evaluators who want to pursue specific methods in more depth.

Data Collection Options: Quantitative

Quantitative data collection methods include tests, performance and portfolio assessments, surveys, goal attainment scaling (GAS), and analysis of secondary data sources. This section examines each of these methods and provides examples from the evaluation literature to illustrate their uses.

Tests

Tests are pervasively used in evaluation. They can provide measurements of a multitude of variables, including knowledge, skills, personality, interests, attitudes, motivation, and other psychological attributes. Tests can be standardized (usually commercially available with uniform directions for administering, scoring, and interpreting) or locally developed (teacher-made or evaluator-developed tests). They can be objective (multiple-choice, true–false) or nonobjective (e.g., open-ended questions, essay tests). Tests can be norm-referenced (a norm group is used for the development of the test, and results are interpreted in reference to that norm group) or criterion-referenced (specific criteria for performance are established, and results of individuals are compared against those criteria). The evaluator must be sure that the tests used:

- Meet the purposes of the data collection and are clear about the variables measured and any subscales included in the instrument.
- Are appropriate in terms of test content and skills tested.
- Are feasible, given the recommended administration procedures (e.g., amount of time required to take the test, expertise of the test administrator, appropriateness of format for participants, scoring processes, and cost).
- Provide appropriate sources of evidence for reliability and validity.
- Are selected in collaboration with knowledgeable persons from the community.
- Do not contain language that is offensive or biased with regard to gender, race/ethnicity, or disability.
- Can be modified if necessary to accommodate diversity within the targeted population.

If modifications of an instrument are necessary, then the evaluator needs to be explicit about the rationale for making the modification, the types of modifications that are allowable in particular contexts, and the meaning of scores obtained under nonstandardized conditions. Pilot-testing of any data collection method is usually recommended; if modifications are made to an existing instrument, pilot-testing is strongly encouraged.

Sources of Information about Tests

In Chapter 7, you have learned about conducting literature reviews and other ways to understand more about the big picture of the attributes that are of interest to you in an evaluation. These strategies can also be used to identify appropriate data collection methods. As noted throughout this chapter, evaluation reports generally include a specific description of data collection methods; if tests were used, you can see whether something used by another evaluator might be appropriate for you. If you are not successful in finding a test through this method, then you can go to databases that contain information about tests. Box 10.4 lists several of these resources.

Universal Design in Learning and Testing

Universal design is a generic term describing design that is intended to simplify life for everyone by making products, communications, and the built environment more usable by as many people as possible at little or no extra cost (Center for Universal Design, 1997). The basic idea behind universal design is that environments and products should be created, right from the start, to meet the needs of all users rather than just an average user. The United Nations included commentary on the need for universal design in its declaration on the rights of persons with disabilities: " 'Universal design' means the design of products, environments, programmes and services to be usable by all people, to the greatest extent possible, without the need for adaptation or specialized design" (United Nations Office of the High Commissioner for Human Rights, 2006). Article 4, under Obligation, states:

1. States Parties undertake to ensure and promote the full realization of all human rights and fundamental freedoms for all persons with disabilities without discrimination of any kind on the basis of disability. To this end, States Parties [promise] ... (f) To undertake or promote research and development of, and to promote the availability and use of new technologies, including information and communications technologies, mobility aids, devices and assistive technologies, suitable for persons with disabilities, giving priority to technologies at an affordable cost. (United Nations Office of the High Commissioner for Human Rights, 2006)

Although many universally designed educational materials and activities have been developed for instructional purposes, the design principles have applicability for data collection in evaluation as well. In a universally designed curriculum, students are presented with a range of options for learning. When tests are used for data collection in evaluation studies, alternative activities allow individuals with wide differences in their abilities (to see, hear, speak, move, read, write, understand English, pay attention, organize, engage, or remember) to demonstrate their achievements. Information can be presented to students through multiple means, such as audio, video, text, speech, Braille, photographs, or images. Likewise, a universal design allows students to use multiple means to express what they know through writing, speaking, drawing, or video recording. Advances in technology have made some universal design strategies much easier to implement. Teachers have access to computers, software, assistive technology, and other tools that can be used to adapt curricula or tests to suit a child's learning style. For example, textbooks and other reading materials can be made available in a digital format that includes audio versions of the text, as well as audio descriptions of visual images and charts. Box 10.5 provides a list of resources on universal design.

Ketterlin-Geller (2005) has listed helpful strategies for the development and pilot-testing of tests using universal design principles. For example, the language and features (such as a read-aloud option) should be appropriate to the individual taking the test. Also, each test taker should be allowed to take a pretest to determine the appropriateness and feasibility of administering the test in the chosen format.

Box 10.4. Sources of Information about Tests and Other Measurement Instruments

Source	Description of source
The *Mental Measurement Yearbooks* (MMY)	The Buros Institute has published the MMY for many years; it is a resource that lists thousands of tests in many categories. The database is made up of tests that have been published, have been revised, or have generated 20 or more references since the last MMY was published. This resource is available at the Buros website (*www.unl.edu/buros*). Information about each test is extensive, and it includes reviews of many of the tests in the database.
Tests in Print	This database is also published by the Buros Institute; it contains a more expansive list of tests, including those that are in print and available for purchase or use, even if they do not meet the criteria to be in MMY. The Buros website allows access to Tests in Print; the website also has a Test Locator search engine, which can be used to search for information on tests with criteria that the evaluator determines are relevant for the study.
PRO-ED, Inc.	This test publisher's website (*www.proedinc.com*) includes tests and reviews of tests in the areas of speech and language pathology, special education and rehabilitation, psychology and counseling, occupational and physical therapy, and early childhood.
American Psychological Association (APA)	Evaluators can find a test locator database at APA's website (*www.apa.org*); this database includes both published and unpublished tests. The website also provides information about appropriately selecting and using tests.
Educational Testing Service (ETS)	ETS maintains an extensive database that includes tests published by ETS as well as tests published elsewhere. Access to the tests is screened according to publisher restrictions (e.g., some tests require that a user be a licensed psychologist). Information is available at the ETS website (*www.ets.org*).
PsycINFO	This database is managed by the APA. It can be accessed at its own section of the APA website (*www.apa.org/pubs/databases/psycinfo/index.aspx*).
Other test publishers	If sufficient information about a test is not available through the previously mentioned sources, an evaluator can write directly to the test publisher to request information needed to make an informed decision.

Box 10.5. Resources for Universal Design in Learning and Testing

- **Center for Applied Special Technology (CAST;** *www.cast.org*). CAST is a nonprofit organization that works to expand learning opportunities for all individuals, especially those with disabilities, through the research and development of innovative, technology-based educational resources and strategies.

- **Parent Advocacy Center for Educational Rights (PACER) Simon Technology Center** *(www.pacer.org/stc)*. The mission of the Simon Center is to expand opportunities and enhance the quality of life of children and young adults with disabilities and their families, based on the concept of parents helping parents. The center is dedicated to making the benefits of technology more accessible to children and adults with disabilities.

- **National Center on Secondary Education and Transition (NCSET)** *(www.ncset.org)* and *(www.ncset.org/topics/udl/?topic=18)*. NCSET coordinates national resources, offers technical assistance, and disseminates information related to secondary education and transition for youth with disabilities, in order to increase the success of their futures.

- **National Center on Accessible Information Technology in Education** *(www.washington.edu/accessit/index.php)*. This center provides access to training for the development of fully accessible web-based materials in educational settings.

- **National Instructional Materials Accessibility Standard at CAST** *(nimas.cast.org)*. This section of the CAST website contains information about a standard approach to making print resources accessible through Braille, Talking Books, and other strategies.

Source: Based on Mertens (2009, p. 274).

· · · · · · · · · · EXTENDING YOUR THINKING · · · · · · · · · ·

Universal Design

Watch the Colorado State University (CSU) video about best practices in universal design for learning for college students *(www.youtube.com/watch?v=j7eUf_7dZVM)*. Note all the different adaptations depicted there.

1. Who benefits from universal design for learning?

2. The video shows many different techniques used by instructors for their students to learn better. Could any of the adaptations or techniques you see in the video be used by you in collecting data? If so, which ones and with which stakeholders?

3. For whom did CSU create this webpage, and why? (Go to *accessproject.colostate.edu/udl/video/transcript/transcript.cfm*)

Computer-Based Testing

Much of what has been done under the auspices of universal design and accommodation for people with disabilities has relevance more generally for consideration of the feasibility and logistics of using computer-based testing. Working from a context of universal design in testing, Thompson, Thurlow, Quenemoen, and Lehr (2002) raise the important issue of equity in terms of access to, and familiarity with, computer technology. The cost of the technology can be prohibitive, thus reducing opportunities for access to those with fewer resources. These individuals will then have less experience with answering questions that appear on a computer screen, using search functions, typing and composing on screen, mouse navigation, and other features unique to computer–human interaction.

Performance Assessment

Performance assessment is talked about in two distinctly different ways in evaluation: (1) as a process of collecting information through systematic observations to make decisions about an individual, and (2) as part of performance management or results-based evaluation. In the first instance, performance assessment typically uses direct observation of performance of some behavior, skill, or product. For example, students in an environmental engineering class can be asked to test a water solution for contaminants. Their performance can be assessed against an established procedure and expected outcomes. This type of performance assessment is explored in more depth just below. The second conceptualization of performance measures is more in line with the use of indicators in evaluation; therefore, this topic is discussed in a later section of this chapter.

Portfolio Assessment

Portfolio assessment has become popular as a form of alternative assessment in schools, because it allows for students to demonstrate types of learning that cannot be demonstrated on a test. Roeber (2002) defined "portfolio assessment" as evaluation of purposeful and systematic collections of student work against predetermined scoring criteria. Recall that at the start of the "Tests" section, we have mentioned criterion-referenced tests that specify expectations in terms of performance. This concept is usually applied in portfolio assessment in the form of a scoring rubric that specifies the components needed from the student and the quality of performance associated with different scores on those components. Several websites are dedicated to providing guidance and examples for rubrics to assess portfolios. For example, *www.rubrics4teachers.com* is a website geared toward teachers that gives tips and examples for rubrics, and *electronicportfolios.com* is a site hosted by Helen Barrett that includes many resources for electronic portfolios and assessment of student performance using rubrics. The *rubistar.4teachers.org* website provides options in terms of content, components, and specification of levels, making it easy to develop a rubric. Figure 10.2 is an example of a rubric to assess the quality of oral presentations.

Johnson, McDaniel, and Willeke (2000) have raised questions about the reliability of scores based on the use of rubrics in evaluation. They suggest that reliability of ratings can be improved by training raters and by having more than one rater score each portfolio so that their responses can be compared. Johnson et al. did this for a rubric to measure the effectiveness of a parent education project and were able to achieve reliability coefficients between .69 and .86 for the rubric's various components.

Category	4	3	2	1
Preparedness	Student is completely prepared and has obviously rehearsed.	Student seems pretty well prepared but might have needed a few more rehearsals.	The student is somewhat prepared, but it is clear that rehearsal was lacking.	Student does not seem at all prepared to present.
Content	Shows a full understanding of the topic.	Shows a good understanding of the topic.	Shows a good understanding of parts of the topic.	Does not seem to understand the topic very well.
Comprehension	Student can accurately answer almost all questions posed by classmates about the topic.	Student can accurately answer most questions posed by classmates about the topic.	Student can accurately answer a few questions posed by classmates about the topic.	Student cannot accurately answer questions posed by classmates about the topic.

Figure 10.2. A sample rubric for assessing oral presentations.

Surveys

Surveys are another pervasively used data collection method in evaluation. Because surveys are used so frequently in Western society, it is possible that evaluators can be lured into believing that they are easy to do. They are not easy to do if evaluators do them right. And there are advantages and disadvantages to the use of surveys that evaluators need to be aware of. The fact that surveys are self-report measures constitutes both an advantage and a disadvantage. One advantage is that a survey can be conducted relatively quickly to collect data from a large number of people. The disadvantage of self-reporting is that it does not involve direct observation of the behaviors in question to confirm that what people say is actually what they do (or believe or feel or …). In addition, an evaluator cannot know for certain whether a participant interpreted the questions the way they were intended to be read. Surveys can be quantitative and/or qualitative data collection methods. In this section, we discuss quantitative survey approaches. Qualitative approaches are discussed later in this chapter under "Interviews."

Multiple resources are available that provide instruction on how to develop surveys; a few of these are listed in Box 10.6.

Here is a set of generic steps in survey development. Evaluators would need to adapt these steps to the particular context in which they are working.

- Clarify the purpose of the survey; determine the types of information needed to answer the evaluation questions; determine the appropriate people to respond to the survey.
- Determine appropriate format for administering the survey (print, telephone, in-person, web-based), and for the survey questions (open-ended vs. closed-ended

Box 10.6. Resources about Surveys in Evaluation

Web-based resources

American Association for Public Opinion Research (*www.aapor.org/Home.htm*)	A professional organization of public opinion and survey research professionals in the United States, with members from academia, the mass media, government, the nonprofit sector, and private industry.
National Criminal Justice Reference Service (*www.ncjrs.gov*)	Maintained by the U.S. Department of Justice; contains advice on construction and use of surveys related to criminal justice and substance abuse. It also posts examples of survey studies conducted under its auspices.
Pew Research Center for the People and the Press (*people-press.org*)	An independent, nonpartisan public opinion research organization that studies attitudes toward politics, the press, and public policy issues.
Gallup Research Center (*www.gallup.com/home.aspx*)	A global research-based consultancy, specializing in employee and customer management.
National Opinion Research Center (*www.norc.org/Aboutus/Pages/default.aspx*)	Like the Gallup Center, a global research-based consultancy that provides services spanning the continuum of social science research.

Survey Research Textbooks

Fink, A. (2009). *How to conduct surveys: A step-by-step guide* (4th ed.). Thousand Oaks, CA: Sage.

Fowler, F. (2009). *Survey research methods* (4th ed.). Thousand Oaks, CA: Sage.

Mertens, D. M. (2010). *Research and evaluation in education and psychology: Integrating diversity with quantitative, qualitative, and mixed methods* (3rd ed.). Thousand Oaks, CA: Sage.

The survey research kit. Thousand Oaks, CA: Sage. This kit contains 10 books, each of which is about 120 pages long. It can be purchased as a kit, or each book can be purchased separately.

     Book 1: *The survey handbook* by Fink
     Book 2: *How to ask survey questions* by Fink
     Book 3: *How to conduct self-administered and mail surveys* by Bourque and Fielder
     Book 4: *How to conduct telephone surveys* by Bourque and Fielder
     Book 5: *How to conduct in-person interviews for surveys* by Oishi
     Book 6: *How to design survey studies* by Fink
     Book 7: *How to sample in surveys* by Fink
     Book 8: *How to assess and interpret survey psychometrics* by Litwin
     Book 9: *How to manage, analyze and interpret survey data* by Fink
     Book 10: *How to report on surveys*

questions, level of language, need for translation, need for accommodation for participants). If interviewers are used, train them as necessary.

▪ Develop an item pool; construct draft instrument.

▪ Pilot-test the draft instrument for both content and process.

▪ Make revisions to content and process as necessary.

▪ Implement the survey.

Examples of the use of surveys in evaluation include Taut's (2007; summarized in Chapter 8) evaluation of a capacity-building initiative in an international organization. Taut used a survey that was adapted from Preskill and Torres's (2001) Readiness for Organizational Learning and Evaluation instrument and a similar instrument developed by Cousins et al. (2003). As noted in Chapter 8, the items on the survey asked about the participants' perceptions of evaluation, leadership, structures, communication, and culture; their experiences with and attitudes toward evaluation, monitoring, and reporting activities; and their background and training in evaluation.

The Center for Information and Research on Civic Learning and Engagement (CIRCLE) at Tufts University *(www.civicyouth.org)* uses surveys to measure young adults' civic engagement. This includes data about their registering to vote, actually voting, contributing money to candidates or parties, and community service, as well as about their knowledge, skills, attitudes, and values related to civic engagement. CIRCLE makes its survey instruments available to anyone to use without formal permission. Chi, Jastrzab, and Melchior (2006) of CIRCLE published a survey that can be used to measure elementary school students' knowledge about and attitudes toward civic engagement. CIRCLE's website also contains examples of youth-led survey teams.

Goal Attainment Scaling

GAS is an evaluation methodology that, similar to other methodologies for measuring achievement (e.g., academic achievement scores), can be used both for individual assessment and in aggregate form to evaluate the program that employs it. The advantage to GAS, however, is that within a single study, the assessment can be applied across an infinite range of cultures, age groups, and interventions. This versatility is made possible through a collaborative relationship between practitioner and client, who together identify a unique, customized set of goals and then weight those goals according to their relative contribution to overall achievement.

Progress toward these weighted goals can then be translated into a single composite score, which can in turn be used for more sophisticated statistical analysis and accountability purposes (Marson, Wei, & Wasserman, 2009). Sherow (2000) found GAS beneficial in two adult family literacy programs: GAS promoted cooperative goal setting, was a valuable teaching–learning skill, and clarified and communicated program goals.

Analysis of Secondary Data Sources

 We have already seen a number of examples of the use of secondary data sources in evaluation studies. Recall Bowman's (2005) use of U.S. Census Bureau data in her evaluation of tribal colleges, and Sharma and Deepak's (2001) use of international agencies' databases in their evaluation of a rehabilitation program in Vietnam (both discussed in Chapter 7; see also Chapter 4, Box 4.11, for Sharma & Deepak). Evaluators commonly use secondary data sources during the early stages of an evaluation, especially as a part of needs sensing. However, secondary data sources can be used at any stage of the evaluation. A number of secondary databases maintained by international donor agencies are described in Chapter 7. Evaluators do need to be cautious about using secondary databases, however, because they have not created the data themselves. Therefore, they need to be aware of any limitations in the reliability, validity, and comprehensiveness of these data, as well as to disaggregate the data by relevant dimensions of diversity for the communities in which they serve. For example, major national databases maintained by the U.S. Department of Education allow for disaggregation by gender and by disability, but not by gender and disability.

··········· E X T E N D I N G   Y O U R   T H I N K I N G ···········
Measuring Complex Constructs

Evaluators are often asked to measure complex concepts such as poverty.

1. Before you continue reading, define "poverty."
2. What does a poor person look like? Describe where and how such people live.
3. How would you measure poverty in a developing country or a rural Midwestern American town? Would you measure poverty in the same way for both? Explain.

Typically, measuring poverty has meant looking at one's income. World governments and international lending institutions work to pull people out of poverty, and they measure their success with economic indicators such as the gross domestic product (GDP) and per capita income. But is poverty more than not having money in one's pocket? Two researchers believe that measuring poverty should also include such indicators such as whether people have clean water for bathing, drinking, and cooking; the ability to access and afford a healthy diet; an education; or appropriate health care. Alkire and Santos (2010) have created the Oxford Poverty and Human Development Initiative (OPHI). They ask questions such as these:

- What dimensions and measures of poverty should be considered?
- Which ethical principles are essential (efficiency, equity, sustainability, empowerment), and how can plural principles guide poverty alleviation?
- How can we understand and predict people's economic behavior, adaptive preferences, and thus poverty outcomes?
- How can digital and analytical technologies improve analysis of complex evidence, modeling of outcomes, connection of levels of analysis, and clarification of value judgments?

(cont.)

> ▪ In historical and political-economy contexts that are often hostile to human development, how can both individual and group capabilities be developed and freedoms be realized?
>
> They list five dimensions of poverty data not mentioned in other poverty scales:
>
> ▪ Employment quality.
>
> ▪ Agency (what people are able to do in line with their conception of what is good). People should be able to live within their value systems—no need to be passive, submissive, or forced to act in ways they would rather not.
>
> ▪ Physical safety.
>
> ▪ The ability to go about without shame.
>
> ▪ Psychological and subjective well-being.
>
> 4. In your definition of poverty, did you think to add how safe people may feel, or whether they have psychological well-being? What if a young man is fed well, is clothed, has a place to sleep, but must sell his body in order to obtain these assets? What if children live in homes where they are physically well cared for but emotionally abused? In what other scenarios would Alkire and Foster (2011) find poverty using their measures where others would not? They note that measuring poverty by income alone may produce a very inadequate picture:
>
>> OPHI aspires to build a more systematic methodological and economic framework to underlie poverty reduction, a framework which will seek to consider several dimensions, interconnections and principles simultaneously in a manner that renders the capability approach operational, and well-connected with existing literatures.
>
> 5. How do you measure corruption? Give some thought to this construct and how it might be measured. If you want to see how two different evaluation teams approached the measurement of corruption, review Marra's (2000) study described in Chapter 1, or an OPHI working paper by Foster, Horowitz, and Méndez (2009).

Data Collection Options: Qualitative

Observations

I have a general rule for the evaluations that I do: I only agree to do them if I can observe the program in action. (This is a natural corollary to my reluctance to send a form that the project director can use at the end of the program.) Observation is a powerful evaluation tool and can be conducted formally or informally, but it is difficult to conceive of an evaluator conducting a study in a context in which he/she has not met face-to-face with the community members. Observations can be made by using a field notes approach and/or by noting specific behaviors of interest. For example, I often start my observations by (1) sketching the area to set the notes in context, (2) labeling the people in the observational setting by using codes that protect their identities, (3) noting who is talking to whom, and

(4) noting what is being said. The number and length of observations vary from study to study (Mertens, 2009).

Various roles are possible for observers, ranging from total membership in the community to being actively or peripherally involved. The choice of an observation role, as well as the schedule and venues for observations, should be made in conjunction with the community discussions that precede data collection. Patton (2002b) provides an extensive list of possible things to notice when observing:

▓ *Program setting.* What is the physical environment like? Try to be specific enough that a person who has not been physically present can see the venue.

▓ *Human and social environment.* What patterns of interaction, frequency of interactions, and directions of communication occur? What variations occur on the basis of gender, race/ethnicity, disability, or other observable dimensions of diversity? How do these variations change during the observation?

▓ *Program activities and behaviors.* What is happening at the beginning of the observation? In the middle? At the end? Who is present and involved? How does this involvement change during the observation? What variations are observable? How are participants reacting at different points of time?

▓ *Informal interactions and unplanned activities.* What is going on when no formal activities are underway? Who talks to whom about what?

▓ *Native language.* What is the native language in the setting? This can mean a spoken, printed, or visual language. It can also mean specific terminology and how that is specifically used in the observed setting.

▓ *Nonverbal communications.* What do body language and nonverbal cues suggest? How do people get the attention of one another? What physical activities are observed (e.g., fidgeting, moving around, expressions of affection)? How do people dress and space themselves?

▓ *Unobtrusive measures.* What physical clues are observable (e.g., dust on, or signs of extensive use of, materials)?

▓ *Observing what does not happen.* Based on prior knowledge and expectations, what is *not* happening that might have been expected? For example, a particular person may be absent or uninvolved, or an activity that is scheduled may not occur.

Cautions about Observations

Evaluators need to be cautious when using observations as the data collection methods. Observed behaviors can be interpreted in many different ways. This is especially troublesome in diverse cultural contexts. Evaluators need to consider how their own positionalities influence their access to the observation context, what they choose to record in their observations, and how people in that context interpret their own behaviors. While observing a teachers' meeting to discuss new curriculum in northeast Brazil, I (A. T. W.) was surprised at the strong emotion with which participants shared their own beliefs. Two teachers spoke loudly to one another, waving their arms and looking to me to be very upset. I moved my chair back, afraid that I might find myself in the middle of a fight. Later, at lunch, I saw the two women sharing lunch together, laughing and conversing, enjoying one another's company. Afterward, I learned that strong expression of emotion is a typical communication pattern that does not carry the same negative connotations that I experience in my own culture. In fact, the first time a Brazilian felt comfortable enough to "yell" at me, I felt that I had finally been accepted by her community.

Interviews

I would be hard pressed to identify an evaluation study that did not include interviewing as part of the data collection, because evaluation by its nature requires interaction with stakeholders. (Go back and review the sample studies summarized in Chapters 3–6, and notice how many used interviewing as a data collection method.) This interaction may be informal or formal. When interviewing is specifically identified as a data collection method in an evaluation, it can take many forms. Roulston, deMarrais, and Lewis (2003) identify many types of interviews: general qualitative interviewing, in-depth interviewing, phenomenological interviewing, focus group interviews, oral histories, and ethnographic interviews. Each type of interview is associated with different procedures, and details about these procedures can be found in many good books on qualitative research and evaluation, as well as in the *Handbook of Interview Research: Context and Method* (Gubrium & Holstein, 2002). Roulston et al. (2003) recognize a number of challenges in the interviewing process, including these:

1. Responding to unexpected participant behaviors (e.g., revelation of an emotionally volatile condition, such as when a participant reports having just learned that her husband is having an affair).

2. Dealing with the consequences of your own actions and subjectivities as the evaluator (e.g., having an emotional reaction when an experience of violence is described that mirrors your own past experience). This relates back to knowing yourself.

3. Phrasing and negotiating questions (e.g., allowing the participants' comments to lead the interview process and keeping the focus on the intended topic).

4. Dealing with sensitive issues (e.g., asking about racism or sexism).

Good practices to consider include keeping a reflective journal, as well as listening to audio recordings, watching videos, or reading transcripts of the interview with these challenges in mind (Gubrium & Holstein, 2002).

Steps in the Interview Process

Corbin and Morse (2003) suggest that an evaluator have at least four meetings with a participant in the course of conducting an interview. The first meeting (the preinterview phase) is held to discuss the study with the intended respondent and determine her/his interest in participating. The evaluator should share all the information needed to obtain informed consent, including expectations in terms of time, topics to be discussed, reciprocity for the participant, and the process to be used to record the interview (if necessary). This may culminate in the person's signing the informed consent agreement and in the scheduling of time for conducting the interview itself. During the early part of an interview (the tentative phase), Corbin and Morse suggest that the participant is usually a little wary about being interviewed and may be trying to determine whether the interviewer is trustworthy. Therefore, they suggest that the interviewer spend additional time explaining the background of the study, conveying both verbally and nonverbally that the participant's contribution is valued.

The immersion phase of the interviews comes next, assuming that the participant is comfortable and willing to share thoughts and feelings honestly. The evaluator must be particularly sensitive to any issues that may upset the person, allow time to address the reason for the emotional response, and assure the participant of support. The interviewer brings closure to the interview (the emergence phase) by checking with his/her understanding of what the participant said; this can be done by summarizing or asking for clarification about specific points. I have found that rich data sometimes emerge during this final phase—possibly because respondents become more relaxed when they think the interview is over, or because their neural connections were stimulated by participating in the interview process and they now have more that they want to say. It may be also be that they have enjoyed being listened to and valued for their contribution.

Cultural Factors in Interviewing

Studies that have used interviews with various racial and ethnic groups provide insights into cultural factors that need to be considered with this approach. For example, Guzman (2003; cited in Mertens, 2009) describes the aspect of Latina/Latino culture that views elders and scholars as deserving respect. This attitude may be evidenced in interview situations when Latinas/Latinos do not make direct eye contact or seem reluctant to express their true feelings about how an intervention has affected them, whether positively or negatively. In U.S. mainstream culture, such behavior might be interpreted as meaning that the persons lacked engagement with, or felt no impact from, the program. Guzman suggests that this situation might be remedied by having a member of the Latina/Latino community conduct such interviews.

Community Involvement: Key to Interviews/Observations

Cardoza, Clayson, et al. (2002; cited in Mertens, 2009) describe the importance of community involvement in their work in Hispanic communities. They combined observation and participation in the community with their desire to conduct interviews. Their attendance at a Christmas *Posada* was viewed as essential to the quality of the data collection, as shown in this example (cited in Mertens, 2009, p. 248):

> At one Christmas *Posada* a community member said to us " ... you see [over there] Maria, she knows everything but unless Pedro says you're ok ... she isn't going to talk to you ... people are afraid of La Migra [the Immigration and Naturalization Service; INS]. We have found that the outsider role severely limits the ability of evaluators to identify and understand the more invisible structures, spoken, unspoken, and formal and informal rules that govern complex community initiatives. Attending celebrations, like *Posadas*, while time intensive, is a primary method for information gathering and understanding the generalities and specifics of community functioning.

Cultural Responsiveness and Data Collection Quality (#1)

Analyze the study described below. Identify the contributors to the quality of the data collection that you see in this study.

Nichols and Keltner (2005; cited in Mertens, 2009) interviewed over 140 people in a study of Native American community perspectives on families caring for children with disabilities. They asked the local advisory board to nominate the interviewers. They provided extensive training for the interviewers to ensure the quality of the data and the confidentiality of the participants, and the researchers visited the participating communities regularly to be sure that the data were being collected as planned. The interview guide was developed in collaboration with the local advisory boards in order to be responsive to the participants' culture in context and form. The interviewers took notes and audiotaped the interviews. Each interview consisted of 11 open-ended questions; three sample questions appear below. Interviewers began with general questions about family life and the hopes and worries that families with small children have in their community. They then moved on to ask about the nature of contact that participants had experienced with people with disabilities. Subsequent questions were designed to build on the community tradition of storytelling.

Native Americans' Perspectives on Children with Disabilities: Sample Interview Questions

One of the best ways to learn about community life is through stories that people share with each other. Do you have a story to tell that features someone with a disability? Family stories sometimes include ways siblings or cousins help each other. Tribal stories sometimes tell about people who had a disability but helped the tribe or community in some way. Could you tell us any stories about a person with a disability in your family or tribe?

All of us have heard different people talk about the good things that happen to them and talk about the bad things that happen to them. Most people live their lives in a way that is comfortable for them (doing certain things, at certain times like dancing or special ceremonies, giving a ride to a cousin who needs to go into town, or listening to elders). Sometimes Indians call this living in harmony and teach their children how to live in harmony. Can you tell me some things you know that families can do to help their children with disabilities live in harmony?

Sometimes families need help with meeting the special needs of their child with disabilities. Depending upon what the special need may be, families may try to use a variety of resources or services. Some of these resources may be within the family (grandmother's advice, uncle familiar with Indian medicines, sister who also has a child with a disability) or some of these resources are from organizations like churches or support groups, or some resources may be from the mainstream society (schools, clinics, physicians). In our community, what kind of resources do you think families use? Would you recommend them to a family you know and cared about? If you would not recommend a resource, could you tell us why not? (Nichols & Keltner, 2005, pp. 38–40; cited in Mertens, 2009, p. 249)

Focus Groups

Focus groups are popular as a means of using a group interview setting for data collection in marketing research. Many textbooks are available that discuss the steps in the conduct of focus groups. Chiu (2003) made extensive use of focus groups in her work facilitating change in health services for culturally complex communities. She developed a cyclical approach integrating the steps of action research with focus group methodology for the purpose of radical social transformation. The three basic stages follow:

■ *Stage 1: Problem identification.* Evaluators need to build their knowledge of the community sufficiently to identify stakeholders and build relationships with participants at all levels of the program (service recipients and providers, funders, administrators). Focus groups can be used initially to identify the issues, concerns, and experiences of the various constituencies. In her study, Chiu (2003) used focus groups to study participants' perceptions and experiences with cervical and breast cancer screening. The meetings included discussion guides, along with such items as a speculum and a breast model; they also included video-based demonstrations of the screening procedure. This combination of stimuli enhanced the women's ability to describe their own experiences and enriched the communication between the women and Chiu. The creation of dialogue is designed to encourage critical thinking and awareness of the issues as a basis for later development of solutions.

■ *Stage 2: Solution generation.* Building on the identified concerns and issues, focus groups can then be used to formulate solutions and identify resources needed to support the implementation of the interventions. Service recipients and/or providers may be enlisted as co-researchers for the focus groups. If necessary, workshops can be offered to build the capacities of the participants and providers to implement and evaluate the proposed solutions.

■ *Stage 3: Implementation and evaluation.* During program implementation, focus groups can be conducted for various purposes, such as regular problem solving during implementation and evaluation as a way to reflect on the intervention and its effectiveness. This provides an opportunity for community members to be actively involved in these projects. In the Chiu (2003) study, focus group co-moderators received intensive training to facilitate focus group discussions, in which, when possible, the use of the members' mother tongue was actively encouraged.

MIXED METHODS AND FOCUS GROUPS

Focus groups are effective when it is possible to get people together to discuss a topic or when individual interviews are not possible. At times, one strategy will be more feasible than another. For example, Cross et al. (2000; see Chapter 6, Box 6.8) combined individual interviews and focus groups in their study of mental health services for children in Native American communities. They used individual interviews with key informants such as medicine people, elders, and other important members of the community. They conducted focus groups with parents, children, service providers, community members, and staff from collaborating programs. The focus group meetings lasted from 2 to 3 hours and began with assurances of confidentiality and the informed consent details.

The evaluators followed up with individual interviews for any tribe members who appeared to be uncomfortable in the focus group setting. The evaluators also participated in a campout with the staff, parents, children, and spiritual leaders. The timing of the data collection was suggested by the community members. Group interviews were either taped or recorded with handwritten notes. Individual interviews were taped, except when the participants asked that notes be taken either during or after the interview. The specific adaptation of the focus group and individual interviews to Native American culture came in the form of the use of the four quadrants of the medicine wheel as a basis for the development of the interview questions.

The four quadrants include context, body, mind, and spirit (Cross et al., 2000, pp. 20–21):

- The *context* includes culture, community, family, peers, work, school and social history.

- The *mind* includes our cognitive processes such as thoughts, memories, knowledge, and emotional processes such as feelings, defenses and self-esteem.

- The *body* includes all physical aspects, such as genetic inheritance, gender and condition, as well as sleep, nutrition and substance use.

- The *spirit* area includes both positive and negative learned teachings and practices, as well as positive and negative metaphysical or innate forces.

Sample questions for each quadrant included the following (Cross et al., 2000, pp. 103–104):

- *Context quadrant:* How does your program draw upon extended family and kinship to help parents help their children? (for service providers).

- *Body quadrant:* Have you or your child (children) participated in any cultural activities to improve physical health? Examples include: special tribal celebrations with food served to mark the occasion, herbal or plant remedies for certain illnesses, smudging or other ways of cleansing for special occasions, or tribally-based recreational opportunities such as dancing or playing games.

- *Mind quadrant:* How has the program helped you develop strategies that use Indian ways for addressing the needs of your child? (for parents).

- *Spirit quadrant:* Have you or your family participated in any rituals or ceremonies to help restore balance to your lives, either through the purging of negative forces or the development of positive forces? Do you use any Indian traditional remedies to restore balance in the spiritual area (example: sweat lodge)?

The interviewers and focus group leaders had their guiding questions; however, they encouraged community members to tell their stories in the way that was most comfortable for them. Hence many of their comments departed from the script. The evaluators believe that these departures provided invaluable data for measuring the project's progress.

Examples of other community-based versions of focus group strategies include the *hui* that Māori people host and the *dingaka* in Botswana. Māori hold day-long meetings called *hui*, at which members of the community are invited to read papers and discuss their meanings with the authors—in this case, meanings centered around marginalization and research protocols (Cram et al., 2006). It is important in these gatherings not to silence the voices of those who are less articulate. Some participants are very articulate and present a particular view. However, those who are living the experience, but not articulating it in ways the researcher finds useful, also need to be heard.

The practices of *dingaka* (diviners) (Dube, 2001; cited in Chilisa, 2005, p. 679) are used as a form of data collection in Botswana. The *dingaka* use a set of up to 60 bones that symbolize divine power, evil power, foreign spirits (good or bad), elderly men and women, young and old, homesteads, family life or death, and ethnic groups (including *Makgoa*, or white people) to construct a story about a consulting client's life. The client throws the bones, and the resulting pattern is interpreted in reference to his or her experiences, networks, and relationships with people and the environment. A diviner proceeds to interpret the pattern of the bones, all the while asking the client to confirm or reject the story the diviner is telling. Thus the diviner and client work together to construct knowledge that is placed within the complexity of the current context. This process yields a community-constructed story, rather than one constructed by the evaluator (the diviner). Chilisa (2005) concludes: "It offers alternative ways in which researchers may work with communities to theorize and build models of research designs that are owned by the people, and restores the dignity and integrity that has [*sic*] been violated by First World epistemologies since colonial times" (p. 680).

- - - - - - - - - - E X T E N D I N G   Y O U R   T H I N K I N G - - - - - - - - - -
Cultural Responsiveness and Data Collection Quality (#2)

Analyze the following example. Again, identify those aspects that contribute to the quality of the data collection from a culturally responsive lens.

Wehipeihana and Pipi (2008) evaluated barriers to uptake and issues of access for a tax credit for families with financially dependent children in the Māori community in New Zealand who were eligible for the credit. Given that many Māori families live in remote areas without transport, and they may not have telephone or Internet service, the evaluators had to design their survey to be responsive to this context. Therefore, they chose to use telephone interviews when these were possible and face-to-face interviews when phone interviews were not possible. The interviews were semistructured in nature, and each interview lasted between 45 minutes and 1 hour. The researchers took notes, and some interviews, with respondents' permission, were audiotaped. The researchers were also involved in ongoing "conversations" with respondents as part of the process of helping them work through the process of determining eligibility for the tax credit (or generally encouraging them to "get sorted" on any other tax-related matters).

The researchers found that there was considerable work in "peeling back the layers" to get to a "place" where they could talk about the tax credit with respondents. One respondent commented, "The questions you are asking are really personal. They touch your soul. Knowing you two I trust that what I say will be looked after" (quoted in Wehipeihana & Pipi, 2008, p. 20). As this comment indicates, one of the things the interviews highlighted was that when respondents got to know and trust

(*cont.*)

the researchers, they were prepared to talk about and reveal more of themselves and to be accountable for their actions. This showed that while it was indeed hard to reach some of those eligible for the tax credit, it was not impossible; it simply required a suitable approach to locate them. The researchers managed to reach these respondents mainly by creating networks and by building relationships of trust. The researchers were sometimes known to the respondents, but mostly connections were made through the referrals of others known to the respondents who could vouch for the trustworthiness of the researchers. This highlights the importance of trustworthy guidance for any "hard-to-reach" group, such as this one, when evaluators are designing any communications to reach them.

Personal reflections from one of the evaluators (Wehipeihana) further emphasize the appropriateness and value of this data collection process for the Māori community.

What makes a good "indigenous" evaluation study? In this particular project, I think our contact method was absolutely critical for identifying eligible Māori whānau (for this research) who were a tiny proportion of the population.

Secondly, talking about money and people's finances is very sensitive–and it worked that we were known to participants, or were referred by somebody they trusted.

Their willingness to talk to us when some of them were operating outside of the law (sharing their tax numbers, working over and above the permitted hours when in receipt of a benefit) is an indication of our ways of working to build trust. Indeed, the clients said they don't believe they would have got this hard-to-reach (and tiny proportion) of the population without our whānau (snowball approach to recruitment)–and would recommend us for this type of work again. (Incidentally, we were tapped for this work. I originally did not want to do this work for our tax department, believing it was focused on tax compliance, and inconveniently lost the business card that I was going to use to follow up on.) When they got me on the phone, via another colleague, the value of this research to making a difference to Māori whānau was a no-brainer, and we really loved this project–particularly helping Māori to "get sorted" and to claim significant financial back payment.

Not branding these whānau negatively was really important to me–particularly as this group of participants are the very group for whom this assistance is intended for [and] supposed to reach.

The workshop with policy and operational staff (from Inland Revenue and Ministry of Social Development who administer unemployment and sole parent benefits), [after] the presentation of the report, I believe provided some valuable insight into policy, operational, and communication considerations.

FOCUS GROUPS: COMMUNITY SCORE CARD

Garbarino and Holland (2009) describe an extension of focus group methods to include collection of quantitative data that they call the "community score card" (CSC).

The CSC is described as a 'mixed method' tool because it generates both quantitative and qualitative data and analysis. The quantitative data comprise perception scores of specific qualities of service provision, usually scored on a 4 or 5 point scale. These scores can then be aggregated from all the focus group discussions held and can be compared across groups and over time. The key to a successful CSC session, in contrast with a survey module, is that the scores are not simply elicited as an end in themselves but feed qualitative discussion. The interactive focus group setting of a CSC exercise allows the facilitators to use the scores generated to encourage an in-depth diagnostic discussion by the group. The scoring is used to prompt a discussion of three questions: (a) Defining the problem/issue; (b) Diagnosing the problem; and (c) Identifying solutions. Follow up action might involve service users taking action or engaging with service providers to resolve some of the problems identified during the CSC session. If appropriate, the CSC facilitators can extend their role to facilitating 'interface' sessions between groups of users and service providers in which the results of the CSC sessions are discussed and action agreed. (Holland et al., 2007; quoted in Garbarino & Holland, 2009, p. 16)

Reviews of Documents or Artifacts

For document and artifact data, a wide variety of sources is available. Documents may include hard-copy, electronic, or handwritten items ranging from official records (e.g., marriage certificates, arrest records) to documents prepared for personal reasons (e.g., diaries, letters). Other types of documents and artifacts include photographs, websites, meeting minutes, project reports, curriculum plans, and many others. In making decisions about documents and artifacts, it is important to keep in mind that issues of power and privilege typically result in the preservation of some groups' artifacts and documents, whereas those of others, having been assigned less importance, either are not in a format that can be preserved (e.g., in written form) or have been destroyed.

Documents and artifacts are valuable in that they can provide background that is not accessible from community members. They can also be used as a basis of conversation with community members to stir memories that might not rise to the surface without such catalysts. Researchers and evaluators must be cautious in the use of extant documents and artifacts, however; again, they reflect only those experiences that have been preserved, thereby eliminating the possibility of the viewpoints of those whose data are not accorded that privilege (Mertens, 2009).

Data Collection Options: Participatory

Most Significant Change

The "most significant change" (MSC) method was developed in the mid-1990s through a collaborative partnership between the Christian Commission for Development in Bangladesh and Rick Davies to create a monitoring system that would involve community members in determining what indicators of change are important to them (Davies, 1998; cited in Whitmore et al., 2006). The MSC method was used successfully in Bangladesh. The heart of this method is described as "the sharing of stories of lived experiences, and systematically selecting those most representative of the type of change being sought to share with others. In so doing, the method allows for an open-ended and rich discussion on a range of aspects of change, rather than snippets of reality that are defined through outsiders in the form of indicators" (Whitmore et al., 2006, p. 345). The method has two parts. First, stories of change are identified; the steps involved in this first part are listed below. Second, a communication pathway is constructed to make sure that all involved parties understand the significant stories of change. The first part includes these processes (Davies, 1998; cited in Whitmore et al., 2006, p. 348):

Identify who is to be involved and how. Who will be asked to share stories (where is the lived experience that others need to hear about)? Who will help to identify the domain(s) of change? To whom will information be communicated?

Identify the domains of change to be discussed. These are often related to key goals of the project/organisation/initiative. (For example, in Brazil, each credit group that received money was asked to discuss three areas: changes in people's lives; changes in people's participation; and changes in the sustainability of people's institutions and their activities.) Additionally, the group can report any other type of change enabling field staff to report on other factors that are deemed important.

Clarify the frequency with which stories will be shared and the most significant one selected. (For example, in Brazil, this was initially monthly but later took place less than quarterly, as this proved to be a more feasible rhythm.)

Share stories using a simple question for each of these four types of changes: "During the last month, in your opinion, what do you think was the most significant change that took place in … [e.g., the lives of the people participating in the project]?"

Select the most significant one from among the stories (per type of change).

Document the answer. The answer has two parts: descriptive—describing what happened in sufficient detail such that an independent person could verify that the event took place—and explanatory—explaining why the group members thought the change was the most significant out of all the changes that took place over that time period.

Gujit (as a contributor to Whitmore et al., 2006, p. 346) explains:

A key strength of the MSC method is that it allows participants to make explicit the criteria for success that they value. This occurs as a result of the built-in reflection, not just stating the most significant change but making clear why this was collectively selected as the most significant one. [When] diverse stakeholder experiences and perspectives [are allowed] to meet and [are shared], the emergent criteria for success provide important insights about what is valued about the initiative being monitored.

And Mertens (2009, p. 261) adds:

When the MSC was used with Brazilian farmers, they identified such change events as being able to prepay a loan to a micro-credit group on time and gaining title to their own land. The MSC seems to be more sustainable in contexts that include a stable organizational hierarchy. When changes occur in leadership, support for the method may diminish, and without support, people who are struggling to make a living may not see the benefit of expending additional time on a process that is not valued by those in power.

Collection of Visual Data

Visual media such as photographs, videos, and web-based presentations can be powerful sources of meaningful data, especially in visually rich cultural communities or in circumstances in which printed language is not a prevalent mode of expression (Rose, 2007; Pink,

2007; Stanczak, 2007). Extant visual materials can be collected and analyzed, or the data collection can involve the creation of visual materials by the evaluator and/or community members. If the evaluator is taking the pictures, then he/she can plan to show changes over time, illustrate oppressive social conditions such as those experienced by immigrant farm workers, or give a human face to a global problem.

A tension exists between promises of confidentiality and revelation of individual identities by showing faces and/or bodies. Rose (2007) recommends the use of a collaborative model in research that uses visual images of people; in this model, the photos are based on agreements between evaluators and community members. Permissions should be obtained at the time of making the visual images, as well as at the point of dissemination of the images as part of the study's results in different venues. If a photo is used in a book or website, or a video in a presentation or website, the people in the pictures should be able to grant permission for such use. The copyright for the visual materials legally rests with the person who took the pictures or made the video. If this person is the researcher or evaluator, then a good practice is to provide copies to the people who appear in the visual materials.

Rose (2007) suggests the use of several steps in using photos that are taken by community members in research or evaluation. The evaluator begins by interviewing community members, then gives them cameras along with guidance regarding what sort of photographs to take. Once the photos are in hand, the participants might be asked to write something about each photo. The researcher/evaluator can then interview participants again about their pictures and written remarks. Analysis and interpretation follow, based on strategies discussed for qualitative data in Chapter 12.

Visual Strategies for Rapid Assessments in International Development

When evaluators work in areas affected by natural disasters or in conflict zones, lengthy evaluations may not be possible or may even be counterproductive (McNall & Foster-Fishman, 2007). The provision of timely information can save lives and lead to more effective responses by service providers. Evaluators in international development have responded to this demand for quick turnaround in the provision of information by developing a number of data collection strategies called "participatory rural appraisal," "rapid evaluation and assessment methods," or "rapid ethnographic assessment." Commonalities of these methods include the following (McNall & Foster-Fishman, 2007):

1. The ability to provide information in a short time frame under challenging conditions.

2. The collection of data from several sources, using several methods.

3. Community involvement.

4. Use of teams of evaluators with co-evaluators from the communities.

5. Iterative use of data, with information from the early cycles of data collection feeding into subsequent decisions about data collection.

Evaluators have adapted some of these strategies for evaluations in other contexts that are not in crisis, such as in developing countries in areas of natural resource management, agriculture, poverty reduction, health and social programs, and nutrition programs. The World Bank has developed a guide for the development and conduct of participatory evaluation methods that is applicable across sectors (Tikare et al., 2001; see Chapter 9, especially Box 9.7). Data collection methods for rapid assessments include many of the basic types we have discussed already in this chapter: surveys, interviews, observations, use of secondary data sources, and focus groups. They can also include the more innovative visual data collection methods described below.

Participatory rural appraisal is associated with a number of visual data collection strategies (Rietbergen-McCraken & Narayan-Parker, 1998; McNall & Foster-Fisher, 2007). These strategies are not limited to rural areas, but they arose from a desire to engage local people in research activities in communities where written forms of literacy are not dominant. Thus the strategies can be implemented by using paper or computer screens, but they can also be done by drawing on the ground with sticks, stones, seeds, or other local materials, or using other techniques. Box 10.7 illustrates some of these.

RANKING EXERCISES

Participants can be shown how to rank things such as problems, preferences, or solutions. The community can generate lists of problems and then rank-order them in terms of importance, as shown in Box 10.7. If evaluators develop pictures that represent the problems on cards, then community members can sort them into the categories from most to least important. In addition, the participants can generate criteria for deciding what is most and least important. A matrix can be used in which the horizontal axis plots the problems and the vertical axis plots the criteria. Participants then rank each item in a position in the matrix. Individuals can do their rankings first, and then the group can compare and discuss their rankings.

TREND ANALYSIS

Calendars or daily activity charts can be used for trend analysis. Participants can indicate their level of activity on a calendar, with notations for seasonal variables such as rainfall, crop sequences, income, and food. Daily activity charts can provide a graphic way for individuals to depict how they spend their day. Such charts can provide insights into differences in time use by men and women, or those who are employed and those who are unemployed. Trend analysis is useful for identifying the busiest times of the day, month, or year as a basis for helping the community members make possible changes in time use.

MAPPING

The technique of mapping can be used for a number of different reasons. Historical mapping allows the participants to depict changes that have occurred in the community. Social maps can illustrate characteristics of the community, such as access to resources, school attendance, or involvement in community activities. Personal maps can show different sections of the community, such as where rich and poor people live or where men and women can go. Institutional maps can represent different groups and organizations in a community and their relationships. These maps can be used as a basis for facilitating participation in decision making by a wider range of constituencies.

Box 10.7. Visual Data Collection Strategies in Participatory Rural Appraisal

Some individuals may find it difficult to prioritize, rank, or categorize items. Visual methods will help them respond to such questions. For example, group members can use the wall chart illustrated below to discuss how common certain problems are, how serious they feel the problems are, and how important they think they are.

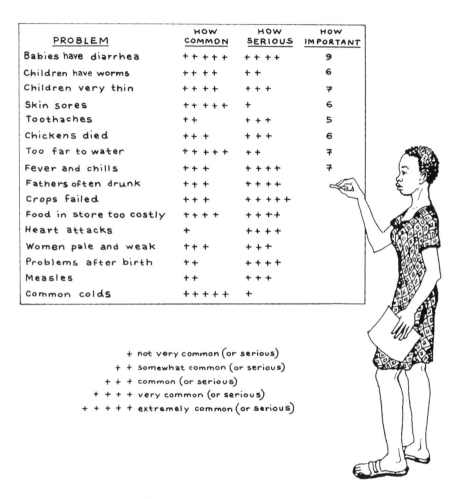

PROBLEM	HOW COMMON	HOW SERIOUS	HOW IMPORTANT
Babies have diarrhea	+ + + + +	+ + + +	9
Children have worms	+ + + +	+ +	6
Children very thin	+ + + +	+ + +	7
Skin sores	+ + + + +	+	6
Toothaches	+ +	+ + +	5
Chickens died	+ + +	+ + +	6
Too far to water	+ + + + +	+ +	7
Fever and chills	+ + +	+ + + +	7
Fathers often drunk	+ + +	+ + + +	
Crops failed	+ + +	+ + + + +	
Food in store too costly	+ + + +	+ + + +	
Heart attacks	+	+ + + +	
Women pale and weak	+ + +	+ + +	
Problems after birth	+ +	+ + + +	
Measles	+ +	+ + +	
Common colds	+ + + + +	+	

+ not very common (or serious)
+ + somewhat common (or serious)
+ + + common (or serious)
+ + + + very common (or serious)
+ + + + + extremely common (or serious)

A wall chart for ranking/prioritizing problems. *Source:* Werner and Bower (1995, pp. 3–14). Copyright 1995 by the Hesperian Foundation. Reprinted by permission.

Another way to assist participants in responding is to use symbols, such as the flannel board symbols shown below for discussing different serious ailments.

(cont.)

Box 10.7 (*cont.*)

SKULLS mean SERIOUS

 Big skulls:
EXTREMELY SERIOUS
deadly

 Middle-sized skulls:
EXTREMELY SERIOUS

Small skulls:
SERIOUS

SAD
FACES   Mean COMMON. The more common a problem is, the more
faces you put next to it.

FACES
WITH      Mean CONTAGIOUS (the illness spreads from one person to
ARROWS   others).

LONG
ARROW   Mean CHRONIC (the problem is long lasting).

Flannel board symbols for discussing serious ailments. *Source:* Werner and Bower (1995, pp. 3–15). Copyright 1995 by the Hesperian Foundation. Reprinted by permission.

Participants can discuss the problems and then indicate how they feel by individually placing the symbols on the flannel board. If participants are unable to read, the words can also be illustrated.

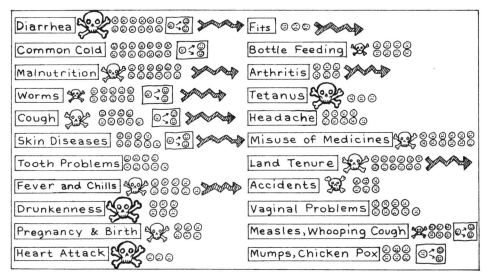

Flannel board discussion of serious ailments. *Source:* Werner and Bower (1995, pp. 3–16). Copyright 1995 by the Hesperian Foundation. Reprinted by permission.

TRANSECT WALKS

Transect walks involve walking through an area while observing and asking questions (e.g., questions about the status of natural resources and how they are preserved and used).

Urban Adaptations of Visual Methods

Collins (2005) adapted some visual strategies from participatory rural appraisal to her study of poverty among women in Niagara Falls, Ontario, who participated in a food co-op. She based her choice of data collection tools on a desire to learn about the daily living experiences of those on low incomes, analyze the role of institutions in their lives, establish an agenda for action to improve their quality of life as a shared task, and give an opportunity for setting local priorities for change. Because many of the women had low literacy skills, she used visual methods such as mapping exercises, seasonality diagrams, timelines, and ranking exercises, because they are nontechnical and accessible. (She also used focus groups and semistructured interviews to gather data.) The visual exercises included asking the women to draw pictures of what it meant to have a good quality of life and then what it meant to have a poor quality of life. The women then used a scale to indicate the relative importance of the factors by drawing a heart around those that were most important for a good quality of life, a circle around things that were somewhat important, and a square around those that were not important. The women indicated that the most important qualities for a good life involved their relationships with family, children, and friends. The women did not indicate a need for an abundance of money, just a cushion to ensure that they would not go hungry and would have a place to live. The women used a seasonality chart to indicate how expenses and the associated stress varied throughout the month and throughout the year. As the end of each month approached, the women expressed greater stress, wondering whether they would have enough food to feed themselves and their families. Winter meant higher utility bills, and thus less money for other needs such as food and medicine.

Visual Data Collection in Children-Centered Research

Barker and Weller (2003) adapted visual data-collection strategies as means of conducting children-centered research. They used photography, diaries, drawings, in-depth interviews, and observation as multiple methods of data collection in two studies: one on children's increasing reliance on cars as a mode of transportation, and the other on citizenship and social exclusion for children in rural areas in England. The researchers gave cameras to the children and asked them to photograph their experiences in the car; they found that parents actually took the pictures. They then discussed the importance of power relations in families and the danger in making assumptions that the intent of children-centered research will be actually operationalized. Hence researchers should not assume that the use of cameras will actually result in children-centered research without active monitoring by the researchers.

Community Mapping with Youth

Amsden and VanWynsberghe (2005) used a community mapping data collection strategy with youths from two groups (a drop-in group for LGBTQ young people, and an education and support group for youths affected by violence) to examine the quality of their health services. Their first step was to establish an atmosphere of trust by asking the youth to identify the ground rules for conduct that would be needed to garner and protect such trust. The second step was to assure the youths that their knowledge and experiences had value, and that each participant would be viewed as an expert in his/her own experience. The evaluators used two templates as visual aids to bring focus to the process. First, they showed a picture that had a baby in one corner and an adult in the other corner, and used this image to generate discussion about the health challenges that youth face as they move from childhood to adulthood. Second, each youth was given a piece of paper with an empty square on it and asked to draw an ideal health service. Amsden and VanWynsberghe (2005) describe the benefits of this process as follows:

> Through this project we found that community mapping offers key strengths as a data collection technique, all of which are based on a respect and valuing of individual and collective voices. Specifically, community mapping establishes an open, unrestricted space in which youth can determine how to represent their voices; the metaphor of a map acts as a clear lens to link the research concepts to the lived, local experience of participants, and the collective nature of the mapmaking process encourages dialogue and collaboration amongst participants. Assuming, shaping, and sharing one's voice must take place within some form of community, however, and so this is the one necessary criteria of community mapping. Finding out how community is defined in each context is the challenge of research and youth facilitators. (p. 369)

Visual Data in Visitors' Studies

"Visitors' studies" is a field of research and evaluation that investigates the broad context of informal learning associated with zoos, museums, and historical sites. Transformative issues of salience in such contexts include the welcoming of diverse visitors; representation of relevant dimensions of diversity; addressing of critical social, historical, and environmental issues in a transformative spirit; and outreach activities that go beyond the exhibits themselves (Mertens, Fraser, & Heimlich, 2008). Historical analysis of the founding of many museums often reveals that the current hegemony of power relations is the same one that was dominant in a society at the time of the founding (Rose, 2007). Hence museums have been criticized because they reflect the white, male, wealthy perspectives of the founders. This historical analysis is useful; however, many museums have made significant strides in addressing issues of cultural complexity and social justice (e.g., the Smithsonian Institution, particularly in its displays on Japanese internment camps in the United States; the Apartheid Museum in Johannesburg, South Africa; the Holocaust Museum in Washington, D.C.; the National Museum of Women in the Arts in Washington, D.C.; the Manchester Museum in Manchester, United Kingdom). The Oregon Museum of Science and Industry has a program designed to bring youth from underrepresented racial/ethnic groups into science fields by training them to be docents at the museum, thus increasing their knowledge and providing role models for others who visit the museum.

Concept Mapping

Concept mapping has been discussed in Chapter 7 as a strategy to develop the context and priorities for an evaluation in a way that helps people think more effectively as a group without losing their individuality, as well as captures the complexity of the group members' ideas (Trochim, 2006).

Appreciative Inquiry

"Appreciative inquiry" is a data collection strategy that specifically focuses on strengths rather than weaknesses in a program, organization, or community. Participants are encouraged to begin their thinking with what is going particularly well in their organization (Coghlan, Preskill, & Catsambas, 2003). The next step is for them to envision a desired future in which "the best of what is" occurs more frequently. They then engage in dialogue about what is needed (tasks and resources) to bring about the desired change. The final step is to implement the needed changes and monitor the effects of those changes.

> A common criticism of Appreciative Inquiry is that it ignores or even denies problems. While at first blush this view may seem understandable, it is nevertheless untrue. Appreciative Inquiry does address issues and problems, but from a different and often more constructive perspective: it reframes problem statements into a focus on strengths and successes. For example, rather than ask participants to list the problems their organization is facing, they are asked to explain what is going well, why it is going well, and what they want more of in the organization. In some Appreciative Inquiry efforts, participants are also asked to state their specific wishes for the organization. This implicitly raises and addresses problems. (Coghlan et al., 2003, p. 6)

Catsambas and Webb (2003) used appreciative inquiry to collect data in an evaluation of the African Women's Media Center (AWMC) in Senegal, West Africa. Here is how they describe the first phase of establishing the focus of the evaluation:

> To develop the evaluation's guiding questions and focus of the evaluation, we conducted a four-hour Appreciative Inquiry process with the executive director, key staff, and board chair. These participants interviewed one another, using the following adapted version of [a] generic appreciative protocol ... :
>
> 1. Reflect for a moment on your involvement with the Africa Program over the last three years, and remember a high point or peak experience—a time when you were most proud and fulfilled to be a member of the IWMF [International Women's Media Foundation] and the AWMC program. Tell the story. What happened? What made this peak experience possible? Who else was important in making this experience happen?
>
> 2. What do you most value about yourself? Your work at IWMF/AWMC?
>
> 3. If you had three wishes to make more of these peak experiences possible, what would they be?
>
> After completing the interviews, the group shared their stories and determined the key themes, core values, and top wishes for the future. They then responded to the question, "What questions should the evaluation answer?" (Catsambas & Webb, 2003, p. 43)

Participants then followed this process: They jotted down their ideas on sticky notes, shared their ideas by displaying their notes on the wall, engaged in group discussion to categorize their ideas, and identified key stakeholders. The evaluators used this information to develop a data collection plan that included interviews of their advisory committee and women journalists in Africa and the United States. The interviews were conducted in pairs as described above, and a large-group assembly was used to share their interview data about the best of AWMC. The evaluators prepared a report that identified the best things that AWMC did, ways to build on those strengths, and needs for resources and tasks to be done to achieve the desired goals.

Other examples of appreciative inquiry in evaluation include Jacobsgaard's (2003) evaluation of a nonprofit agency in Sri Lanka, and Smart and Mann's (2003) evaluation of a program for Girl Scouts whose mothers were in prison.

Gender Analysis

Gender analysis has been discussed in Chapter 8 as one purpose of evaluations that focus on the determination of inequities between women and men. The Danish International Development Agency (DANIDA, 2006) suggests a process for conducting a gender analysis that begins with developing a team of stakeholders; these might include representatives from government agencies, development partners, members of civil society, and the private sector. The purpose is to agree on a management structure and the necessary information that will be required. The second step is to identify existing analyses and data sources, such as national documentation in the form of official reports, reports by the national women's machinery, national MDG reports (see Chapter 1), studies by women's organizations and NGOs, academic reports, and national gender policy or national statistics. Emphasis should be given to the indicators used by the government and others to track gender equality results in the country. International documentation might include country or sector gender profiles and analyses conducted by the World Bank, the United Nations, and international NGOs. Documentation from bilateral development partners might include past project/program reports, evaluations, and similar analyses of country programs.

The third step is to identify what additional information is needed and how that will be collected. This also involves discussions with development partners and government.

The Interagency Coalition on AIDS and Development (2007) suggests a similar process for conducting a gender analysis and labels the analysis of existing data sources as a macro level of data collection. It then recommends the following types of data collection (pp. 2–3):

(1) Data collection techniques used for micro-level analysis include: interviews, focus group discussions, community mapping, program attendance records, project documents, questionnaires, etc. At the micro-level, categories of men and women may be identified by socioeconomics or ethnicity, therefore information collected at the micro level is important to clearly define target groups. It can also provide baseline data for monitoring and evaluation purposes throughout the project cycle.

(2) **Institutional Analysis** reviews the capacity of implementing organizations to contribute to the planned project. Structural mechanisms within the organization, such as gender policies, gender committees or gender monitoring frameworks indicate a commitment to gender issues. Information to consider includes perceptions and attitudes of staff, skills for gender programming, management support for integrating gender issues and the gender balance in the overall staffing and decision-making processes. Weaknesses in the organization may be addressed through formal and informal links with partners.

(3) **Project or Proposal Analysis** assesses the impact of proposed and existing programs on women and men by using the information collected in the previous three phases. This section demonstrates how gender analysis can improve the project design if it is integrated

into all stages of project cycle management rather than simply added onto the evaluation of on-going projects.

(4) **Project Identification.** Then identify an issue that the project can address. Regardless of the project field (e.g., agriculture, environment, etc.) the macro- and micro-level gender analyses outlined above are integral to the project identification process because they help to describe the context of the identified problem. By understanding the level at which a problem originates (e.g., federal policy, community response to laws), project planners are better able to define the problem and suggest possible solutions. Proposals should contain a gender statement to explain the implications of the analysis results.

Delay (2004) provides an example of the types of data needed for a gender analysis of HIV/AIDS programs (Box 10.8). This listing provides a glimpse into the complexity of data collection within a specific sector in international development.

Bradshaw (2000) has developed a comprehensive list of data collection questions for conducting a gender analysis in the context of an evaluation of response to natural disasters. She originally presented this list as a tool for evaluating the response to Hurricane Mitch (which devastated large portions of Nicaragua in 1999), but it has applicability to broader contexts as well. An outline of data collection phases and methods based on her list is provided in Box 10.9.

For additional ideas for gender analysis data collection, UN Women, the International Monetary Fund, the World Bank, the International Training Centre of the International Labour Organization, the OECD, and the United Nations Educational, Scientific and Cultural Organization (UNESCO) offer many resources at their websites.

Network Analysis

The Annie E. Casey Foundation recognizes the importance of community involvement to bring about and sustain change in high-poverty neighborhoods. As part of the evaluation of projects that this foundation funds, network analysis is used as a tool to evaluate the quality of community networks. Ahsan (2009, p. 17) describes the process as follows:

As these approaches are implemented, there is a need to look at the process; to assess the structure of the network, what the value propositions are, how information flows, what the members do, the goals of the network, and how they are linked to local theories of change and to outcomes. It's also important to try and assess approaches to managing the network in a way that supports creativity and initiative among members but is not so loose that it lacks definition or value.

There is an array of evaluation and diagnostic tools available to help sites, including Geographical Information System (GIS) mapping to show geographic clusters of networks or outreach activities, and specialized software that can visually display the relationships, or flow of information or other resources among individuals and networks, organizations, and systems, using data collected from surveys of members. These tools are fairly simple for small groups to use and implement but can be fairly labor intensive when the number of actors is large. They are useful for testing assumptions about the effectiveness and reach of strategies, and they can also inform the next generation of strategy development and data collection activities.

Cross, Dickmann, Newman-Gonchar, and Fagan (2009) provide an example of mixed methods network analysis data collection for an evaluation of interagency collaboration.

Box 10.8. Types of Data Collection for Gender Analysis of HIV/AIDS Programs

Type of data	Description	Methods of data collection
Biological data	Number of people who: Are infected with HIV Have AIDS symptoms Die from the disease	Sentinel surveillance methods (read description here: *www.cdc.gov/STD/Program/surveillance/4-PGsurveillance.htm*) Biological testing as part of community population surveys
Policy environment data	Policies that: Increase access to services Protect vulnerable groups' rights Provide resources	Data tools such as: National Composite Index AIDS Programme Effort Index Key interviews of officials, service providers, and persons affected by the disease
Behavioral surveillance data	Measures of: The level of risk for HIV transmission Changes in risk levels over time	Major population surveys: Demographic health surveys Behavioral Sentinel Surveillance Surveys
Resource flows data	Tracking contributions from external donors, national expenditures, and spending by families and persons affected by HIV/AIDS	Global resource-tracking databases: OECD National Health Accounts National AIDS Accounts
Tracking commodities data	Proxy data that document program implementation	Donor community reports of commodities: Drugs Condoms HIV diagnostic kits
Prevention and treatment services data	Tracking services for prevention and treatment, and the quality of these services	Health facility surveys
Disease and death data	Numbers of births, deaths, and causes of death	Vital records registration

Source: Based on Delay (2004, pp. 1979–1980).

Box 10.9. Gender Analysis and Data Collection after a Natural Disaster

Needs assessment

- What are the priority needs of women and men?

- What factors are causing these needs?

- How can we meet these needs?

- What capabilities exist in the community?

- What type of intervention is necessary (training, money, etc.)?

Activity profile

- What did men, women, and children formerly do, and what are they doing currently?

- What is the division of labor on gender lines like?

- Is it flexible or not?

- What is the significance of the labor division, power relations, the vulnerability of individuals, and so on?

Resources, access, and control profile

- What resources are used by men and women to carry out their activities?

- Have they lost these resources?

- What resources (land, skills, money, savings, loan arrangements, etc.) are available to men and women?

- Do men and women have control of resources, the ability to decide how and when to use them, and the like?

Limitations and opportunities

- What vulnerabilities do the various groups of people in the community have? What differences exist in terms of power, access, and control of resources?

- What capabilities, skills, knowledge, and strategies do various groups of people in the community have?

Source: Based on Bradshaw (2000, p. 21), who adapted it from a study by Moser (1996).

> Network analysis examines the relationships between a set of objects and uses graphs to demonstrate the structure of those relationships. In a network graph, objects, called nodes, are connected to each other with a line, called an edge, which represents the direction or strength of the relationship. In this study, we are interested in the relationships (edges) between agencies and service provider groups (nodes). (pp. 315–316)

Their qualitative data consisted of transcripts of discussions that occurred during the development of the network analysis data, written accounts by individuals who participated in the discussions, and semi-structured interviews with the organization's leaders. Results of the network analysis are displayed in Figure 10.3.

Social Network Analysis

"Social network analysis" (SNA) is "the study of relationships within the context of social situations" (Durland, 2005, p. 35). The collection of data for SNA might begin with a survey or a question such as "Who are your friends?" or "Who do you work with on this project?" Data for SNA can also be collected through observations, interviews, surveys, artifacts, documents, and records. Surveys can be conducted in different formats (e.g., paper and pencil, online) and can present a list of selected options, or respondents can list names of members or categories or persons. Networks can be established in other ways, such as via snowball sampling (discussed in Chapter 11).

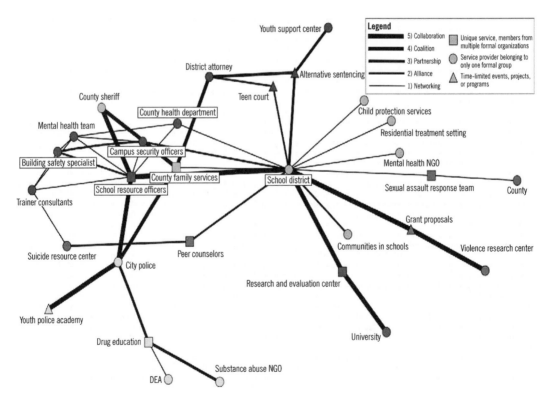

Figure 10.3. Example of interagency network analysis. *Source:* Cross, Dickmann, Newman-Gonchar, and Fagan (2009, p. 321). Copyright 2009 by the American Evaluation Association. Reprinted by permission.

Fredericks and Durland (2005; cited in Mertens, 2009, p. 267) describe an SNA study in which the goal was to reduce 12-year-olds' gang involvement through a mentoring program. Children were asked to name their best friends and who they hung out with at the start of the program and at various intervals during the project. The SNA allowed them to use this data to determine which children were cultivating friendships inside and outside known gangs, and whether leadership roles were being assumed by any of the children in the gangs. The authors used numerical data and sociograms (i.e., social maps or visual images depicting the relationships among individuals) to explore the relationships and how they changed during the study.

Members of the International Network for Social Network Analysis (INSNA, 2008) come from many disciplines, including anthropology, biology, communications science, economics, history, human geography, political science, sociology, and other fields of study. Researchers have used SNA in diverse settings to gather data about how HIV spreads through sexual contacts from person to person, or how friends and families' opinions affect one's choice of a personal digital assistant, as well as to define relationships between members of organized crime or within and between gangs. An example of a popular software analysis tool that illustrates networks from the data collected is Pajek. Examples of Pajek network analyses can be found by searching the Web using the terms "Pajek" and "network analysis."

· · · · · · · · · · · E X T E N D I N G   Y O U R   T H I N K I N G · · · · · · · · · · ·

Social Network Analysis

An SNA tool recommended for use with participants with little education living in rural communities is a low-tech, low-cost tool called Net-Map. Net-Map is an interview-based mapping tool that helps people understand, visualize, discuss, and improve situations in which many different actors influence outcomes. By creating influence network maps, individuals and groups can clarify their own views of a situation, foster discussion, and develop a strategic approach to their networking activities. More specifically, Net-Map helps players to determine:

- What actors are involved in a given network.
- How they are linked.
- How influential they are.
- What their goals are.

Determining linkages, levels of influence, and goals allows users to be more strategic about how they act in these complex situations.

Go to the Net-Map website *(netmap.wordpress.com)*. In a small group, create a question that you can work through together, both to get a feel for the tool and actually to work through an issue. Perhaps you can work on who can influence your success in a particular course, in your graduate studies generally, in a project at work, or in a neighborhood program. Although this tool is recommended for use in rural programs in developing countries, it is also quite useful in a more urban, Western setting.

Mixed Methods Data Collection: Strategies and Challenges

You will have already noticed that several of the data collection strategies listed in this chapter lend themselves to inclusion in a mixed methods design. Evaluators commonly use interviews to establish the focus of an evaluation, followed by quantitative measures of intended outcomes. These might be combined with observations and document reviews during the course of the project. Here are some additional examples of mixed methods data collection in evaluation:

- Brady and O'Regan's evaluation of the youth mentoring program in Ireland (see Chapter 3, Box 3.2) used mixed methods.

- Trochim, Marcus, Mâsse, Moser, and Weld (2008) evaluated the research activities of major federal agencies, using these methods: concept mapping; logic modeling; a detailed researcher survey; content analysis and systematic peer evaluation of progress reports; bibliometric analysis and peer evaluation of publications and citations; and financial expenditures analysis.

- Jewish youth had an opportunity to learn about their cultural heritage in a program of "Israeli experience" tours. The evaluators for this study (Kadushin, Hecht, Sasson, & Saxe, 2008) used the following methods: observer quantitative ratings on guide performance and group dynamics; observer qualitative narratives on program content; participant observer diaries; and participant questionnaires.

If evaluators have clarified their assumptions as suggested earlier in this book, then data collection decisions can be justified on the basis of congruence with philosophical principles, theoretical frameworks, and alignment with the evaluation purposes and questions. Mixing methods requires awareness of the implications of epistemological and ontological beliefs. In order to capture the complexity of reality in the complexity of context, multiple methods are probably needed. Evaluators need to work with stakeholders to determine the types and timing of data collection methods.

Performance Indicators and Data Collection

How do the stakeholders know whether the evidence presented to them from data collection indicates the extent to which a program succeeded or failed? To answer this question, evaluators encourage stakeholders to give thought to the performance indicators that they would accept as evidence of the program's success or failure.

> An indicator is a pointer. It can be a measurement, a number, a fact, an opinion or a perception that directs attention to a specific condition or situation. It measures changes in that condition or situation over time. In other words, indicators provide a close look at the results of initiatives and actions. The difference between an indicator and a statistic is that using indicators should involve comparison with a norm. For example, a statistic would be "30 per cent of women are literate," whereas an indicator would be "30 per cent of women and 70 per cent of men are literate." (UNIFEM, 2009, p. 29)

Performance indicators are sometimes also called performance targets or benchmarks. They specify the level of outcome attainment stakeholders expected or hoped for (e.g., the percentage of participants enrolled in postsecondary education; how many grade-level increases in reading ability) (WKKF, 1998, p. 34). Recall the use of performance indicators associated with achieving the MDGs related to reduction of poverty, increase in literacy, improvement of gender equity, and so on (see Chapter 1, Box 1.3).

It is often best to set performance targets based on past performance. Therefore, you may want to wait until you have some baseline outcome data before determining performance targets. However, if you do not have the luxury of waiting to collect baseline data, you can set initial performance targets based on levels attained in comparable or related programs.

Perhaps one of the most remarkable indicators of success is the Bhutan government's "gross national happiness" (GNH) index, which it uses to gauge the success of its policies and services. The GNH is made up of several happiness domains, including psychological well-being, ecology, health, education, cultural diversity and resilience, living standards, time use, community vitality, and good governance. Each domain includes its own indicators. For instance, indicators for psychological well-being include a general psychological distress indicator, an emotional balance indicator, and a spirituality indicator; for cultural diversity and resilience, indicators include a dialect use indicator, a traditional sports indicator, a community festival indicator, an artisan skill indicator, a value transmission indicator, and a basic precept indicator. Surveys of randomly selected representatives of various communities are conducted; a cutoff score is determined that indicates a person has reached a level of sufficient happiness; and the results can be used to calculate one number that is an indicator of GNH or can be disaggregated on the various dimensions. Here is a description of the Bhutan government's process for determining who is happy:

> The sufficiency cut-offs are set so that any person who had achieved full sufficiency in every dimension would be regarded as fully happy. The measure seems to be *understandable and easy to describe,* because it relies on a cutoff approach which is widely used in policy already. It can reflect *common sense notions of happiness* in that the dimensions and indicators directly were chosen because of their relevance in the Bhutanese context. Furthermore this measure is specifically geared not just to notice incremental changes over time, but also to *target, track changes, and guide policy.* This is because the measure is actually developed by considering the sector of the population who does *not* enjoy a sufficient quality of life at present and scrutinizing the dimensions in which they fall short. The measure *can be decomposed* by variables such as district or language group, and the quality of life can then be broken down by dimension to *identify which dimensions show the highest shortfalls* in different regions or groups. This last characteristic makes it a good tool for tracking changes across time, or for guiding policies to address specific needs of different groups efficiently. It is *technically solid,* enjoying properties of dimensional monotonicity and decomposability. (Ura & Galay, 2004; emphasis in original)

The GNH is interesting on a number of levels: It is innovative, takes on a complex measurement challenge, and has intuitive appeal. Who could be against people being happier? As in most evaluation contexts, however, issues of power are present in who decides on the indicators of happiness. Given that the Bhutan government has a goal of preserving the country's culture and that Bhutan is a Buddhist kingdom, government officials view the precepts of Buddhism as the foundation of happiness. Thus they have outlawed the practice of other religions; Christians and Hindus must flee the country or practice their religions underground. Also, since 1990, police have the right to fine any man not wearing the official national dress of the robe-like *gho,* and women can be fined for not wearing the apron-like *kira* (Public Broadcasting Services, 2010).

DANIDA (2006) and UNIFEM (2009) recommend the development of gender-sensitive indicators, because data needs to be disaggregated to reveal the differences in men and women's experiences. For example, national indicators rarely take into account areas of work typically done by women, such as child care and housework. "Gender-sensitive indicators are important because they can measure changes in gender equality—a definition of a gender-sensitive indicator is an indicator which measures gender-related changes in society over time" (UNIFEM, 2009, p. 29). Examples of gender-sensitive indicators appear in Box 10.10.

DANIDA (2006) also identifies several limitations of indicators when these are used without additional contextual awareness:

- It is difficult to find indicators that provide dynamic information on gender relations, how they were shaped, and how they can be changed.

- Indicator data are often based on census surveys, which are prone to sex biases (e.g., collected by people who lack gender awareness and use imprecise definitions of key gender-related terms).

- Measurements may not be comparable internationally, due to country-, language-, or culture-specific definitions, which often have very different implications (e.g., the exact meaning of "economic activity" and "literacy").

- It is often not thought through or made clear what changes should be measured against. For example, when a study is examining women's status in a specific country, would the benchmark or target be the situation of men in that particular country, the situation of women in other countries, or another measure altogether?

- Indicators are often developed by experts in a nonparticipatory manner, and as such might not include cross-cultural dimensions or reflect a general consensus. Women and men from the target groups might measure changes against crucial cultural or local elements that are likely to be overseen by experts formulating the indicators on their behalf. In that case, important indications of changes in gender relations, or in the position of women in society, the household, or the community might be neglected.

- There are few indicators measuring the quality of gender equality—the process that brings it about and the nature of its outcome. Achieving numerical equality is clearly important in a world where even this goal has yet to be attained. However, unless indicators are also developed for measuring the quality of change, too much importance may be attached to mere quantitative change, as opposed to the way in which it is achieved.

- In many developing countries, statistical data are outdated or imprecise, and the capacity to collect, analyze, disseminate, and store the data is often inadequate. Introducing gender-disaggregated data collection can be a great burden on an already overloaded system.

When performance measurement is seen as part of performance management or results-based evaluation, data collection occurs on specified quantitative outcomes that are measured routinely (daily, weekly, monthly, or quarterly to monitor progress) through surveys or information systems (Nielsen & Ejler, 2008). An example from a U.S. Department of Justice (2009) anti-gang funding initiative (see Box 10.11) illustrates the use of performance measurement for results-based evaluation.

Box 10.10. Examples of Gender-Sensitive Indicators at Different Levels

Macro level

Typical indicators used to measure the following gender equality issues at the macro level:

- Changes in legislation/policy frameworks affecting gender equality.

- Changes in national/sector budget allocations in favor of gender equality issues.

- Access to productive assets (land, credit, vocational training).

- Access to basic services (education, health, water) by women/men, girls/boys; rates of employment/unemployment (female and male) in different sectors at different levels.

Meso level

Typical indicators used to measure the following issues:

- Changes in quantity/quality of gender-competent staff in partner government, NGOs, and other donors.

- Changes in recruitment practices in favor of equal opportunities.

- Changes in budget allocation in favor of gender at this level.

Micro level

Typical indicators at this level are needed in order to measure the following:

- Met/unmet practical and strategic needs of women and men (compared with changes in project budget allocation in favor of gender at this level.

- Changes in project staff's capacity to mainstream gender equality.

- Emergence of new gender issues in the project or as a result of the project.

Source: Adapted from UNIFEM (2009, pp. 31–32).

Box 10.11. Performance Measures for Two Goals in an Anti-Gang Funding Initiative

Goals	Performance measures	Data from grantee
Reduce the occurrence of violent gang-related incidents through both reactive and proactive efforts supported by enforcement planning coordinated with federal, state,	The percentage of combined homicides, aggravated assaults, and	▪ The total number of gang-related homicides that occurred during the current reporting period. ▪ The total number of gang-related aggravated assaults that occurred

(cont.)

Box 10.11 (*cont.*)

Goals	Performance measures	Data from grantee
and local law enforcement and informed by data and real-time intelligence.	robberies that are gang-related.	during the current reporting period.
Reduce the occurrence of youth gang-related incidents and increase positive outcomes for youth at high risk for gang involvement through targeted, evidence-based gang prevention (for grantees using funding for prevention programming).	The percentage of youth completing program requirements.	▪ Total number of youth participating in the program during the current reporting period. ▪ Number of youth that completed the program during the current reporting period. ▪ Number of youth that exited the program during the current reporting period without completing the program.

Source: U.S. Department of Justice (2009, pp. 2–3).

· · · · · · · · · · E X T E N D I N G   Y O U R   T H I N K I N G · · · · · · · · · ·
Performance Indicators in Evaluation

1. Read the following paragraph about the relation between GDP and human flourishing; then examine the table of human development indicators cited in this paragraph. What is the value of the indicators that are used?

   Assumption 1: A high GDP per capita is necessary for human flourishing

   The first assumption is that economic growth is desirable, in part, because it raises people's income, hence their quality of life. In many circumstances this is true, but not always and not necessarily. Empirical evidence shows no *automatic* connection between a high GDP per capita and the ability of people to flourish. [The] table [below] illustrates the link between GDP and some dimensions of human flourishing such as health, education and political freedom, in the case of Saudi Arabia and Uruguay, the Russian Federation and Costa Rica, and Vietnam and Morocco. Uruguay has a much lower GDP per capita than Saudi Arabia. Yet people live longer. Women are more literate. Fewer children die prematurely, and basic political rights and civil liberties (such as the right to vote and the freedom of expression and association) are fully respected. The contrast between the Russian Federation and Costa Rica yields similar conclusions: Russia is wealthier, but its inhabitants live much shorter lives in a much more constrained political environment. While Morocco has a higher GDP per capita than Vietnam, its illiteracy and infant mortality rates are much higher. The discrimination against women, as measured by the difference between the adult literacy and adult female literacy rate, is also much higher. When countries are arranged according to the

Human Development Index—a composite index which measures progress in economic conditions, life expectancy and literacy—the wealthier countries in terms of GDP per capita are not necessarily better off when human dimensions such as health and education are taken into account. Saudi Arabia and Russia, the two richest countries of [the] table … in terms of economic development, are ultimately poorer than Uruguay and Costa Rica in human development terms. (Alkire & Deneulin, 2009, p. 15)

Some Human Development Indicators

	Saudi Arabia	Uruguay	Russia	Costa Rica	Vietnam	Morocco
GDP per capita ([purchasing power parity,] US$)	15,711	9,962	10,845	9,481	3,071	4,555
Adult literacy rate (%)	82.9	96.8	99.4	94.9	90.3	52.3
Female literacy rate (%)	76.3	97.3	99.2	95.1	86.9	39.6
Life expectancy (years)	72.2	75.9	65.0	78.5	73.7	70.4
Under-5 mortality	26	15	18	12	19	40
Political rights/civil liberties[a]	7/6	1/1	6/5	1/1	7/5	5/4
Human development index	0.812	0.852	0.802	0.846	0.733	0.646

Source: Data from *Human Development Report 2007/2008* (see *www.undp.org*), except as noted.

[a]Data from Freedom House 2008 (with 1 being most free and 7 less free; see *www.freedomhouse.org*).

2. Another example shows that the language of indicators matters. The U.S. Department of Agriculture used to use as an indicator "number of people who are hungry." It recently changed that indicator to "number of people who have low food security." What does this change imply as an indicator of not having enough to eat?

Planning Your Evaluation: Data Collection and Indicators

Now that you have an evaluation plan that includes a description of the evaluand, identification of stakeholders, and lists of evaluation questions, you need to specify how you will collect the data to get answers to the questions. Add a piece to your plan about data collection that aligns with your evaluation questions and design. Add another column to the plan for the indicators that you will use to judge the success (or not) of the results that you will get from your collected data.

 ### Moving On to the Next Chapter

Once you have completed this part of the plan, you will need to develop a plan for how to select people (or things) from whom (or which) to collect data. That is the topic of Chapter 11.

Preparing to Read Chapter Eleven

As you prepare to read this chapter, think about these questions:

1. The *Literary Digest* mailed 10 million surveys to voters to learn who they believed would win the 1936 election between Franklin D. Roosevelt and Alfred E. Landon. The voters' names were selected randomly from lists of automobile and telephone owners throughout the United States (Squire, 1988). The *Digest* was off by 19 percentage points when it predicted that Landon would win; in actuality, Roosevelt won by a landslide. Why do you think the *Digest* made such a poor prediction?

2. Imagine that you are about to begin planning an evaluation. You and the stakeholders discuss from whom you will collect data. You are the expert and must guide the group. Are you ready for these questions?

   ■ How will you decide from whom to collect data?

   ■ How can you be assured that those you have chosen to collect data from are the appropriate people?

   ■ How do you make sure that the people you are collecting data from will remain anonymous and safe throughout the process, if this is a promise that was made?

   ■ How many people do you have to include in your study so that the sample size is adequate?

   ■ How would someone working in the Methods Branch work, in comparison with someone selecting participants in the Use, Values, or Social Justice Branches?

CHAPTER ELEVEN

Stakeholders, Participants,

and Sampling

The ubiquitous mentions of stakeholders throughout this text testify to their importance in an evaluation study. In Chapter 7, we have seen that different branches of evaluation look differently at who needs to be included and how to include them; yet all evaluators recognize the need to identify the stakeholders and involve them appropriately in the process of planning, implementing, and using evaluations. In some ways, stakeholders constitute a larger universe than is typically thought of as a "population" or a "sample" in a research study. In research, the population is the larger group from which a researcher selects a sample to collect data. For example, an evaluation of a health services initiative may collect data from 10% of its participants. The population is all of the service recipients; the sample is the 10% from whom data are collected. Stakeholders include everyone who has a stake in the study: funders, administrators, service providers, and program participants and nonparticipants.

In many evaluation studies, data are collected from the entire stakeholder group. In such situations, sampling strategies are irrelevant, and hence you might think that you can skip this chapter. However, evaluators sometimes find themselves engaged in studies with large groups of stakeholders that decrease the feasibility of collecting data from everyone. Under such circumstances, evaluators will choose selected individuals from the larger groups to provide data. Besides, this chapter also includes valuable information about ethics and other interesting aspects of working with people in evaluation studies. Therefore, we encourage you *not* to skip this chapter.

In this chapter, the rationale for sampling is explained. Issues surrounding conceptual and operational definitions of populations and samples are discussed in the evaluation context. Particular attention is given to dealing with ethical issues, especially with regard to cultural issues related to informed consent, confidentiality, and anonymity. Challenges in identifying sample members when definitions are not clear-cut (e.g., race, disability) are also examined. A framework for sampling options is presented in terms of probability-based sampling and purposeful/theoretical sampling. Sampling is looked at from the perspectives of the four evaluation branches. The importance of understanding relevant subgroups within populations and extending invitations to participate in culturally appropriate ways is illustrated through examples of social justice evaluation studies. In addition, strategies for sampling in mixed methods studies are presented (Collins, Onwuegbuzie, & Jiao, 2007). Options for sample size decisions are presented. We also provide you with opportunities to engage in activities to clarify issues of sampling, and to make use of web-based resources that support sampling decisions.

Rationale for Sampling

The simplest rationale for sampling is that it may not be feasible because of time or financial constraints, or even physically possible, to collect data from everyone involved in an evaluation. Sampling strategies provide systematic, transparent processes for choosing who will actually be asked to provide data. As you can easily imagine, decisions about sampling need to be given careful consideration, in order to avoid potential bias in the results from using data collected from a nonrepresentative group. If particular groups are not represented in the sample, this can lead to an inaccurate picture of needs to be addressed, adequacy of implementation, or effectiveness of the program.

Defining Populations and Samples

Populations and samples can be thought of in two ways: conceptually and operationally. Conceptual definitions use other constructs to describe who will be in the study (e.g., "fourth-grade deaf students"). Operational definitions describe exactly how the evaluator will determine who will be in the study (e.g., "all fourth-grade deaf students at the Model Elementary School for the Deaf"). Technical terminology related to populations and samples is presented in Box 11.1.

· · · · · · · · · · · **EXTENDING YOUR THINKING** · · · · · · · · · · ·

Populations and Samples

After reading the conceptual and operational definitions in the following example, what are your ideas for who might be named in the categories: target population, experimentally accessible population, sampling frame, and population validity?

Terminology	Definition	Example
Conceptual definition of a sample	What a concept means in abstract or theoretical terms	Unmarried immigrant mothers living in the United States
Operational definition of a sample	What you will observe and/or measure; links the concept you want to sample to the real world	Unmarried immigrant mothers who have obtained social services from NGOs in Phoenix, Arizona

Terminology	Definition	Example
Target population	Group to whom you wish to generalize your results	
Experimentally accessible population	List of people who match the conceptual definition	

Terminology	Definition	Example
Sampling frame	List of people in the experimentally accessible population	
Population validity	Match between accessible population and target population	

Box 11.1. Population and Sampling Definitions

Terminology	Definition	Example
Conceptual definition of a sample	What a concept means in abstract or theoretical terms	Gang members in middle school
Operational definition of a sample	What you will observe and/or measure; links the concept you want to sample to the real world	All gang members known to the police or school officials in a particular school

Knowing the conceptual and operational definitions will then help you determine the target population, the experimentally accessible population, the sampling frame, and the population validity.

Terminology	Definition	Example	
Target population	Group to which you wish to generalize your results	Gang members in middle school	Gang members in middle school
Experimentally accessible population	List of people who match the conceptual definition	Gang members in a particular county middle school	Gang members Babson Middle School
Sampling frame	List of people in the experimentally accessible population	Actual names of known gang members in a data base	Names of 21 students in the Skeleton Crew gang
Population validity	Match between accessible population and target population	Actual list that is reflective of target population	17 students are still in middle school and still members of the gang

In evaluation, population and sampling definitions are complicated by these factors:

██ Populations are sometimes determined by default; in other words, the population is the community that receives the services. Sometimes sampling is a moot point, in that the number of people involved in the program is not large, and it is possible to collect data from everyone.

██ Evaluations can be conducted solely to inform decision making at a local level. When this is the case, sampling is not viewed as a vehicle to be able to generalize results to another setting.

██ Lists of participants or eligible participants may not be up to date or accurate; evaluators should inquire to determine who might be missing and for what reasons.

██ Willingness to be identified as a member of a group or to come forward publicly may be affected by the target population's circumstances (e.g., drug users, gang members, illegal immigrants).

Ethical Issues in Sampling

Although ethical concerns are pervasive throughout the course of an evaluation, they are particularly salient when the topic of sampling is raised. This is a point of intersection between the evaluator and the people in the study that historically has received attention. Recall from Chapter 1 that ethical review boards are established to protect humans (and animals) who participate in studies. Some ethical review boards provide exemptions for evaluation studies if the board members determine that the evaluation is part of accepted educational practices (e.g., classroom testing) or if no unique identifiers would allow the data to be traced back to an individual. However, evaluators should pay attention to the ethical principles designed to protect human beings (and animals); in particular, they should examine issues of informed consent, confidentiality, and anonymity through a cultural lens. In addition, challenges associated with determining who has the characteristics to be included in the sample must be with dealt with when operational definitions are not clear-cut (e.g., race, disability).

Informed Consent

One of the norms for ethical research discussed in Chapter 1 is the need for participants to provide **informed consent** prior to participation. Informed consent can be defined as voluntary consent without threat or undue inducement; it includes knowing what a reasonable person would want to know before giving consent (informed), and explicitly agreeing to participate (consent). In the United States, the most common way to obtain informed consent is to provide each potential participant with a letter that explains the study processes, demands on participants, compensation for participation, potential risks, and the right of the individual to withdraw from the study at any time. Each individual is then asked to sign the letter of informed consent. Most institutions have a specific format for the informed consent letter, so evaluators should check with their home institutions about this. An example can be found in the general guidelines for writing informed consent documents from the National Institutes of Health's (2006) Office of Human Subjects Research.

In some institutions, the standard informed consent format is very legalistic and may be difficult for people with low literacy, lack of expertise in English, or low education levels to understand. Evaluators need to consider how information can be presented to such participants in ways that are appropriate to the people in the study. Advice is provided here regarding particular groups: children, older people, people with mental illness, and indigenous and postcolonial peoples.

Children

In the United States, anyone under the age of 18 is legally considered a child. Children cannot sign an informed consent form (even if they are old enough to write their own names) because they are not of legal age. Ethical review boards generally require a signed informed consent form from a child's parent and assent from the child. Assent involves explaining the study to the child in language he/she can understand and asking the child whether he/she is willing to participate. The requirement of parent signature can be problematic if the topic is sensitive (e.g., the evaluation is of a program for LGBTQ individuals and the child has not told the parents about his/her sexual identity). Dodd (2009) suggests that in such circumstances, another person could be asked to sign the consent form for the child (e.g., a school counselor or a local service provider). She also recommends having an ethics board made up of members of the LGBTQ community to guide evaluators who work in this community.

Vargas and Montoya (2009) describe challenges when children are from nondominant cultural or linguistic groups. They worry that parents might sign or not sign the consent forms for the wrong reasons. For example, undocumented immigrant parents might sign because they are afraid to alienate the teacher or authority figure who asks them to do so. Or they might not sign because they are afraid the person asking for the signature will have them deported.

> A meaningful informed consent and assent procedure must be carried out in a context that considers the knowledge base of the participants and their families; the experiences that the participants, families, or prior generations have had with research; the language and customs of the participants, families, and communities, and the parents; views about values such as independence and collectivism as pertains to their children. (Vargas & Montoya, 2009, p. 500)

In cultures where participation in research and informed consent are not common, the researcher may need to conduct an educational session to explain the study. Even this may not be sufficient; Vargas and Montoya recommend forming partnerships in communities, so that there can be ongoing relationships based on mutual trust.

Older People

Older people may be able to read, understand, and sign a consent form. However, it is possible that their mental acuity could decline, suggesting a need to revisit informed consent in studies that involve this population (Szala-Meneok, 2009). If signs of dementia appear, an evaluator could ask a significant other (such as a family member or service provider) to affirm the informed consent.

People with Mental Illness

The many possible variations of mental illness prevent evaluators from adopting a single strategy to obtain informed consent from this population. However, if a person is severely mentally ill (lacking mental competence to execute legal documents), how can the person give consent to participate in evaluation studies? The American Psychiatric Association (2009) recommends several possible approaches, such as asking the person to give an advance directive when symptoms do not impair her/his ability to do so, or asking family members, advocates, or surrogates to safeguard the person's interests. Evaluators need to work with service providers to ensure that treatments are not resulting in a worsening of symptoms. An evaluator can also ask about the necessity of exploring other treatments, strategies to withdraw from the study, and providing support for anyone who does leave the study.

Indigenous and Postcolonial Peoples

Indigenous and postcolonial peoples have historically been excluded from the power to make informed decisions about choosing to participate in evaluation studies on their own terms. American Indians (LaFrance & Crazy Bull, 2009), Māori (Cram, 2009), and Africans (Quigley, 2006) have developed ethical review boards that are rooted in their cultural traditions. Chapter 7 provides insights into some of the ethical conditions for conduct in these indigenous communities, along with ideas for forming partnerships and relationships with members of these communities. Informed consent in indigenous contexts can be affected by a myriad of cultural and power-related issues. For example, Wilson (2005) evaluated services provided to deaf people in a Caribbean nation by international donor agencies. She was interested in how the deaf people felt they were viewed by the donor agencies. She explained the purpose of her study in the local sign language, and was a bit surprised to find that people would not sign the informed consent form. Yet, at night, under cover of darkness, they would tap on her window and tell her that they wanted to be interviewed, but they did not want to sign the form. They felt that the donor agencies viewed them as helpless children who needed to be taken care of by hearing people, but they did not want anyone to know that they were saying such things. They feared that the little bit of support they did receive from the donors would be cut off if it was known that they were complaining. In Kenya, Wilson (2005) also found that many people who did not know how to read or write had learned how to sign their names in order to sign documents to borrow money from banks or to purchase land. Therefore, signing their names to an informed consent form took on tremendous significance and brought great fear to the participants. Individuals agreed to participate in the study only after others in the community explained the importance of the study and their participation in it, and what their signatures signified.

    Ntseane (2009) described another situation in which the participants were willing to be interviewed, but they were not willing to sign the informed consent form. Ntseane was evaluating an entrepreneurship initiative for women in Africa in her home country. She explained that the purpose of the study was to give the women a chance to tell their own stories. However, when she asked them to sign the form, she received a surprising response. The women told her that they had given her their word that they agreed to participate; if she insisted that they sign the form, this was an insult—as if she did not believe them and take them at their word.

Anonymity and Confidentiality

In the Belmont Report (National Commission for the Protection of Human Subjects of Biomedical and Behavioral Research, 1979), the ethical principle of respect is interpreted as ensuring the confidentiality of the participants. **Confidentiality** means collecting, analyzing, storing, and reporting data in such a way that the data cannot be traced back to the individual who provides them. **Anonymity** means that no uniquely identifiable information is attached to the data; no one, not even the evaluator, can trace the data to the individual. Both these concepts are more challenging to ensure in evaluations than in some research studies, because of the interaction between evaluators and the participants/stakeholders.

In some evaluation studies, it may not be possible to interview the participants alone. In a rural India, the entire village followed the American researcher (Wilson, 2005) to the home of the participant who was to be interviewed. The only enclosed parts of the home were the kitchen and a small sleeping area for the participant and her child; all other activities took place on a cloth placed on the dry ground alongside the kitchen. Children and adults circled Wilson, her interpreter, and the mother to be interviewed, and it was inappropriate in that community to ask them to leave.

Sometimes participants in evaluation studies reject the idea of maintaining confidentiality. For example, in Ntseane's (2009) study in Africa, the women told her that if she was supposed to be telling their stories, they wanted their names to be attached to those stories. Not only did they want their own names made known, but they wanted the names of their family members and other people who helped them build their businesses to be given as well. This is reflective of the African valuing of collectivism over individualism. Conducting group interviews or having others present in an interview also negates the possibility of confidentiality among those present.

In another instance, Jacobs (personal communication, May 21, 2005) interviewed parents of deaf children in rural areas of India. She realized that the standard informed consent form was incomprehensible to the mothers. Jacobs rewrote it, tested it, and found that her new version was understood much better. Her revised statement read as follows:

> My name is Namita Jacobs. I am a teacher of young children who have trouble seeing. Currently, I am doing higher studies. As part of my studies, I am trying to understand the situation of families like yours who live in villages and who have young children who have trouble seeing.
>
> We have very little information about the situation in villages. It is important to get this information from people like you who live here and can speak of the hardships as well as the help you receive in raising your child. I would like to ask you and the people here questions about your child, your family, your village and about your experiences in raising this child. Later, with your permission, I may return again to speak to you and others who care for your child.
>
> This conversation should take less than an hour. So that I can pay attention to what you are saying, I will record our conversation. This way, I can be sure that I am not missing anything you have said. In writing my reports, I will make sure that your family and child cannot be identified in any way. I will not use your real names or the name of your village. However, you do not have to talk to me at all. It will not affect any services you are receiving in any way. After we begin, you can change your mind and ask me to stop.
>
> __ I have understood what you have told me and agree to participate.
>
> __ You have my permission to return again to speak to me and others who care for my child.

There are times when the social positioning of the respondents needs to be protected because of real risks of danger if they are revealed. This can occur in any evaluation focusing on persons who engage in illegal behaviors or who suffer from social stigma. Evaluators have an ethical responsibility to report individuals who disclose that they have committed a crime or that they intend to do so. However, evaluators who report the activities of drug users, sex workers, or illegal immigrants will probably find that they no longer have participants from those communities. Dodd (2009) has discussed the dangers of revealing identities in the LGBTQ community. Evaluators can pursue certificates of confidentiality to protect participants from being subpoenaed for legal proceedings. In the United States, these certificates can be obtained from National Institutes of Health Office of Human Subjects Research.

Although evaluators have an obligation to promise that they will attempt to keep the names of participants confidential, they also have to acknowledge that they may not be able to keep this promise fully (Wiles, Crow, Heath, & Charles, 2006). In cases of illegal behavior, such as abuse of children or other vulnerable people, the identities of the perpetrators must be reported. In small communities, such as the deaf community, an evaluator has to be cognizant of the fact that members of that community may know each other well enough to infer identities that may not be obvious to the evaluator (Harris et al., 2009). In such circumstances, the evaluator may need to delete personally identifying information, use pseudonyms, or change details. The evaluator can share the quotes with the participants before they are shared with a wider audience, and may also need to discuss the potential of harm if identities are disclosed.

Identification of Sample Members

Identification of sample members can be incredibly simple: You walk into a classroom or clinic, and there are the sample members. However, it can also be a bit more challenging if the criteria for determining who is eligible for services are ambiguous or ill defined. Two examples of categories that fit this latter description include race/ethnicity and disability. In addition, within-group heterogeneity requires awareness of relevant dimensions of diversity within these categories.

Race/Ethnicity

Race and ethnicity have long been contentious variables in the U.S. research world. What does it mean to be black, white, Hispanic, Latina/Latino, or Asian? Although race is defined as a biogenetic variable, physical differences associated with race may be very difficult to pin down. Also, the term "race" is sometimes used interchangeably with "ethnicity"; however, race is usually categorized, rightly or not, in terms of physical characteristics (e.g., skin color or facial features), and ethnicity is usually defined in terms of a common origin or culture resulting from shared activities and identity based on some mixture of language, religion, race, and ancestry (C. D. Lee, 2003). Use of race and ethnicity as explanatory variables should be critically examined to determine whether they are standing as proxies for other causal variables, such as poverty, unemployment, or family structure. In addition, use of broad categories such as "African American" or "Asian American" hides the diversity within these populations—for example, if some members of these groups are recent immigrants, have different experiences in their home countries, or have different levels of education or economic security. The American Psychological Association (APA) Joint Task Force of Divisions 17 and 45 (2002) has published guidelines for working in four racial/ethnic communities: persons of African descent, Hispanics, Asian American/Pacific Islander populations, and American Indians. One of their guiding principles specifically addresses the need to recognize diversity within communities:

> Recognition of the ways in which the intersection of racial and ethnic group membership with other dimensions of identity (e.g., gender, age, sexual orientation, disability, religion/spiritual orientation, educational attainment/experiences, and socioeconomic status) enhances the understanding and treatment of all people. (APA Joint Task Force, 2002, p. 1)

Heterogeneity based on race, ethnicity, and country of origin escalates when we consider the extent of globalization that is occurring across the world (Banks, 2008; Stake & Rizvi, 2009). In many places, previously fairly homogeneous communities have become multicultural venues with the influx of people from different countries because of war, violence, drought, or famine, or just the desire for a better quality of life. Kien Lee's (2003) work on communities of immigrants to the United States uncovered important differences in the conditions under which the immigrants left their home countries. If immigrants came from a country with a repressive style of government, they were less inclined to accept the promises of authorities that they were there "to help them." Instead, they preferred to create their own networks of people from their home country to learn how to cope in their new situation and to find support in terms of obtaining needed services.

Disability

In the United States, the federal Individuals with Disabilities Education Improvement Act of 2004 (IDEA 2004; Public Law 108-446) defines 13 categories of disabilities (U.S. Department of Education, 2009).

- Specific learning disability
- Speech or language impairment
- Mental retardation
- Emotional disturbance
- Multiple disabilities
- Hearing impairment
- Deafness
- Orthopedic impairment
- Other health impairment
- Visual impairment
- Autism
- Deaf-blindness
- Traumatic brain injury

Some of these categories are fairly straightforward, such as hearing impairment and visual impairment. Some are considered to be insulting to people who would be so labeled (e.g., mental retardation). Some are so broad as to seriously challenge the evaluator who would try to identify such individuals (e.g., other health impairment or multiple disabilities). All the categories represent a challenge for appropriately identifying individuals who fit into them, as well as for recognizing the relevant dimensions of diversity (as discussed above under "Race/Ethnicity") that need to be taken into consideration. Mertens and McLaughlin (2004) provide conceptual and operational definitions of the 13 categories of disabilities contained in the IDEA legislation.

Heterogeneity in the federal definitions reveals the challenges faced by evaluators who wish to select individuals who fit in the various categories. The definition of "specific learning disability" in the IDEA legislation illustrates this challenge. The legislation lists seven areas in which the learning disability can be manifested: imperfect ability to listen, think, speak, read, write, spell, or do mathematical calculations. This conceptual definition leads to challenges in identifying an appropriate operational definition. Evaluators often accept a school's records stating that a student has a learning disability. However, researchers recognize that methods of identifying a learning disability are not necessarily reliable or valid (Aaron, Joshi, Gooden, & Bentum, 2008). Sometimes children who exhibit characteristics similar to learning disabilities are not identified as having such disabilities; the reverse is equally true.

The U.S. Department of Education (2009) suggests that learning disabilities be identified through a process known as "response to intervention" (RtI), rather than relying on a single test or a battery of tests. The National Association of State Directors of Special Education (Batsche et al., 2005) describes RtI as containing these components:

1. Use of a multitier model of service delivery.

2. Use of a problem-solving method to make decisions about appropriate levels of intervention.

3. Use of evidence-based interventions.

4. Student progress monitoring to inform instruction and intervention.

5. Use of data to make decisions regarding student response to intervention.

6. Use of assessment for three different reasons: screening, diagnostic, and progress monitoring.

This example based on learning disabilities is just the tip of the iceberg. Individuals working in all disability communities need to have in-depth understandings of the complexities associated with these populations.

Sampling Strategies

A framework for sampling options is presented here in terms of (1) probability-based sampling and (2) purposeful/theoretical sampling. Evaluators from different branches hold different views on appropriate strategies for sampling. Methods Branch evaluators tend to focus more on probability-based approaches; Use Branch evaluators focus on those who can provide the most useful information; Values Branch evaluators use theoretically or purposeful sampling strategies; and Social Justice Branch evaluators can use a combination of strategies, but they always sample with an eye to providing equity of representation and appropriate support for marginalized groups to ensure sufficient and accurate inclusion.

Probability–Based Sampling

Probability-based sampling involves the selection of a sample from a population in a way that allows for an estimation of the amount of possible bias and sampling error.

   ▪ **Sampling error** is the difference between the sample and the population.

   ▪ **Random samples** are those in which every member of a population has a known nonzero probability of being included in the sample.

   ▪ "Random" means that the selection of each unit (person, classroom) is independent of the selection of any other unit.

There are multiple methods for doing probability-based sampling. These range from putting all the names of people in the population in a hat and drawing them out at random, to using a table of random numbers to identify who is selected, to having a computer generate a list of random numbers or names. Theoretically, a randomly selected sample will be representative of the larger population. Specific probability-based sampling strategies are illustrated in Figure 11.1 and explained in Box 11.2. The rationale for probability-based sampling is to obtain a sample that is representative of the population so that the results from the sample can be generalized to the population. If the results of the evaluation can be generalized to the larger population, then the study is said to have external validity (see Chapter 9).

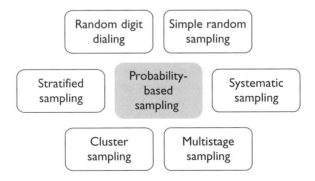

Figure 11.1. Probability–based sampling strategies.

Box 11.2. Probability-Based Sampling Strategies

Strategy	Definition/example	Requirements
Simple random sampling	Every member of the population has an equal and independent chance of being selected.	You must have an accurate and complete list of members of the population.
Random digit dialing	Use in telephone surveys; computer generates a random list of phone numbers.	You need telephone exchanges for the desired geographic area; solves the problem of out-of-date directories or unlisted numbers.
Systematic sampling	Take every nth name off a list. Suppose you have 1,000 names on the list and you need a 10% sample. You pick a random number between 1 and 10, start there, and then take every 10th name on the list.	You need a full list of the population; however, you need to be cognizant of any particular order that the list is in and of the impact this might have on any systematic bias.
Stratified sampling	If there are different groups (strata) that you want to be sure to include, then you can divide the population into subgroups first and then randomly sample from the subgroups.	Strategy allows for obtaining representation from smaller subgroups; you must decide whether you will sample proportionally or disproportionately to the groups' representation in the population.[1]
Cluster sampling	Use with naturally occurring groups (e.g., classrooms, school districts, city blocks). Units are randomly selected from full list of possible sites. Then you can collect data from the members in the randomly selected unit.	Need a full list of classrooms, school districts, or blocks. Useful when site visits are needed and money can be saved by collecting data at a limited number of sites. At the analysis stage, the mean for each cluster replaces individual means, resulting in less precision in measuring effects.
Multistage sampling	Use a combination of sampling strategies over the course of the study (e.g., start with cluster sampling, then use simple random sampling within clusters).	Statistical analysis can be complicated with multistage sampling; clusters may need to include as many as 30–50 units for statistical analysis purposes.

Source: Based on Mertens (2010, pp. 317–319).

[1]"Proportional representation" means that individuals are sampled based on the same fraction that they represent in the population. This results in different sample sizes for each stratum. But it might yield sample sizes too small for analysis when a subgroup is very small in the population. "Disproportional representation" is used when the sizes of the subgroups differ significantly in the population. A different fraction of each subgroup is selected (e.g., 50% of a small group, 10% of a large group). When disproportional representation is used, weights need to be used in analysis. Most computer programs will calculate the necessary weights to use in calculations.

Example of Probability-Based Sampling

Brady and O'Regan's (2009) study of youth mentoring (see Chapter 3, Box 3.2) provides good insights into the challenges of probability-based sampling. Here is how they describe their sampling strategy:

> In relation to sample size, we were supported in our work by members of our EAG, who had particular experience in experimental design. This group advised that a minimum sample size of 200 would be required in order to potentially identify the expected effect size of a Cohen's d of just under .2. However, the recruitment of 200 study participants would represent a challenge for the program. At the time, Foroige, the service provider, was supporting 60 mentoring pairs in the western region and had just received funding to roll out the program nationally. Given, as mentioned earlier, that programs undergoing RCT [randomized controlled trials] should be well established, the decision was made to restrict the study to the western region where the BBBS program was in operation for 5 years. This meant the program had to grow exponentially from supporting 60 matches to supporting an additional 100 to conduct the study.... The youth in the control group would be placed on a waiting list for support. However, as a result, the target sample age group would have to be reduced from 10–18 years to 10–14 years, so that the young people on the waiting list would have a chance to be matched and benefit from a mentor's support before being ineligible for the program when they reached the age of 18 years. (p. 272)

> Another factor of relevance at this stage was the difficulty associated with recruitment of the sample. The search for sufficient numbers of participants took longer and was more difficult than anticipated. The data collection time points had to be extended, and the eventual final sample size was reduced to 164. The fact that the projected sample size would limit the statistical impact of the study gave us renewed focus on considering how we could strengthen the study through a strong combination of both quantitative and qualitative approaches. (p. 273)

Purposeful/Theoretical Sampling

Theoretical sampling or **purposeful sampling** grew out of the constructivist paradigm (associated with the Values Branch), because in qualitative research, samples are selected that have the potential for yielding information-rich cases that can be studied in depth. The goal of purposeful/theoretical sampling is not to be able to generalize from a sample to a population; rather, it is to make clear the specific uniqueness of an individual case, as well as to inform discussion about the case as a general example of that phenomenon. Lincoln and Guba (2000) suggested that qualitative researchers use the term "transferability" instead of "generalizability." Transferability is achieved by an evaluator's providing enough of a description for readers to understand the contextual richness of the phenomenon under study; we call this **thick description.** The onus of responsibility for the evaluator is to provide a sufficiently thick description that readers can make a judgment about the transferability of the individual cases studied to their own situations. Evaluators who use purposeful/theoretical sampling also have the responsibility of making clear the criteria they use to determine from whom to collect data. Patton (2002b) has identified a number of possible categories of criteria for evaluators to consider when planning purposeful/theoretical sampling. These are illustrated in Figure 11.2 and explained in Box 11.3).

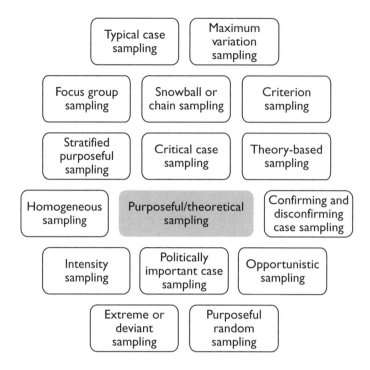

Figure 11.2. Purposeful/theoretical sampling strategies.

Box 11.3. Purposeful/Theoretical Sampling Strategies

Strategy	Definition/example	Requirements
Extreme or deviant sampling	Choose unusual or special individuals (e.g., highly successful or unsuccessful school principals).	This strategy makes the assumption that studying the unusual will illuminate typical cases. Criterion for selection: From whom can you learn the most? Criticism: Extremeness or deviance may present a distorted picture.
Intensity sampling	Identify instances where the phenomenon of interest is strongly represented. Look for rich cases that are not necessarily extreme.	You need to be knowledgeable about the community, so as to recognize appropriate individuals who fit the criterion of providing a rich data source. This may require exploratory fieldwork.

Strategy	Definition/example	Requirements
Maximum variation sampling	Choose individuals that represent maximum variation of the phenomenon (e.g., teachers in isolated rural, suburban, and inner-city areas).	This strategy can reveal uniqueness of phenomena in different contexts (e.g., in terms of retention rates, access to resources), and commonalities that the different contexts share.
Homogeneous sampling	Identify strongly homogeneous cases; find individuals who share relevant characteristics and experiences.	People who share experiences can yield a picture of that experience (e.g., parents whose children participate in an early childhood intervention program in a local neighborhood).
Focus group sampling	In most cases, use homogeneous groups (e.g., if service providers and participants are included in the same focus group, this might yield biased results).	Sometimes in heterogeneous focus groups, members of a dominant group monopolize the discussion time.
Typical case sampling	This is the opposite of the extreme or deviant sampling strategy; you want to identify the typical or average person participating in the program.	You can ask for recommendations from individuals familiar with the program, or rely on demographic or programmatic data to identify the typical cases.
Stratified purposeful sampling	Strategy combines the identification of strata of relevant subgroups with purposeful selection from those subgroups.	You can divide programs into highly, moderately, and less successful categories and then purposefully select individuals from each of those stratum.
Critical case sampling	Use cases that can make a point dramatically or are important for other reasons. Patton (2002b) says that the key to identifying a critical case is "If it's true of this one case, it's likely to be true of all other cases" (p. 243).	When evaluating an agricultural program, you might choose an area where the conditions are very challenging because of extreme poverty, natural disaster, or limited water access.
Snowball or chain sampling	Start with key informants who are then asked to recommend others you should talk with—some who agree with them and some who disagree with them.	Useful strategy when the individuals with the desired characteristic are few in numbers and difficult to find; a few contacts can snowball into a larger group from whom to collect data.

(cont.)

Box 11.3 (*cont.*)

Strategy	Definition/example	Requirements
Criterion sampling	Set up criteria to specify what characteristics people in the study need to have.	You might want people with lengthy experience or newcomers in a program. You might want people who can hear and people who cannot. Criteria are contextually dependent.
Theory-based sampling	If the evaluation is focused on a theoretical construct such as creativity, you need to describe the meaning of that construct, and then identify individuals who theoretically exemplify that construct.	Students who participate in the art fair may theoretically be expected to exhibit higher levels of creativity than students who participate in dirt bike racing.
Confirming and disconfirming case sampling	Look for cases that both confirm and disconfirm emerging hypotheses.	Used particularly in grounded theory; as theory emerges, you look for cases that challenge or confirm the emerging theory.
Opportunistic sampling	Selection of individuals emerges as the study progresses; you do not know a priori who will need to be included.	As theory emerges, you may need to make up your mind on the spot regarding the need to include an individual in the study sample.
Purposeful random sampling	Randomly choose individuals from a purposefully defined group.	Purpose is not for representation and generalization; rather, it is to avoid bias if individuals are recommended by someone who has a stake in making the program look good.
Politically important case sampling	Determine whether there is a political reason for including particular areas and individuals for the credibility and perceived usefulness of the study.	If a program is funded by a government grant, you might want to make sure to include individuals in the sample from the district of the legislator who sponsored the legislation.

Source: Based on Patton (2002b).

··········· **E X T E N D I N G   Y O U R   T H I N K I N G** ···········

Purposeful/Theoretical Sampling

Brainstorm two scenarios in which you would choose a purposeful/theoretical sampling strategy sample over a probability-based sampling strategy. Describe why theoretical sampling was a better choice than probability-based sampling in these scenarios. Under what conditions would you choose to do probability-based sampling rather than theoretical sampling?

Case Study Sampling

As discussed in Chapters 5 and 8, Stake (2004) has contributed a great deal of knowledge and wisdom on the use of case studies in evaluation. Any of the sampling strategies in Box 11.3 can be used in a case study evaluation. Stake provides advice in sampling that is geared more to the case as bounded system than to the individuals from whom data are collected. For any type of case study, evaluators needs to be clear about the purpose of the study and match their sampling strategy to the study. Three strategies for sampling of cases are these:

1. *Intrinsic case study.* Sometimes a case is selected by default or intrinsically. If the evaluation is of a specific case (e.g., a school or clinic), then that is the case. In such circumstances, the focus is on developing a rich understanding of that one particular case, not on trying to generalize to other situations.

2. *Instrumental case study.* If the goal is to use a case to understand a concept more broadly, then an instrumental case study strategy can be used. Here is how Stake (2004) describes this approach:

   The researcher examines various interests in the phenomenon, selecting a case of some typicality but leaning toward those cases that seem to offer opportunity to learn. My choice would be to choose the case from which we feel we can learn the most. That may mean taking the one most accessible or the one we spend the most time with. Potential for learning is a different and sometimes superior criterion to representativeness. Sometimes it is better to learn a lot from an atypical case than a little from a seemingly typical case. (p. 451)

3. *Collective or multiple case studies.* Several cases can be chosen if the need is to examine a phenomenon in different contexts. The evaluators may start with one case and discover something that merits examination in another context. Hence all the cases may not be known at the beginning of the study.

· · · · · · · · · · · **EXTENDING YOUR THINKING** · · · · · · · · · · ·
Sampling Strategies

1. The president of the Colorado Schools of Massage wishes to identify the attitudes of instructors in massage schools toward the idea of introducing aromatherapy into their curriculum. She will be asking some of the instructors to fill out a survey. To identify who fills out the survey (sample subjects), she uses a three-step procedure:

   a. *Step 1:* She first divides Colorado into rural versus urban areas.

   b. *Step 2:* She then lists the massage schools located in both the rural and urban areas. Using a table of random numbers, she selects an equal number of urban and rural schools (6 urban and 6 rural).

   c. *Step 3:* She sends surveys to all of the mind–body instructors in all 12 schools.

   ▒ This is an example of what kind of sampling?

   ▒ Do you think this will give her the information she needs? Explain.

2. What if the president pretargets *only* those instructors who have earned an advanced certificate in aromatherapy?

   ▒ What kind of sampling is this?

   ▒ Do you think this will give her the information she needs? Explain.

3. What if the president also tries to nonrandomly keep the female–male ratio the same as it is found among massage school instructors throughout Colorado (three females for every male)?

   ▒ What kind of sampling is this?

   ▒ Do you think this will give her the information she needs? Explain.

4. What if, instead, the president tries to do this survey quickly and cheaply, and only surveys the schools close to her office?

   ▒ What kind of sampling is this?

   ▒ Do you think this will give her the information she needs? Explain.

5. What if the president begins with one instructor who is most accessible (e.g., expresses interest), has that interested instructor pass out the survey in her school, and asks those in the school who express interest to fill out the survey, too?

   ▒ What kind of sampling is this?

   ▒ Do you think this will give her the information she needs? Explain.

6. What if the president pregroups the state into rural versus urban, and then chooses every fifth school within both the rural and urban areas?

- What kind of sampling is this?
- Do you think this will give her the information she needs? Explain.

7. What kind of sampling would you suggest the president conduct if she is hoping to discover why some instructors who enroll in aromatherapy training fail the course? Why?

8. Which sampling strategy would you suggest if the president is evaluating Colorado's state government economic grant for training massage therapists to use essential oils produced in Colorado flower fields? Why?

9. Can you imagine a scenario where the president might be encouraged to use a homogeneous sample strategy? Why do you suggest that strategy?

10. In what scenario can you imagine the president might want to use an extreme or deviant sampling strategy? Why do you suggest that strategy?

Example of Purposeful/Theoretical Sampling

 Barela's (2008) evaluation of high-poverty schools and interventions in Los Angeles (see Chapter 5, Box 5.2) provides an example of sampling for a case study approach:

We selected 12 [Los Angeles Unified School District, or LAUSD] schools based on their status as either California Title I Academic Achievement Award (AAA) schools or as Watch List (WL) schools in 2004–2005. AAA and WL status is based on meeting Adequate Yearly Progress (AYP) criteria as stipulated by NCLB. AYP criteria consist of school-wide participation and performance targets in English/language arts and math. If there are numerically significant subgroups of students, a school must then meet participation and performance requirements in English/language arts and math for each subgroup. Relevant subgroups are organized on the basis of student ethnicities, socioeconomically disadvantaged status, English-learner status, and disability status. For a school to meet its AYP targets, it must meet all of its criteria ...

The sample included 8 AAA elementary schools selected from a population of 43 LAUSD AAA elementary schools and 4 WL schools selected from a population of 138 LAUSD WL schools. In this study, WL schools were considered for inclusion if they did not meet their school-wide English/language arts–performance criterion and their socioeconomically disadvantaged and English learner subgroup, English/language arts–performance criteria. WL schools were matched to AAA schools by percentage of students living in poverty, overall school population, and proportion of socioeconomically disadvantaged students and English learners. More than 65% of a school's population must be living in poverty to receive the maximum amount of Title I funding from the LAUSD. All sample schools had a poverty percentage of at least 65% and ranged from 68% to 97%. The overall school populations of the sample schools ranged from 400 to 950 students. The proportion of socioeconomically disadvantaged students ranged from 63% to 96%. The proportion of English learners ranged from 34% to 85%.

In total, we observed 131 days of instructional practice from 66 randomly selected teachers (43 AAA and 23 WL) and 66 relevant meetings (e.g., grade-level, school-wide professional development, parent, intervention). We interviewed 61 teachers and 37 administrators, such as principals, assistant principals, and Title I coordinators. (Barela, 2008, pp. 532–533)

Sampling and the Use Branch

Not surprisingly, Patton (2008) argues that sampling, like other decisions in evaluation, should be made in collaboration with stakeholders. The evaluator's role is to present possible options along with potential consequences of choosing one option over another, and then to engage in dialogue with the stakeholders about the sampling strategy that they believe will give them usable information. The hallmarks of UFE sampling strategies (see Chapter 5) are appropriateness and credibility. Decision makers may not be accustomed to being asked to participate in decision making about something they think is technical, like sampling decisions. However, Patton claims that the more the decision makers know about the possible sampling strategies, the more comfortable they will feel about discussing the options. The more involvement they have in the development of sampling strategies, the more inclined they will be to use the results. (In addition, they may have ideas that the evaluator may not. Perhaps there is a group of participants that the evaluator may not have thought of and should be included—single fathers, recently retired teachers, etc.)

Example of Use Branch Sampling

Sharma and Deepak's (2001) evaluation in Vietnam about persons with disabilities (see Chapter 4, Box 4.11) provides an example of sampling within the Use Branch. They conducted six focus groups with committee members at the provincial and district levels for a total of 33 participants. They used a different sample for interviews with persons with disabilities (PWD in the quotation below).

> Interviews were conducted at this level in only 5 districts of three provinces that were chosen randomly at the national level for visits. The district level personnel selected the actual communes. All the PWD and personnel involved in the commune were contacted for the interviews. Three CBR supervisors (all males) working at the commune level, five CBR workers (4 females, 1 male), and five adult PWD (3 males, 2 females), and six children (2 males, 4 females), and two parents of infants with disability (both females) were interviewed. (p. 354)

Sampling and the Social Justice Branch

The assumptions of the transformative paradigm and the Social Justice Branch lead to several implications for sampling: Beware of the myth of homogeneity; understand culturally relevant dimensions of diversity; and be aware of theoretically important constructs in relationships with people (e.g., trust, reciprocity) and the impact of labels that could be demeaning or self-defeating (e.g., at risk) (Mertens, 2009). Sampling within the Social Justice Branch involves overcoming barriers to inclusion, issuing invitations that are viewed as authentic, and supporting people as necessary so they can participate meaningfully.

The **myth of homogeneity** means assuming that all people within a particular subgroup are similar to each other in terms of their other background characteristics, or at least sufficiently similar that you do not have to focus on those differences. When you read journal articles, you often see the divisions of people into groups (e.g., deaf, hard of hearing; and hearing, or black, Hispanic, and white. This myth has been discussed earlier in this chapter, in regard to the identification of sample members. Here the discussion is expanded to demonstrate ways that knowledge of diversity within cultural groups can lead to a better understanding of issues of importance in sampling. Mertens (2009, pp. 200–202) makes these points:

> Because the transformative paradigm is rooted in issues of diversity, privilege, and power, recognizing the intersection of relevant dimensions of diversity is a central focus. Researchers and evaluators raise questions to program personnel and participants to consider the relevant dimensions of diversity, especially with regard to traditionally underserved groups—whether based on race/ethnicity, gender, socioeconomic class, religion, disability status, age, sexual orientation, political party, or other characteristics associated with less privilege—and ways to structure program activities and measure appropriate outcomes, based on those dimensions. For example, if the central focus of a program is race and ethnicity, what other dimensions need to be considered? Gender, disability, SES [socioeconomic status], reading level, or home language other than English? Length of time with HIV/AIDS infection, role in the family, access to medications, presence of supportive community? Participation in various political parties that have a history of adversarial relationships?
>
> Cultural competence is a necessary disposition when working within the transformative paradigm in order to uncover and respond to the relevant dimensions of diversity. Some semblance of cultural competence is required to identify those dimensions that are important to the specific context. Who needs to be included? How should they be included? How can they be invited in a way that they feel truly welcome and able to represent their own concerns accurately? What kinds of support are necessary to provide an appropriate venue for people with less privilege to share their experiences with the goal to improve teaching and learning? Or health care? Or participation in governance? Or reduction of poverty? What is the meaning of interacting in a culturally competent way with people from diverse backgrounds? How can relevant dimensions of diversity be identified and integrated into programs designed to serve populations characterized by a diversity that is unfairly used to limit their life opportunities? Understanding the critical dimensions of diversity that require representation in order for transformative research or evaluation to contribute to social change is dependent on the realization that relevant characteristics are context dependent. Important questions include:

■ What are the dimensions of diversity that are important in this study?

■ Who is on the program team?

■ Who is on the research or evaluation team?

■ How reflective are team members of the targeted community?

■ How can stakeholders be identified and invited to participate in a truly welcoming manner?

■ What support is needed?

■ What sampling issues need to be addressed?

■ To what extent do underrepresented groups (disaggregated) have input into decisions about what and how issues will be addressed and how the impact of the interventions will be measured?

- How is resource distribution affecting the ability of stakeholders to benefit from the innovations?

- Who cannot participate and why?

- How can power differences be safely acknowledged and accommodated?

Example of Social Justice Branch Sampling

The WKKF funded a project to determine how to improve the accessibility of courts for deaf and hard-of-hearing people across the United States (Mertens, 2000). The sampling strategy used in this study illustrates sampling implications derived from the transformative paradigm (see Box 11.4). Because this was a study of court access, it was important to acknowledge that each of these dimensions of diversity was relevant to the provision of appropriate support for individuals to be included in the study. Glossing over these differences would have led to an inappropriate conclusion that if a court provides an interpreter, all is well. Other relevant dimensions of diversity that this study included were race/ethnicity, gender, and status within a court (jurist, witness, defendant, or complainant).

The way people are invited to participate in an evaluation can influence their decisions to share their experiences with another person. In a study of a tax credit program in New Zealand, the evaluators described the process they used to invite Māori participants:

> In seeking to identify possible research respondents, the researchers were proactive in utilising all forums, opportunities and networks to "seek out" potentially eligible respondents. This meant "working the crowd" at a major event or *hui* or simply asking all *whānau* and friends if they were receiving [the tax credit]. It also meant providing sufficient information to *whānau* and friends to determine whether they knew of people who the researchers might follow up with. This generated a list of potential respondents. Sometimes their contact details were given directly to the researchers and at other times *whānau* members initiated contact and provided contact details to the researcher or the potential respondent contacted the researchers directly. (Wehipeihana & Pipi, 2008, p. 19)

People can be suspicious when asked about their experiences with government programs, especially if there is a history of betrayal between their communities and the government. Thus evaluators need to be prepared to go out into the communities and use their networks to make contact with individuals in different types of settings. Wehipeihana and Oakden's (2009) invitation process provides an example of culturally appropriate ways to invite indigenous people to participate in an evaluation project. In this study, given the Māori's history of not feeling welcome at schools and perhaps having had negative experiences there themselves, Māori adults needed to receive an invitation that they believed was genuine to participate in a school-based program evaluation. In addition, meeting with the adults needed to be scheduled around the Māori's other commitments to work, family, and community. Some also required support for transportation. These are the strategies that Wehipeihana and Oakden used in their evaluation of the reading program:

Box 11.4. Relevant Dimensions of Diversity and Support in a Transformative Evaluation

Type of hearing loss and communication mode	Support needed
Highly educated American Sign Language (ASL) users; sign, but no voicing	Hearing and deaf ASL-using co-moderators; ASL interpreters signing for the deaf; voicing for the hearing; real-time captioning
Low-literacy ASL users	Same as above
Deaf persons without sign language skills; communication with minimal signs, gestures, and pantomimes	Deaf interpreter who watches ASL interpreter, then conveys meaning to deaf participant using signs, gestures, and pantomime
Deaf-blind individuals	ASL interpreter who signs into the hands of a deaf-blind person
Mexican Sign Language (MSL) users, low-literacy	ASL interpreter who knows MSL
Deaf persons, using cochlear implants (CI)	ASL or English word order interpreter; technological support for use of CI
Deaf persons, no sign language; reading lips, voices	Hearing interpreter who enunciates what is being said to make the language visible on the lips and face
Hard-of-hearing persons, no sign language	Technological support through FM antennae in room to enhance voices

Source: Based on Mertens (2000).

- Used the school newsletter to promote the Reading Together Programme, making clear that all *whānau* were invited.

- Worked with teachers to be sure they would respond positively to inquiries to participate in the workshops.

- Made a particular effort to spell the names of the adults and children correctly, and to learn with whom each child was living.

■ Employed a personal approach to invitations—approaching parents in school playgrounds, home visits, and phone calls if face-to-face invitations were not possible.

■ Trained workshop leaders to emphasize with *whānau* that the program was not based on the perspective that they were the "problem."

Mixed Methods Sampling

Evaluators commonly use mixed methods (i.e., combining the collection of quantitative and qualitative data, either sequentially or concurrently). They may involve different groups of people in different ways. Therefore, it is important to give some thought to the implications of sampling within a mixed methods context. Several scholars have addressed this issue (Collins et al., 2007; B. Johnson & Christensen, 2008; Teddlie & Tashakkori, 2009; Teddlie & Yu, 2007). They identify the following design options and sampling strategies for mixed methods studies:

■ Identical samples for both the quantitative and qualitative parts of the study (i.e., the same people are used).

■ Parallel sampling (i.e., different people are in the quantitative and qualitative portions of the study, but they are from the same population).

■ Nested sampling (i.e., data are collected from a large group with one method; then a subset of that group is chosen to provide data from the other method).

■ Multilevel sampling (i.e., different people from different populations are chosen for data collection for different parts of the study).

Mertens et al. (2007) illustrate an identical, parallel, multilevel sampling strategy in their evaluation of a teacher preparation program (see Chapter 6, Box 6.10). The evaluators began with a qualitative portion of the study, in which all the graduates of the program who had returned to campus for a reflective seminar were engaged. They followed this by interviewing this same set of individuals based on the evaluators' observational data (identical, sequential). The data from the interviews were used to develop an online quantitative survey to be sent to all program graduates who had not been able to attend the seminar (parallel). The data from the observations, interviews, and survey were combined to serve as a basis for interviewing the university faculty and staff from the cooperating schools (multilevel).

- - - - - - - - - - E X T E N D I N G   Y O U R   T H I N K I N G - - - - - - - - - -
Feelings about Being Interviewed

Let's turn the tables. Imagine that you have been approached by an evaluator and requested to participate in a one-on-one interview about your workplace. You have worked in your current position for 3 years and are grateful to be working, but you also know that the working conditions are not the best for you. Your employer has told you that an evaluation of the company would begin this week, so you are not surprised to be approached about an interview.

1. What characteristics would you like the evaluator to have that would make this invitation an inviting and safe one for you to participate in? Why do these characteristics "work" for you?

2. What characteristics of an evaluator would make you feel that this invitation would not be safe or comfortable for you to participate in? Why do these characteristics not "work" for you?

3. If you were initially wary about an evaluator's request for an interview, is there anything the evaluator could do that would make him/her more trustworthy to you?

4. In the future, when you are working in the field, is there anything you will consciously do when the participants in your evaluation are recognizably different from you?

Sample Size

Sample size, like other aspects of sampling, may be determined by default. If you are working with everyone in a program, then there is no need to worry about calculating the needed sample size. In this situation, the sample size is the total number of people in the program. However, if you do plan to select a sample from a larger group, there are several ways to determine how many people you need: rules of thumb, sample size tables, formulae used to calculate sample size, and recommendations by scholars who have expertise in this field.

Rules of Thumb and Formulae for Probability-Based Sampling

In conducting quantitative evaluations, evaluators can refer to the work of Onwuegbuzie, Jiao, and Bostick (2004) or Gall, Gall, and Borg (2007). They recommend the sample sizes listed in Box 11.5 for different evaluation approaches.

The numbers in Box 11.5 are derived through the use of formulae to calculate sample sizes. Specifically, the formulae are used to determine the minimum sample size needed to detect a statistically significant difference between groups, assuming that there is a difference between the two groups that is greater than chance. This type of analysis is called a "power analysis." Lipsey (1990) defines "power" as "the probability that statistical significance will be attained *given* that there really is a treatment effect" (p. 20; emphasis in original). If you know the expected mean differences between groups—for example, from previous research on a similar sample and the level of significance that you need to have

Box 11.5. Recommended Sample Sizes for Different Evaluation Approaches

Evaluation approach	Recommended sample size
Correlational[1] (looking at strength and direction of relationship between two or more variables)	64 participants for one-tailed hypotheses[2]; 82 participants for two-tailed hypotheses
Multiple regression (looking for strength and direction of relationship for multiple independent variables)	At least 15 observations per variable[3]
Survey research	100 for each major subgroup; 20–50 for each minor subgroup
Causal comparative (comparing groups based on inherent characteristics—e.g., hearing status, gender, race/ethnicity)	51 participants per group for one-tailed hypotheses; 64 for two-tailed hypotheses
Experimental or quasi-experimental designs	21 individuals per group for one-tailed hypotheses

[1]Onwuegbuzie et al. (2004) provide estimates for correlational, causal comparative, and experimental or quasi-experimental designs.

[2]One-tailed and two-tailed hypotheses refer to the statistical testing of group differences. One-tailed tests make it easier to obtain statistical significance than do two-tailed tests. That is, using a two-tailed test requires a bigger sample to obtain statistical significance when it is present in the population. This is explained further in Chapter 12.

[3]Gall et al. (2007) provide the estimates for multiple regression and survey research.

before you accept that there is a significant difference (explained in Chapter 12)—then you can use a table to determine the recommended sample size. Statistical texts often include such tables; they are also easily accessible through the World Wide Web. (When I did a Google search using the terms "sample size formula," I got 3,350,000 hits. A very good website is *www.surveysystem.com/resource.htm*.) Web sources often provide the formulae that they used to calculate the recommended sample sizes if you want to do the calculations for yourself. Box 11.6 displays a short list of recommended sample sizes for different sizes of populations and levels of precision (statistical significance) in probability-based sampling.

Box 11.6. Recommended Sample Sizes for Probability-Based Sampling

Size of population	Sample size (n) for precision (e) of:		
	±5%	±7%	±10%
500	222	145	83
600	240	152	86
700	255	158	88
800	267	163	89
900	277	166	90
1,000	286	169	91
2,000	333	185	95
3,000	353	191	97

Source: Based on Israel (2009).

Recommended Sample Sizes for Qualitative Research

Rules for selection of sample size in qualitative research are a bit more complicated than for probability-based sampling. There are no formulae; evaluators may not even know exactly how many people they will need to sample when they begin their study. The number of people in the study is dependent upon the particular qualitative approach, the size of the community from which the participants come, the length of time available for data collection, and the types of issues that surface during the early stages of the study. If new lines of thought are opened up on the basis of early data collection, the evaluators may need to expand the sample pool. Scholars have provided rules of thumb for sample sizes in different qualitative approaches. These are not sufficient justification for final sample sizes, but they can give you an idea of the number of people you might need to include (see Box 11.7).

Sampling decisions can be as simple as saying, "I'm going to collect data from all the participants," or as complex as needing to understand the relevant dimensions of diversity, appropriately approaching communities to determine how best to do sampling, and recognizing that invitations for some participants need to be accompanied by appropriate provision of support to allow them to have meaningful participation. Sample sizes can be as simple as saying, "I'm going to collect data from everyone," to complex statistical formulae, to looking up information in a sample size table. Evaluators need to be cognizant of the ethical implications of all their sampling decisions.

Box 11.7. Sample Sizes Recommended in Qualitative Studies

Qualitative approach	Recommended sample size
Ethnography	Approximately 30–50 interviews
Case studies	Can be only 1 case or multiple cases
Phenomenology	Approximately 6 participants
Grounded theory	Approximately 30–50 interviews
Participative inquiry	Small working team; whole community for meetings; samples for surveys (see Box 11.5).
Focus groups	6–9 people per group; 4 groups for each major audience

Sources: Morse (2000) provided the sample size estimates for ethnography, phenomenology, and grounded theory; Krueger (2000) provided them for focus groups.

- - - - - - - - - - E X T E N D I N G   Y O U R   T H I N K I N G - - - - - - - - - -

Sampling Strategies in Practice

1. Find three evaluations done in your field of interest. Identify how the evaluators sampled the population. What sampling strategy did the evaluators use? How and why did they decide to use this sampling strategy? Do you think the strategy was appropriate? Explain. Would you have selected the sample in a different manner?

2. Throughout the world, many people do not have access to health care. A nonprofit organization, the Hesperian Foundation, creates materials that are written "so that people with little formal education can understand, apply and share health information. Developed collaboratively with health workers and community members from around the world, our books and newsletters address the underlying social, political, and economic causes of poor health and suggest ways groups can organize to improve health conditions in their communities" (Hesperian Foundation, 2010a). Imagine that you have been asked by a large donor to this foundation to evaluate its Gratis Fund program (Hesperian Foundation, 2010a), to discern whether the thousands of books given away are arriving in the appropriate hands overseas. From reading a brief description of the program *(www.hesperian.org/gratis),* whom do you think you would sample and why? What sampling techniques would you use, and why?

Planning Your Evaluation: Sampling Plan

Add a sample plan to your evaluation plan. Make sure that you align the needed samples with the evaluation questions, designs, and data collection strategies. For each evaluation question, from whom will you collect data? What sampling strategies will you use? How many people will you include in your samples?

 ### *Moving On to the Next Chapter*

Once the participants are identified for each portion of an evaluation study, and data collection strategies are selected for each sample, then decisions can be made about appropriate ways to analyze the data. Chapter 12 describes options for data analysis.

Preparing to Read Chapter Twelve

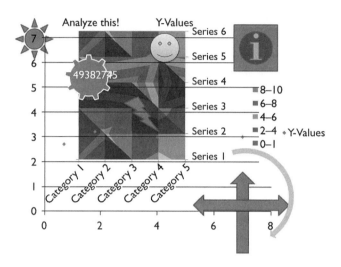

As you prepare to read this chapter, think about these questions:

1. What is your knowledge of statistics? When you hear people talk about "average performance," do you have a good idea of what they mean? If they say there is not much "variability" in a group's skill levels, do you understand what they are saying? If you can answer yes to these two questions, you already have a basic understanding of descriptive statistics.

2. What do you understand about qualitative data analysis? Do you recall having a long conversation with someone, and then when someone else asks you what you talked about, you identify the major themes of your conversation? This is the basic process of qualitative analysis. You will learn ways to systematize your analysis of this type of data, as well as various theoretical lenses that can help you identify important questions to use when conducting the analysis.

3. What do you do if you have both quantitative and qualitative data? How do you handle that type of analysis? What if the two sources of data result in conflicting findings? What do you do?

4. What types of people do you think can be involved in data analysis? Are they only statistical experts or professors at universities? What added value is found when stakeholders are involved in the interpretation of the findings?

CHAPTER TWELVE

Data Analysis

and Interpretation

Data analysis can be viewed as a mysterious process conducted by expert statisticians with quantitative data, or as a mystical process conducted by those with sufficient wisdom and insight to see patterns emerging in qualitative data. In this chapter, we hope to demystify data analysis and interpretation by situating this part of an evaluation within the context that should be familiar to you by now. We acknowledge that we cannot present the equivalent of several statistical books or books on qualitative data analysis in one chapter. Therefore, our discussion of data analysis and interpretation is anchored in a conceptual understanding of data analysis strategies and of evaluators' relationships with stakeholders.

Within the framework of responsiveness to stakeholders, we discuss strategies for data analysis (quantitative, qualitative, and mixed methods) at a conceptual level, to enhance your abilities to make decisions about appropriate analysis choices. Web-based resources are provided to support this decision-making process. Major categories of statistical analysis are reviewed, along with challenges associated with these approaches. In addition, innovative analytic strategies that engage quantitative and qualitative data together are examined, as these are emerging from the scholarship in mixed methods. This chapter also presents strategies to enhance involvement of stakeholders in the interpretation of data.

Involving Stakeholders in Data Analysis

Involving stakeholders in data analysis may seem far-fetched to those who think that only experts with high levels of statistical sophistication or spirituality can engage in this process. Data analysis does require specific skills that may be lacking in some stakeholder groups. However, evaluators work with very diverse communities, and all these communities can understand the process of data analysis at some level. For example, explaining quantitative data with graphs or other visual means can help audiences understand the data analysis process. Evaluators can also explain the basis for analyzing qualitative data in terms of identifying codes and themes, and can engage with stakeholders during this process. What is required is a commitment to meeting the stakeholders on their own terms and to making sufficient effort to communicate effectively about the data analysis strategies.

As is evident throughout this text, evaluators from different branches of the discipline interpret the strategies of stakeholder involvement differently. This is true also in the process of data analysis and interpretation. Evaluators in the Methods Branch tend to emphasize the evaluators' expertise in data analysis as being indicative that sharing this part of the process with those with less or no expertise would threaten the quality of the evaluation's outcomes. Evaluators from the other branches tend to explore ways to include stakeholders in more substantial ways. However, when it comes to data analysis, most evaluators do not pay sufficient attention to mechanisms for meaningful involvement of stakeholders. Mercado-Martinez, Tejado-Tayabas, and Springett (2008) conducted a review of literature from 21 Spanish and Portuguese-speaking countries on the involvement of stakeholders in evaluations that are allowed to evolve throughout the course of the project, called **emergent evaluations** (i.e., participatory, qualitative, critical, hermeneutical, bottom-up, collaborative, and transdisciplinary approaches). They provide us with a glimpse into this problem:

> One of the main assumptions of emergent evaluation is that key participants should be involved in all aspects of the process, including data analysis. The ultimate goal is to incorporate as many stakeholders as possible to increase their sense of ownership, responsibility, and motivation and thus to achieve long-term sustainability for the project (Platt, 1996). It is, however, in data analysis where the greatest contradictions and lack of information can be observed in the publications reviewed and where the traditional model tends to prevail.... All indications point to analysis being an issue that remains in the hands of the experts, the evaluators, or the academics, which puts the participatory, democratic, or collaborative nature of the process into question and contradicts any participatory work done in prior stages. This is not surprising because sharing the analysis between researchers and other participants is a complex challenge. Collective analysis is not only time-consuming but also demands the use of innovative strategies, which tend not to be supported by the working conditions of researchers and evaluators in the Iberoamerican[1] region. Those who carry out the analysis as academics or evaluators usually are subject to time constraints because of demands related to efficiency and productivity, an issue also facing evaluators in other regions.... This is important because most studies were concerned with learning, understanding, or incorporating the perspectives of others in the evaluation of programs. It would therefore seem to be vital to bring to any debate the incorporation of other analytical strategies, such as ... critical discourse and dialogic analysis ... to explore the stakeholders' worlds (Cheek, 2004; Mercado & Hernández, 2007). (Mercado-Martinez et al., 2008, p. 1284)

During the data analysis, evaluators should ensure meaningful involvement of stakeholders.

Capacity Building and Data Analysis

Just as in other aspects of evaluation, evaluators can accept responsibility to build the capacity of the stakeholders with regard to data analysis. Suarez-Balcazar, Harper, and Lewis (2005) trained stakeholders how to use a database and how to do simple data analysis. They suggested that evaluators train more than one person in these skills, because staff turnover may cause a problem if the one person with the skills leaves. They also discuss this strategy as part of the reciprocity they bring to the evaluation. They leave the stakeholders with new skills that can be used in other contexts.

Huffman, Thomas, and Lawrenz (2008) worked with teachers in an evaluation in which the teachers were trained as data collection and data analysis representatives. The teachers had responsibility for developing a database for survey data, student achievement, and instructional practices. The teams met monthly to analyze the results and make decisions about needed instructional changes. These evaluators note that engaging in this process changed the culture of the school to one that used data to inform decision making:

> The structural changes also reflect a cultural change in the school, and anyone new to the school would be incorporated into the new culture for evaluation. As the reliance on evaluation continues to permeate the school culture, it would be helpful if the schools hired an internal evaluation capacity practitioner to assist staff with evaluation activities, in the development of evaluation skills, and in creating even more structural changes in evaluation processes in the schools. However, in most school districts, evaluation is an activity that is conducted by the district office, not by school-level personnel. In the collaborative immersion project, we moved evaluation into the realm of teachers in the schools. This provided a way to think about extending capacity beyond sending individuals to workshops or individualist training. The immersion approach creates a complex, collaborative immersion experience as a means of developing evaluation capacity and, more important, helping to move evaluation into the day-to-day work of teachers in our schools. (Huffman et al., 2008, p. 367)

Stakeholders can be trained in data collection and analysis.

Qualitative Data Analysis

Qualitative data analysis can occur within a specific theoretical framework, as a means of building a theory, or simply as a way to identify emergent themes in the data. The essential strategies include the following:

- Engage in continuous and ongoing data analysis from the beginning of the study to the end.
- Reflectively read interview transcripts, field notes, and relevant documents, to gain a holistic picture of the phenomenon under study.
- Decide whether you want to use a computer program to support your data analysis, or not.
- If you use a computer program, then transcribe the data in the required program format; if not, then transcribe the data in word processing.
- Determine codes for the data that suggest emergent concepts.
- Order the codes into thematic units.

As simple as this sounds, the actual doing of qualitative data analysis is anything but simple. Below, we list texts that focus specifically on qualitative data analysis.

Bernard, R., & Ryan, G. (2010). *Analyzing qualitative data: Systematic approaches.* Thousand Oaks, CA: Sage.

Charmaz, K. (2006). *Constructing grounded theory: A practical guide through qualitative analysis.* Thousand Oaks, CA: Sage.

Miles, M. B., & Huberman, A. M. (1994). *Qualitative data analysis: An expanded sourcebook* (2nd ed.). Thousand Oaks, CA: Sage.

Rogers, R. (2004). *An introduction to critical discourse analysis in education.* Mahwah, NJ: Erlbaum.

An example of how evaluators describe their qualitative data analysis process provides insight into the complexity of the process. Sutherland's (2004, p. 281) evaluation of school reform (see Chapter 4, Box 4.9) began with recorded interviews. She writes:

> The audiotaped interviews were transcribed into verbatim transcript (data) files. Through classroom observations, we were better able to understand whether, and how, the reform designs were being implemented and adapted by teachers. . . . Observation logs and field notes were added to the data file. Using Folio Views 4.2[2] information management software, the data files were assigned codes to reflect the variables associated in the conceptual framework; however, close attention was paid to the existence of new variables and unanticipated effects. Using the aforementioned software, the coded transcript files were analyzed using a thematic approach (Miles & Huberman, 1994). A data display table was created in an attempt to assemble a sample of prototypical quotes into an immediate and accessible form.

Within this example, we can see the incremental building of the database—starting with interview data, moving to observations, and then moving to field notes.

· · · · · · · · · · E X T E N D I N G   Y O U R   T H I N K I N G · · · · · · · · · ·
Transcription of Data

Transcription of data raises a number of questions. Hesse-Biber and Leavy (2006) identify these decisions that need to be made:

1. Will you transcribe all the data or only some of it? How will you decide what to include and what to exclude?

2. How will you do the transcription? Word for word? With all the "hmm's," laughter, crying, and pauses? Will you include the speech pattern of the person speaking or change it to standard English?

3. How will you deal with nonverbal behaviors? Hand gestures?

4. What if the language used is not English? How will you handle translation issues?

5. What if the language used does not exist in a print form (e.g., American Sign Language or Hmong language)?

6. Will you do the transcription yourself or hire someone else to do it?

Examine an evaluation report that used qualitative data analysis; what evidence do you see that they gave consideration to these issues?

Now think about the context in which you will collect data for an evaluation. How would you answer these questions?

In her study, Sutherland (2004) chose to use computer program Using Folio Views 4.2 to organize and analyze the data. Coding proceeded by examining the data for references to her conceptual framework, as well as dealing with data that did not reflect that framework. Then the coded transcripts were thematically analyzed. This is where the mystery arises. Let us take a closer look at steps in qualitative data analysis.

Computer Programs versus Manual Analysis

You need to decide whether you will use a computer program to support your data analysis, or will do it by hand (manually). Factors that may influence which you choose are described on a website called Online QDA (see below):

- The amount of time you have available for analysis of the data.
- The amount of time it will require for you to learn and use a method—the more complex, the more time-consuming,
- The amount of data you have collected and will be analyzing.
- The training and support that may be available to you at your institution, online at websites, or via email or phone from the software seller.
- The availability of technological equipment or software in your institution.
- Budget to pay for equipment or software and training; both could be cost-prohibitive.

Qualitative data analysis has been transformed by the use of computer-based software packages that have been developed explicitly for that purpose. Some evaluators use word-processing or spreadsheet programs for their qualitative data analysis; however, several programs exist that are specifically designed for qualitative data analysis:

- AnSWR—a program developed by the CDC that is free to use and incorporates only text data *(www.cdc.gov/hiv/software/answr.htm)*.
- ATLAS.ti—one of the more complex programs for qualitative data analysis. It will incorporate both text and visual data; it also allows for hierarchical analysis. Purchase price can be found at the website *(www.atlasti.com)*.
- Ethnograph—easier to learn than ATLAS.ti, but does not accommodate visual data; cost is available at website *(qualisresearch.com)*.
- HyperResearch—a user-friendly program that accommodates both text and video data; price is available at website *(researchware.com)*.
- NVivo—allows for use of both text and visual data; price is available at website *(www.qsrinternational.com)*.
- MAXQDA—allows for combination of quantitative and qualitative data; available at website *(www.maxqda.com)*.
- QDA Miner—allows for combination of quantitative and qualitative data; available at website *(www.provalisresearch.com)*.
- ELAN (European Distributed Corpora Project [EUDICO] Linguistic Annotator)—a program developed by linguists. It allows for direct transcription from video- or

audio-based data that includes time alignment between the video/audio and the transcript. It can be downloaded for free *(www.lat-mpi.eu/tools/elan)*.

Because computer software changes quickly, the reader will be pleased to know that there is a qualitative data analysis website called Online QDA, which updates comparisons of qualitative data analysis programs regularly *(onlineqda.hud.ac.uk/Introduction/index. php)*. The advantages of using computer-based software are that you only have to enter the data once, and you can go through many different types of sorting activities as your understanding of the phenomenon changes. You can select data for particular individuals or for groups of individuals who share particular characteristics to see a subset of the coded data. The disadvantage is that you might not be as totally immersed in the data as you would be if you were doing manual analysis. See Box 12.1 for an excerpt from an evaluation study (Saulnier, 2000) that used computer-based software for data analysis.

Box 12.1. Example of the Use of Computer-Based Software in Qualitative Data Analysis

The collaborative approach offered an opportunity for research committee members to learn about analysis. Equally important, it provided the benefit of multiple perspectives. Interrater agreement determines level of reliability (Stewart & Shamdasani, 1990). In this case, the research committee honed interrater agreement in relationship, that is, in groups, through consensus rather than the usual approach used in standardized research whereby coders independently conduct analyses then quantify consistency of interrater agreement. In working collaboratively, the research committee viewed alternative interpretations as a strength rather than a weakness, thus taking advantage of multiple perspectives to formulate an assessment of findings. Transcripts were entered into HyperRESEARCH, a qualitative program that allowed the researcher to analyze transcript content through a system of coding, organization, storage, and retrieval. Analysis was assisted by manipulation of portions of researcher-coded source material. HyperRESEARCH recorded the location of selected text along with the specified code name assigned by the researcher. Coding facilitated analysis by allowing the researcher to cluster all data on a particular topic under one heading, thus making the study of source material more manageable for analysis purposes (Franklin & Bloor, 1999). With HyperRESEARCH, as with several qualitative data analysis programs, any previously coded passage of text can be coded in multiple ways and displayed alone, in the context of the full transcript, or as part of a report. This ability to access coded segments in their original location ensured that no data were lost in the coding process (Franklin & Bloor, 1999). Segments of the transcript were often assigned multiple nonexclusive codes because at this stage, it was premature to rule out any of the analytic topics to which a segment related. Final interpretation came much later than the initial coding. At this stage, the researcher was posing several possible interpretations, postponing final interpretive decisions until the coded segments had been systematically compared with all other segments similarly coded (Franklin & Bloor, 1999).

Source: Saulnier (2000, p. 516).

In a national evaluation of early intervention services for children who are deaf or hard of hearing, the evaluation team decided to use Ethnograph as the computer program to support the qualitative data analysis (Meadow-Orlans, Mertens, & Sass-Lehrer, 2003). All the data were text-based, and Ethnograph allowed for disaggregation by identified subgroups (e.g., parents who were deaf; children who had a disability in addition to deafness).

If you decide to go the manual route for qualitative data analysis, it is still a good idea to use a word-processing program to transcribe all the data. Then you can read through the data, and as you begin to see codes and themes emerge, you can organize the data by using folders for each code or cutting and pasting codes into separate documents.

Coding

Codes are the building blocks of qualitative data analysis. Codes are usually developed after careful, reflective reading of transcripts. Each code is applied to selected passages of text or video that are illustrative of the particular code. In the Meadow-Orlans et al. (2003) evaluation (see above), the evaluation team members first read through all the interview transcripts several times. They developed a tentative list of codes based on this preliminary reading. A codebook was developed that included each potential code and a brief description of the meaning of that code. Then the three team members began a cyclical process of coding and checking with each other as they proceeded.

> One team member coded the first interview and shared her coded transcript with the other team members. A second interview was coded by all three of the team members, who discussed their codes and made additions and revisions to the codebook. The three then coded two interviews independently and compared the coded results. They discussed these until they agreed on codebook categories and definitions. After coding three pilot interviews, the team found the coding decisions to be reliable. Two of the three senior team members independently coded the remaining transcripts in alternate pairs, comparing and discussing for coder agreement. (Meadow-Orlans et al., 2003, pp. 190–191)

· · · · · · · · · · EXTENDING YOUR THINKING · · · · · · · · · ·
Transcription and Coding

Read this partial transcript and make up codes that you might use to capture what is happening in this interview of a mother with a young deaf child who was also diagnosed with attention-deficit/hyperactivity disorder.

Person speaking	Comments
Interviewer	OK, great, um, my first question is, um, if you could tell me about your son and how would you describe him and how is he doing?
Mother	OK, I can tell you at first I had two with different—he was my second baby. And then after him, I had another baby.
Interviewer	Uh-huh.

(cont.)

Mother	And there was four years between 'em, the first two, and he was, um, a boy and she was a girl. He was different from a baby, like, than she was. And I—from six months old I kept telling the doctor I thought that he was different. Something was just not right, he didn't respond or whatever.
	Till he was, let's see, this went on—I went to the pediatrician twice, so he was three and a half. In May I took him at three years old and he was going to turn four in July. And then I took him to the school for the deaf to be tested. And when I took him they said, "Oh God, yes, his left ear is completely gone, and his right ear—he has a little bit of hearing, but we're going to try to use hearing aids."
	He was a behavior problem from the get-go. Screaming, yelling, fighting, um, trying to hurt my two little babies all the time. He was just a mess. And we did not understand what all this was, and we saw them at the school and they said, "Yes, he's deaf and frustrated."
	We had to wait three months to get two hearing aids—to put two hearing aids on him. When I got him into school, he was four and a half.
	Big difference. He learned how to sign, he learned how to communicate, and behavior at home was much better.

Now look at this excerpt from a codebook that was developed as part of the analysis strategies in this study of parents' early experiences with their deaf children (Meadows-Orlan et al., 2003):

Behavior	Reasons for or descriptions of behavior problems
CommSchool	Refers to communication strategies used at school
Delay	Reasons for delay of diagnosis or services
Diagnosis	Information about circumstances of diagnosis (e.g., age, who diagnosed loss, strategies to detect loss)
HearAids	Any reference to hearing aids (e.g., use of, availability, age when received)
Siblings	Reference to siblings, interaction, birth order
Warning	Warning signs, who suspected hearing loss, and reasons for suspecting it

Compare the codes you came up with yourself with those listed in the codebook. What is similar? What is different?

Now use the codes from the codebook to code the data in the transcript excerpt above, without looking at the following example. When you complete your own coding, then look at the coding found in the following table. Compare your own coding with what you see in the table. What was similar? What was different? Do you disagree with any of the codes that you see in the table? Would you recommend adding additional codes, and if so, what would they be?

Person speaking	Comments	Code
Interviewer	OK, great, um, my first question, is, um if you could tell me about your son and how would you describe him and how is he doing?	
Mother	OK, I can tell you at first I had two with different—he was my second baby. And then after him, I had another baby.	Siblings
Interviewer	Uh-huh.	
Mother	And there was four years between 'em, the first two, and he was, um, a boy and she was a girl. He was different from a baby, like, than she was. And I—from six months old, I kept telling the doctor I thought that he was different. Something was just not right, he didn't respond or whatever.	Warning
Mother	Till he was, let's see, this went on—I went to the pediatrician twice, so he was three and a half. In May I took him at three years old and he was going to turn four in July. And then I took him to the school for the deaf to be tested. And when I took him they said, "Oh God, yes, his left ear is completely gone, and his right ear—he has a little bit of hearing, but we're going to try to use hearing aids."	Delay Diagnosis
Mother	He was a behavior problem from the get-go. Screaming, yelling, fighting, um, trying to hurt my two little babies all the time. He was just a mess. And we did not understand what all this was, and we saw them at the school and they said "Yes, he's deaf and frustrated."	Behavior
Mother	We had to wait three months to get two hearing aids—to put two hearing aids on him. When I got him into school, he was four and a half.	HearAids
Mother	Big difference. He learned how to sign, he learned how to communicate, and behavior at home was much better.	CommSchool Behavior

Theoretical Frameworks for Qualitative Data Analysis

In Chapter 6, you have been introduced to a number of theoretical frameworks that are commensurate with the transformative paradigm and the Social Justice Branch of evaluation. Evaluators who begin their work using such theoretical lenses continue to use those lenses in the data analysis stage of the study. Recall that the theoretical frameworks include CRT, indigenous theory, culturally responsive theory, feminist theory, transformative participatory theory, human rights theory, disability and deaf rights theory, and queer/LGBTQ theory. There are, of course, other theoretical lenses that can be brought to bear on the analysis of qualitative data, such as theories of literacy development, attitude change, or motivation.

Postcolonial and Indigenous Theories

Native Americans, Māori, Aboriginal peoples, and Africans have contributed greatly to developing the postcolonial and indigenous lenses that can be brought to qualitative data analysis. One of the keys to using a postcolonial or indigenous lens in data analysis is appropriate involvement of members of the community under study. Horn et al. (2008) provide one example of data collection and analysis that was framed by the use of the Native American medicine wheel for a smoking cessation program evaluation. Wehipeihana and Oakden (2009) used an indigenous approach in their evaluation of a literacy development program focused on culturally appropriate support for Māori families helping their children learning to read. The evaluation team was composed of Māori evaluators who understood the importance of recognizing the value and legitimacy of Māori culture. They involved members of the Māori community in defining the meaning of engagement in the program and the cultural responsiveness of the invitation process before they collected and analyzed data about the effects of the program. In Bowman's (2005) evaluation of tribal colleges, indigenous theory also provided guidance in terms of having a Native American evaluator and an all–Native American evaluation team. The Native American community was included, respected, and consulted throughout the study, including during the data analysis stage.

> The data analysis process was an extensive one that included data cleaning, data description and reduction, triangulations, and data comparisons through a constant comparative, multi-level, and participatory method. After each focus group or day of individual interviews, the evaluation team convened at the home office to discuss the day's events, share notes and insights, and review written, visual, or audio files. Data was then turned over to project staff to be cleaned, entered, and coded into the data collection system (Excel). Codes were given for Tribal affiliation, study activity (focus group or interview), age (elder, youth, adult), gender (m/f), political status (employee, elected, or community member), industry or sector representation, and student or non-student. Data during phase one [were] analyzed and findings discussed by the evaluation team, stakeholder team, and evaluation lead for the focus group and interview phases. Prior to and after each phase an on-site planning session (½ or full day) was completed with the stakeholder group at NATC to delve deeper into the initial findings, challenge questionable findings, and modify the next process or phase to clarify findings. Additionally weekly phone calls and online discussions ensued with key participants on the stakeholder team which provided further guidance, scheduling confirmations, and feedback from the field that came as a result of individual or community feedback after the evaluation team had been in a community collecting data. A final analysis was completed looking at all of the data to confirm through three data sets or more (triangulation) by a constant comparative method if themes and grounded theories could be substantiated according to the evaluation questions guiding the overall study. (Bowman, 2005, pp. 13–14)

Feminist Theory

Many versions of feminist theory are found in the literature. Ghertner (2006) situated her study of the effectiveness of a cookstove project in India (see Chapter 1) within a gender analysis framework that was commensurate with the principles of feminist theory. Using this framework, she was able to analyze the data to reveal inequities between men and women that resulted from a well-intentioned introduction of a new type of cookstove. The rationale for the project was that women who used cookstoves would be freed from the burden of searching for fuel (which can take up to 4 hours a day), and thus would have more time to engage in revenue-producing activities. The project started off well enough, with some women being hired to build the stoves and others purchasing them. However, finding funds to purchase the stove was difficult, and husbands rarely supported use of funds for a stove purchase, because their wives had traditionally been finding fuel for cooking; paying for a stove to give the women more time did not seem reasonable to them. The project staff then decided that it would offer the stoves at a 50% subsidy to encourage adoption. However,

> At the same time that the 50 percent subsidy came into place in Nada, the NPDIC started distributing *chulhas* in villages at 100 percent subsidy. This undercut the income-generating opportunities for the women masons and resulted in universal acceptance of the improved *chulha* where available (because it was free) and the refusal by other households to pay for improved *chulha*s. When available at no cost, husbands happily accepted the *chulha*s. Sarin found that the materials from the free *chulha* were somewhat valuable to the men. In particular, the chimneys were made of sheet metal and had alternative uses for which the men dismantled the *chulha*s. The men thus appropriated the stoves for non-cooking related activities, clearly removing any material benefit that would have gone to women. (Ghertner, 2006, p. 295)

Thus the analysis of the data through a feminist/gender analysis lens allowed for the revelation of the power dynamics between men and women that doomed the project to failure.

Queer/LGBTQ Theory

Just as feminist theory focuses on gender inequities, queer/LGBTQ theory focuses on inequities based on sexual orientation (lesbian, gay, bisexual) and gender identity (transgender). Abes and Kasch (2007) provide this succinct description of queer theory: "critically analyzes the meaning of identity, focusing on intersections of identities and resisting oppressive social constructions of sexual orientation and gender" (p. 620). Renn (2010) recently reviewed the status of the academic world with regard to use of LGBTQ theory as a theoretical framework for data analysis and found that there is a significant gap between theory and practice. The academic world produces a great deal of literature about queer/LGBTQ theory, but not a great deal of literature in which this theory is used as a framework for data analysis.

Critical Race Theory

A CRT lens in data analysis provides support for identifying issues of power, discrimination, and oppression on the basis of race or ethnicity. Fierro's (2006) study (see Chapter 6, Box 6.7) illustrates the application of a CRT lens as she analyzed data concerning the reasons why mothers faced challenges in trying to get their children back after the state had taken custody of them. Madison (2005; cited in Mertens, 2009, p. 285) provides these questions to guide evaluators in the use of CRT in qualitative data analysis:

1. How does race function as a barrier between the powerful and the marginalized?

2. What is the role of racial prejudice as an explanatory lens for the research findings?

3. How does racism operate through unconscious habit, naturalized practices, and beliefs of white supremacy?

4. How are people in the setting constructed as racial beings and what assumptions are associated with their race and that of others?

5. How is white privilege influencing behaviors, attitudes, and social relations in the setting?

Disability and Deaf Rights Theory

Sullivan (2009; Mertens et al., 2011; Mertens, Bledsoe, Sullivan, & Wilson, 2010) has examined the use of a disability rights lens in the analysis of qualitative and mixed methods data. The following questions are based on May and Raske's (2005) disability discrimination model; they provide guidance in using disability and deaf rights as a filter for qualitative data analysis:

1. How is impairment associated with disability understood? As social construction or as a consequence of disability?

2. How does impairment associated with disability connected to discrimination, poverty, or marginalization?

3. How is impairment associated with disability connected to people's making claims for what they need?

4. How do people with disabilities, as well as deaf people who do not regard themselves as disabled, assert their rights as equal citizens under the law?

The major emphasis of disability and deaf rights in terms of analysis and interpretation of data is on making sure that people with disabilities or deaf have a voice in the process and outcomes.

· · · · · · · · · · E X T E N D I N G   Y O U R   T H I N K I N G · · · · · · · · · ·

Theoretical Lenses in Data Analysis

Find an example of an evaluation in which data were analyzed and interpreted through one of the following lenses: CRT, queer/LGBTQ theory, feminist theory, postcolonial and indigenous theories, disability and deaf rights theory, or human rights theory.

1. What lens was used?

2. Were the stakeholders involved in the data analysis process?

3. How were codes identified?

4. What themes emerged, and would these themes have emerged if the theoretical framework was not employed? Explain.

5. Do you think that applying another or an additional lens to this study would have revealed different themes? Explain.

Specific Qualitative Strategies: Discourse Analysis and Constant Comparison Methods

So far we have discussed a generic qualitative data analysis strategy and theoretical frameworks that can be used to bring a social justice lens to the analysis. There are many other approaches to qualitative data analysis, each associated with different theoretical frameworks, such as conversation analysis (see ***www-staff.lboro.ac.uk/~sscal/sitemenu.htm***), narrative analysis (see ***onlineqda.hud.ac.uk/resources.php#Narrative***), content analysis, discourse analysis, and constant comparison methods. In this section, we discuss discourse analysis and constant comparison methods.

Discourse Analysis

Two distinct types of discourse analysis are used to analyze qualitative data: generic discourse analysis and critical discourse analysis (CDA).

In generic discourse analysis, evaluators tend to focus on analyzing smaller amounts of data, rather than coding the full body of data as in the general qualitative method described earlier in this chapter (Lewins, Taylor, & Gibbs, 2005). The evaluator may code the data, but not for the purpose of identifying themes. Rather, the analysis focuses on the patterns and structures used in language. Leech and Onwuegbuzie (2008) state that discourse analysis

> involves selecting representative or unique segments of language use, such as several lines of an interview transcript, and then examining them in detail. Discourse analysts treat language as being situated in action. When people use language they perform different social actions such as questioning or blaming. Language then varies as a function of the action performed. Thus, *variability* can be used as a tool to show how individuals use different discursive constructions to perform different social actions. Words can be examined to see how people use *accountability* for their versions of experiences, events, people, locations, and the like. (p. 591; emphasis in original)

Gee (2005) suggests a generic set of questions to consider in doing discourse analysis:

1. How does the speaker indicate the significance of what they are saying (e.g., tone of voice, body language)?

2. What is the activity that the language is being used to facilitate (e.g., make an argument; support a position)?

3. What is the identity of the speaker in terms of language use (e.g., power broker, facilitator, subordinate)?

4. What are the implications from the language that is used with regard to the speaker's relationship with the audience?

5. How does the language reflect the politics of the situation (e.g., set the agenda; reveal who is in charge)?

6. What can be inferred about the connections and relevance of people and concepts from the use of the language?

7. How does the language privilege certain ways of knowing? (Who is the expert? Who is the novice?)

CDA is a variation of discourse analysis that uses the transformative theoretical lens to bring meaning to the data.

> CDA departs from discourse analysis and sociolinguistic analyses in its movement from description and interpretation to *explanation* of how discourse systematically constructs versions of the social world. Furthermore, critical analyses position subjects in relations of power (both liberatory and oppressive aspects of power) rather than analyzing language as a way of explaining the psychological intentions, motivations, skills, and competencies of individuals (Luke, 1995/1996). (Rogers, Malancharuvil-Berkes, Mosley, Hui, & Joseph, 2005, pp. 371–372)

CDA encompasses the transformative theories already discussed in this chapter and integrates those with the analysis of language. CDA "was an attempt to bring social theory and discourse analysis together to describe, interpret, and explain the ways in which discourse constructs, becomes constructed by, represents, and becomes represented by the social world" (Rogers et al., 2005, p. 366). The focus of CDA is on the use of language as a tool of oppression or transformation. There is no one specific method for CDA. Rogers et al. describe various levels in the analysis procedure, including a linguistic analysis of textual data, an examination of data from interactions, and bridging from the text and interactional data to wider social issues. The wider focus is on subtleties of power and privilege and on the use of language to maintain historical power structures. Much of CDA examines how power is reproduced, rather than how language can be used to challenge the status quo and bring about social transformation.

Fox and Fox (2002) examined the power issues that allowed deception to prevail in faculty meetings about overcrowding at a university in Croatia. A candidate for the dean's position promised to address the overcrowding by limiting enrollment and making sure there was a chair for every student. After being selected as the dean, the person did not keep his promise. The person with power (the dean) used language to deactivate faculty requests for additional classroom space. The dean circumvented this request by stating that someday things would be better. Faculty members maintained silence, thus indicating acceptance of the deception. The authors explain this acceptance in terms of hierarchical structures of power that could be challenged only at the faculty members' risk.

· · · · · · · · · · E X T E N D I N G   Y O U R   T H I N K I N G · · · · · · · · · ·

Critical Discourse Analysis

Barker's (2003) CDA of the self-identities of two youth subcultures, Goths and Pagans, illustrates several ways the participants used language to construct versions of their experiences. For example, she noted that some of those she interviewed put on dumb or silly voices when they imitated other people making comments about their clothing. This voicing showed that they regarded other people's views as ridiculous. Also, one participant recounted someone's comments about her using ungrammatical English, in a way showing her view of the other person as ignorant.

1. For the next day or so, play close attention not only to what people say, but also to how they say it.

2. List additional ways in which you are receiving information (winks, facial expressions, gestures, etc.).

3. What additional information are people giving you, other than just the words they are speaking or signing?

4. What would you miss or misunderstand if you were not critically analyzing their discourse?

Constant Comparison Analysis and Grounded Theory

Grounded theory is a theoretical framework consistent with the Values Branch. In keeping with the "Global Conveyor Belt" metaphor introduced in Chapter 2 (see Figure 2.3), grounded theory provides strategies for qualitative data analysis within the Use and Social Justice Branches as well. Glaser and Strauss (1967) initiated grounded theory as a systematic method for analyzing data for the purpose of constructing theories. Corbin and Strauss (2008) explain that theoretical propositions are not stated at the outset of the study; rather, they emerge out of the data themselves. Thus the name "grounded theory" indicates that the theories are grounded in the data as they are analyzed in that particular study.

Corbin and Strauss (2008) and Charmaz (2007) suggest the use of a constant comparison data analysis strategy in grounded theory:

1. Constantly interact with the data, asking questions, generating hypotheses, and making comparisons. Revise your thinking as needed, and sketch out preliminary theoretical frameworks.

2. Use these preliminary theoretical frameworks to guide you in pursuit of additional data that will help illuminate or refute your theoretical concepts.

3. Code the data in reference to your emerging theory. Corbin and Strauss (2008) label two steps in coding: "Open" and "axial" coding. Charmaz (2007) labels these same steps as "initial" coding and "focused" coding. Initial coding involves attaching codes to words, lines, and segments of text. Focused coding involves testing the initial codes by comparing them to a larger set of data to reveal relationships among the codes and develop the theoretical frameworks further.

4. Write memos in the database to indicate your thinking and feeling, and how these change throughout the process of the theory construction.

5. Continue to ask questions of your data to capture the complexity, diversity, and nature of the relationships among the variables. Questions to ask: Who? When? Where? What? How? How much? Why? Identify gaps in the theory, and seek additional data to address those gaps.

6. Use the constant comparison of codes and the relationships that emerge among them to refine the theory.

Charmaz (2007) adds questions that can be useful in examining the data for issues of social justice. She suggests asking about available resources; differential access to resources; presence of hierarchies, benefits and oppressive impacts of hierarchies; control over who makes the rules; differential impacts of rules and practices; points of resistance and contestation; and facilitation of social justice.

Evaluators sometimes use constant comparison analysis even when they are not interested in generating theory. Under those circumstances, the steps can be reduced to identifying codes and checking those codes against the larger body of data in a process of comparison throughout the analysis process.

· · · · · · · · · · · **EXTENDING YOUR THINKING** · · · · · · · · · · ·

Qualitative Data Analysis

 Often, details about data analysis are omitted. For example, in Sharma and Deepak's (2001) evaluation of community-based services in Vietnam, the authors provide this description of their data analysis:

> The data were recorded in the form of notes in a field book. Then the data were collated in three categories: (1) village and commune level; (2) district and province level; and (3) national level in the four identified themes of: (1) strengths; (2) weaknesses; (3) opportunities; and (4) threats. Each idea expressed by participants was written down. If the statements supplemented an existing idea it was added to the already written statement. Efforts were taken to document all the ideas mentioned by the participants. Finally, the data were re-collated across levels along the four themes. The data analysis was done by transcribing the field notes on a computer word processor. (Sharma & Deepak, 2001, p. 354)

What information is given in the example above about the qualitative data analysis? What additional information is needed to judge the quality of the data analysis?

Pilot Studies and Qualitative Data Analysis

Evaluators who conduct qualitative studies should give consideration to conducting a small-scale pilot study before they implement the study on a large scale. This allows them not only to test their methods of sampling and data collection, but also to gain insights into potential themes that might emerge in the study. Goodman et al. (2004, p. 816) provide this description of how their large-scale evaluation was changed after their analysis of pilot interviews:

> As a result of this methodology, our view of the work was transformed following pilot interviews with community members and service providers. We expected to learn about the problems with existing services and how to make them more culturally competent. After speaking with community members, however, it became clear to us that providing adequate services for Haitian immigrant women would require more than "cleaning up" or adding to existing ser-

vices. Instead, community members wanted to reflect on alternative strategies for addressing intimate-partner violence that did not even involve the mainstream system of service provision.

Quantitative Analysis Strategies

Quantitative data analysis generally takes the form of some type of statistical analysis. Statistics can be useful because they reduce a large data set into more meaningful terms, such as average performance or amount of variability in a sample. Evaluators need to be aware of potential dangers associated with the misuse of statistics as well. It is not possible to provide an in-depth treatment of quantitative statistical strategies in this chapter; if you are interested in pursuing this topic further, we direct you to the resources listed below. In this section, we review some of the basic terminology of statistics, guidance for selecting statistical procedures, and issues that affect the interpretation of the numbers.

Elliott, A. C. (2007). *Statistical analysis quick reference guidebook*. Thousand Oaks, CA: Sage.

Field, A. P. (2009). *Discovering statistics using SPSS* (3rd ed.). Thousand Oaks, CA: Sage.

Frankfort-Nachmias, C., & Leon-Guerrero, A. (2011). *Social statistics for a diverse society* (6th ed.). Thousand Oaks, CA: Pine Forge Press.

Meyers, L. S., Gamst, G., & Guarino, A. J. (2006). *Applied multivariate research*. Thousand Oaks, CA: Sage.

Salkind, N. J. (2007). *Statistics for people who (think they) hate statistics* (4th ed.). Thousand Oaks, CA: Sage. (Available as a regular book and for use with Excel)

Sirkin, R. M. (1999). *Statistics for the social sciences* (2nd ed.). Thousand Oaks, CA: Sage.

Steinberg, W. (2011). *Statistics alive!* (2nd ed.). Thousand Oaks, CA: Sage.

Wagner, W. E. (2010). *Using SPSS for social statistics and research methods* (2nd ed.). Thousand Oaks, CA: Pine Forge Press.

Warner, R. M. (2007). *Applied statistics: From bivariate through multivariate techniques*. Thousand Oaks, CA: Sage.

Most statistics can generally be thought of as falling into three categories: (1) descriptive statistics, such as means and standard deviations, which allow the evaluator to describe the overall average and amount of variability in a sample; (2) correlational statistics, which indicate the strength and direction of relationships between or among variables; and (3) *inferential statistics,* which provide a test of the statistical significance of the results of a statistical test (e.g., group comparisons). Brief descriptions of various types of statistics and suggestions for their use are displayed in Box 12.2.

Statistical Terminology

Number of Participants

In statistical terminology, the number of people from whom data are collected is commonly depicted with the letter n. In Moss and Yeaton's (2006) evaluation of a developmental English program, they indicated their sample size as follows: "From an initial cohort, participants were divided into two groups: one group required by the college to take developmental English ($n = 782$) and a second group not required to take developmental English ($n = 994$)" (p. 219).

Box 12.2. Statistical Methods and Their Uses

Type of statistic	Recommended uses[1]
For descriptive evaluation questions	
Measures of central tendency	
Mean: Arithmetic average	For interval or ratio data
Median: The middlemost point in the data	For interval, ratio, or ordinal data
Mode: The most frequently occurring score	For interval, ratio, or nominal data
Percentages	For ratio, interval, ordinal, or nominal data
Measures of variability	
Range: Highest to lowest values	For interval or ratio data
Standard deviation: Dispersion of scores around the mean	For interval or ratio data
Variance: Standard deviation squared	For interval or ratio data
For visual displays of data	
Graphs, tables, figures	For all types of data
For relationship evaluation questions	
For two variables	
Pearson product–moment coefficient of correlation	
Spearman rank-order coefficient of correlation or Kendall rank correlation	For ordinal data
Point biserial correlation coefficient	For interval, nominal, or ordinal data
Contingency coefficient	For nominal data
Ordinary least-squares regression analysis	For interval, ratio, or nominal data
For more than two variables	
Multiple-regression analysis	For interval, ratio, or nominal data
Kendall partial rank correlation	For ordinal data
Discriminant analysis	For nominal data
Factor analysis (to determine the structure of variables)	For interval or ratio data

[1]The terms used in this column for various levels of data are explained in Box 12.3.

Type of statistic	Recommended uses[1]
For group differences evaluation questions	

For two variables and for related samples

t-test for correlated samples (allows for comparison of two groups with one independent variable; related groups are the same people measured twice or matched samples)	For interval or ratio data
Wilcoxon matched-pairs signed-ranks test	For ordinal data
McNemar test for the significance of changes	For nominal data

For two variables and for independent samples

t-test for independent samples (similar to *t*-test for correlated samples, except the two groups being compared are independent of each other)	For interval or ratio data
Mann–Whitney *U*-test or Kolmogorov–Smirnov two-sample test	For ordinal data
Chi square test	For nominal data

For more than two variables and for related samples

Repeated-measures analysis of variance (ANOVA) (used to compare two or more groups or when you have more than one independent variable)	For ratio or interval data
Friedman two-way ANOVA	For ordinal data
Cochran *Q*-test	For nominal data

For more than two variables and independent samples

ANOVA	For interval or ratio data
Kruskal–Wallis one-way ANOVA	For ordinal data
Chi-square test for independent samples	For nominal data

For more than one dependent variable

| Multivariate analysis of variance (MANOVA) | For interval or ratio data |

For evaluation questions to predict group membership

| Discriminant function analysis | For all data types |

(*cont.*)

Box 12.2 (*cont.*)

Type of statistic	Recommended uses[1]
For evaluation questions about complex theoretical models	
Structural equation modeling (SEM) (used to test theoretical models or confirm factor structures by assessing relationships between manifest [observed] and latent [theorized] variables)	For ordinal or ratio data
Multidimensional scaling	For concept mapping
Hierarchical cluster analysis	
Regression discontinuity design (combines the features of ANOVA and regression analysis to test for trend differences based on preestablished criteria)	

Descriptive Statistics

The most commonly reported descriptive statistics are the mean and standard deviation and percentages. Two common symbols for means are an $\overline{X}$ (with a bar over it) or the capital letter *M*. Standard deviations are often labeled as *SD* or *sd*. For example, Moss and Yeaton (2006) compared the grade point averages for students who were in the developmental program with those who were not in the program. They reported that the developmental group had a mean of 2.74 (*SD* = 0.90) and the nondevelopmental group had a mean of 2.96 (*SD* = 0.98).

Correlational Statistics

Correlation coefficients are usually denoted with an *r*. Moss and Yeaton (2006) examined the correlation between the number of terms it took nondevelopmental students to take their college-level English class and their grade in the class (*r* = –.02). The correlation between the number of terms for the developmental students and their English grade was also low (*r* = –.01). The evaluators interpreted these results to mean that there was no evidence that students who delayed taking college-level English courses had systematically lower grades. If a regression analysis is used to determine relationships among variables, then the statistic that results is called beta and appears as the Greek letter ß; the weights for each variable are standardized, and then they are labeled beta. Here is an excerpt from the Moss and Yeaton (2006) study:

> Those with the lowest pretest scores who completed developmental English coursework significantly increased their English achievement over what was predicted by the linear trend in nondevelopmental students.... This interpretation is confirmed by the significant linear

interaction term in the model (β_3 = – 22, p < .01). Hence, the treatment was found to have a greater positive influence on English achievement for those who were the most underprepared. (p. 224)

Inferential Statistics

Inferential statistics are used to determine whether the samples' scores differ significantly from the population values or from each other. Moss and Yeaton (2006) used a t-test for independent samples to determine whether people who dropped out before completing their college-level English classes differed on their pretest of English skills from students who stayed and completed the courses. They reported that there was no significant difference between the two groups (t = .88, p = .38). They are used for testing group differences and strengths of relationships. A common inferential statistic is the analysis of variance (ANOVA). The statistic that results from ANOVA is depicted as F. There are many variations of ANOVA. Evaluators can enter variables to control (such as background variables) before the ANOVA is conducted. These variables are called covariates, and when this procedure is used, it is called an analysis of covariance, or ANCOVA. If the data set includes more than one independent variable, then the multivariate analysis of variance (MANOVA) is used.

ANOVA and its variations test an overall difference between groups or variables. However, if there are more than two groups or variables, then it is common for evaluators to do post hoc analyses to see where the differences among the groups and variables lie. Such tests can be selected from a statistical program and have names such as Scheffe's, Bonferroni's, or Tukey's.

Evaluators make certain assumptions about their data when they use inferential statistics. These include (1) that the characteristic is normally distributed in the population; (2) that the level of measurement is ordinal or ratio; and (3) that the participants in the study were randomly selected from the population. If these assumptions are not met, then evaluators need to think about several things. First, they can make an assumption that the inferential statistical tests are robust and go ahead and use them anyway. Second, they can decide to use a different type of statistic that does not require these assumptions to be met—nonparametric statistics.

Nonparametric Statistics

Nonparametric statistics do not require that the rigorous assumptions for inferential statistics be met. They can be applied to ordinal and nominal data. Because they are not as commonly used as inferential statistics, reports usually include the full name of the statistical test (with the exception of the chi-square test, which is sometimes identified only by the Greek symbol χ^2).

Statistical Significance

Statistics that are used to determine differences between samples and populations, two or more groups, or two or more variables are usually reported in terms of the level of statistical significance. Statistical significance is based on probability theory and indicates the probability that the results could have been achieved by chance, rather than reflecting a stable difference or relationship. Evaluators set up hypotheses and test these by using statistical tests. If a hypothesis states that there is no difference between the scores of the experimental group and the control group, then that is called a "null" hypothesis. If the hypothesis states that there will be a difference, then that is the "alternative" or "directional" hypothesis. We have seen several examples in the preceding explanations of evaluators reporting the t value and then its associated p value. The p value indicates the level of probability associated with the statistical significance. For example, a p value less than .05 indicates a 5% possibility that you are rejecting the null hypothesis when it might indeed be true. (This is known as a "Type I error.")

Choice of Statistics

The choice of statistics is dependent on several variables:

1. What is the evaluation question? Are you interested in describing a phenomenon (descriptive), determining relationships (correlational), comparing groups (inferential or nonparametric), or doing more complex types of analyses?

2. What types of groups do you have? Do the data points come from the same people at different points in time or from matched groups (related samples)? Do they come from different individuals in each group (independent samples)?

3. How many independent and dependent variables do you have?

4. What is the scale of measurement used for the variables? (See Box 12.3 for an explanation of different scales of measurement.)

5. Can you satisfy the assumptions required for use of inferential statistics?

Box 12.3. Scales of Measurement

▪ The nominal level is used for categorical data like colors, genders, races, or languages.

▪ The ordinal level is the arrangement of data into an order dependent on the increasing or decreasing of a characteristic (e.g., from tallest to shortest, from oldest to youngest).

▪ The interval level is a scale in which the increments between data points are equidistant from each other, but the scale does not have a meaningful zero point. For instance, when the thermometer says that the temperature is 0 degrees, this does not mean that we have no temperature.

▪ The ratio level also has equidistance between data points, but it also has a meaningful zero point. For example, 2 pounds of cheese is twice as much as 1 pound of cheese. If I have 0 cheese, I don't have any cheese.

After answering these basic questions, you can use Box 12.2 to make your selection of appropriate statistical analysis procedures.

Mixed Methods Data Analysis Strategies

Mixed methods data analysis strategies are partially determined by the mixed methods design that is employed. If one type of data is collected first, followed by another type, then the strategy is to clarify the relationship between the two data sets. How does the first stage of data analysis influence decisions in the second stage of data analysis? If the two types of data are collected simultaneously, then the data analysis seeks to integrate data analysis strategies. The *Journal of Mixed Methods Research* has many examples of strategies for analyzing mixed methods data. Jang, McDougall, Pollon, Herbert, and Russell (2008) provide one such example: They describe the data analysis strategies used in a concurrent mixed methods study of academic success in schools in high-poverty areas with a high percentage of English language learners as students. The evaluators conducted a survey that they quantitatively factor-analyzed to determine relevant constructs in the determination of school success. They also conducted individual interviews and focus groups with principals, teachers, parents, and students during the same period of time (concurrently). They analyzed the qualitative data via standard qualitative analysis strategies, identifying codes and ending up with 11 themes that were inductively derived. Box 12.4 presents a description of how Jang et al. (2008) integrated the two data sets; all page numbers in the box refer to their article.

Box 12.4. An Example of Integrated Mixed Methods Data Analysis

Independent Quantitative and Qualitative Analyses

At the outset, qualitative interview and focus group data and quantitative survey strands of data that were collected concurrently were analyzed independently. The qualitative data from 80 interviews with principals and teachers and 40 focus groups with students and parents were analyzed inductively. The results of the qualitative data analysis resulted in 11 themes associated with school improvement. The surveys of 440 teachers and principals were factor analyzed to reduce the observed variables into a smaller number of factors underlying the school participants' perspectives about school improvement. (pp. 228–229)

Integrated Analysis and Data Transformation

We agreed that the results from the independent analyses of the qualitative and quantitative data provided both overlapping and different aspects of the characteristics of school improvement. For example, five themes associated with distributed leadership—professional learning, positive school culture, data-based decision making process, and community outreach—were supported by both the interview and survey data. General descriptions of these factors from the generic survey data were enriched

(cont.)

Box 12.4 (*cont.*)

by contextually rich accounts of the themes from the interviews. The results from the interview data also provided new insights into the characteristics of school improvement. To make data comparison more transparent, we transformed the results from the quantitative data by creating narrative descriptions of the nine factors based on the graphs and descriptive tables. The transformed data were compared with the qualitative themes in a matrix....

Themes from the interviews, associated with parental involvement, communication capacity, access to extracurricular programs and resources, diversity in learning, building literacy and numeracy skills, and child's SEB [social, emotional, and behavioral] development, were not clearly present in the survey results. These characteristics seemed unique and context specific to schools facing challenging circumstances. For example, the theme of child's SEB development reflected on the common perspective that ensuring students' social, emotional, and behavioral stability was viewed as a significant factor leading to academic success in schools with challenging circumstances....

Although the results from the survey pointed to nine factors associated with school improvement, they were limited to the perspectives of the teaching staff. The results from the interviews allowed us to obtain an enriched understanding of the characteristics of school improvement from multiple perspectives. The comparison of the findings from the qualitative and quantitative data through data transformation brought forward not only overlapping but also nonoverlapping aspects of school improvement in these schools facing challenging circumstances. (p. 233)

Blended Analysis: Data Consolidation

To further our understanding of the characteristics of school improvement, we utilized an additional data consolidation analytic strategy (Bazeley, 2006; Caracelli & Greene, 1993) by combining the results from both qualitative and quantitative data to create blended data for further analysis. First, we jointly reviewed the results from the qualitative and quantitative data. We reviewed the 75 survey items to examine the extent to which the 11 themes that emerged from the qualitative data were present in the survey data. Out of 75 items, 63 were identified as addressing constructs similar to the 11 themes from the qualitative data analyses. We concluded that 3 themes, including access to programs and resources, building literacy and numeracy, and use of data for improvement, were not present in the survey instrument. The research team independently recoded the 63 items using the themes brought by the qualitative data. Then we met and shared our reassignments to the new 8 themes. Whenever we disagreed, we discussed the survey question and how it related to the theme. We continued to deliberate until we all agreed on the new allocation. In this way, we created a new set of thematic variables out of the joint use of both data types and quantified it by distributing the 63 items into 1 of the 8 themes. (p. 236)

Case Analysis

The integrated mixed methods case analysis approach took place in two steps. We first identified school cases that showed a statistically significant difference from the overall mean of the 20 schools. We repeated this procedure for each of the eight consolidated themes. Next, we revisited the qualitative interview and focus group data for identified schools. We reread the portion of the data related to themes that identified the schools.

The results were integrated into a narrative school case profile.

For each theme, we created bar charts that graph the mean and 95% confidence interval for the mean of each school. We compared the mean score of each school on each of the eight consolidated themes to the scores for all 20 schools in the project. We identified schools that differed significantly from the average score of all of the 20 schools on the basis of the nonoverlapping confidence interval approach (Thompson, 2002). [The evaluators plotted the mean scores of the 20 schools to identify those that were significantly different on each of the themes.] ... Once we identified schools that differed from other schools, we revisited the qualitative data from those schools to provide a contextually rich narrative of the nature of each theme and unique challenges. (p. 238)

Source: Jang et al. (2008). Reprinted by permission of Sage Publications.

Bazeley (2009a, p. 205) has identified a number of strategies for integrating quantitative and qualitative data during the analysis stage. The strategies are derived from various sources (Bazeley, 2009b; Caracelli & Greene, 1993; Creswell & Plano Clark, 2007; Greene, 2007; Miles & Huberman, 1994; Teddlie & Tashakkori, 2009):

- Intensive case analysis (e.g., using the quantitative data to select a smaller subsample of cases to describe in great detail using qualitative data).

- Employment of the results from analysis of one form of data in approaching the analysis of another form of data (referred to by some as typology development (e.g., using categories identified through quantitative data collection as a basis for coding qualitative data).

- Synthesis of data generated from a variety of sources, for further joint interpretation (e.g., combining quantitative demographic and performance data with qualitative data derived from interviews and observations).

- Comparison of coded or thematic qualitative data across groups defined by categorical or scaled variables, and matched, where possible, on an individual basis (e.g., conducting qualitative analysis on subgroups identified through quantitative analysis).

- Pattern analysis using matrices (e.g., entering qualitative data into theoretically derived matrices, and then comparing patterns in the data).

- Conversion of qualitative to quantitative coding to allow for descriptive, inferential, or exploratory statistical analysis (e.g., creating frequency counts of types of utterances).

- Conversion of quantitative data into narrative form, most often for profiling (e.g., using quantitative data to describe the average participant in qualitative terms).

■ Creation of blended variables to facilitate further analysis (e.g., creating variables derived from both quantitative and qualitative data that can be used to explore the meanings in the data further).

■ Extreme and negative case analysis (e.g., using quantitative data to identify extreme or negative cases, and then analyzing the qualitative data for that subset).

■ Inherently mixed data analysis, where a single source gives rise to both qualitative and quantitative information, such as in some forms of SNA (e.g., having individuals provide quantitative data on their social networks, as well as qualitative data that expand on the meaning of those social networks).

■ Often flexible, iterative analyses involving multiple, sequenced phases where the conduct of each phase arises out of or draws on the analysis of the preceding phase (e.g., using survey results to develop qualitative data needs; when the qualitative data are analyzed, this is done with a consciousness of the relationship between the two data analysis strategies).

Garbarino and Holland (2009) also suggest possible strategies for the combined use of qualitative and quantitative data analyses in an international development context:

1. A survey is used to select a qualitative investigation sample.

2. A survey highlights priority issues to be covered in qualitative research.

3. Qualitative analysis identifies knowledge gaps to be filled by surveys. White (2008) describes how crucial information was not collected before a quantitative baseline survey took place, and consequently no information was collected on one key explanatory variable.

4. Qualitative analysis enables surveys to predict more accurately which issues (sectoral, cross-sectoral, or other) and which options are of importance to local people, and what explanations they might give. This improves the definition of survey modules and questions, and the categories of choice of answer available.

5. Qualitative analysis identifies what is highly contextual information, and therefore what should *not* be subjected to standardized quantitative methods.

6. Qualitative research suggests the importance and means of constructing indicators that usefully complement or replace existing indicators. There has been considerable recent activity in constructing indicators of qualitative (nonmaterial) development impacts, including governance, empowerment, social capital, and social exclusion.

7. Insights from qualitative and quantitative studies help to define population subgroup sampling frames.

8. Qualitative analysis (including that of key informants) helps determine "appropriate" stratification of the quantitative survey, and subsequent disaggregation of survey cross-tabulation analysis (e.g., along gender, age, socioeconomic, political, sociocultural, or ethnic lines).

Computer Programs for Mixed Methods Analysis

Some of the software packages listed earlier in this chapter can be used to integrate quantitative and qualitative data analysis (e.g., NVivo, MAXQDA, and QDA Miner). Use of these computer programs allows for expeditious mixed methods data analysis, because an evaluator can quickly identify potential cases to "mine" qualitatively by their linkage with the corresponding quantitative data.

Mixed Methods Analysis as a Dialectical Process

Greene (2007) provides food for thought about mixed methods data analysis; her suggestions emanate from her dialectical stance (see Chapter 9). She recognizes that evaluators whose work is situated within one branch or another will bring differences in strengths and interests to the analysis of qualitative and quantitative data. These differences can sometimes be viewed as barriers to effective communication or integration of data in a mixed methods study. However, the dialectical stance supports conversations across paradigms and branches. Through such conversations, mixed methods can bring a

> better understanding of the phenomena being studied than can a single method as all methods each offer but one perspective, one partial view. And [I] believe that better understanding takes its most important form as generative insights, which are in turn best attained through a respectful conversation among different ways of seeing and knowing. Our rich tradition of philosophical paradigms and even richer array of multiple mental models offer many different ways of seeing and knowing, many different conversational partners. (Greene, 2007, p. 79)

Thus Greene suggests that mixed methods data analysis as a process of reflective conversations across differences of perspectives has the potential to yield greater insights.

· · · · · · · · · · EXTENDING YOUR THINKING · · · · · · · · · ·

Mixed Methods Data Analysis

Lindsay (2002) noted that past evaluations of public health programs have used quantitative approaches such as epidemiological and statistical techniques to make judgments about program effectiveness based on predetermined outcomes. However, public health program evaluators have begun to use qualitative techniques, such as rapid ethnographic assessments and focus groups. Lindsay conducted a mixed methods study, using both quantitative and qualitative methods to evaluate the outcomes of a community health workers' program "to assess the impact of child survival interventions in reducing infant mortality and inadequate weight gain in children among municipalities in the state of Ceará, Northeast Brazil" (p. 570). She used quantitative techniques such as ecological analysis; her data consisted of infant mortality rates, diarrhea-specific infant mortality rates, inadequate weight gain in children, breast-feeding rates and duration, access to clear water and sanitation, female illiteracy, and use of prenatal and child health care. And she used qualitative

(cont.)

techniques such as in-depth interviews and verbal autopsies. The interviews were conducted with service providers and recipients about such topics as factors that might have prevented neonatal deaths, the circumstances of the infants' deaths, timing and place of deaths, and mothers' health-care-seeking behaviors during their infants' illnesses. The quantitative data were analyzed via multiple-regression analysis to test the strength and direction of effects of the independent variables (e.g., amount of breast feeding) on the dependent variables (e.g., infant mortality). Lindsay (2002) described the qualitative data analysis as follows: "The transcripts were analyzed inductively to identify recurring themes, from which we generated a list of categories of themes based on the most frequent answers cited by respondents. The qualitative data were coded into three main categories of problems: delay in seeking medical care; delay in receiving medical care; and timely, but ineffective care" (p. 575).

The quantitative results indicated that a strong relationship existed between three independent variables (i.e., exclusive use of breast feeding, female literacy, and increased seeking of health care for sick infants) and three dependent variables (i.e., a lower rate of infant mortality, diarrhea-specific mortality, and inadequate weight gain). The qualitative data on circumstances of death revealed that 60% of the infants died at home after being taken to a health care center. The mothers' comments indicated that they did take their children to the health care center, but they said the treatments prescribed were ineffective or that they arrived at the hospital too late in the day to be seen and had to make several trips to the health center, thus delaying treatment.

1. What do you see as the added advantage to conducting a mixed methods study in this context?

2. How did the evaluator integrate the findings to increase her understanding of the complexity of the issues?

3. What recommendations for action would you consider, based on the summary of this study?

4. Choose another study that used mixed methods analysis. Examine how the evaluators integrated the two types of data and how the knowledge gained from one set of data informed analysis of the other set of data. Possible choices might be these:

   a. Arango, Kurtines, Montgomery, and Ritchie (2008) studied the effect of a program for adolescents that was designed to promote healthy life choices.
   b. Garbarino and Holland (2009) analyzed quantitative and qualitative data in a study of poverty and its social impact.
   c. Yoshikawa, Weisner, Kalil, and Way (2008) explained their mixed methods analysis strategies in an evaluation of programs designed to enhance child development.

   Search on the topic "community score card" (the CSC is used in international development evaluations; see Chapter 10) to explore this as a mixed methods strategy and to determine which analysis techniques are used in this type of study.

Data Interpretation

A number of issues arise in the interpretation of both quantitative and qualitative data. These issues are discussed in this section, along with strategies to address the issues. Particular attention is given to the involvement of stakeholders at the data interpretation phase of the evaluation. In quantitative studies, the issues include the effects of being able to randomize or not; threats to validity because of the use of intact groups; the influence of the sample size on analysis process and outcomes; and the difference between statistical and practical significance. In qualitative studies, issues of selectivity that reflect the evaluators' biases need to be addressed. In both types of studies (and in mixed methods studies), issues arise about cultural bias and generalizability. Qualitative evaluators develop codes and themes and select segments of data to illustrate their use of these. Quantitative evaluators use scales with the purpose of reducing the complexity of a situation and may well do damage to salient cultural issues.

Quantitative Issues

Randomization

Recall that the use of inferential statistics is premised on the assumption that the participants in the study were randomly selected from the population and that they were randomly assigned to treatment groups. If these conditions hold, then there is no need for concern. However, in many evaluation contexts, it is not possible to use random selection or assignment. Therefore, evaluators may decide to use inferential statistics anyway, relying on their robustness. "Robustness" means that the assumptions can be violated within certain parameters, and the statistical techniques have still been found to be accurate. Furthermore, random selection of a sample from a population is used in the Methods Branch as an indicator of the representativeness of the findings from the sample back to the population. If randomized selection does not occur, this has implications for generalizability (discussed below).

Using Intact Groups

In many evaluations, the evaluator is faced with collecting data from intact groups. This means that there is no real selection process beyond that used to determine who will be in a program. This decision is sometimes based on who goes to a particular school, lives in a particular area, or has a certain condition. When a sample is an intact group, it is difficult for the evaluator to know whether the sample is representative of any larger group. In such a situation, the evaluator should collect relevant data that describe the individuals in the group sufficiently that he/she can consider possible biases based on the uniqueness of that group. This also allows readers of the report to determine the potential applicability of results from the evaluation to other contexts.

Sample Size

There is an inverse relationship between the size of a sample and the ease of obtaining statistical significance. In other words, if the sample size is very small, it is harder to get statistical significance. If the sample size is very large, it is easier to get statistical significance. How does the evaluator know whether statistical significance is the result of an overly large sample? How does the evaluator know whether a lack of statistical significance is because of a too small sample? As mentioned in Chapter 10, evaluators can use power analysis to determine the appropriate sample size needed to obtain a specified level of statistical significance.

Statistical and Practical Significance

Because of the ease of getting statistical significance with very large groups, statisticians have recommended looking at two concepts: statistical significance and practical significance. Suppose I compare the outcomes of two different reading programs and find that the new program yields a statistically significant improvement in achievement scores, compared to the traditional program. If I compare the effect size of the programs, and it indicates that the new program raises scores the equivalent of 1 month over a 2-year period, whereas the traditional approach only raises them 1 week, is this enough practical significance to recommend that the school district adopt the new program? Other variables to consider for practical significance include the cost of the program and the logistics of implementation. If the new program costs five times as much as the old program, what would you recommend? If the new program requires an entire school reorganization, what would you do?

Qualitative Issues

Representation

Qualitative evaluators often struggle with the issue of representation, that is, who speaks for whom. Representation is a factor in the sources of information as well as in the evaluator's decision in who will be heard. The evaluator has a responsibility to report the source of the information while safeguarding the identity of the source. You can identify the source as observation, field notes, document review (possibly specifying the document's name), or interview notes. You can also include the date that the data were collected. It is advisable to include the position of the person speaking, such as "parent of a deaf child with a cochlear implant" or "teacher in a third-grade classroom."

Qualitative evaluators need to consider how much raw data (i.e., quotations from interviews, field notes, or documents) versus how much interpretation is being provided. In our opinion, the evaluator should provide a balance of raw data and interpretation. Evaluators have a responsibility to bring an interpretive lens to the data, rather than publishing great numbers of direct quotes and leaving the interpretation to the reader. Evaluators have valuable knowledge about context and theoretical framing and can provide insights that the outside reader may not have. Evaluators also have a responsibility to provide a clear explanation of the contextual and theoretical concepts that framed their interpretation of the data.

Selectivity

Generally, in qualitative research, there is far more data than can be presented in a written report of the research. Therefore, you need to be clear about how you select the data you present in the report. If you organize the report by themes that emerged from the data, then you can explain that the selected quotations were chosen to be illustrative of the theme that is discussed. If a quotation is unique, then explain the reason for choosing that particular quote to represent an unusual opinion in the sample.

Qualitative and Quantitative Issues

Cultural Bias

We have discussed cultural bias as an issue that circulates throughout evaluation work— from the methods used to determine the evaluation focus, to concerns about data collection, to the analysis and interpretation of data. In Chapter 10 on data collection, we have described processes that qualitative evaluators can use to check their cultural biases. These include progressive subjectivity checks in the form of journaling or memos, peer debriefing, member checking, and thick description.

Generalizability

Generalizability has been discussed in terms of sampling and in terms of the impact of using intact groups to collect quantitative data. This concept has relevance for qualitative data analysis as well. Generally, qualitative data analysis involves smaller samples; the goal is to have a "representative" sample in the same sense as quantitative evaluators define this concept. However, qualitative evaluators need to analyze their data within the constraints of the sample from which they collect their data. This means acknowledging limitations, as well as providing sufficient details that readers can make up their own minds about the applicability of results to another context (thick description).

Community Involvement in Data Interpretation

Social justice evaluators have been at the forefront of involving community members in the interpretation of data. Recall the use of the medicine wheel (Horn et al., 2008) as a framework for discussing the interpretation of the data from the smoking cessation evaluation conducted in a Native American community. Māori (Cram, 2009) use community gatherings called *hui* to engage community members in discussions of the meaning of evaluation findings. Other cultural groups provide additional examples of these approaches. Goodman et al. (2004) evaluated domestic violence services for Haitian immigrants, using open-ended interviews. Here is how they described their data analysis:

> Data analysis was content derived, indicating that preconceived categories were not superimposed on data. Rather, categories emerged from the data as coding proceeded. Also, data collection and analysis occurred simultaneously so that each could influence the other.... Finally, to ensure the credibility and validity of the findings, we established a Haitian advisory board, which was made up of Haitian community leaders. The advisory board was given a detailed summary of the findings, interpretations, and conclusions of the research and encouraged to give feedback regarding the accuracy and credibility of the research.... (Goodman et al., 2004, pp. 815–816)

Uses of advisory boards have been discussed in the section of Chapter 7 on bringing focus to the evaluation. Recall that Dodd (2009) recommended using members of the LGBTQ community to parallel reviews of institutional review boards. This type of advisory board could be used in the interpretation of data as well.

··········· E X T E N D I N G   Y O U R   T H I N K I N G ···········
Community–Based Data Analysis

Bardwell et al. (2009) trained 152 adolescents to conduct community-based research about obesity and diabetes in their medically underserved home region of Appalachia. The evaluators described conditions that existed before the work began:

> If our observation of the lack of base knowledge among these maturing adolescents is representative of their communities, the information divide between health care givers and this community concerning diabetes and its prevention is enormous. It also became apparent that aspects of culture, language and behavior specific to rural West Virginians needed to be catered to in order for the participants to understand the concepts involved. Beyond acquaintance with what the words mean, there was essentially no comprehension of energy balance, obesity was a trait to be made fun of, and diabetes represented a dreaded diagnosis to be feared. (p. 342)

1. Read the article and note who the participants/researchers were, how they were chosen, how they were trained, and what work they accomplished.

2. How was the data analysis simplified for the students yet still in a valid format?

3. Bardwell et al. were unabashedly excited about the data they collected. What did they learn about diabetes and obesity? What did they learn about community-based participatory research with adolescents?

4. Would you want to train community members to do participatory research? If yes, with whom and on what topic?

Planning Your Evaluation

At this point, your evaluation plan is nearing completion. You have determined your worldview, described the evaluand, identified stakeholders, and decided on data collection and sampling strategies. Now you need to add the data analysis plan and align it with the data collection part of the plan. How will you analyze the data that you collect?

 ### In Part IV

In Part IV of this text, you will be introduced to how evaluators manage and implement their evaluations. You will add a management plan and budget to your evaluation plan, based on the material presented in Chapter 13.

Notes

1. Iberoamerican is a term used for nations colonized by Spain and Portugal in the Middle Ages, including Andorra, Portugal, South America, and parts of North America.

2. Folio Views used to be a free software package for qualitative data analysis. It has since been acquired by a commercial vendor that markets it primarily to businesses (see ***www.rocketsoftware. com***).

IMPLEMENTATION IN EVALUATION

Communication and Utilization of Findings,

Management, Meta-Evaluation, and Challenges

Evaluations typically consist of the various components that we have discussed so far in this text: identification of the evaluator's worldview; description of the context and the evaluand; and determination of stakeholders, approaches, participants, data collection strategies, and data analysis strategies. In Part IV, we take up three more aspects of the evaluation plan, which move into the territory of evaluation implementation. In Chapter 13, we discuss communication and utilization of findings. In Chapter 14, we present the final components of an evaluation plan: project management and meta-evaluation. These are both part of the evaluation plan and are integrally related to the implementation of the evaluation. In Chapter 15, we address issues that arise in the implementation of evaluations and that represent perennial or emerging challenges in this field.

Part IV includes the following chapters:

Preparing to Read Chapter Thirteen

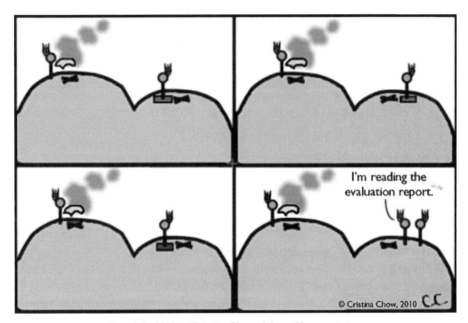

Copyright 2010 by Cristina Chow. Adapted by permission.

As you prepare to read this chapter, think about these questions:

1. How will the findings of the evaluation be communicated to stakeholders?

2. Who will be involved in writing the evaluation report?

3. How will you or others use (or not use) the report's findings?

4. Where can you learn how to write a report?

5. How do you publish a report in a professional journal?

6. What alternative formats for disseminating the findings should you consider?

7. What do you think about using a theatrical production to disseminate evaluation findings?

CHAPTER THIRTEEN

Communication

and Utilization of Findings

Evaluators need to plan for use from the beginning of an evaluation throughout the entire process. Thus the topics of communication and utilization of findings have already surfaced at various places earlier in this text. In this chapter, specific options for reporting are examined, including assorted language-based options (written, oral, signed); visual displays (tables, charts, graphs, maps); and presentations and performances. Reporting in evaluation needs to be seen as part of a dynamic process, in which information is provided to stakeholders at key points during the evaluation. Use of evaluation-generated information is also part of this ongoing, dynamic process, which is designed to give feedback at critical stages and to facilitate use of that information by those in positions to make course corrections. Recall that evaluations can have multiple purposes. They may start with an assessment of context, input, needs, and assets; move to a process evaluation (monitoring, formative, developmental); and conclude with some kind of outcome or impact assessment. Sometimes they include evaluation for the purpose of replication or sustainability. And some evaluations have a specific focus on furthering social justice and human rights. Therefore, report planning needs to be conducted within the framework of the evaluation's purpose.

Communication and utilization of findings represent one of the synergistic dimensions of evaluation work; therefore, decisions about what and how to report to whom are integrally connected with the intended uses of the reports. These decisions need to be directly linked with the purpose of the evaluation (Chapter 8) and the data collection methods (Chapter 10). This chapter opens with an explanation of options for reporting, and then moves to consideration of uses and lessons learned in light of evaluation purposes and data collection.

Communication of Evaluation Findings

Reporting in evaluation is sometimes narrowly perceived as writing a report at the end of the evaluation. However, because evaluation studies often involve ongoing assessments and interactions with stakeholders in an attempt to improve a program, reporting needs to occur throughout the course of the study. In this section of the chapter, we present a wide variety of options for reporting: not only the preparation of final reports, but also small-group presentations, focus groups, web-based reporting, and performances as strategies for reporting. In addition, use of visual presentation strategies is highlighted.

In my early days as an evaluator, I (Donna M. Mertens) faithfully prepared a final report for each major phase of the projects with which I worked. I produced thick reports that carefully explained my methodology and all the findings. Once I submitted those reports to the "feds," I did not think much more about their use. It was something that I had been trained to do well and that was expected as part of the contract. The evaluation field has progressed considerably over the last 40 years, as you will see in this chapter.

Language-Based Options for Communicating Evaluation Findings

Formal Written Reports

An evaluator exercises a certain power when deciding to write a formal report, as writing is a creative, interpretive, and selective process. Evaluators bring their own judgment to how they choose to write and what content they choose to include in the writing. In evaluation, a report can be written by a single evaluator or by a team of people who serve different roles in the writing process. Greenwood, Brydon-Miller, and Shafer (2006) described their experiences in developing reports throughout the course of a multiyear project. When an internal report was needed for decision making in the early stages of the project, the evaluators wrote it themselves. As the evaluation progressed, they involved a writing team to review outlines for potential reports and to accept responsibility for writing various sections of the reports. This involved working to give one-on-one support to some of the team members who had less experience in writing of this type. Such a situation also raises questions about shared authorship. Whose names should be on the report as authors? Evaluators should recognize this as an issue that merits discussion whenever multiple writers collaborate. Some evaluators will include qualitative data in their reports to illustrate points. Box 13.1 describes an approach used to determine which stories to include in the evaluation report.

Written reports in evaluation can take many different forms—from scholarly academic reports to more narrowly focused technical reports to flyers, brochures, webpages, news releases, and memos. Each option needs to be considered in light of the intended readers and the purposes of sharing the information. For scholarly academic writing, there is a traditional format that is used in many publications. It consists of the following sections:

- Introduction (this establishes the broader context of the report and situates the study in extant literature)
- Evaluand (this describes the intervention or program)
- Methodology (this includes a description of stakeholders, data collection strategies and instruments, participants, and data analysis)
- Results (this presents the findings of quantitative, qualitative, and mixed methods data analysis)
- Conclusions (this presents an explanation of the findings and their implications, usually with recommendations for next steps)

Academic reports are often written for the purpose of publication in scholarly journals. Writers interested in this avenue should check the webpages of the journals to which they intend to submit reports, to determine their mission and requirements for manuscripts.

Box 13.1. Group Process in Writing: Choosing the Stories

The stories were selected at meetings with the help of a facilitator. Story titles were recorded under the respective domains. When all the stories had been read out, each domain was considered in turn. The facilitator then asked questions to encourage debate before moving on to a vote by show of hands. Each committee member was given one vote for each domain. If there was no consensus, which was common, further discussion was facilitated until those meeting could agree on which story should be selected. Agreement was normally achieved by an iterative voting and discussion process. If no agreement could be reached, either two stories were selected, or none. Some stories were selected with the proviso that a caveat be attached to the story explaining additional factors, or indicating that not all committee members agreed about the value of the outcome. The idea was to come to an agreement as a group. In addition to selecting a story, committee members were also asked to state why that story had been selected above the others. Much of the discussion revolved around explanations of why committee members thought one story was particularly valuable or misleading. This discussion was recorded on tape or by a note-taker.

Source: Dart and Davies (2003, p. 144).

· · · · · · · · · · E X T E N D I N G   Y O U R   T H I N K I N G · · · · · · · · · ·

Publishing in Journals

What style of writing do you use when you write papers? (APA? *The Chicago Manual of Style*?) And what style will you need to use when you write for a journal? What topics are journals looking to publish, and how long can submitted articles be? How long will a journal hold your manuscript before its editors inform you if they have accepted it for publication?

1. Read the publication specifications for a few journals, such as the following:

   a. *American Journal of Evaluation*

   b. *New Directions for Evaluation*

   c. *Journal of Mixed Methods Research*

   d. *Educational Researcher*

   e. *Disability and Society*

2. Which journal would you be interested in writing for? What differences do you notice in the journals' submission guidelines?

Technical reports often include similar sections, although it is not unusual for the literature review section to be more abbreviated than in scholarly academic reports. Technical reports also tend to be quite a bit longer, because they usually include examples of instruments and more details about findings. Stufflebeam et al.'s (2002) technical report on the Hawaiian housing evaluation study (see Chapter 4, Box 4.3) is 185 pages long. The table of contents for this report is displayed in Box 13.2.

· · · · · · · · · · E X T E N D I N G   Y O U R   T H I N K I N G · · · · · · · · · ·

Organizing an Evaluation Report

The Asian Development Bank (2010) finances projects in resource-poor Asian countries meant to improve the quality of life of those living in poverty. You can read summaries of the evaluations of these projects on its website, and then download the accompanying technical report as a .pdf file. Select a topic that interests you, read the summary, and then glance through the accompanying .pdf file. Read through the table of contents and note how these technical reports are written. What is included in this technical report that you don't find in other written evaluation reports? Would writing this kind of detail for an evaluation you have done interest you?

News Releases

Writing for the general public in the form of news releases is not a skill that most evaluators have. It requires writing more like a journalist than like an evaluator. Journalists tend to use the "inverted pyramid" format—presenting the most important facts first, followed by supportive evidence and subsidiary points in decreasing order of importance (United Nations, 2009). This format is based on the premise (supported by communication researchers) that readers read the beginning of the text to learn the most important facts and to determine whether it is worth their while to read the rest of the article. This is quite different from most scholarly writing, which provides a literature base and extensive methodological descriptions before the findings. In news releases, less complex descriptions of methods are recommended, perhaps together with sources where interested readers can go for more detail. News releases also usually avoid the use of overly technical jargon and use simple writing, in the form of covering one idea per sentence and starting each paragraph with an important idea. The United Nations (2006) provides these suggested steps for the preparation of a news release:

- It tells a story about the data.
- It has relevance for the public and answers the question "Why should my audience want to read about this?"
- It catches the reader's attention quickly with a headline or image.
- It is easily understood, interesting, and often entertaining.
- It encourages others, including the mass media, to use statistics appropriately to add impact to what they are communicating.

Box 13.2. Table of Contents for a Technical Evaluation Report

Source: Stufflebeam et al. (2002, p. vi). Reprinted by permission of Daniel L. Stufflebeam.

Box 13.3 contains a press release that announces the success of the U.S. government's Children's Health Insurance Program. The press release is accompanied by a fact sheet (Box 13.4) with bulleted points and a link to the full report online.

··········· E X T E N D I N G   Y O U R   T H I N K I N G ···········
News Releases

1. We are able to find the results of many reports written as news releases in our newspapers. Peruse the Sunday edition of the major newspaper in your area and find one example. How does it follow or not follow the United Nations (2009) suggestions for writing news releases?

2. Project ALERT "is a school-based prevention program for middle or junior high school students that focuses on alcohol, tobacco, and marijuana use. It seeks to prevent adolescent nonusers from experimenting with these drugs, and to prevent youths who are already experimenting from becoming more regular users or abusers" (***www.promoteprevent.org/publications/ebi-factsheets/project-alert***).

Memos, Flyers, Brochures, and Web-Based Reporting

Partially because of concerns about the seeming lack of use of evaluation data, evaluators began to give consideration to other types of evaluation reporting that are smaller in scale than academic or technical reports. These might include memos that are used as interim reports, in which evaluators present formative data at various stages of an evaluation. They can also use flyers or brochures that contain both text and graphics. In addition, web-based distribution of knowledge is flourishing and offers many options in terms of combining text and graphics, as well as linkages to other relevant resources. Web-based technologies also offer many emerging strategies for disseminating reports, as well as obtaining feedback on reports. For example, blogs and web-based chat rooms provide means both to disseminate findings and to obtain feedback from large groups of people in very short time frames. As technology is a fast-developing area, ethical issues may emerge that we cannot even begin to perceive at the moment (Burbules, 2009).

The U.S. Department of Health and Human Services has developed Research-Based Web Design and Usability Guidelines, which will help you share your reports with the public through creating effective and easy-to-use websites. You can download the 292-page noninteractive file to read and follow offline (***www.usability.gov/guidelines/guidelines_book.pdf***), or you can build your website while following an interactive .pdf file online; downloading is also an option (***www.earlham.edu/~markp/design/Usability_guidelines.pdf***). Designing a website can feel like a daunting task, but these guidelines break the process down into several sections (i.e., design, organization, accessibility consideration, navigation), which make developing your webpages straightforward and motivating. The Usability Guidelines suggest that you design your pages so that they are easily navigated and accessible to all users; that you use colors wisely (keeping in mind color-blind browsers);

Box 13.3. Sample News Release

FOR IMMEDIATE RELEASE

Thursday, February 4, 2010

Contact: HHS: (202) 690-XXXX

USDA: (202) 720-XXXX

Sebelius, Vilsack Celebrate One-Year Anniversary of Children's Health Insurance Law, Highlight Campaign to Cover Kids

Sebelius Promotes the Secretary's Challenge: "Connecting Kids to Coverage"

Exactly one year after President Obama signed the Children's Health Insurance Program Reauthorization Act, HHS [Health and Human Services] Secretary Kathleen Sebelius and Agriculture Secretary Tom Vilsack today announced that 2.6 million more children were served by Medicaid or the Children's Health Insurance Program (CHIP) at some point over the past year and released the Children's Health Insurance Program Reauthorization Act One Year Later: Connecting Kids to Coverage, a comprehensive review of the past year's accomplishments in finding and enrolling children in health coverage.

Sebelius also highlighted The Secretary's Challenge: Connecting Kids to Coverage, a five-year-long campaign that will challenge federal officials, governors, mayors, community organizations, tribal leaders and faith-based organizations to build on this success and enroll the nearly five million uninsured children who are eligible for Medicaid or CHIP but are not enrolled.

As part of the Secretary's challenge, Vilsack and Sebelius announced plans to work with state Supplemental Nutrition Assistance Programs (SNAP, formerly the food stamp program), to encourage them to work with their state's Medicaid and CHIP programs to share data and identify uninsured children who are potentially eligible for coverage through Medicaid or CHIP. Leaders from the Departments of Agriculture and HHS will provide guidance to state officials on how to better share data and reach families in need.

"One of President Obama's first actions as President has proven to be a tremendous success," said Sebelius. "Now we must build on our accomplishments. Today, I am calling on leaders across the country—from federal, state and local officials to private sector leaders—to join our effort to insure more children. We all have a stake in America's children and together, we will ensure millions more children get the care they need."

While Medicaid and CHIP have helped bring the rate of uninsured children to the lowest level in more than two decades, an estimated five million uninsured children are thought to be eligible for one of these programs yet not covered.

The Secretary's Challenge: Connecting Kids to Coverage will support efforts to reach more children by providing leaders with critical information and support as they work to insure more children in their communities and by closely monitoring progress.

"State policymakers have demonstrated their commitment to improving children's health, even as they face economic challenges," said Cindy Mann, director of the Center for Medicaid and State Operations within the Centers for Medicare and Medicaid Services (CMS). "Now, we will work with leaders at every level to help cover more children."

More information about CHIP can be found at *www.insurekidsnow.gov*.

Box 13.4. Sample Fact Sheet Providing More Information

Fact Sheet: Children's Health Insurance Program Reauthorization Act (CHIPRA)

New State Strategies to Boost Enrollment

Given new flexibility under CHIPRA, states have adopted several new strategies to ease enrollment. Since CHIPRA was enacted on February 4, 2009, states have sought CMS approval for the following program improvements:

- 17 states have submitted plans to CMS to streamline their enrollment and renewal processes;

- Three of these states have received approval for the new Express Lane Eligibility option in Medicaid and/or CHIP. Express Lane Eligibility allows states to enroll children into one of the programs based on information obtained through other state programs and data bases;

- 15 states have expanded income eligibility levels in their CHIP and/or Medicaid programs;

- 19 states have lifted the five-year waiting period for eligible children and/or pregnant women who are lawfully residing in the United States; and,

- All 50 states set up data agreements with the Social Security Administration to verify citizenship for purposes of Medicaid and CHIP eligibility.

Funding enhancements have led all but two states to covering children in families earning at least 200 percent of the federal poverty level, or $48,100 for a family of four in 2009. Families at this income level contribute to the cost of coverage through monthly premiums and other out-of-pocket expenses.

The full report and more information about CHIP can be found at *www.insurekids-now.gov*.

---

and that graphics and images should each have a purpose and should be used sparingly. Some additional considerations from these guidelines include the following:

- The design process should be collaborative as you are deciding on goals, designing ideas, and creating and evaluating possible prototypes.

- The website design should establish levels of importance; this will reduce the user's workload when visiting the site. Feedback should be given as the user explores your page.

- The content should be organized by level of importance and utility, and presented in short sentences and as brief paragraphs.

- Your titles, headings, and links should be clear and concise.

- Pages should be consistent from page to page, all important information located at the top of the page, and all empty space utilized.

- Text size, font size, and print/background should make the visit a comfortable reading experience for the user.

- Use text as links (not graphics), use descriptive link labels, repeat text links, and avoid "mouse-overs."

- Navigation aids should be consistent, grouped together, and placed on the right side of the webpage.

· · · · · · · · · · · E X T E N D I N G   Y O U R   T H I N K I N G · · · · · · · · · · ·

Web-Based Reporting

Many of us may be guilty of creating websites without any guidance other than following the instructions offered by the companies that have sold us the sites. Read the online version of the Research-Based Web Design and Usability Guidelines (see the URL above), and study the suggestions for designing a webpage. Then visit the page "Biggest Mistakes in Web Design 1995–2015" on the Web Pages That Suck website (*www.webpagesthatsuck.com*), which illustrates why you need to follow the Usability Guidelines.

1. Find two websites that illustrate good website design, and describe how they follow the Usability Guidelines.

2. Find two websites that illustrate poor website design and describe how they do not follow the Usability Guidelines.

Many multilateral organizations use flyers or brochures to present their results to their stakeholders because they represent a way to communicate with shorter, more focused messages. A sample page of an eight-page brochure published by three United Nations agencies on HIV/AIDS and women appears in Box 13.5. The full brochure can be viewed at the United Nations Population Fund (UNFPA) website (*www.unfpa.org/hiv/docs/women-aids.pdf*).

Reporting in a Short Time Frame: Mixed Methods

McNall and Foster-Fishman (2007) discuss the need for reporting information in real time, especially when evaluators are working in settings in which natural disasters have occurred. In these settings, information is needed as soon as possible to assess the extent of damage, identify needs, and design, implement, and evaluate interventions. Lives depend on quick action. These authors have extended ideas from participatory action research and rapid

Box 13.5. A Sample Page from a United Nations Brochure

About 200 million women become pregnant each year and need information, counselling and services to help the 99% who are HIV negative remain so, and address the needs of those who are HIV positive. By preventing HIV infection in pregnant women, prevention of transmission to children is assured.

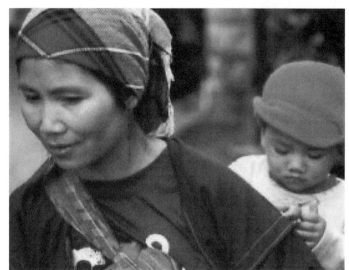

Photo: UNFPA

Women confront a number of gender-based obstacles to prevent becoming infected with HIV, and if positive, to prevent transmission to their offspring:

- Women may be unable to negotiate safe sexual practices, including condom use to prevent infection and/or unintended pregnancies.

- Women may be unable to access pre-natal health services as their partners often control the household financial or transportation resources, as they cannot take time off work, or because they cannot leave their dependents to travel to a clinic or hospital.

- Fear of rejection, stigmatization, violence or abuse may prevent women from utilizing HIV voluntary counselling and testing services, disclosing their HIV status, accessing HIV prevention programmes targeting pregnant women, mothers and their children, or engaging in safer infant feeding practices.

WOMEN, WORKPLACE AND HIV/AIDS
The workplace provides an opportunity to instill positive norms and standards to safeguard employees from HIV infection and care for those who are infected or affected by HIV/AIDS. Employers can effectively address HIV infection within the work community by avoiding work patterns that separate workers from their families for prolonged periods of time; providing education on HIV/AIDS; enforcing non-discriminatory hiring practices and 'zero tolerance' policies on violence or harassment against women; supporting STI diagnosis and treatment; and providing antiretroviral drugs to workers and their families.

Source: UNFPA, UNAIDS, and UNIFEM (n.d., p. 5). Reprinted by permission of UNIFEM.

rural appraisal (see Chapter 10) to formulate **rapid evaluation and assessment methods** (**REAM**). The typical kinds of data collection are used (e.g., review of extant data, observations, interviews, focus groups, mapping, transect walking). However, data collection, analysis, and reporting are done through participatory methods that are designed to share information in real time. The REAM process is an iterative one, with decisions about the need to collect more data or different data being made at each juncture of the process. Preliminary findings can be used to guide decisions, while the evaluation cycle continues to provide more refined information or information about new needs that surface. The combined process can take from a few weeks to a few months. Representatives of the local population are considered essential for the process to work successfully. A team is formed that includes evaluators, decision makers, and local populations.

Dart and Davies (2003) have developed a form of reporting that emanates from the use of the MSC method (see Chapter 10). Recall that this method can be used both to identify desirable outcomes to guide development of interventions and to determine what participants determine to be the most significant outcomes after the program implementation. Dart (2008) has expanded the MSC method to include participatory performance story reporting. She explains that performance story reports are short reports (no more than 20 pages, or possibly even in brochures) that portray the outcomes of an evaluation. The written part of the report includes five elements:

1. A narrative section explaining the program context and rationale.

2. A "results chart," which summarizes the achievements of a program against a program logic model.

3. A narrative section describing the implications of the results (e.g., what was learned, and what will be changed as a result of what has been learned).

4. A section that provides a number of vignettes illustrating instances of significant change, usually first-person narratives.

5. An index providing more detail on the sources of evidence.

Each of these elements is developed through a participatory process. The logic model is developed collaboratively (see Chapter 7). Data collection can be undertaken as a team, and capacity development can be provided as necessary. Once the results chart is compiled, this is provided to an outcomes panel consisting of representatives of various stakeholder groups, who then are asked to assess how the intervention contributes to meeting goals, given the available knowledge. Finally, a summit workshop is held to review the chosen significant changes. These are then used to develop recommendations. The summit also includes a broad array of stakeholders, funders, service providers, and community members. Dart (2008) acknowledges that participatory performance story reporting is good for reporting outcomes, but is not appropriate for other purposes, such as cost analysis.

Issues Related to Written Reports

Chilisa (2005) has raised questions about the use of written reports from an indigenous postcolonial perspective. She critiques the privilege that is traditionally given to the written format, suggesting that First World researchers have enjoyed the privilege of the written word and have used the written text as the forum for debate and for legitimizing knowledge.

> Unfortunately, the majority of the researched, who constitute two-thirds of the world, are left out of the debate and do not, therefore, participate in legitimizing the very knowledge they are supposed to produce. The end result has been that ethics protocols of individual consent and notions of confidentiality have been misused to disrespect and make value judgments that are psychologically damaging to communities and nations at large. But, above all, the production of knowledge continues to work within the framework of colonizer/colonized. The colonizer still strives to provide ways of knowing and insists on others to use these paradigms. In the postcolonial era, however, it is important to move beyond knowledge construction by the Western First World as the knower. Resistance to this domination continues and it is attested, among other things, by the current African Renaissance. (Chilisa, 2005, p. 677)

Even when all participants collaborate in writing the final report, it may be published in a format inaccessible to many, such as on websites, in Western journals, or in an electronic format that requires a computer to read. Porter (1995) supports publishing in local journals and with local book publishers, but warns of the economic precariousness that threatens the sustainability of print media in Africa.

Ladd (2003) raises similar issues in his reflections on the privileging of written English over the use of American Sign Language:

> Each discourse contains its own unspoken rules as to what can or cannot be said and how, when and where. Each, therefore, constructs canons of "truth" around whatever its participants decide is "admissible evidence," a process that in the case of certain prestigious discourses, such as those found in universities, medical establishments and communication medias, can be seen as particularly dangerous when unexamined, for these then come to determine what counts as knowledge itself. (p. 76)

Working with Languages That Are Not Written: Challenges

As mentioned at several points in this book, some languages either do not have a written form or include expressions that do not translate well into a written form. Consider, for example, Twesigye's (2005) discussion of problems translating the Bantu language into a written form:

> The academic task of translating oral literatures into written, accurate, and formal texts is a serious challenge in most of Africa. There are forms of oral poetry and literature which were created to be "spoken" and "heard" and will die if written. "Sound," being an essential and symbolic component of the oral tradition, often defies adequate linguistic rendition when written down. For instance, among the Bantu—especially the Banyankore, Bakiga, Batorro, Banyoro, and Bagisu—there are sounds made to indicate disgust, defiance, annoyance, accent, joy, amazement, and the like, which are untranslatable into English or other languages. They are meant to be heard. They speak for themselves. Likewise, oral stories cannot be adequately translated into English or Swahili. This includes p'Bitek's *Song of Lawino*. It was originally writ-

ten in Luo and then later translated into English. Luo cultural nationalists and literary critics both agree that the original text in Luo was better than the English translation. (p. 238)

He continues:

> There is always something lost or added into the text or speech being written from the oral tradition, or translated from one language into another. In some cases, the interpreter may say the very opposite of what the original speaker intended. Some metaphors, expressions, imageries, words, sounds, symbols, ideas, and gestures in one culture may not have equivalents to transfer and translate them in another dissimilar culture, language, world-view, and set of symbolic systems. Imbo (2002) identifies some other factors that complicate the cross-cultural translation of both oral and written texts: (1) the motives of the speaker and interpreter; (2) the age and skill of the interpreter; (3) the number of languages involved; and (4) the conceptual framework of all speakers. (Twesigye, 2005, p. 238)

We have elsewhere discussed challenges associated with working with languages that do not have a written form, such as the Hmong language and American Sign Language. A journal has recently been launched that is completely published online in American Sign Language: *Deaf Studies Digital Journal* (**dsdj.gallaudet.edu**).

Ethics and Reporting

Evaluators sometimes experience pressure to report more favorable (or more unfavorable) results than are warranted by the data. A program director may wish to show the program in its most favorable light to ensure that it will be continued or to have access to increased funding. It is also possible that an agency wants to cut a program, and therefore that staff members will ask for a report that emphasizes the less favorable findings. Here is the description of an experience (adapted from a letter by a real evaluator who will remain nameless) in which the evaluator found that the superintendent of the school district was using the evaluation results to present a far more positive picture of the program than was warranted by the data:

> I am currently facing a situation that I have not encountered before, and I am hoping you can offer some wisdom based on *The Program Evaluation Standards* and the *Guiding Principles for Evaluators*. I completed a report on one of our alternative schools last year that painted a dismal picture of academic performance among students. They came in at risk and left the school, on average, about one grade equivalent lower across various measures. The longer they stayed, the worse their performance. The school is run by a private, for-profit entity, that guaranteed certain academic outcomes for students who stayed one full academic year. There were 4 out of 1,200 who met this criterion. Recently, at a presentation for other educators, our superintendent, in cooperation with the private company, declared the intention of taking this program to the national level based on the strong performance of students. He cited data demonstrating two-plus-grade-equivalent gains in less than one year. I've no idea where he got this data, unless the negative gain signs in my report were altered to be positive. I'm furious; yet, as an in-house evaluator, I'm probably taking a chance even sending this plea. I feel betrayed, and I'm wondering if you can give me any advice.

··········· E X T E N D I N G   Y O U R   T H I N K I N G ···········
Balanced Reporting

1. Review *The Program Evaluation Standards* (Joint Committee on Standards for Educational Evaluation, 2011) and the *Guiding Principles for Evaluators* (AEA, 2004), discussed in Chapter 1. Which of the standards or principles would you cite as appropriate for analyzing this ethical dilemma?

2. Describe what action you would take if you were the evaluator in the situation described in the quotation above. Would you hire a lawyer? Would you seek a meeting with the superintendent? Which other persons would you bring into this conversation, and what would you say to them?

Visual Displays of Results: Tables, Charts, Graphs, and Maps

Some visual strategies for displaying data are also very familiar to academicians, such as the use of bar charts, scatter plots, maps, and (more recently) animated population pyramids and charts (see Google Public Data Explorer: ***www.google.com/publicdata/home***).

The United Nations (2009) document cited earlier in this chapter also leads evaluators through the preparation of tables, charts, maps, and other visual devices for the display of statistical data. A checklist for the development of good visual displays for statistical data is presented in Box 13.6.

Tables

Evaluators use tables to present data in a concise fashion. A few tips for developing tables include these: (1) Provide a meaningful title that answers "what," "where," and "when." (2) Be sure to label all the rows and columns so the reader can easily see the source of the data. Box 13.7 displays a table that was created in the evaluation of the program for teachers of children who are deaf or hard of hearing and who have a disability (Mertens et al., 2007; see Chapter 6, Box 6.10). The title of the table as it was displayed in the report is found at the top. Then columns appear. The first is a list of topics; this is followed by a 5-point scale labeled from "Not at all prepared" to "Very prepared." The data in these columns shows the frequency and percentage of people who responded for each scale point. There is also a column to show how many participants did not answer each item. Two more columns show the average rating of each item and how many people responded to the item.

Charts, Graphs, and Maps

Charts and graphs serve a function similar to that for tabular displays of data, but in a more visually friendly form. Charts and graphs display data in the form of bars or lines that are visually communicative. They are useful to show comparisons of groups, changes over time, frequencies of occurrence, correlations between variables, and comparison of a

Box 13.6. Checklist for Developing Good Data Visualizations

When producing visual presentations, you should think about these things:

- **The target group.** Different forms of presentation may be needed for different audiences (e.g., business vs. academia, specialists vs. the general population).

- **The role of the graphic in the overall presentation.** Analyzing the big picture or focusing attention on key points may require different types of visual presentations.

- **How and where the message will be presented** (e.g., a long, detailed analysis or a quick slideshow).

- **Contextual issues that may distort understanding** (e.g., expert vs. novice data users).

- **Whether textual analysis or a data table would be a better solution.**

- **Accessibility considerations:**

  - Provide text alternatives for nontextual elements, such as charts and images.

  - Don't rely on color alone. If you remove the color, is the presentation still understandable? Do color combinations have sufficient contrast? Do the colors work for color-blind users (e.g., red/green)?

  - Ensure that time-sensitive content can be controlled by the users (e.g., pausing of animated graphics).

- **Consistency across data visualizations.** Ensure that elements within visualizations are designed consistently, and use common conventions where possible (e.g., blue to represent water on a map).

- **Size, duration, and complexity.** Is your presentation easy to understand? Is it too much for the audience to grasp at a given session?

- **Possibility of misinterpretation.** Test your presentation on colleagues, friends, or some people from your target group to see whether they get the intended messages.

Source: Based on United Nations (2009, p. 11).

---

part to the whole (e.g., pie charts). As with all visual displays, your choice of which type of chart or graph to use should be based on the audience and the message you intend to convey. Bar charts are good for presenting comparisons of frequencies, such as the number of deaf people in different countries or the number of math courses taken by ethnicity or race. Line charts are better for displaying trends or changes over time. Pie charts are good for showing frequencies in different parts of a population, but they should not be used if there are numerous segments (usually not more than six slices of a pie are recommended).

Box 13.7. Sample Table That Depicts Quality of Preparation for Teaching on Specific Topics

15. How well prepared were you in your teaching job in the following areas?

	Not at all prepared				Very prepared	N/A	Rating average	Response count
Diverse home languages	6.7% (1)	0.0% (0)	**46.7% (7)**	13.3% (2)	26.7% (4)	6.7% (1)	3.57	15
Deaf culture	0.0% (0)	0.0% (0)	6.7% (1)	6.7% (1)	**86.7% (13)**	0.0% (0)	4.80	15
Program development	0.0% (0)	0.0% (0)	33.3% (5)	13.3% (2)	**40.0% (6)**	13.3% (2)	4.08	15
Special education	6.7% (1)	0.0% (0)	13.3% (2)	26.7% (4)	**53.3% (8)**	0.0% (0)	4.20	15
Learning disabilities	6.7% (1)	0.0% (0)	20.0% (3)	**46.7% (7)**	26.7% (4)	0.0% (0)	3.87	15
Autism	13.3% (2)	0.0% (0)	26.7% (4)	26.7% (4)	33.3% (5)	0.0% (0)	3.67	15
Cerebral palsy	6.7% (1)	6.7% (1)	6.7% (1)	**40.0% (6)**	**40.0% (6)**	0.0% (0)	4.00	15
Severe multiple disabilities	13.3% (2)	0.0% (0)	13.3% (2)	**40.0% (6)**	33.3% (5)	0.0% (0)	3.80	15
Behavior management	0.0% (0)	6.7% (1)	13.3% (2)	**60.0% (9)**	20.0% (3)	0.0% (0)	3.93	15
IEP development	0.0% (0)	13.3% (2)	13.3% (2)	33.3% (5)	**40.0% (6)**	0.0% (0)	4.00	15
Working with parents	0.0% (0)	13.3% (2)	13.3% (2)	**40.0% (6)**	33.3% (5)	0.0% (0)	3.93	15
Working with multi-disciplinary specialists	6.7% (1)	13.3% (2)	20.0% (3)	26.7% (4)	33.3% (5)	0.0% (0)	3.67	15
Working with school faculty/staff/administrators	6.7% (1)	20.0% (3)	20.0% (3)	26.7% (4)	26.7% (4)	0.0% (0)	3.47	15
Diverse communication modes (e.g., ASL, PSE, cued speech, oral, CI)	0.0% (0)	0.0% (0)	33.3% (5)	33.3% (5)	33.3% (5)	0.0% (0)	4.00	15

Source: Mertens, Harris, Holmes, and Brandt (2007, p. 9).

Scatter plots are recommended when the purpose is to show the relationship between two variables (e.g., income and nutrition). With the advent of sophisticated graphics programs built into many word-processing programs, evaluators are no longer limited to these traditional visual displays. Box 13.8 provides a list of suggestions for developing charts.

Box 13.8. Checklist for Developing Good Charts

When producing charts, you should think about these things:

- The **chart title** should give a clear idea of what the chart is about. It has to be short and concise. You can have two types of titles:

  - An **informative title** provides all the information needed to understand the data. It should answer the three questions "what," "where," and "when."

  - A **descriptive title** is a caption that highlights the main pattern or trend displayed in the chart. It states in a few words the story that the chart illustrates.

- The **axis labels** should identify the values displayed in the chart. The labels should be displayed horizontally on both axes.

- The **axis titles** should identify the unit of measure of the data (e.g., "in thousands," "%," "age (in years)," or "$"). You do not need to include an axis title when the unit of measure is obvious (e.g., "years" for time series).

- **Gridlines** can be added in bar and line charts to help users read and compare the values of the data.

- The **legend and data labels** should identify the symbols, patterns, or colors used to represent the data in the chart. The legend should not be displayed when only one series of values is represented in the chart. Whenever possible, you should use data labels rather than a legend. Data labels are displayed on or next to the data components (bars, areas, lines) to facilitate their identification and understanding.

- A **footnote** may be used to provide definitions or methodological information.

- The **data source** should be identified at the bottom of the chart.

Source: Based on United Nations (2009, pp. 23–24).

Figure 13.1 shows a simple bar chart. Figure 13.2 shows a more complex bar chart. Figure 13.3 shows a variation of a bar chart known as a stacked bar chart. Figure 13.4 shows a map as a visual method of displaying data. Figure 13.5 shows a line graph that displays trends over years for math scores. Figure 13.6 displays a pie chart of HIV infection rates broken down by men, women, and children globally. And Figure 13.7 displays another pie chart based on costs of a project.

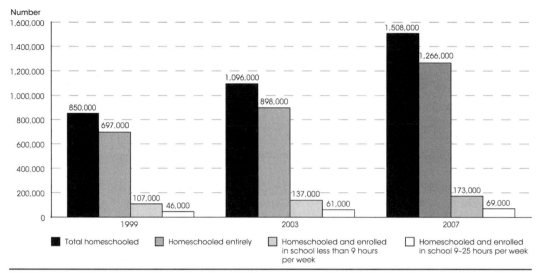

NOTE: Homeschooled students are school-age children (ages 5–17) in a grade equivalent to at least kindergarten and not higher than 12th grade. Excludes students who were enrolled in public or private school more than 25 hours per week and students who were homeschooled only because of temporary illness. For more information on the National Household Education Surveys Program (NHES), see *supplemental note 3*.
SOURCE: U.S. Department of Education, National Center for Education Statistics, Parent Survey of the 1999 National Household Education Surveys Program (NHES), Parent and Family Involvement in Education Survey of the 2003 and 2007 NHES.

Figure 13.1. Percentage of school-age children who were homeschooled, by reasons parents gave as the most important reason for homeschooling: 2007. *Source:* Planty et al. (2009, Figure 6-2).

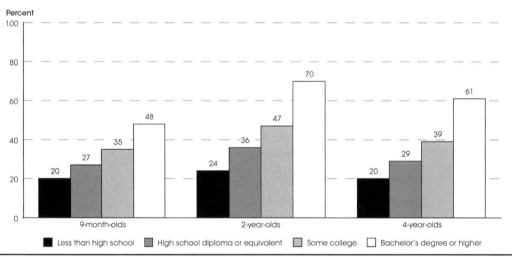

NOTE: The Early Childhood Longitudinal Study, Birth Cohort (ECLS-B) sampled children born in 2001. Each age variable corresponds with the year of the estimate. For example, the 9-month estimates for "Read to" reflect the percentage of children whose parents read to them daily in a typical week at the time of the 9-month data collection. For more information on parents' education, see *supplemental note 1*; for more information on the ECLS-B, see *supplemental note 3*.
SOURCE: U.S. Department of Education, National Center for Education Statistics, Early Childhood Longitudinal Study, Birth Cohort (ECLS-B), Longitudinal 9-month–Preschool Restricted-Use Data File (NCES 2008-034).

Figure 13.2. Percentage of 9-month-olds, 2-year-olds, and 4-year-olds read to, told stories, and sung to daily in a typical week by a family member, by mother's education: 2001–02, 2003–04, and 2005–06. *Source:* Planty et al. (2009, Figure 2-1).

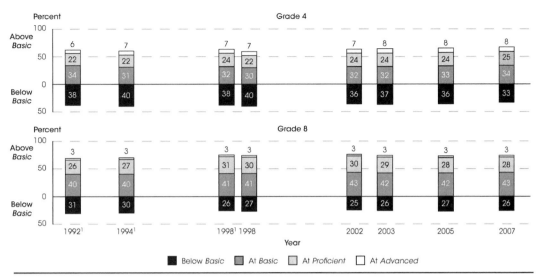

¹ Testing accommodations (e.g., extended time, small group testing) for children with disabilities and limited-English-proficient students were not permitted.
NOTE: The National Assessment of Educational Progress (NAEP) achievement levels define what students should know and be able to do: *Basic* indicates partial mastery of fundamental skills; *Proficient* indicates demonstrated competency over challenging subject matter; and *Advanced* indicates superior performance. For more information on NAEP, see *supplemental note 4*. Detail may not sum to totals because of rounding.
SOURCE: U.S. Department of Education, National Center for Education Statistics, National Assessment of Educational Progress (NAEP), selected years, 1992–2007 Reading Assessments, NAEP Data Explorer.

Figure 13.3. Percentage distribution of 4th- and 8th-grade students across NAEP reading achievement levels: Selected years, 1992–2007. *Source:* Planty et al. (2009, Figure 2-1).

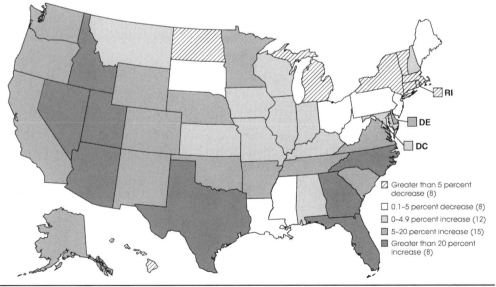

NOTE: The most recent year of actual data is 2006, and 2018 is the last year for which projected data are available. For more information on projections, see NCES 2009-062. For a list of states in each region, see *supplemental note 1*.
SOURCE: U.S. Department of Education, National Center for Education Statistics (NCES), Common Core of Data (CCD), "State Nonfiscal Survey of Public Elementary/Secondary Education," 2006–07; and Public State Elementary and Secondary Enrollment Model, 1980–2006.

Figure 13.4. Projected percent change in public school enrollment in grades prekindergarten through 12, by state: Between fall 2006 and fall 2018. *Source:* Planty et al. (2009, Figure 4-2).

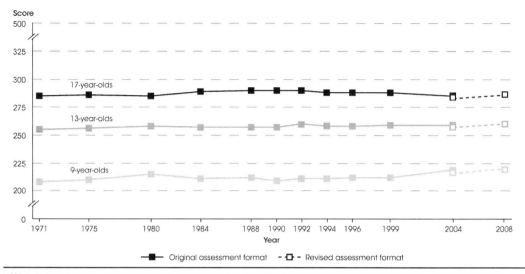

NOTE: Includes public and private schools. NAEP scores range from 0 to 500. Scores for the revised assessment format reflect the inclusion of and accommodations for students with disabilities and English language learners. For more information on NAEP, see *supplemental note 4.* SOURCE: Rampey, B.D., Dion, G.S., and Donahue, P.L. (2009). *NAEP 2008 Trends in Academic Progress in Reading and Mathematics* (NCES 2009-479). National Center for Education Statistics, Institute of Education Sciences, U.S. Department of Education, Washington, DC.

Figure 13.5. Average reading scale scores on the long–term trend National Assessment of Educational Progress (NAEP), by age: Various years, 1971 through 2008. *Source:* Planty et al. (2009, Figure 14-1).

Women are increasingly becoming infected with HIV:

In 1997, 41% of adults living with HIV/AIDS worldwide were women; by 2001, this figure had risen to 50%.

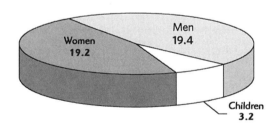

Figure 13.6. Proportion of men, women, and children infected with HIV worldwide (in millions). *Source:* UNFPA, UNAIDS, and UNIFEM (n.d., p. 8). Reprinted by permission of UNIFEM.

Presentations and Performances

Concerns about the fact that written reports often go unused, as well as about inappropriate uses of written reports to exclude and possibly oppress important constituencies, have led to the development of presentation- and performance-oriented reporting. These are described next.

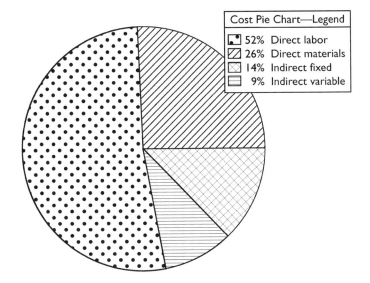

Figure 13.7. Pie chart showing the cost percentages associated with the four-cost categories: direct materials, direct labor, indirect variable, and indirect fixed. *Source:* Linton et al. (1994, Figure 11). Copyright 1994 by Sage Publications Ltd. Reprinted by permission.

Presentations

Some of the presentation strategies for evaluation reporting are taken directly from the world of academia, in which formal presentations are made at conferences or to groups assembled for the purpose of the presentations. The use of PowerPoint slide shows is common in professional presentations. Box 13.9 contains a list of suggestions from AEA for professional presentations.

Several books have been written that also will help you spice up your presentations (Duarte, 2008; Reynolds, 2008; Tufte, 2001).

Slide shows and videos can also be used in community-based reporting. Cardoza Clayson, Castañeda, Sanchez, and Brindis (2002) used a 20-minute slide presentation on civic engagement to disseminate information about effective strategies for recent immigrants to become involved in the government in their communities. Lai (2009) used a video of indigenous peoples from Hawaii to disseminate the results of his evaluation in their native language.

Evaluators can also use focus groups to present reports, as well as to get feedback on their findings. In addition, as mentioned in Chapter 12 on data analysis, community-based meetings can allow for interpretation of findings and for commentary on the reports themselves.

Other presentation forms are anchored in some of the data collection strategies discussed in Chapter 10. For example, community-based data collection methods yield immediate results that can be viewed by everyone present. Visual data that are collected by means of "photovoice" (when participants are given voice by using cameras to take pictures of things that are important to them) can be used in conjunction with interviews with the photographers to elicit their interpretations of the data. The reporting of the results can include the display of pictures.

Box 13.9. Suggestions for Professional Presentations

■ **Prepare your presentation:** Consider the time available, the audience's likely desire to ask questions, and the multiple learning styles of attendees (auditory, visual, etc.), when preparing to create a memorable and valuable presentation.

■ **Identify the time allocated:** As part of the ongoing preconference discussion, clarify the time to be allocated to your presentation. If you are presenting a paper [at an AEA meeting], you will have 15 minutes. However, if you are part of a panel, demonstration, think tank, etc., then you will need to determine among the presenters how much time is to be devoted to what content.

■ **Determine when questions and discussion will take place:** Again, as part of the preconference discussion, identify the time to be devoted to questions and discussion and whether you will take questions during your presentation or only afterwards. If you are presenting a paper, you may choose to take questions during your 15-minute presentation time; however, you must cede the floor at the end of 15 minutes, and there will be an open question time at the end of the session.

■ **Plan your presentation:** Create an outline for yourself of the key points to be conveyed and then develop notes regarding what you wish to share relating to each key point. Develop visual aids (see below) to illustrate your key points and serve as an outline to the session.

■ **Prepare visual aids:** The vast majority of presenters use overhead transparencies, PowerPoint slides, or other visual aids as part of their presentation. Each room [at an AEA meeting] is equipped with a traditional transparency projector for plastic transparencies, an LCD projector, a computer, and a screen.

■ **Type:** Use at least 24-point type so that it may easily be read from across the room. Avoid *italics* and ALL CAPS for more than a few words as they are difficult to read.

■ **Bullets:** Limit yourself to at most 6 bullets per slide and 10 or so words per bullet. Describe details verbally and use the bullet points to provide an outline of key concepts.

■ **Number:** A rough rule of thumb is to prepare no more than one slide for every two minutes you will be presenting. This is an upper limit. The slides are an aid, not the presentation itself.

■ **Avoid acronyms, jargon, and abbreviations:** Past evaluations have clearly indicated that one frustration, in particular for new and international attendees, is the use of "insider" language, acronyms, and abbreviations that make it difficult to comprehend readily a presentation.

■ **Contact information slide:** Prepare one slide that you can put up at the beginning and end of the presentation with your presentation title, name, and contact information. In case you do not have enough handouts, encourage attendees to write down this information for follow-up.

Source: American Evaluation Association (2010).

Use of photographs needs to be negotiated very carefully, to protect the identity of all those who might be made more vulnerable if their identities were revealed. For example, Frohmann (2005) conducted a study of an art therapy intervention for battered women that included having the women take pictures that depicted their experiences in battering relationships, how they extricated themselves from those relationships, and how they kept themselves safe now. The pictures they took included the following:

> Participants photographed safety strategies, which included their zones of safety, such as the bathroom and bedrooms where they sought refuge from the battering, and lookout posts to watch for signs of impending violence, such as a chair a participant sat in that provided her a clear vantage point from which to see all the doors and rooms of the house. Others documented preparations for leaving, such as one woman's photograph of her grabbing her coat and keys that always hung at the back door for easy escape. They also photographed zones of violence, such as the kitchen, or the house where a participant and her husband lived when the battering first began. (p. 1413)

Reporting took place at the individual and community levels. The women first put their pictures in a logical order to tell their story; they then narrated their stories. Frohmann (2005) noted that in telling their own stories, many of the women gained insights that stimulated them to make changes in their lives. A second phase of the study involved displaying the pictures to the wider community. The individual women decided what pictures would be displayed and the extent to which they wanted to mask their identities. Some chose to use their own names, others to use pseudonyms, and still others to be anonymous. The women also controlled the amount of detail that they revealed in conjunction with their photographs. The purpose of the public display was to educate the community about the experience of living in an abusive relationship. Here is the description of the exhibits:

> The exhibits have been held at a social service agency, the Mexican consulate, a café, and a conference. Efforts were made to widely publicize the events through such avenues as sending invitations to all the domestic violence service agencies in the metro area, and announcements in all Spanish- and English-language area newspapers and entertainment guides. Having one exhibit at the Mexican consulate gave high level official recognition of battered women's situations and was empowering to the women. It also brought the exhibit to a much broader audience. For example, persons waiting in line at the consulate for visas and other documents were taken in groups to view the exhibit. Thus, at least 1,000 people viewed the exhibit over the 2-month period it was on display. (Frohmann, 2005, p. 1410)

The women in the study engaged in ongoing meetings with a counselor during the exhibition period, to deal with their changing emotional states. The visual displays served as a reporting mechanism as well as a stimulus for social action. This study also serves as an example of the use of a feminist lens throughout the study. From the conceptualization to the reporting, the author was aware of feminist theory informing her work.

Performance: Ethnodrama

The first time I became aware of ethnodrama as a method of reporting evaluation results, I was organizing a strand of sessions for the International Sociological Association on nondiscriminatory and emancipatory methods. We received a submission from James Mienczakowski in which he proposed to present on a method called "ethnodrama," using his work on changing conditions in a hospital that served patients battling drug and alcohol addiction. I rejected the proposal because it did not look like the traditional scholarly reporting that I was used to. Fortunately, Mienczakowski had the wisdom to submit his proposal to another subsection, and fortunately, that subsection had the wisdom to accept it. When I attended the conference, a number of people attended Mienczakowski's presentation and told me how impressed they were with this method of reporting, which actually attracted large audiences and stimulated changes. Not being one to wallow in my mistakes, I approached Mienczakowski about submitting a chapter based on his work for a book on research and inequality about the ethnodrama approach to reporting results. Fortunately for all of us, he agreed.

Mienczakowski (2000; Mienczakowski & Morgan, 2001) said that he adopted this approach because he was aware of how few people actually read most academic reports. Therefore, he combined ethnography and drama to share data with various constituencies in a way that facilitated discussion about the results and development of strategies for change. Mienczakowski and Morgan (2006) used ethnodrama as a reporting mechanism for a study of recovery from sexual attacks. They developed a script that used the data collected during their ethnographic study, and then shared the script with the stakeholders for validation. The script was made up of narratives from the qualitative data that were organized according to the emergent themes. Then the evaluators scheduled a performance of the script with the stakeholder group as the first audience, in order to ensure that the script as implemented was also viewed as a valid portrayal of their experiences. The change-directed part of the ethnodrama comes in the form of a detailed performance guidebook that staff can use to prepare the audience before the production and to lead discussions after the performance. The cast and audience can engage in discussions together as well. The point is for the audience members to leave the performance with ideas on how to modify their practice.

Ethical issues also surface with the use of ethnodrama, especially with such emotionally charged topics as drug or alcohol abuse or sexual attacks. It may be necessary to have counselors on hand, just as Frohmann (2005) did in the study of battered women described above.

Bridging Data Analysis, Interpretation, and Utilization: Lessons Learned

As others have noted, sometimes we do not know what we understand or how we interpret data until we sit down to write about it. Eisner (1979b) offers a set of questions that evaluators can use to move from data analysis to interpretation to use of findings in evaluation:

> Such participation makes it possible for readers to know that aspect of classroom life emotionally. Through it they are able to know what only the artistic use of language can provide.
>
> Educational criticism, however, is not limited to the artistic description of events. It also includes their interpretation and appraisal. Interpretation as we conceive it is the process of applying theoretical ideas to explain the conditions that have been described. Why is it that this classroom functions in this particular way? Why do these side effects occur? How does the

reward structure of this classroom shape the relationships students have with one another? How is time used in this classroom and why does it mean what it means to students? Questions such as these require answers that are more than descriptive, they require the application of relevant theory in the social sciences. The application of such theories to the qualities that have been described constitutes the second important phase or aspect of educational criticism.

The third phase or aspect of educational criticism is concerned with appraisal or evaluation. What is the educational significance of what children have learned? What is the educational import of what has transpired? What are the educational trade-offs among the pedagogical devices that the teacher has used and were there alternatives that could have been selected? Please note that this last question begins to soften the distinction between appraisal and supervision and/or "coaching." When an educational critic appraises in a way which is designed to provide constructive feedback to the teacher, evaluation begins to perform its most important function: providing the conditions that lead to the improvement of the educational process. In some respect this function of educational evaluation is analogous to the function the conductor performs when guiding an orchestra in the performance of a symphony. The conductor's task is first to hear what the orchestra is playing and to assess it against the schema of the music that he holds. Second, the conductor must locate the discrepancy between the schema and the performance and then provide feedback. (p. 16)

Consideration of the Intended Users and Intended Uses

In the very early days of evaluation, this section might have been titled "Consider the Audience." However, Patton's (2008) groundbreaking work on uses of evaluation shifted attention from a *passive* portrayal of an audience to the *dynamic* portrayal of intended users. Evaluators in all four branches would agree that the intended users for and intended uses of information need to be considered in the preparation and delivery of reports.

Recall that *The Program Evaluation Standards* (Joint Committee, 2011) list "utility" as the first category for judging the quality of an evaluation (see Chapter 1, Box 1.5). However, differences surface in the various branches as to the meaning of use and the responsibility of evaluators to ensure use. Part of the confusion in this discourse is based on definitions of the term "use." Patton (2008, pp. 102–104) offers five nonexclusive categories of use; the listing below is based on his five categories.

1. *Instrumental use*, in which evaluation findings directly inform decision making or problem solving. If a school decides on the basis of evaluation data to adopt a new curriculum, then this is an example of instrumental use. Marra's (2000) study of corruption included analysis of instrumental use, in that she and her colleagues interviewed decision makers to determine whether they took direct action to achieve their goals as a result of the evaluation. Examples of instrumental use that they discovered included revision of training materials for journalists reporting on corruption so that these reflected actual conditions in different regions of Africa, as well as translation of materials into French for Francophone countries. The decision makers also hired local consultants to develop simulation exercises that reflected local conditions.

2. *Conceptual use*, in which evaluation findings influence how key people think. For example, policy makers may understand an issue better after an evaluation although it may not lead to direct action. Weiss (2004) has labeled this category "enlightenment" and suggested that exposure to evaluation findings may percolate over an indefinite amount

of time and resurface as directives for action at that time. Marra (2000) and her colleagues also looked at enlightenment use to determine whether the evaluation generated findings that eventually emerged as a stimulus for action. They found that the program developers engaged in deep discussions about various theories of corruption and the prevention of corruption and that these discussions influenced their theory about the program. They produced a strategy paper that outlined their understandings of the different theories. They planned to use this paper as a basis for redesigning the curriculum.

3. *Symbolic use*, in which the evaluation is primarily conducted for the sake of appearances and the decision makers have no intention of actually using the results to change anything. This might have been the case with the Mertens et al. (2007) evaluation of the teacher preparation study if the team had not devised ways to bring the findings to a wider community.

4. *Persuasive use*, in which the evaluation findings are used selectively to support a previously held position. For example, the Just Say No program to prevent early pregnancies (discussed in Chapter 15) is not effective, but it conforms to some people's views of morally correct behavior; therefore, they will select those portions of the reporting to bolster their case to continue funding such a program. If the data actually support the position, then there is no problem with using the data to persuade others of its merits.

5. *Legitimate utilization*, in which evaluation data are used to support a program that the decision makers have already decided to support. Leviton (2003) and Owen and Rogers (1999) have all described this type of use. The decision makers simply use the data to legitimize the continuation of the program. There is no problem with this unless the data are manipulated to make a case that does not exist.

As you can see, some of the recognized uses of evaluations might be more accurately labeled "misuses." This raises questions about evaluators' responsibilities in terms of the uses or misuses of their findings.

Concerns about lack of use of evaluation findings are not new; they have been discussed for all the many years that I have worked as an evaluator. Although Patton has written about this topic since the early 1970s and has contributed much to the understanding of this topic, concerns continue to be expressed by evaluators, funding agencies, and communities. Several evaluators have conducted research on how decision makers use data and what factors influence use of the data. Johnson et al. (2009) reviewed 25 years of research on use of evaluation studies. They concluded from the empirical data that

> stakeholder involvement is a mechanism that facilitates those aspects of an evaluation's process or setting that lead to greater use. More than just involvement by stakeholders or decision makers alone, however, the findings from this literature review suggest that engagement, interaction, and communication between evaluation clients and evaluators is key to maximizing the use of the evaluation in the long run. (p. 389)

In addition, they found that the perceived competence of the evaluator was also an important factor that influenced use.

Christie (2007) explored how decision makers use data. She created a simulation exercise that asked participants to indicate which three types of data would influence their decision making: large-scale study, case study, and anecdotal accounts. The participants were advanced graduate students in educational leadership departments who had prior experience and were currently working in leadership positions. They were told that a specific decision needed to be made. Participants then indicated the extent of influence that each of the types of data had on their decisions. Overall, decision makers were influenced more by large-scale and case study data than by anecdotal accounts. However, different groups of decision makers were influenced more by one type of evaluation data than by the other two. Participants working in K–12 public schools or district offices were less likely to be influenced by large-scale study data than were those working in other organizations. Christie (2007) suggests that evaluators ask decision makers about the type of evaluation information that would be most influential in their particular social and political context.

How Do Lessons Learned from Evaluations Influence the Impact of Evaluations?

On February 8, 2010, Samuel Norgah asked a question about the use of evaluation findings and the nature or quality of the lessons learned as a partial determinant of the use of those findings. These results stimulated an interesting discussion on the AfrEA (see Chapter 1) listserv about these topics. Box 13.10 contains the text of Norgah's email, which is reproduced with his permission.

The United Nations Environment Programme (UNEP) maintains a database of lessons learned from the evaluations that it sponsors. Spilsbury, Perch, Norgbey, Rauniyar, and Battaglino (2007) reported on the quality of the lessons learned from this database. They used the Organization for Economic Cooperation and Development (OECD) with the Development Assistance Committee's (DAC) (n.d., p. 5) definition of lessons learned: "Generalizations based on evaluation experiences with projects, programs, or policies that abstract from the specific circumstances to broader situations. Frequently, lessons highlight strengths or weaknesses in preparation, design, and implementation that affect performance, outcome, and impact." Box 13.11 displays examples of lessons learned from an evaluation of international development programs for people with disabilities (Albert, 2005).

Note that the OECD DAC (n.d.) makes a distinction between recommendations (project-specific suggestions for actions) and lessons learned (generalizations of conclusions applicable for wider use). Not every agency makes this distinction; for example, the Catholic Relief Services (n.d.) organization includes project-specific recommendations as lessons learned. Spilsbury et al. (2007) went on to define the characteristics of a good statement of lessons learned as follows: It should

- Concisely capture the context from which it is derived.

- Be applicable in a different context (generic), have a clear "application domain," and identify target users.

- Suggest a prescription and guide action.

The results of their analysis, however, suggested that 50% of the lessons learned in the UNEP database did not meet these minimal requirements for quality. Spilsbury et al. suggested that the reasons for suboptimal impact of UNEP evaluation lessons could be categorized as follows:

Box 13.10. Lessons Learned in Evaluation

De: "Norgah, Samuel"
AfrEA Listserv <afrea@yahoogroups.com>
Envoyle: Lun 8 Février 2010, 14 h 33 min 25 s
Objet: [AfrEA] Lessons Learnt

Dear friends,

I've been struggling to understand what 'evaluators' mean by 'lessons learnt' whenever they conduct evaluations for us. To a large extent, what is captured as lessons are just obvious statements and observations, please see examples below which I captured from an evaluation which was recently conducted for one of our offices.

Child-Centred Community Development (CCCD): Lessons Learned

- Orchestrating the evolution of CCCD as a rights-based approach requires continuous support and consistent leadership and communication.

- Most Plan-supported communities and partners have not been adequately engaged in a dialogue to understand the concepts and implications of Plan's CCCD approach, making effective partnership a challenge.

- A stronger and more regular engagement with partners' and sub-contractors' activities is needed to better ensure that project objectives and targets are met.

- Identifying and engaging with grass-roots civil society organizations and groups demands a proper mapping of such organizations and groups, and going beyond working exclusively with established local leaders.

As you can see from the examples above, most of the statements above are very obvious. I will like to know what people think about 'lessons learnt' and what should be captured. I'm also wondering whether this 'development expression' is being abused!

Samuel Norgah
Westlands, Nairobi (Kenya)

- Imperfect project design (lack of ownership and shared vision with stakeholders during the design and implementation of the projects).

- Inefficient project management (delays in implementation due to slow recruitment of project staff, poor coordination, ineffective communication, poor fund management, inadequate dissemination and outreach, and high transition costs because of lack of capacity building with local experts).

- Suboptimal processes for realizing impact (lack of ownership and legitimacy of proposed outcomes because of lack of stakeholder involvement; avoidance of difficult but important issues; lack of a "critical mass" because of too many project activities during too short a time frame).

Rick Davies (2009a) suggests that evaluators consider a half-day workshop to derive meaningful lessons learned. The structure could involve distribution of materials before the meeting; a short presentation highlighting key findings; small-group discussions, possibly organized by stakeholder groups, to identify lessons learned that the groups view as useful; and then a report back to the larger group for discussion of recommendations of lessons learned. Evaluators can facilitate the process by providing possible categories for the lessons learned and by providing examples of good lessons learned from other studies. See Davies (2009b) for more resources about lessons learned.

Box 13.11. Lessons Learned from an Evaluation of International Development Programs for People with Disabilities

Lesson 1: Supporting local DPOs [Disabled people's organizations]:

With an increasing proportion of aid being provided in ways which limit the ability to impose micro-level conditions, one of the most potent ways for DFID [the U.K. Department for International Development] to ensure disability gets included in development is by supporting disabled people's organisations (DPOs). Among other things, this gives disabled people the capacity to lobby for their rights and hold their governments to account. The Disability Policy Officer makes a strong case for this in all her reports. Practical examples of how this plays out are also detailed in the Disability KaR [Knowledge and Research] reports. *The Role and Effectiveness of Disability Legislation in South Africa—Promoting Inclusion: Disabled People, Legislation and Public Policy* asks "are disabled people's voices from both South and North being heard in the development process?"

Lesson 2: Ensuring disability issues are included in all processes relating to new aid instruments:

DFID engages in and supports efforts to collect data for such studies as Poverty Social Impact Analyses (PSIAs) which help prepare the ground for aid interventions. It is, therefore, in a position to make sure that disability is explicitly included in such processes.

Besides giving general support to DPOs, the Disability Policy Officer also sees a more specific role for DFID. This role is to include DPOs in consultations on Country Assistant Plans (CAPs) as well as providing assistance so that DPOs can participate effectively as part of civil society in formulating Poverty Reduction Strategy Papers (PRSPs). A case study of this is offered in the Disability KaR report *Participation of Disabled People in the PRSP Process in Uganda*.

Source: Miller and Albert (2005, p. 38).

··········· **E X T E N D I N G   Y O U R   T H I N K I N G** ···········
Lessons Learned

UNICEF (2009b) distinguishes among innovations, lessons learned, and good practices:

> Innovations are summaries of programmatic or operational innovations that have or
> are being implemented under UNICEF's mandate. These innovations may be pilot proj-
> ects or new approaches to a standard programming model that can demonstrate initial
> results.
>
> Lessons learned are more detailed reflections on a particular programme or opera-
> tion and extraction of lessons learned through its implementation. These lessons may
> be positive (successes) or negative (failures). Lessons learned have undergone a wider
> review than innovations and have often been implemented over a longer time frame.
>
> Good practices are well documented and assessed programming practices that pro-
> vide evidence of success/impact and which are valuable for replication, scaling up and
> further study. They are generally based on similar experiences from different countries
> and contexts.

Since 2000, UNICEF has annually compiled lessons learned in its five focus
areas: (1) young children's survival and development, (2) basic education and gender
equality, (3) HIV/AIDS and children, (4) protection of children from violence and
abuse, and (5) policy advocacy and partnerships for children's rights. Open UNI-
CEF's (2009a) compendium of lessons learned from its 2007 program (*www.uni-
cef.org/evaluation/files/llcompexternal2007_17feb09.pdf*). Select one of the five focus
areas and read the brief summary, including the lessons learned.

1. Which program did you pick? Do the lessons learned fit UNICEF's own
   description of a lesson learned?

2. Does the lesson learned fit the OECD DAC's definition of a lesson learned
   (see text above)?

3. Identify an innovation and a good practice in the program you have
   selected.

Sustainability and Evaluation Use

We have discussed sustainability in Chapter 8 in connection with evaluation purposes. In
this section of this chapter, we examine sustainability as an indicator of evaluation use
for considering long-term consequences once project funding from an outside source is
removed. The EU has required social programs to demonstrate sustainability for many
years; its member nations sponsor a conference and training on this topic annually (see
www.sustainability.at/easy).

Sometimes sustainability is conceived of as continuing a program after external funds
are no longer available. However, Rogers and Williams (2008) have identified several other

possible aspects of sustainability, such as improved skills within the community, improved systems for delivery of services, and capacity building of program participants. Therefore, sustainability can be considered in contexts in which project activities themselves are not sustained. Rogers and Williams suggest that evaluators engage in planning activities with the stakeholders to prioritize the parts of the project that may need to be sustained. They offer the following as possible ways to improve sustainability:

- Identify organizations that could support activities in the future (e.g., identify a funding stream for the project or incorporate its activities into another organization). If this is to be accomplished, the project staff and evaluators need to begin planning early, before the original funding ends. The selection of a partner organization needs to consider the alignment of missions and goals of the project and the intended partner.

- Develop networks and partnerships to nurture potential partnerships and community ownership (e.g., begin sharing tasks with partners, build relationships, create opportunities for people from the community to become involved, and formalize the network or partnership through such means as a memorandum of understanding).

- Support skills development in fund raising and in project management (e.g., train local people to manage and implement the program, teach them to advocate for themselves, and alert partners to possible funding sources).

- Demonstrate results and promote the project, both within the community to enhance ownership and outside the community to generate wider support (e.g., plan for promotional events, and disseminate reports in a variety of formats and venues).

- Create an overall strategy that incorporates sustainability by creating an awareness of the importance of sustainability early in the project's life (e.g., begin discussions with community members about the importance of sustainability based on addressing a critical need; give consideration to sustainability of some aspects of the project if it is not feasible to continue it in its entirety; and possibly consider establishing a specific group to address sustainability, such as a task force).

- Respond to external factors such as changes in policies at all levels of government (e.g., maintain contact with legislators to inform them of the importance and results of the project and the need for continued funding, capitalize on opportunities that appear from other sources, and revise the project without sacrificing its integrity to appear to meet emerging political priorities).

Recall from Chapter 8 the sustainability evaluation of social service projects in Israel (Savaya et al., 2008). This evaluation confirmed the importance of a project's finding a host organization that shared the project's mission, saw the importance of the services provided, fought for its survival, and developed a network of support for the project in the broader community. Savaya et al. write:

> What emerges ... is that the key to program sustainability is the human factor—namely, the leadership of the host organization. The heads of the host organization of the programs that survived fought hard to keep the programs alive and understood what was needed to do so.

Appreciating the paramount importance of funding, they had the foresight not to wait for funds to come to them and the drive and interpersonal skills to actively market the program to raise funds from a variety of sources and to cultivate champions in the community and in government agencies to help in these endeavors. When problems or obstacles arose, they exercised determination, ingenuity, and flexibility to overcome them in many ways, for example, cutting costs, lobbying, or mounting public protests. They had the patience to maneuver within the government bureaucracy. It was also the decisions of the host organization leadership that ensured sustenance of the surviving programs by giving them high priority and integrating them into the organization's structure. (p. 490)

·········· E X T E N D I N G   Y O U R   T H I N K I N G ··········

Sustainability

1. What characteristics of Savaya et al.'s (2008) findings confirm the factors related to sustainability that were reported by Rogers and Williams (2008)?

2. How can evaluators contribute to the following:

    a. Procurement of alternative funding sources?

    b. Demonstration of effectiveness?

    c. Communication of a project's effectiveness?

    d. Planning for future sustainability?

    e. Development of partnerships and community ownership?

3. Explore other resources about sustainability, to determine how you can include this concept in your evaluation plan.

Influencing Policy[1]

Policy analysis is a discipline unto itself, and it is not possible to address this topic in all of its complexity. Rather, we focus here on the link between evaluation and policy. The evaluator's role may not have traditionally included influencing policy; however, given the potential for evaluators to engage in this type of activity, Benjamin and Greene (2009) suggest that the evaluator's role be reconceptualized to include this dimension. This might also include expanding the notion of the evaluand as a bounded system to make it more inclusive of the wider social and political context. "The complex reasons for this shift include the recognition that effective solutions to problems depend on the coordination of many actors—nonprofit, for profit, and public organizations, working at the local, state, national, and international levels" (Benjamin & Greene, 2009, p. 297). They recommend focusing and describing such efforts in economic terms—the language of policy makers. Based on their work evaluating a collaborative to strengthen the field of early care and education, they framed their own work in this way: "Driving the team's work was the explicit assumption that reframing [early care and education] in economic terms would spur new action and investment in this sector, leading to a high-quality, accessible, and affordable early care and education system in the United States" (Benjamin & Greene, 2009, p. 297).

Two U.S.-based organizations have developed materials that provide guidance to evaluators in working with other stakeholders to influence policy: the California Endowment, a foundation that supports equity in access to health services, and the Work Group on Health Promotion and Community Development at the University of Kansas in Lawrence, a grassroots organization. Both of these organizations developed their materials within the U.S. context; therefore, some limitations in transferability to other contexts need to be acknowledged.

Guthrie, Louie, David, and Foster (2005; cited in Mertens, 2009) wrote a report for the California Endowment and other foundations to guide their work in assessing projects that addressed policy change and advocacy. I adapted their principles to focus more on the community members' role in policy and advocacy projects (Mertens, 2009, pp. 337–338):

Step 1: Adopt a conceptual model for understanding the process of policy change. Involvement of key stakeholders is critical to ensure that contextual factors are understood and strategies for making change are articulated through a communal effort.

Step 2: Develop a theory about how and why planned activities lead to desired outcomes (often called a "theory of change"). Continued stakeholder involvement is needed to clarify how the group's activities are expected to lead to the desired change, to build a common language, and to reach consensus on the desired outcomes.

Step 3: Select benchmarks to monitor progress (benchmarks are outcomes that indicate change or progress). Because policy change is a complicated process, benchmarks need to be developed that address such issues as constituency and coalition building, conduct of necessary research, education of policy makers, and media and public information campaigns. In addition, outcomes need to be included that indicate the capacity building of the community members themselves in their role in policy and advocacy projects.

Step 4: Prepare a policy change proposal and bring it to the attention of the policy makers. Recognize the complexity of the policy environment and the many factors that influence policy decisions. Because timing is of the essence in the policy world, policy initiatives need to be introduced at the right time of the policy-making cycle.

Step 5: Collect data and measure progress toward benchmarks. Additional capacity building and resources may be needed to (a) support the collection of data that document changes in policy or (b) create advocacy activities to that end.

The following links provide additional information on the California Endowment's resources on policy and advocacy:

- *www.calendow.org/Article.aspx?id=1800&ItemID=1800* (California Endowment publications)
- *www.calendow.org/Category.aspx?id=342&ItemID=342* (California Endowment and advocacy)

The Work Group on Health Promotion and Community Development at the University of Kansas has developed a Community Tool Box (CTB) in collaboration with AHEC/

Community Partners in Amherst, Massachusetts. This information is available at the CTB website (*ctb.ku.edu/en/tablecontents/index.aspx*), which contains a list of core competencies and toolkits. These toolkits are organized to help communities gain access to frameworks within which to organize their work. They also provide examples of how the work could be accomplished, as well as links to specific tools in the CTB and to the CTB Learning Community, which includes forums and chat rooms for individual support. The CTB begins with a framework for community development and includes many useful steps for agenda setting, promotion of ideas through the media, development of a strategic plan, and leadership skill building.

Evaluation and Public Policy in International Development

The use of evaluation to influence policy is evident in the international development communities' commitment to the reduction of poverty. For example, each country formulates a Poverty Reduction Strategy (PRS) that is reviewed by the World Bank and the International Monetary Fund to determine the extent of funding it will approve. The PRS is the primary policy document for a country to obtain funding for poverty reduction. The PRS papers are reviewed on a periodic basis as a means to implementing iterative, evidence-based policy making. Thus evaluators, working in concert with country representatives, have an important opportunity to influence decisions in all sectors.

UNIFEM (2010) has published a guide to involvement of evaluators in the PRS process. This guide identifies possible entry points for evaluation information to be fed into the development, implementation, and review of PRS policies. These could include diagnosis and analysis of poverty in terms of the extent of the problem and policies to address it; capacity development during implementation stages; and development of a monitoring and evaluation framework that allows for progress reports and for formulation of lessons learned. The UNIFEM (2010) guidebook also includes additional resources, suggestions on how to set up an effective advocacy or lobbying strategy, and many examples of successful cases.

Box 13.12 lists several relevant web-based resources on influencing the development and revision of poverty reduction policies.

Here is an example of using evaluation results to make policy recommendations:

> Since the mid-90s, the government of the Indian state of Andhra Pradesh has been encouraging women-only grassroots organisations at the village level called Self-Help Groups (SHGs). By 2007, over 700,000 such groups had been formed, partly facilitated by two externally funded programmes supported by [the U.K. Department for International Development] and the World Bank which provided funds and technical training to SHGs. [The World Bank Independent Evaluation Group's] evaluation of these programmes utilised panel data collected in 2005 and 2007. Responses to the village questionnaire, which listed all the SHGs in the village, confirmed a continued rise in the number of these organisations but the individual-level data showed a drop in participation in SHGs. This apparent discrepancy was readily explained by the qualitative data collected alongside the quantitative survey which revealed the build up of non-functioning SHGs—through a lack of skills, non-payment, factionalism and so on—which nonetheless remained on the books. Had the researchers anticipated this attrition of SHGs—through preceding qualitative research—the survey could have included questions regarding the reasons for dropouts. SHG dropout had affected the poor most, with participation rates for the upper deciles over twice those of the lower deciles. The qualitative fieldwork pointed to some possible policy responses to this problem, including support to illiterate groups in

Box 13.12. Resources for Evaluators on Influencing Poverty Reduction Policies

- The World's Bank *Poverty Reduction Strategies Sourcebook*, Chapter 10, Annex I, Technical Note I.1 ("Engendering Participation")

- The OECD's *Guide for Non-Economists to Negotiate Poverty Reduction Strategies*

- Disability International's online handbook on how to make PRS policies inclusive

- Oxfam's guide to influencing PRS policies

record-keeping (and adoption of simpler bookkeeping systems suitable for semi-literates), finding alternative payment arrangements for the poorest households (lower payments or not requiring payment on a monthly basis), the need for animal insurance to accompany livestock loans, and defining a different (social protection) model to assist those unable to engage in productive activities. Further policy implications came from the quantitative analysis of the membership decision. Households with multiple eligible female members were not receiving a higher level of loans and so were not participating. The policy implications were clear: either to revise the goal of 100 percent coverage downwards or attempt to change village-level behaviour so that households with multiple members did receive multiple loans. (White, 2008; cited in Garbarino & Holland, 2009, p. 14)

Planning Your Evaluation: Communication and Utilization of Findings

Throughout this chapter, you should have noticed how an evaluation plan is one evolving unit that depends heavily on earlier decisions, such as purpose and data collection. At any point during the planning, you can revisit earlier components of the plan and make revisions as necessary. You now have almost completed your evaluation plan. Add a plan for communication and utilization of findings. Be sure to align the reporting with the data collection part of the plan.

 ### Moving On to the Next Chapter

In Chapter 14, we examine how to develop a management plan and budget, as well as a plan for monitoring the quality of an evaluation as it is implemented (i.e., meta-evaluation). Hanssen, Lawrenz, and Dunet (2008) argue that serious and continuous attention to meta-evaluation is also an integral part of increasing the potential for use of an evaluation.

Note

1. This section is adapted from Mertens (2009, pp. 337–338). Copyright 2009 by The Guilford Press.

Preparing to Read Chapter Fourteen

As you prepare to read this chapter, think about these questions:

1. What is a meta-evaluation, and why do you need to do one?

2. How will you personally benefit from a meta-evaluation?

3. What do these two terms suggest to you: "critical friend" and "smart enemy"?

4. What software tools are available to help you plan the management of your evaluation?

5. Where will future employers look for you in order to hire you to do an evaluation?

6. How much should you charge for your work as an evaluator?

7. How do you plan a budget for an evaluation?

CHAPTER FOURTEEN

Meta–Evaluation
and Project Management

Once your communication and utilization plan has evolved to this point, then you can add the final components to your evaluation plan: a plan for evaluating the evaluation (meta-evaluation) and a plan for managing the evaluation, along with an evaluation budget. First, you need to plan for meta-evaluation (i.e., strategies for ongoing monitoring and evaluation of the evaluation itself to ensure its quality). Reflection on the quality of evaluation is an important part of the evaluation process. In the first part of this chapter, the methods for meta-evaluation are described, and strategies for implementing a meta-evaluation are illustrated.

Evaluations also need to be planned and implemented in ways that allow for tracking the evaluation's progress. In the remainder of this chapter, we introduce practical methods for management of evaluations. Various examples of tools for management planning are provided, such as charts for personnel responsibilities, time frames for task accomplishment, checklists for developing a management and budget plan, and budgeting for evaluations. Walker and Wiseman (2006) provide a framework for evaluation management that recognizes the roles of policy makers and program developers, service users, evaluators, and the media. Their model reflects a recursive nature of the relationships between the development of programs and policies and the development of the evaluation plan. This dynamic relational model provides a framework for discussing management issues for evaluators in terms of personnel, staffing, resources, and time constraints.

Meta–Evaluation

"Meta-evaluation" first came into the lexicon of the evaluation community when Michael Scriven (1969) coined the term in a project for the Urban Institute to help it evaluate the quality and comparability of its evaluations (see also Scriven, 2009). As testament to its importance in evaluation, meta-evaluation was added as a major category as an indicator of an evaluation's quality with the most recent revision of *The Program Evaluation Standards* (Joint Committee, 2011). Recall from Chapter 1 that the meta-evaluation standard should be used to determine the extent to which

- The purpose of the evaluation served the intended users' needs.
- Appropriate standards of quality were identified and applied.
- The meta-evaluation was based on adequate and accurate documentation.

The idea of meta-evaluation—especially allowing an outside expert to scrutinize the quality of an evaluation—may leave some of us evaluators feeling uncomfortable. After all, which of us wants to make our mistakes public? However, Scriven (2009) argues that meta-evaluation is the equivalent of the peer review process that is used for proposal reviews or publication decisions. If we view external meta-evaluation as an opportunity of obtaining feedback on the strengths and areas in need of improvement from another set of eyes, then we can see it as a necessary part of the process to ensure the quality of the evaluation. If we are evaluators, shouldn't our work be evaluated too? The use of both external and internal meta-evaluation should be part of standard evaluation practice, and time and money should be included in the budget to support this activity.

Checklists and Qualitative Analysis as Meta-Evaluation Tools

To make life easier with regard to the use of meta-evaluation, Daniel Stufflebeam created a meta-evaluation checklist that relied on the use of an earlier version of the *Standards* (Joint Committee, 1994). Box 14.1 contains excerpts from the Program Evaluations Meta-evaluation Checklist developed by Stufflebeam (1999c). He and the Western Michigan University Evaluation Center team developed checklists based on the CIPP model, the *Standards*, and AEA's (2004) *Guiding Principles for Evaluators*. Scriven (2007) developed a similar checklist called the Key Evaluation Checklist. The idea in both checklists is to review the evaluation and rate it on the various standards or principles. Each checklist includes a scale that allows for a quantitative calculation depicting the overall quality of the evaluation. Stufflebeam et al. (2002) applied the Stufflebeam's checklist to their work in the Hawaiian housing evaluation study (see Chapter 4, Box 4.3).

Scriven (2009) says that a checklist is a good idea; however, evaluators should not look upon the task of meta-evaluation only as the completion of a checklist. Evaluators need to think broadly, holistically, and critically about the underlying assumptions of the evaluation before plunging into the details represented in a checklist. This is in accord with our own position, stated throughout this text, that evaluators do need to be explicit about their assumptions throughout the evaluation process.

Helga and Ribeiro (2009) recommend the use of qualitative data analysis strategies (discussed in Chapter 12) as tools for conducting meta-analysis. By identifying patterns in the study and emergent themes, an evaluator can take a more holistic look at an evaluation's quality. They emphasize that this approach is particularly critical when working with evaluation of projects in complex contexts such as those found in Brazil.

> The Brazilian social reality has structural problems, which produce hunger, poverty and social disaggregation.... The social programs are created to intervene in these situations; however, due to their originating complexity, the possibility of action is limited and may cause both advances and regressions. An advance is considered when these programs transcend governments and become continuous services. This way their execution becomes independent of the government policy.... The social reality in which the social programs are inserted present challenges for the management of programs, both in the effectiveness of actions and in program evaluation. Hence the social reality being fluid and mutable supports the drawn programs that need constant evaluation and monitoring. These evaluations also need to be meta-evaluated. (p. 219)

Box 14.1. Excerpts from the Program Evaluations Metaevaluation Checklist

To Meet the Requirements for Utility, Program Evaluations <u>Should</u>:

U1 Stakeholder Identification

- ❏ Clearly identify the evaluation client
- ❏ Engage leadership figures to identify other stakeholders
- ❏ Consult stakeholders to identify their information needs
- ❏ Ask stakeholders to identify other stakeholders
- ❏ Arrange to involve stakeholders throughout the evaluation, consistent with the formal evaluation agreement
- ❏ Keep the evaluation open to serve newly identified stakeholders

❏ 6 Excellent   ❏ 5 Very Good   ❏ 4 Good   ❏ 2–3 Fair   ❏ 0–1 Poor

To Meet the Requirements for Feasibility, Program Evaluations <u>Should</u>:

F2 Political Viability

- ❏ Anticipate different positions of different interest groups
- ❏ Be vigilant and appropriately counteractive concerning pressures and actions designed to impede or destroy the evaluation
- ❏ Foster cooperation
- ❏ Report divergent views
- ❏ As possible, make constructive use of diverse political forces to achieve the evaluation's purposes
- ❏ Terminate any corrupted evaluation

❏ 6 Excellent   ❏ 5 Very Good   ❏ 4 Good   ❏ 2–3 Fair   ❏ 0–1 Poor

To Meet the Requirements for Propriety, Program Evaluations <u>Should</u>:

P4 Human Interactions

- ❏ Consistently relate to all stakeholders in a professional manner
- ❏ Honor participants' privacy rights
- ❏ Honor time commitments
- ❏ Be sensitive to participants' diversity of values and cultural differences
- ❏ Be evenly respectful in addressing different stakeholders
- ❏ Do not ignore or help cover up any participant's incompetence, unethical behavior, fraud, waste, or abuse

❏ 6 Excellent   ❏ 5 Very Good   ❏ 4 Good   ❏ 2–3 Fair   ❏ 0–1 Poor

(cont.)

Box 14.1 (cont.)

To Meet the Requirements for Accuracy, Program Evaluations Should:

A2 Context Analysis

❑ Describe the context's technical, social, political, organizational, and economic features

❑ Maintain a log of unusual circumstances

❑ Report those contextual influences that appeared to significantly influence the program and that might be of interest to potential adopters

❑ Estimate the effects of context on program outcomes

❑ Identify and describe any critical competitors to this program that functioned at the same time and in the program's environment

❑ Describe how people in the program's general area perceived the program's existence, importance, and quality

❑ 6 Excellent   ❑ 5 Very Good   ❑ 4 Good   ❑ 2–3 Fair   ❑ 0–1 Poor

A12 Metaevaluation[1]

❑ Budget appropriately and sufficiently for conducting an internal metaevaluation and, as feasible, an external metaevaluation

❑ Designate or define the standards the evaluators used to guide and assess their evaluation

❑ Record the full range of information needed to judge the evaluation against the employed standards

❑ As feasible and appropriate, contract for an independent metaevaluation

❑ Evaluate all important aspects of the evaluation, including the instrumentation, data collection, data handling, coding, analysis, synthesis, and reporting

❑ Obtain and report both formative and summative metaevaluations to the right-to-know audiences

❑ 6 Excellent   ❑ 5 Very Good   ❑ 4 Good   ❑ 2–3 Fair   ❑ 0–1 Poor

Source: Stufflebeam (1999c). Reprinted by permission of Daniel L. Stufflebeam.

[1]This checklist was developed in 1999 and based on the 1994 *Standards*. A revision based on the latest version of the *Standards*, including a special category and instructions for meta-evaluation, was not available at the time the present book went to press.

Qualitative tools allow for the consideration of these contextual variables in ways that are not possible with a quantitative checklist.

Who Should Do an External Meta–Evaluation?

A wise evaluator engages in meta-evaluation throughout the planning and implementation of the evaluation, reflecting on the evaluation and being aware of the need to make changes. However, meta-evaluation is usually an activity in which an external reviewer is involved as well. Options for an external meta-evaluator include a "critical friend" or a "smart enemy." Scriven (2009) worries that a critical friend would not be ruthless enough, and so recommends a smart enemy on the grounds that this person would be inclined to give a more honest appraisal. However, I (Donna M. Mertens) have used critical friends and found that they are more than happy to point out weaknesses in my evaluation work. Perhaps we have different kinds of relationships with our friends.

When Should Meta–Evaluation Be Done?

I have found it helpful to commission a meta-evaluation at three points during the evaluation (see Figure 14.1). The first review is conducted after the planning stage of the evaluation is complete, before the implementation phase begins. This review point allows you and the external evaluator to make early corrections in the evaluation strategies. The second point is midway through the evaluation, as a check to see whether the evaluation is proceeding as planned or whether midcourse adjustments are necessary. The final meta-evaluation review is conducted as the study nears its end. The external meta-evaluator can be provided with a draft of the final report and asked to review it to determine the overall quality of the evaluation and any corrections that need to be made before the final report is considered to be final. This is but one possible model for conducting a meta-evaluation.

Cooksy and Caracelli (2009) conducted a review of the meta-evaluation literature. They reported that meta-evaluations are infrequently conducted, and that it is more common to do a summative meta-evaluation than a formative one. They reviewed 17 meta-evaluation studies over a 30-year period and found that only one had a formative purpose. The most common methods used included reviewing reports and other documents, and

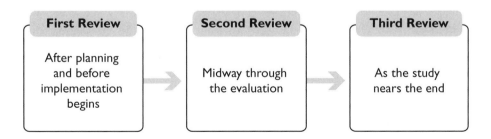

Figure 14.1. When to do meta–evaluation reviews.

conducting meetings with the evaluation team and other stakeholder groups. The meta-evaluations were defined by establishing their purpose (summative or formative), identifying criteria for judging quality (e.g., predetermined checklists or emergent categories), and making decisions about data collection strategies. Some of the meta-evaluations used qualitative approaches, such as case studies, expert panel reviews, and audit procedures that involved the examination of procedures and results against a set of criteria for judging quality (Schwandt, 1989). These criteria parallel those examined in Chapter 12 on qualitative data analysis, such as credibility, dependability, and confirmability. The others used the quantitative checklist approach.

Hanssen et al. (2008) conducted what they called a "concurrent" meta-evaluation that involved a larger role than simply reviewing plans, midpoint accomplishments, and final reports. They were asked to evaluate a U.S. federal agency's evaluation technique as it was being developed and implemented. Hence they were continuously involved in the evaluation, even attending data collection events and verifying the quality of the data collected. They started with three questions:

1. What are the strengths and weaknesses of the evaluation process, including each of its components in terms of producing its intended results? How can the evaluation process be improved?

2. How efficacious is the evaluation process for producing its intended results?

3. To what degree does the evaluation framework enable an evaluator to produce an evaluation that satisfies accepted program evaluation standards?

They used a framework based on the two sources mentioned previously: the Joint Committee's (1994) *Standards* and Scriven's (2007) Key Evaluation Checklist. In addition, they used a checklist that was germane to the specific domain of the study (i.e., health care). The Society for Prevention Research (2004) developed a checklist called Standards of Evidence that provides additional guidance, particularly with respect to the use of practical procedures in the health care context. The meta-evaluators' roles were quite ambitious. They participated in regular conference calls with the project evaluator and accompanied the evaluator on site visits in which they observed the evaluation team in action and gave them feedback. They reviewed interview transcripts and provided feedback in short time frames. They also interviewed members of an expert panel who had been involved in rating various sites to determine their perceptions of the quality of the information collected. The meta-evaluators engaged a separate panel of experts to rate the programs as a reliability check of the ratings done by the original panel. They also interviewed project team members and personnel from the various sites to determine their perceptions of the quality of the evaluation. "All of this work was covered under a separate contract with the federal agency that sponsored the effort. This contract was for approximately US$50,000, although the total project cost was roughly US$490,000. Work took place over a period of 20 months, beginning in April 2005 and ending in December 2006" (Hanssen et al., 2008, p. 577).

Box 14.2 provides a generic example of a meta-evaluation plan.

Box 14.2. Generic Meta-Evaluation Plan

Meta-evaluation stage	Who?	When?	Strategies/tools
First round	Evaluation team; decision makers	End of second month	Evaluation plan; Joint Committee's *Standards*; email dissemination, followed by virtual conference to discuss; revision of plan as necessary
Second round	Evaluation team; decision makers; participants	Midway through evaluation	Interviews with decision makers; online survey of participants; revision of evaluation implementation as necessary
Third round	Evaluation team; decision makers; representatives of participants	As the project comes to a close	Dissemination of draft evaluation report; focus groups to discuss findings; revisions to final report

· · · · · · · · · E X T E N D I N G   Y O U R   T H I N K I N G · · · · · · · · · ·

Conducting a Meta-Evaluation

This activity is based on one described by Randall Davies (2009).

As you learn to be a trained evaluator, or an informed consumer of evaluation, you must be able to judge the quality of an evaluation. To do this properly, you should have an understanding of the purpose of evaluation in general, various approaches to doing evaluation, and (most importantly) an understanding that evaluations are value-driven. Clearly an evaluation must be accurate and useful; it should be conducted systematically by competent evaluators; it should be done in an ethical and efficient manner; but it must also consider values in terms of what is important. This can be a challenge, in that value and what is considered important vary (sometimes drastically) from person to person. Meta-evaluation also requires a set of standards (i.e., criteria) by which the evaluation will be judged. The standards you should use are the Joint Committee's *Standards* and the AEA's *Guiding Principles for Evaluators*.

This task is an opportunity for you to become better acquainted with evaluation standards and to develop your skills as a meta-evaluator. I would suggest you follow the following steps.

(cont.)

1. Select an evaluation report on a topic of interest to you.

2. Select a meta-evaluation checklist (*www.wmich.edu/evalctr/checklists/meta-evaluation* for examples).

3. Read the report, and then use the checklist you selected to evaluate the quality of the report. Make sure to document (record) your thoughts, reasoning, and rationale for each aspect on the evaluation checklist. If a portion of the evaluation report is less than satisfactory, make a judgment of its importance to the goals (completeness or quality) of the overall evaluation.

4. Write a reflective summary. This should include the following:

   a. A brief statement of the evaluation purpose, and a brief description of the evaluand.

   b. Your overall judgment of the quality of the evaluation being evaluated.

   c. A clear but concise statement (a paragraph or two) justifying your decision. This may include reasons and examples of where the evaluation excelled (strengths) and where the evaluation was inadequate (weaknesses).

   d. If appropriate, include recommendations for how the evaluation might have been improved.

· · · · · · · · · · · E X T E N D I N G   Y O U R   T H I N K I N G · · · · · · · · · · ·
Creating a Meta–Evaluation Plan

Following the example of the generic meta-evaluation plan displayed in Box 14.2, create a meta-evaluation plan for your own evaluand. Include who will be involved, what strategies and instruments will be used, and the time frame. If the meta-evaluation is to occur several times during the study, include this information for each of those occurrences. Here is a template, based on Box 14.2.

Template for a Meta–Evaluation Plan

Meta-evaluation stage	Who?	When?	Strategies/tools
First round			

Second round

_____

Third round

_____

Management of Evaluations: Management Plan and Budget

Management plans generally consist of two components: a timeline with associated tasks and responsibilities, and a budget for the evaluation. As important as this topic is, it is one of those parts of evaluation planning and implementation that seems to be described simply as "Then you just develop the management plan and budget," as if this is an intuitive skill. Fortunately, AEA's Topical Interest Group for Evaluation Managers and Supervisors has noted the lack of attention given to this topic. Two of its members described the state of knowledge about managing evaluations as follows:

> Managing evaluation is an almost invisible practice, one little studied and little written about. Illuminating everyday practice and perspectives on it serves to make the taken-for-granted, the seemingly invisible and often ineffable, available. In so doing, much of what is seen seems obvious, too often boring. Everyday managing is precisely about the ordinary, mundane work of managing evaluation studies, evaluators and other workers, and an evaluation unit. This is the ground of the work and it is what must be noticed, studied, taught, and learned. (Baizerman & Compton, 2009a, p. 8)

Baizerman and Compton's (2009a) work makes clear the variation in levels of management expertise that occur in evaluation, ranging from an individual evaluator's managing a single project to an evaluation shop in which a manager oversees multiple evaluation projects and evaluators. They offer both a conceptual and a practical definition of effective management in evaluation:

> *Conceptual Definition*
>
> The phrase *effective managing* refers to the *everyday, mundane action* necessary in each *organizational context and moment* to make possible one or more evaluation studies, the work of evaluators, and the collective workings of an evaluation unit for the purpose of using quality evaluation for program improvement, accountability, or evaluation capacity building, among other intentions. (p. 13; emphasis in original)

Practical Definition

The phrase *effective managing of evaluation* means the practical, everyday, professional expertise necessary to bring about the implementation and use of quality studies, the development of productive workers, and the sustaining of a well-run, ongoing, and influential evaluation unit. (p. 13)

At the practical level, Bell (2004) suggests consideration of the following factors in planning project management of an evaluation study: Clarify the evaluation purpose and goals; determine staffing needs and organizational resources; make appropriate assignments of tasks to persons; and use the plan to monitor progress and enhance the quality of the final product. Remember the learning organization theory of evaluation developed by Preskill and colleagues (Preskill & Torres, 1999; Russ-Eft & Preskill, 2001) and discussed in Chapter 4? As a part of a learning organization's metamorphosis, use of a management plan is essential to determine personnel and budget needs, to develop timelines for activities to be accomplished, and to monitor progress in terms of task achievement and budget expenditures.

Managing the Study, Staff, and Unit

Evaluation management can be thought of in terms of managing the study, managing the staff, and managing organizational units (Baizerman & Compton, 2009a). Resources for managing the study itself include checklists from the Western Michigan University Evaluation Center (see Box 14.4) and the OECD DAC's (2006b) *Guidance for Managing Joint Evaluations* for evaluations of international development projects. For large-scale evaluations, the OECD DAC recommends having both a higher-level management steering committee and on-the-ground managers who conduct the day-to-day management activities. Larger-scale evaluations also involve the management of staff, a topic that is rarely addressed in the evaluation literature. Finally, management in a setting with an evaluation unit embedded in a larger organization means that the manager needs to be cognizant of the politics of the organization and of the ways these impinge on the unit's ability to conduct and manage the evaluation. This requires building relationships with members of other units and devising effective communication strategies to keep them informed about the evaluation work.

Baizerman and Compton (2009b) describe expert managers as evaluators whose expertise

> shows itself in the "already known," "done that before," "know how to do this." They have set up systems, procedures, rules, and practices that institutionalized the work so there is a standard way to do it, albeit one that is flexible and responsive to situation, context, politics, and personality. More than anything, they are systematic and in this way, using their standardized templates, they are able to effectively respond to the never-ending demands from above, below, and alongside them; this is how they work to order or control the omnipresence and simultaneity of the demands characterizing their everyday work world; there is always something, and usually many "somethings" at once. In more typical terms, their expertise is in knowing which systems to set up, modify, sustain, and defend (to get the work done), and in knowing whom they need to do this. Systems and people in place, their expertise is seen as managing workflow, the worker–research–study nexus in time. They are and see themselves as jugglers, even when their workplace is to them not quite a circus! (pp. 82–83)

Box 14.3. Checklists for Managing and Budgeting Evaluations

Checklist	Author(s)/date
Evaluation Plans and Operations Checklist	Stufflebeam (1999b)
A Checklist for Developing and Evaluating Budgets	Horn (2001)
Evaluation Contracts Checklist	Stufflebeam (1999a)
Evaluation Design Checklist	Stufflebeam (2004)
Negotiating Agreements	Stake (1976b)
Feedback Workshop Checklist	Gullickson and Stufflebeam (2001)
Evaluation Report Checklist	Miron (2004)
Making Evaluation Meaningful to All Education Stakeholders	Gangopadhyay (2002)

Source: Western Michigan University Evaluation Center Checklist Project (*www.wmich.edu/evalctr/checklists*).

Steps in Developing the Management Plan

Walker and Wiseman (2006) provide a framework for understanding the broad context in which program management occurs. The steps they identify for developing a management plan include consideration of the policy context and stakeholders, including policy makers, project staff, organizational personnel, and program participants.

■ *Step 1.* Identify the constraints of the project from the request for proposal (RFP) or through discussions with the project funders and staff. Find out exactly what is required by the client and in what form that information needs to be presented.

■ *Step 2.* Determine the parameters within which the evaluation is expected to occur. If the client has a predetermined idea about the design of the evaluation, examine it critically. At this stage of the process, it may be possible to promote an alternative approach that is justified on the basis of cost or data quality.

■ *Step 3.* Identify the tasks that are needed to complete the evaluation, based on your understanding of the evaluand, its timelines, and the available funding. This involves examining past evaluation management plans to see the list of tasks typically involved and the level of effort needed to accomplish the tasks. Individuals who have completed such tasks in the past can be asked to provide estimates of the time needed to complete them. Once estimates are provided, the evaluation team can meet to discuss those and to determine their appropriateness for the new project. It may also be possible to review time sheets from previous projects to add information to the decision-making process.

■ *Step 4.* Determine the expertise needed to accomplish the tasks. Is that expertise

Box 14.4. Sample Evaluation Management Plan

Project name	Person(s) responsible	Days	Start	End	9 Jul	16 Jul	23 Jul	30 Jul	6 Aug	13 Aug	20 Aug	27 Aug	3 Sep	10 Sep	17 Sep	24 Sep
Evaluation Management Plan	Evaluation manager	**70**	**9 Jul**	**25 Sep**	■	■	■	■	■	■	■	■	■	■	■	■
Scope definition phase		10	**9 Jul**	**19 Jul**	■	■										
Define objectives	Evaluation Team	3	9 Jul	12 Jul	■											
Define requirements	Evaluation team	7	10 Jul	17 Jul	■	■										
Determine in-house resource or hire vendor	Evaluation manager	2	15 Jul	17 Jul		■										
Implementation phase	**Evaluator**	**47**	**9 Aug**	**25 Sep**			■	■	■						■	
Develop data collection strategies for needs sensing	Evaluator and evaluation assistant	2	9 Aug	11 Aug					■	■						
Interview stakeholders to determine their information needs	Evaluator and evaluation assistant	2	11 Aug	13 Aug						■	■					
Document information needs	Evaluator and evaluation assistant	1	13 Aug	14 Aug						■						

Task	Resource	Duration	Start	End	Gantt
Identify information to be gathered in evaluation	Evaluator and evaluation assistant	2	16 Aug	18 Aug	
Identify source of information	Evaluator and evaluation assistant	1	18 Aug	19 Aug	
Identify evaluation method (primary or secondary)	Evaluator and evaluation assistant	1	19 Aug	20 Aug	
Identify evaluation participants	Evaluator and evaluation assistant	1	20 Aug	21 Aug	
Identify evaluation technique (focus group or survey)	Evaluator and evaluation assistant	1	23 Aug	24 Aug	
Identify timing requirements and budget	Evaluator and evaluation assistant	1	24 Aug	25 Aug	
Refine evaluation plan	Evaluator and evaluation assistant	1	25 Aug	26 Aug	
Develop evaluation information-gathering tool	Evaluator and evaluation assistant	2	26 Aug	28 Aug	
Conduct evaluation	Evaluator and evaluation assistant	10	30 Aug	9 Sep	
Analyze data	Evaluator and evaluation assistant	5	13 Sep	18 Sep	

Box 14.4 (cont.)

Project name	Person(s) responsible	Days	Start	End	9 Jul	16 Jul	23 Jul	30 Jul	6 Aug	13 Aug	20 Aug	27 Aug	3 Sep	10 Sep	17 Sep	24 Sep
Develop evaluation report	Evaluator and evaluation assistant	3	20 Sep	23 Sep											■	
Review report with stakeholder group	Evaluator and evaluation assistant	2	23 Sep	25 Sep											■	■
Conduct meta-evaluation	Consultant	6	9 Jul	25 Sep		■				■					■	■

Source: Adapted from Unger (2009).

Note: Shading indicates in which months the activities noted in the first column will occur.

present in the evaluation team? If not, should a consultant be brought into the process for that purpose? Or, is it possible to do capacity building within the team to obtain the needed expertise? This is a task that needs to be included in the management plan and budget.

▨ *Step 5*. Include consideration of additional resources that may be needed, such as overhead (costs of running the project in terms of the physical structure, lights, heat, water, etc.), required travel, and support staff.

▨ *Step 6*. Submit the entire evaluation plan, complete with management and budget plans. Be prepared for the negotiations that follow, to discuss possible changes in activities and budget.

▨ *Step 7*. Once the award is made for the evaluation, you are in a position as the manager to focus on the many relationships that need to be nurtured or developed in order for the evaluation to proceed smoothly.

A sample management plan for a short-term, 70-day project is displayed in Box 14.4. Unger provides other examples of management plans in a presentation she made at the 2009 AEA annual meeting (this is available at the AEA website; go to "Reading," then go to "Public eLibrary" and search "Unger"). The key elements are the major phases of activities, delineation of specific tasks, identification of who is responsible for those tasks, the number of days needed to accomplish the tasks, the starting and ending dates for each task, and a bar chart that shows when the tasks will be completed against the project timeline. Such charts can be created in Microsoft Word or Excel, using the chart function.

There are also some free, open-access software products that can be used for this purpose. Here are a few examples:[1]

▨ GanttProject (***ganttproject.biz***) is a cross-platform desktop tool for project scheduling and management. It runs on Windows, Linux, and Mac OS X; it is free; and its code is open-source. It can create Gantt charts (bar charts that show task loads against a calendar) and PERT charts (a management tool developed by the U.S. Navy in the 1950s, see below; PERT stands for "program evaluation review technique"). It also allows you to share your projects with others who are using this software. Gantt charts are named after Henry Gantt (1910/1974) who popularized them in the early 20th century.

▨ NetMBA (***www.netmba.com/operations/project/pert***) is a website with instructions on how to create PERT charts, as well as useful examples of this management tool. A PERT chart shows a network of activities that communicates the necessary sequencing of these activities. The network is made up of activities and events. An activity is a task (e.g., develop instruments); an event is a milestone, marking the completion of that activity that needed to be accomplished before moving on to the next activity. Sometimes the activities are listed on the arrows that connect the nodes and the nodes are used to represent the time period by which the activity needs to be completed. Another variation is to use circles or rectangles with text included. This is the strategy used in the sample PERT chart displayed as Figure 14.2.

▨ Managers developed the critical path analysis (CPA) or critical path method as a modification of the basic PERT method (***www.mindtools.com/critpath.html***). The CPA shows which tasks have to be completed on time in order for other tasks to be

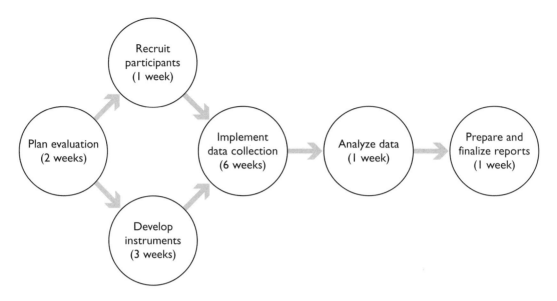

Figure 14.2. Sample PERT chart.

started. This allows for the identification of critical paths (i.e., those activities that need to be given priority so the work can advance).

▇ Open Workbench is an open-source, Windows-based desktop application that can be used for scheduling and management and is free to distribute.

▇ PHProjekt (***phprojekt.com***) is a modular application for coordinating group activities and for sharing information and documents via the Web. OpenProj (***source-forge.net/projects/openpro***) is another free, open-source, Windows-based desktop application. Both of these applications work similarly to Microsoft Project (***office. microsoft.com/en-us/project/default.aspx***), a software management tool one buys separately from Microsoft Office. Both applications have tools for planning, budgeting, reporting, tracking, and analysis.

· · · · · · · · · · · E X T E N D I N G   Y O U R   T H I N K I N G · · · · · · · · · · ·
Software Tools

Visit the websites of the software products listed above. Some of the sites have videos you can watch to get a feel for the products. It is interesting to note how some of the free software is as robust as the software that must be purchased. It is exciting to see how your plan actually looks when you plug the data into some of these programs. Try them out and see what works for you. Everyone has different preferences in software tools. Which of these tools do you think you could use with your evaluation plan? Why does it "feel right" to you?

Management Challenges

One of the first challenges for a new evaluator who needs to manage an evaluation is learning how to do it. The information in this chapter and in the other resources discussed here is good for that purpose. However, the actual practice of effective management may best be learned from a mentor who can guide a novice through the learning experience.

> Managing is difficult to do and seemingly difficult for practitioners to describe, analyze, and teach, except by example. What is needed is a vocabulary and skill in its use. Until then, being mentored seems to be the best way for a novice to grasp managing as ordinary, mundane professional work. (Baizerman & Compton, 2009b, p. 84)

In keeping with the spirit of learning from experience, we can also turn to experts who write about challenges they have encountered. Knowing about such challenges makes it possible to anticipate and plan strategies for addressing them. Walker and Wiseman (2006) provide us with a list of challenges that I have also encountered in my years as an evaluator.

▓ Sometimes the funding comes later than expected, creating the challenge of recruiting participants and staff in the limited time frame of the project. I experienced this in an evaluation of a summer program for gifted deaf adolescents in marine biology. The funding arrived late. The consequence was that the project director hired only one sign language interpreter for the entire 6-week program. Interpreters usually work in pairs and switch off with one another every 20 minutes or so to prevent fatigue. This interpreter was overworked and stressed; she was also a graduate student in the project director's program at the university, so she did her best. This situation resulted in a great deal of chaos in the program, as staff members who could not sign were unable to control the adolescents' behaviors. Another implication of the late funding was that the program accepted some deaf students who were not in the gifted range because of their late start on recruitment. As the evaluator, I communicated with the project director about these concerns. He was distressed, but resolute about going forward. The happy ending came in the second year of the project, when he was able to hire two interpreters, dorm staffers who could sign, and two instructors who could sign. There were still three staff members who could not sign, but things went much smoother the next year.

▓ Recruitment of participants can also be a problem if the program is voluntary, not mandatory. Walker and Wiseman (2006) found it difficult to recruit for a work support program for families living in poverty, because it was voluntary and involved random assignment. They experienced various challenges in explaining the design, and they encountered some hostility from community members. Through perseverance, they were able to successfully recruit and assign to groups a sufficient number of participants. Borman et al. (2007) reported a similar problem with recruitment of schools for an evaluation of a new reading program. In past evaluations of the program, schools had paid $75,000 for the program in its first year, $35,000 in the second year, and $25,000 the third year. None of the schools in the 2007 study would agree to that level of expenditure. Finally, Borman et al. agreed to pay the schools a one-time lump sum of $30,000 each for both control and experimental studies. Then they found that none of the schools wanted to be in the control group, so they compromised and allowed the control schools to use the program in grades 4–7 and did their experimental study on grades K–3, comparing schools that used the program with those who did not. Such necessary compromises certainly have implications both for management of the evaluation and for its budget.

■ The idea of keeping the independent variable (i.e., the program) constant and unchanged over a period of years in order to test its effects is problematic. Changes can enter into the program either as responses to formative evaluation that indicates needed changes, or as results of external changes in policies that are germane to the evaluand. In Walker and Wiseman's (2006) example, they note that the agency in which the work program was situated changed its policies to increase barriers to accessing funds. These changes affected both the experimental and the control group.

■ Political factors are ever present in evaluation; they can also have direct implications for evaluation management and budget. If a state or the federal government makes a change relevant to the program, this can influence delivery of services and eligibility for participation. When there is a change in administration at the highest level (e.g., the United States elects a new president or a state elects a new governor), it is not unusual for the incoming president or governor to make cuts in programs that were supported by his predecessor. I have been on phone calls to revise federal management and budget plans when a new president came into power and issued a directive to everyone who was funded under a particular federal initiative to make a 25% budget cut. At that point, the leadership team needs to work together to establish priorities and make realistic decisions about what can be accomplished effectively under the new constraints. Political challenges also include possible shifts in objectives, indicators, and timelines.

■ A budget submitted in a proposal is rarely the budget that is funded. Negotiations about budget typically result in less money than was initially requested. Thus the ability to negotiate effectively is an important skill, as is the ability to think creatively when money that was requested is denied. In one evaluation that I did, which involved all 50 states and 154 universities, the funding agency decided to fund everything we asked for except travel for regional directors and participants. We decided to do as much as possible virtually, using video conferencing. (It was a project to improve the use of technology for the preparation of teachers of deaf students.) We also created ways for the regional directors and participants to request "mini-grants" to develop specific applications of technology. The regional directors and participants could use their funds at their own discretion, but many chose to use them to attend meetings related to the project. We also scheduled major meetings for the project to coincide with the time of the annual professional conference for this group of educators. Thus people could attend their conference and also participate in project-related activities.

■ In studies that involve experimental and control groups, evaluators need to be aware of the threat to validity of treatment contamination. People will talk about something, particularly if they really like or dislike it. If the people in the control and experimental groups are in close proximity, it is possible that people from the control group might adopt some of the experimental treatment strategies. Borman et al. (2007) visited the control classrooms in their reading study and found that this did happen on a limited basis. They found some of the experimental materials in the control classrooms. They met with the teachers and reinforced the necessity of control group teachers not using these materials until the study was complete.

······· E X T E N D I N G   Y O U R   T H I N K I N G ·······

Developing Your Management Plan

Review your evaluation plan in its current form. Develop a management plan, using one of the strategies that are discussed in this chapter. Share your management plan with a peer, and then ask the peer to explain it to you. If parts of the plan are not clear, make the needed revisions. You might find it useful to use the following template, or to follow the example of the more complex management plan displayed in Box 14.4.

Template for an Evaluation Management Plan

Activity	Person(s) responsible	Days	Start	End	First quarter	Second quarter	Third quarter	Fourth quarter
Plan								
Implement								
Report								
Meta-evaluation								

Identifying an Evaluator

When organizations are searching for an evaluator, where do they begin? How do they go about finding you? Dubose (2008) suggests that organizations follow these steps:

> First, you must determine the needs of your program and your funder. Then, ask yourself: Why am I seeking an evaluator? What are my expectations, and what are the requirements of my grant funder? Answers to these and other questions are contained in a Request for Proposals (RFP) to evaluate a specific grant program. If you have not developed a specific grant- or program-driven RFP, you can issue a Request for Qualifications (RFQ) asking interested parties to submit résumés, price estimates for evaluations, and other supporting materials demonstrating their capacity to evaluate programs in a given area. Then, when a third-party evaluation is required in the future for any given program, you will have an assortment of evaluators

from which to select the most qualified. For example, you may select three evaluation firms or consultants to provide services to your organization: Vendor 1, who works with school districts and education; Vendor 2, whose expertise lies in criminal justice; and Vendor 3, who specializes in programs concerning alcohol and drug abuse. If your organization received a GEARUP grant to help high school students continue their education in college, then you would select Vendor 1 as your evaluator. If you received a crime reduction grant for a community, then you would employ Vendor 2. Regardless of whether you issue an RFP or an RFQ, knowing what you are seeking and why will go a long way toward ensuring the best fit between your needs and the evaluator's abilities.

After organizations decide what abilities they hope to find in an evaluator, where can you be "seen" in the evaluation world so that you will be considered? As there is no agency or organization that certifies evaluators and thus would be a place to begin, the U.S. Department of Health and Human Services (2005) suggests that you be found among other evaluation experts who respect your work and who are willing to recommend you for the work. Therefore, networking with your colleagues at professional conferences, in school, and out in the field is important. Your future employers can obtain referrals from professional associations such as AEA or AERA, or from postings in professional publications/newsletters or on professional websites such as LinkedIn Xing (*www.xing.com*). After collecting curricula vitae (CVs) and other documentation, organizations can develop a list of criteria to assess and compare all of the candidates and score them according to their training, knowledge, experience, references, quality of work, cost, and (if interviewed) interpersonal skills.

Budgeting for an Evaluation

Usually project staffers prepare a budget for the overall project and have a dollar figure in mind for the evaluation portion of the project, but not always. They sometimes depend on the evaluator to provide an estimate of the cost of the evaluation and then proceed to negotiate from there. The evaluator generally provides the details of how the money is spent specifically for evaluation activities. Horn's (2001) checklist for developing a budget for evaluation is listed in Box 14.3.

How Much Do Evaluators Get Paid?

An answer to the question of how much evaluators get paid will be helpful in preparing a budget. This topic is raised periodically on EvalTalk, AEA's listserv. The official policy of AEA is that it cannot collect such information because of the potential threat of legal action under price-fixing legislation. However, evaluators can discuss how much money they charge, and some are willing to do so. Hence the latest news on evaluation pricing is that a new evaluator might be in the $100–$300/day range, a somewhat experienced evaluator in the $300–$800/day range, and a very experienced evaluator in the $900–$2,000/day range. Sometimes new evaluators will work only for expenses in their first few jobs, just to get the experience and/or to help out an NGO that may not have the funding to pay for evaluation services. Of course, there are some evaluators who do some of their work pro bono (for free, usually for a nonprofit or other worthy cause when resources are not available or could be put to better use). There are probably superstar evaluators who get paid a lot more than $2,000/day, but no one has admitted that to me yet.

Box 14.5 contains a typical advertisement for an evaluation position, along with a salary range. The AEA website also has an ongoing job bank that lists evaluation opportunities all over the world—some short-term, some long-term positions. Several other listservs (e.g., *AfrEA@yahoogroups.com, IAEVAL@yahoogroups.com,* and *XCeval@yahoogroups. com*) list employment opportunities for evaluators, usually in the international development context.

Determining Costs of an Evaluation

The budget checklist developed by Horn (2001; again, see Box 14.3) provides good ideas about what needs to be considered in developing a budget. The evaluator needs to be clear about the type and source of funding (e.g., grant, contract, or cooperative agreement), the condition of payment (cost reimbursement or fixed price), and the funding period. Much of this information is usually available from the RFP that solicits the work; however, it is also possible and appropriate to explore these topics with the designated contact in the funding organization. The evaluator can also find out whether there is a specified form in which the budget needs to be provided for both the funding agency and their home institution. Sometimes budgets need to be broken down to show a relationship between tasks and money. It is good practice to include notes that explain the amount of money requested (e.g., number of copies of reports and lengths of reports).

Factors to consider in calculating personnel costs include the different types of personnel (management, evaluators, student assistants, support staff), the basis for costing (e.g., by hours, days, or products), the need for possible merit increases over time, and the need for fringe benefits. Travel costs need to be justified in terms of purpose, mode of transportation, allowable expenses, and local costs of housing and meals. Supplies, materials, and equipment can include typical office supplies, as well as specialized materials that might be needed (e.g., web cameras, computer software, or computers). Another factor to consider is whether any materials are explicitly excluded in the RFP. It is not unusual for federal grants to disallow expenditures for computers and other pieces of hardware, based on a belief that organizations should acquire those as part of their regular business expenses and they should not be purchased with federal monies designed for provision of services. Communication expenses include those related to telephones and Internet services, as well as copying and printing of reports and promotional materials.

Another expense that needs to be considered is that of consultants. What consultants might be needed? What is the general cost of hiring a consultant? What about their expenses if travel is involved? Many granting agencies require either in-kind or cost sharing. This means that the management team needs to calculate the value of services that are being provided to the grant and that are not being reimbursed. Finally, indirect costs need to be calculated. These are sometimes fixed by the federal agency and the home organization. However, it may be necessary to negotiate with both groups if there is no agreement on what this rate should be. "Usually the indirect rate is a percentage of the total direct costs and a percentage of all salaries and wages with the possible exclusion of such costs as equipment or subcontracts" (Horn, 2001, p. 6).

The development of budget plans has been greatly simplified by the availability of software for this purpose (e.g., Microsoft's Excel program). See Box 14.6 for a sample of an evaluation budget template.

Box 14.5. Sample Advertisement for an Evaluation Position

The Department of Health's Center for Health Promotion is seeking a full-time evaluator to work on "healthy eating in schools" efforts. The position is a 2-year position. The closing date is April 30. Salary information is as follows:

$25.51–$37.93 hourly, $53,265–$79,198 annually

Working title: Evaluator
Hiring agency: Health Department, Healthy School Meals

Location: [City, State,] USA

Job description: This position exists to plan, design, implement, analyze, interpret, and report on assessment and evaluation research, data sources, systems, and activities relevant to a healthy eating grant. This position also provides expertise in scientific research, methodology, and analysis. The activities include planning, designing, and implementing the evaluation systems to measure the progress and impact of the grant; conducting a cost–benefit analysis on the health impact of a statewide certification policy; and developing a potential legislative proposal on statewide certification policy for consideration in the 2012 legislative session. The work carried out by this position will enable the Health Department to accomplish work specified in the grant and other internal and external collaborative obesity-related data and evaluation initiatives.

Minimum qualifications: Master's degree in one of the behavioral or social sciences, public health, neuropsychology, epidemiology, health services research, or closely related field;

AND

Three years' professional experience in designing, planning, organizing, implementing, directing, or evaluating data-related projects, and including (but not limited to) needs assessments, program evaluation, research studies using primary or secondary database linkage efforts, data analysis and interpretation, management information systems or data collection, and monitoring systems in health-related programs.

A PhD in one of the areas above will substitute for one year of professional experience.

Ability to conceive, organize, and carry out research projects independently.

Preferred qualifications: Considerable knowledge in programmatic evaluation design and methodology.

Considerable knowledge in scientific, experimental, statistical, and research design and methodology.

Strong knowledge of chronic disease surveillance data sources, methodologies, and literature.

Strong experience in analyzing and interpreting program evaluation data.

Strong experience in computers, statistical software (i.e., SAS, SPSS), and database management.

Knowledge of public health principles.

Knowledge of epidemiology and prevention of obesity.

Knowledge and background in health economics.

Ability to present evaluation and research results clearly and effectively in writing, and effectively organize and synthesize material from diverse sources into comprehensive reports for a variety of audiences.

Ability to build and develop ongoing working relationships and to collaborate with a variety of organizations, professionals, and lay citizens. (This is essential.)

Manage work load and work independently.

Source: Minnesota Department of Health (personal communication, April 27, 2010). Adapted by permission of Laura Hutton, Obesity Prevention Evaluation Coordinator, Minnesota Department of Health.

Unger (2009) has provided a guide for pricing evaluations from the Evaluation Solutions consulting firm (*www.evaluationsolutions.com*). The specific examples included in her presentation are helpful in regard to using Gantt charts, establishing timelines, and creating progress reports. She suggests that evaluators consider a pricing strategy that allows for one-third of the funds to pay personnel; one-third to cover overhead costs, such as equipment, rent, and supplies; and one-third of the funds for profit.

Unger also warns evaluators to beware of "price creep" (i.e., agreeing to a fixed amount and then finding that a client wants more than is covered by the previously agreed-upon price). I have found myself in this position several times. Sometimes the client agrees to pay more, sometimes not. Then my decision is to go with some unpaid services and my integrity, or not. I have sometimes gone without pay for the additional work needed to do an effective job with the evaluation.

· · · · · · · · · · · E X T E N D I N G   Y O U R   T H I N K I N G · · · · · · · · · · ·

Planning a Budget

Create a budget for your evaluation. Be sure to include all the relevant components, and use realistic cost estimates (e.g., for travel, you can go to the Web and obtain costs for plane travel, hotels, and other expenses). Provide justification for the numbers in your budget. Use the "Planned expense" column in Box 14.6 as a template.

Box 14.6. Sample Evaluation Budget Template

Expense category	Planned expense	Actual expense	Variance
Building rent/lease			
Salaries			
Project manager			
Evaluator			
Research assistant			
Consultant for meta-evaluation			
Supplies/equipment			
Computer/printer			
Coffee			
Other			
Marketing expenses			
Brochure			
Website			
Business cards			
Advertising			
Other			
Administrative expenses			
Fax/copies			
Postage			
Office supplies			
Other			
Travel expenses			
Flights			
Meals			
Housing			
Mileage			
Parking			
Other			
Operating expenses			
Utilities			
Insurance			
Miscellaneous			
Indirect costs			
Total expenses			

Moving On to the Next Chapter

Now your evaluation plan is complete. You should also have developed insights into challenges and opportunities that arise in the implementation of the evaluation. Chapter 15, the final chapter of this book, addresses issues of perennial interest in evaluation. Smith and Brandon (2008) describe these as fundamental issues—that is,

> those underlying concerns, problems, or choices that continually resurface in different guises throughout evaluation work. By their very nature, these issues can never be finally solved but only temporarily resolved. Fundamental issues underlie all areas of evaluation, whether it be communication with clients, ethical dilemmas, cultural differences, preparation of new evaluators, work with special populations, governmental service, methodological difficulties, social justice, evaluation influence, or economic survival as a professional. (p. viii)

With this quotation as a segue, we trust you are ready to read the final chapter.

Note

1. Many of these sources are courtesy of Bob Williams's resource page for evaluators (***www.bobwilliams.co.nz/Resources.html***).

Preparing to Read Chapter Fifteen

As you prepare to read this chapter, think about these questions:

1. How has evaluation evolved from the history of its very beginning until today, and why?

2. Evaluation will continue to evolve. What issues do you think will face evaluators in the next decade?

3. What should you as an evaluator do in order to be culturally responsive and culturally competent throughout an evaluation in a culture different from your own?

4. The U.S. government has supported experimental design as a means to "effectively and efficiently" capture data to create federal policy. How could one argue that a mixed methods approach would improve an evaluation's capacity for producing credible evidence of a program's effectiveness?

5. Why would stakeholders be resistant to evaluations? List several reasons.

6. Is it a great time to be an evaluator?

CHAPTER FIFTEEN

Perennial and Emerging Issues in Evaluation

On the topic of politics and evaluation, Greene and McClintock (1991) refer to a piece written by Cronbach and his associates in 1980. Their extension of Cronbach et al.'s earlier recognition of the political context in which evaluators work is a powerful and prescient description of tensions in the evaluation field that have existed throughout its history, currently, and into the future. They wrote:

> evaluators now do their work with a 'recognition that politics and science are both integral aspects of evaluation' (Cronbach et al., 1980, p. 35) and that values inhere even in the methodological choices evaluators make. [And] … that politics and values are inherent in evaluation and that diverse methods can enable evaluators to develop more complete understanding of how programs work within particular cultural contexts. (p. 13)

Encapsulated in this small quotation are many of the perennial and emerging issues in evaluation. These include the inherency of politics and values in evaluation; deliberation about appropriate evaluator roles and methodologies; and the need for evaluators to be responsive to the cultural context in which they find themselves. In particular, political factors and recognition of diverse value positions serve as a basis for looking back at the history of perennial issues—or "fundamental issues," as Smith & Brandon (2008) call them. They also provide a framework for understanding contemporary and emerging issues in the field.

In this chapter, we discuss a broad range of issues faced by evaluators in the implementation of their evaluations. Many of these issues are discussed in reflective articles written by evaluators to illustrate strategies deemed either effective or challenging during the conduct of evaluations. These include a revisiting of political and contextual issues, ethical issues, human relationships, working with stakeholders, partnerships, and other issues firmly grounded in the experiences of front-line evaluators. Again, these issues are discussed under the overarching theme of politics and values in evaluation.

Politics and Values: Extending the History of Evaluation to Current Times

Earlier chapters of this text have provided you with brief glimpses into the history of evaluation from its early years in the 1950s and 1960s into the present moment. The chapters in Part II have described many of the important theorists, as well as the approaches that have been evolving since evaluation's early beginnings. We have also alluded to periods of upheaval in the evaluation community in the 1970s, when Guba and Lincoln introduced the constructivist paradigm and qualitative methods. This period was sometimes referred to as the "paradigm wars" (see Chapter 5). A period of relative calm ensued through the 1980s and 1990s, with general acceptance that both methods could have potential to serve stakeholders' needs. However, the seemingly placid evaluation waters became turbulent again in 2001, with the U.S. Congress's passage of the No Child Left Behind (NCLB) Act, which reauthorized the Elementary and Secondary Education Act.

The Controversy over Defining Scientifically Based Research

The NCLB Act placed priority on the provision of scientific evidence as the basis for educational funding and practice. The legislation defined "scientifically based research" (SBR) as "research that involves the application of rigorous, systematic, and objective procedures to obtain reliable and valid knowledge relevant to education activities and problems" (Title IX, Part A, §9109[37]; NCLB Act of 2001). Although common sense suggests that demonstration of effectiveness should be required and that evaluation is well situated to provide this evidence, the rub came with the framing of SBR exclusively in terms of experimental and quasi-experimental design: SBR was further defined as research that "is evaluated using experimental or quasi-experimental designs in which individuals, entities, programs, or activities are assigned to different conditions and with appropriate controls to evaluate the effects of the condition of interest, with a preference for random-assignment experiments, or across-condition controls" (Title IX, Part A, §9109[37]; NCLB Act of 2001). This is congruent with the precepts of the positivist and postpositivist paradigms and the Methods Branch. However, it ignores the complexity and sometimes impossibility of implementing a randomized controlled trial in social settings, and it effectively dismisses developments in the field of evaluation over the last 40 years that arose because of the limitations of a strictly methods-based approach to evaluation.[1]

The situation was exacerbated when the National Research Council (2002) issued a report in which the definition of SBR recognized experimental designs as the preferred strategies and dismissed qualitative approaches as not having the potential to establish causality. This report proclaimed experimental designs as the "gold standard" for evaluations when the goal is to establish causality.

This prioritization of experimental designs and dismissal of other approaches led to a flurry of responses from various professional associations, including AEA, AERA, the National Education Association, and the European Evaluation Society (EES). These organizations' statements were similar in sentiment. AEA's (2003) statement read in part: "While we agree with the intent of ensuring that federally sponsored programs be 'evaluated using scientifically based research ... to determine the effectiveness of a project intervention,' we do not agree that 'evaluation methods using an experimental design are best for determining project effectiveness.'" (AEA's statement was not accepted as reflecting the views of all its members, however. Box 15.1 contains information from one group of evaluators who strenuously objected to AEA's position.)

An excerpt from the EES's (2007) statement read as follows:

> The European Evaluation Society (EES), consistent with its mission to promote the 'theory, practice and utilization of high quality evaluation', notes the current interest in improving impact evaluation and assessment (IE) with respect to development and development aid. EES

Box 15.1. Objection to AEA's Policy Statement on Experimental Designs

The following statement was signed by Leonard Bickman, Robert F. Boruch, Thomas D. Cook, David S. Cordray, Gary Henry, Mark W. Lipsey, Peter H. Rossi, and Lee Sechrest:

> This statement is intended to support the [NCLB Act's] definition and associated preference for the use of such designs for outcome evaluation when they are applicable. It is also intended to provide a counterpoint to the statement submitted by the AEA leadership as the Association's position on this matter. The generalized opposition to use of experimental and quasi-experimental methods evinced in the AEA statement is unjustified, speciously argued, and represents neither the methodological norms in the evaluation field nor the views of the large segment of the AEA membership with significant experience conducting experimental and quasi-experimental evaluations of program effects.

Source: Mark W. Lipsey, "NOT the AEA statement on Scientifically Based Evaluation." EvalTalk post of December 3, 2003, 13:22:10-0600. Retrieved from *tinyurl.com/y5v2fg9*

however deplores one perspective currently being strongly advocated: that the best or only rigorous and scientific way of doing so is through randomized controlled trials (RCTs). In contrast, the EES supports multi-method approaches to IE and does not consider any single method such as RCTs as the first choice or as the 'gold standard.' (p. 1)

Another use of experimental designs as "gatekeepers" for what is considered credible evidence came in the establishment of the What Works Clearinghouse (WWC) by the U.S. Department of Education's Institute of Education Sciences in 2002. The WWC's mission is to review the evidence base for educational interventions and rate them as to the quality of that evidence. According to the Institute of Education Sciences (2008), the WWC reviews each study that passes eligibility screens to determine whether the study provides

- strong evidence (*Meets Evidence Standards*),
- weaker evidence (*Meets Evidence Standards with Reservations*), or
- insufficient evidence (*Does Not Meet Evidence Standards*) for an intervention's effectiveness.

Currently, only well-designed and well-implemented randomized controlled trials (RCTs) are considered strong evidence, while quasi-experimental designs (QEDs) with equating may only meet standards with reservations; evidence standards for regression discontinuity and single-case designs are under development. (Retrieved from *ies.ed.gov/ncee/wwc/*)

Interestingly, the National Research Council (2004) took exception to the narrow view of acceptable methods for producing evaluation evidence. It called for a combination of content analysis to review the curriculum content against standards; comparative studies that examined group differences for students who were exposed to different instructional experiences; and case studies to answer how and why questions about a program's functioning. Nevertheless, the council still maintained its previous requirement that a methodologically acceptable study needs to use experimental or quasi-experimental comparative designs.

Impact Evaluation in International Development

The World Bank (Legovini, 2010) and other international organizations also chose to emphasize impact evaluation and the use of randomized controlled trials for that purpose. The World Bank established the Development Impact Evaluation Initiative, which was tasked with increasing the number of projects with impact evaluations. It too recommended the use of experimental or quasi-experimental designs, requiring that impact evaluations include a "counterfactual" (a comparison group).

AEA's Proactive Contribution to U.S. Federal Policy about Evaluation

AEA took a proactive step in 2009 by composing a "roadmap" for evaluation, which it shared with senior administrative officials of the U.S. federal government. This roadmap lists the following functions that evaluation can serve (AEA Evaluation Policy Task Force, 2009, p. 2):

> The new administration would benefit significantly by using program evaluation to

> - address questions about current and emerging problems
> - reduce waste and enhance efficiency
> - increase accountability and transparency
> - monitor program performance
> - improve programs and policies in a systematic manner
> - support major decisions about program reform, expansion, or termination
> - assess whether existing programs are still needed or effective
> - identify program implementation and outcome failures
> - inform the development of new programs where needed
> - share information about effective practices across government programs and agencies

It also emphasizes the need for evaluation to be given a higher profile in the government, and for evaluations to be conducted throughout the life cycle of projects and programs. The issue of methodology is addressed in the roadmap as well (AEA Evaluation Policy Task Force, 2009, p. 5):

> Over the years, the evaluation field has developed an extensive array of analytic approaches and methods that can be applied and adapted to various types of programs, depending upon the circumstances and stages of the program's implementation. For example, surveys are among the bedrock tools for evaluation. But there are many ways in which they can be used, and this method, just like all the others, has evolved to address new and emerging policy interests....

Fundamentally, all evaluation methods should be context-sensitive, culturally relevant, and methodologically sound. A complete set of evaluation approaches and methods would include but not be limited to:

- case studies
- surveys
- quasi-experimental designs
- randomized field experiments
- cost–benefit and cost-effectiveness analyses
- needs assessments
- early implementation reviews
- logic models and evaluability assessments

Thus AEA is arguing for breadth in the development of credible evidence, with methods that are driven by the purpose, context, and intended use of the evaluation findings. I (Donna M. Mertens) would argue that consideration also needs to be given to the assumptions that drive the evaluation decisions. Erickson (as a contributor to Moss et al., 2009) agrees with me on this point. This has been a consistent theme throughout this book and is demonstrated by the book's organization around paradigms and branches that guide evaluation thinking.

Pluralism in Evaluation Approaches

Tarsilla (2010a) has identified the values underlying the divergence in viewpoints with regard to recommended (or required) methodological choices as being related to concerns with bias and objectivity. He raises several interesting questions that stimulate thought about values in evaluation:

1. "[To what degree does] distance from the evaluand enhance validity and reliability of evaluation findings?" (p. 200)

2. "What is the evaluator's main responsibility? Is it really to identify the public truth and unmet needs? If so, is the evaluator's isolation instrumental in achieving the envisaged evaluation purposes?" (p. 202)

3. "Whose responsibility is it to turn evaluative judgments into concrete public actions with a social significance?" (p. 202)

Tarsilla contrasts the Methods Branch evaluation theories (which are based on the assumption that distance from the evaluand is desirable) with the theories associated with the other branches (which are based on the assumption that closeness to the evaluand is necessary to develop rapport in evaluation contexts, especially those evaluands that are complex and involve a variety of stakeholders).[2] Tarsilla clearly argues for a pluralistic approach that includes developing a close relationship with the evaluand and stakeholders. His rationale is based on an ontological assumption that there are multiple realities, and that evaluators need to engage appropriately with stakeholders to capture those various realities. Epistemologically, he argues for the need to be closely involved with the community and build rapport and trust in order to determine whose needs are being met and how well, as well as whose needs are not being met. Axiologically, evaluators need to avoid putting themselves in the "God position," meaning that they consider themselves above and not involved in the fray. This requires that evaluators immerse themselves in the stakeholders' reality and develop a deep understanding of the contextual factors therein. Without this level of involvement, evaluators can find themselves in a position that limits the potential use of their findings.

The pluralistic approach is commensurate with the transformative paradigm in terms of the philosophical assumptions put forth by Tarsilla (2010a).[3] He argues that evaluators need to address the concept of advocacy in their work, making clear the value positions that they hold (i.e., advocating for social justice, advocating for the best interests of participants). He states that evaluators should strive for a participatory approach, because it "can effectively coexist with advocacy, so long as the evaluators clarify their stances vis-à-vis the social, economic, and political issues associated with their evaluand. This is the case of transformative evaluators, who address power imbalances in society as part of their work by pushing further for social change and equity (Mertens, 2009)" (Tarsilla, 2010a, p. 204).

Ongoing Developments: Cultural Responsiveness and Mixed Methods

Cultural Responsiveness Revisited

An increase in concerns about representation and voice has led to increased awareness of issues in evaluation when the targeted stakeholder group has experienced discrimination or oppression on the multiple dimensions of diversity that are used to deny people access to services and to diminish their stance as people who are worthy of respect. The topics of cultural responsiveness and competence have been discussed in Chapter 6. Here we extend that discussion to include advice from evaluators about what to do when you attempt to conduct an evaluation in a culture that is not your own.

Three evaluators from New Zealand and one from the United States have addressed this issue by reviewing literature related to culture and cultural contexts in evaluation (Wehipeihana, Davidson, McKegg, & Shanker, 2010). Wehipeihana is a Māori woman who lives and works in New Zealand; Davidson and McKegg are Pakeha (New Zealanders of European descent) women who also live and work in New Zealand. The fourth author is Shanker, whose family emigrated from India; she was born in the United States, where she currently lives and works. Davidson's position is that she is not qualified to bid on requests for proposals that call for culturally based evaluations in the Māori or Pasifika (New Zealand people whose origins include Samoa, Tonga, Niue, Cook Islands, Fiji, and Tokelau) communities, because she is not from those communities. Davidson points out that selection of evaluators who are from the community is crucial if the evaluation is to have validity and credibility. Māori or Pasifika know their language and culture and have the relationships that give them legitimacy in the eyes of the stakeholders. Their involvement as evaluators is needed throughout the life of the evaluation, from the design to data collection to analysis and interpretation to use. Genuine fluency in the language is critical; as we have noted earlier, translation is not a simple task. In some languages, there are concepts that simply do not translate into other languages. Being bilingual is not enough.

To do an effective job of translating ideas and experiences across cultural boundaries, you really have to understand not just the language and culture, but also the subject matter you are trying to explore, and what exactly you are trying to find out or convey. It's not about having any person from the target community involved in the project; it's about having people with both the cultural knowledge, language competence, and community connections and the evaluation skills and experience to get the job done well. (Davidson, as a contributor to Wehipeihana et al., 2010, pp. 185–186)

In her contribution to the 2010 article, Wehipeihana agrees with Davidson regarding the importance of this deep level of experience with the targeted community, and adds that the evaluator also needs a methodological evaluation theory and practice "toolkit" that is grounded in that cultural understanding. She places priority on appropriately engaging with stakeholders throughout the evaluation process. In order to accomplish this, she asserts that the evaluation should be led by Wehipeihana if that is the targeted community. At the same time, she reminds evaluators that all contexts are multicultural, and that representatives of those diverse cultures should be tapped to lead evaluations in their communities. This is particularly important for making sense of the data that are collected, analyzed, and interpreted. She references the work of Symonette (2004) and Kirkhart (2005) as it relates to the importance of the evaluator knowing who they are, how they are perceived by the stakeholders, and the nature of their identity in relation to that community. Rather than seeing evaluation work in Māori communities as the sole domain of Māori evaluators, Wehipeihana holds that Māori evaluators should be the lead evaluators, but that there is a place for team members who are Pakeha or members of other cultural groups.

· · · · · · · · · · **EXTENDING YOUR THINKING** · · · · · · · · · ·

Community Membership Issues

1. Shanker (as a contributor to Wehipeihana et al., 2010) reflected on the idea of having evaluators who were not from the targeted community. She wrote: "It is laughable that [an evaluator] thought s/he could design an evaluation *for* another community and then receive assistance *from* them in delivering it *to* them. But it happens all the time, right in front of my face" (p. 190; emphasis in original). What is your reaction to this statement?

2. What is your stance with regard to the need for the evaluator (or the lead evaluator) to be from the targeted community?

3. Recall that Mertens et al. (2007) (see Chapter 6, Box 6.10) viewed the transformative paradigm as one framework that encouraged a team approach between deaf and hearing evaluators/researchers. What is your stance in regard to working in teams of evaluators, some of whom are from the community being evaluated and some of whom are not?

(*cont.*)

4. Sullivan (2009) has argued that the combination of members and nonmembers of the disability community on the evaluation team actually works to reduce the marginalization of the members of the disability communities. What do you think of his position?

5. What kinds of strategies would enhance the quality of teams of evaluators working together? What can be done to address issues of power and privilege in the evaluation team?

Mixed Methods Revisited

Mixed methods are receiving increased attention and interest in the evaluation community. As evaluators look for ways to respond to the political factors discussed earlier in this chapter, mixed methods offer one potential strategy to gather evidence that is viewed as credible and valid. In Part II and in Chapter 9, we have explained that three positions on mixed methods have emerged from the research and evaluation communities. The first one is consistent with the Use Branch, and the second with the Social Justice Branch. The third position is the dialectical stance advocated by Greene and Maxwell. Recall that this stance involves adherence to the beliefs of the methods and Values Branches, with opportunity for dialogue across these branches as a way of extending the understandings that emerge from each one. In 2010, AEA approved a topical interest group (TIG) called Mixed Methods in Evaluation. Its mission statement reads:

> The Mixed Methods in Evaluation TIG will examine the use of mixed methods in evaluation through the reflective analysis of the philosophy, theory, and methodology that is developing in the field of mixed methods. AEA members will be encouraged to submit both theoretical and empirical papers on the topic of mixed methods. Mixed methods is viewed as the combination of more than one methodological standpoint in the same study. The mixing can occur at the level of inquiry purpose, philosophical assumptions, methodological design, and/or specific data gathering technique. Evaluators have commonly used a mix of methods in their work; however, there has not been a concentrated opportunity to examine what that means theoretically and practically for the evaluation field. Hence, this TIG would contribute to the improvement of evaluation practices, method and use because it will focus on the contributions that a better understanding of mixed methods has to offer (Mertens & Yamashita, 2010).

This TIG provides one venue for evaluators who are interested in pursuing mixed methods as a means to address the challenges regarding what is considered credible evidence.

The U.S. government's reliance on randomized controlled trials as the sole method capable of producing credible evidence appears to be the result of work undertaken by the private, nonprofit Coalition for Evidence-Based Policy (***evidencebasedprograms.org/wordpress***). The Coalition developed the tiered system that we have seen illustrated for review of projects for the WWC. In response to Congressional inquiries about this tiered system, the U.S. Government Accountability Office (U.S. GAO, 2009), which serves as Congress's watchdog for evaluation of federal programs, issued a report to Congress entitled *Program Evaluation: A Variety of Rigorous Methods Can Help Identify Effective Interventions*. This agency recognized the problem that "The Top Tier initiative's choice of broad topics (such as early childhood interventions), emphasis on long-term effects, and use of narrow evidence criteria combine to provide limited information on what is effective in achieving specific outcomes" (U.S. GAO, 2009, p. 15). It noted that other criteria for evidence credibility can be appropriately used to determine an intervention's effectiveness. Its statement reveals its support for randomized experiments when these are possible, but for the appropriateness of other standards of evidence when these are not:

> The program evaluation literature generally agrees that well-conducted randomized experiments are best suited for assessing effectiveness when multiple causal influences create uncertainty about what caused results. However, they are often difficult, and sometimes impossible, to carry out. An evaluation must be able to control exposure to the intervention and ensure that treatment and control groups' experiences remain separate and distinct throughout the study. (U.S. GAO, 2009, p. 15)

It went on to note that various alternatives to experimental designs, such as quasi-experimental designs, statistical analysis of observational data, and in-depth case studies, can also be used to construct credible evidence of program effectiveness.

· · · · · · · · · · · E X T E N D I N G   Y O U R   T H I N K I N G · · · · · · · · · · ·

Evaluation and Policy

1. How do you understand the influence of broad national policy on evaluation practice?

2. What are your thoughts with regard to the use of randomized experimental designs as the sole method for producing credible evidence of program effectiveness?

3. What other roles can evaluation play with regard to informing national policies?

4. Think about the advice from AEA and the U.S. GAO about use of multiple methods. How would you use this advice to attempt to influence federal policy?

5. Erickson (as a contributor to Moss et al., 2009, p. 505) reacted to the focus of the federal government on effectiveness and efficiency by writing about the need to ask a question about the values that underlie choice of programs:

> A prior question lurks: "Do we want to do this in the first place?" (i.e., Is this a means or an end that is worth pursuing?). Such questions can be addressed indirectly by evidence from empirical study, whether quantitative or qualitative, but ultimately they involve also considering value choices directly: whether to teach for basic skills or for understanding; whether children should be able to use calculators in doing arithmetic or use invented spelling in learning literacy; whether racially segregated schools are inherently demeaning and unjust; whether differential spending levels between schools in high- and low-income neighborhoods are wrong or right; whether charter schools are a potential blessing or a curse; whether mother tongue instruction in bilin-

(cont.)

gual education should be encouraged or discouraged. These and many other questions involve issues of value (and of political interest) most fundamentally rather than of simple instrumental utility.

What is your reaction to Erickson's call for an additional, prior question to the questions of effectiveness and efficiency?

6. Floden (also a contributor to Moss et al., 2009, p. 505) offered these thoughts, which seem to suggest that a mixed methods approach can be used to engender improved understanding:

> Discussions about research quality often cast the issues, for rhetorical reasons, in an either/or framework. A scholar, for example, either is interested in understanding the meanings participants attach to particular events or is interested in generalizations about associations among variables. I think making such sharp dichotomous divisions is not helpful. Scholars often have interests in mixtures of meaning, events, behaviors, actions, and causes. The quality of research encompasses multiple dimensions, with gradations of quality, rather than classifications as good or bad.

7. Lather (as another contributor to Moss et al., 2009, p. 506) argues that the basic assumptions that claims of causality must be based on experimental designs are flawed. She does not see the overtures to find common ground and common language persuasive as a strategy to improve the evaluation of interventions. Rather, she suggests a need to recognize "the power struggles over who gets to set the terms of debate and what it means to court interruption/counter narratives [as] a move toward better work all the way around." Respond to Lather about her position with regard to rejecting the fundamental assumptions that guide the Methods Branch. Compare her position with those of Erickson and Floden (see questions 5 and 6, above).

Credible Evidence: Need for More Research on Evaluation

In some respects, the many issues discussed so far as perennial and emerging issues in evaluation come down to a question of what is considered credible evidence. In 2006, a group of evaluators assembled at a conference at Claremont Graduate School in California to address this topic. This meeting resulted in a book entitled *What Counts as Credible Evidence in Applied Research and Evaluation?* (Donaldson, Christie, & Mark, 2009). The majority of the book is devoted to separate sections written by representatives of the Methods and Values Branches, based on Christie and Fleischer's (2009) assertion that most evaluators align themselves with two paradigms: postpositivism (Methods Branch) and constructivism (Values Branch). They barely mention mixed methods, which is curious, given the interest in mixed methods in the broader evaluation community.[4] In some respects, the contributors simply continue to repeat age-old arguments that elevate one approach over the other, except that they also recommend some additions to randomized controlled trials (e.g., regression discontinuity designs). Having evaluators who represent these two viewpoints exchange ideas is healthy, but it does not get us past the division that has plagued the evaluation community for decades.

Mark and Henry (2004) write about the need for additional research on theories of evaluation as a means of addressing this divisiveness. The lack of agreement on the meaning of credible evidence and the potential for various branches to contribute to the construction of such evidence inhibits our ability to make definitive statements about appropriate methods and uses of evaluation. Schwandt (2009) offers a framework for considering a theory of credible evidence that is not anchored in either the methods or Values Branches:

> Clearing out the underbrush of the quantitative–qualitative debate and the thicket of scientism makes it possible to frame the discussion of what constitutes credible evidence in evaluation in potentially more educative and enlightening ways.... [Schwandt proposes] a potential theory of evidence for evaluation that attends to questions of the credibility, relevance, and probative value of evidence while embracing a range of methods. At minimum, an adequate theory of evidence includes analyses of several kinds—the character of evidence, the ethics of evidence, the contexts of the application of evidence, and the nature of rationality and argumentation. (p. 199)

With regard to the character of evidence, Schwandt argues that we use many different types of evidence derived from many different sources to reach conclusions about important issues. In addition to evidence generated by randomized controlled trials, he notes that analyses of speeches, memos, historical documents, legal cases, and other documents, as well as interviews and observations, are used to make claims of causality. For example, I recently broke my arm; the doctor examined X-rays of my bone as evidence of its progress in healing. My sister is a judge; she uses legal precedents and evidence (presented in the form of documents and testimony from witnesses and experts) to determine guilt or innocence.

The critical questions about evidence are these (Schwandt, 2009, p. 201):

- *Relevance*—Does the information bear directly on the hypothesis or claim in question?

- *Credibility*—Can we believe the information?

- *Probative (inferential) force*—How strongly does the information point toward the claim or hypothesis being considered?

Of course, these still leave the sticky questions of the rigor of the methods used to create the evidence and the need to interpret the evidence once it is gathered. Claims of causality can be bolstered by having multiple sources of evidence. However, in the social world, no evidence can support claims of causality infallibly. There is always a margin of error, and competing explanations can never be completely ruled out. In addition, there are ever-present concerns about who is in the position of power to create the evidence, and what that means in terms of whose perspectives are not represented in the evidence that is created.

Discussion of power, representation, and interpretation lead directly to questions of ethics in evaluation, especially in terms of acceptance of credible data as the bases for action. Actions based on evaluation findings have the potential to change lives, for better or worse. These implications lead to the need for evaluators to be conscious of the ethical issues involved in the interpretation, dissemination, and use of evidence by various stakeholder groups. Schwandt (2009) concludes his argument by discussing the importance of context in the valuing of different types of evidence:

> The basis on which we substantiate the use of any method in evaluation is not a hierarchy of method—with RCTs at the highest level—and expert opinion at the lowest level—but a judgment of the aptness of a given method to generate the kind of information needed to produce empirical evidence in support of a judgment of value of an evaluand. (p. 207)

Schwandt (2009) offers evaluators a way to overcome differences and to value appropriate types of evidence in specific contexts. There is much room for additional thought and research on this issue.

· · · · · · · · · · E X T E N D I N G   Y O U R   T H I N K I N G · · · · · · · · · ·

Evaluation Theory

1. Consider Schwandt's (2009) arguments for a practical theory of evaluation that sweeps away questions of methodology as the basis for divisiveness. How do you respond to these ideas?

2. Think about the nature of making decisions. To what extent are decisions based solely on one piece of evidence, even if that evidence is produced through randomized controlled trials? What are the other factors that need to be considered in analyzing the process of decision making?

3. Greene (2009) argues that evaluators have a responsibility to understand "the inherent *complexity* of human phenomena in contrast with evidence that both denies and simplifies the wondrous and diverse panorama of the human species" (p. 155; emphasis in original). Discuss this idea in the context of credible evidence and decision making in evaluation.

4. Think about the four paradigms and branches of evaluation explained throughout this text. What is their usefulness in light of the possibility of Schwandt's proposed practical theory as a means of unifying evaluation theory about credible evidence?

5. All this talk of the need for high-quality evaluations in order to influence policy and program decisions is not altogether straightforward. For example, there are programs that do not have evidence of their effectiveness, yet they continue to be funded and implemented. Two examples are the Drug Abuse Resistance Education (D.A.R.E.) program to keep youth off drugs (Berman & Fox, 2009) and the Just Say No program to prevent teenage pregnancies.

    a. Berman and Fox (2009) reviewed over 30 evaluation reports of D.A.R.E. that either showed little or no effect on teen drug use or actually showed a slight increase over several years. Yet "D.A.R.E. is alive and well, taught in about 75% of school districts across the country. Over 15,000 police officers participate as D.A.R.E. instructors, providing educational sessions about drugs and drug abuse largely targeted at 5th and 6th graders" (p. 1).

b. Just Say No is a program supported by the U.S. government that teaches students to avoid teenage pregnancies and STDs by "just saying no" to sex prior to marriage. The U.S. government has allocated $50 million dollars annually to support the Just Say No program since 1998. This type of program is also called an "abstinence-only" program, as compared to a comprehensive sex education program that includes instruction about STDs and birth control strategies. An evaluation sponsored by the U.S. Department of Health and Human Services was conducted by Mathematica Policy Research Corporation (Trenholm et al., 2008). This study used an experimental design with randomized groups that received either the Just Say No program or comprehensive sex education. The results were as follows:

> Findings indicate that youth in the program group were no more likely than control group youth to have abstained from sex and, among those who reported having had sex, they had similar numbers of sexual partners and had initiated sex at the same mean age. Contrary to concerns raised by some critics of the Title V, Section 510 abstinence funding, however, program group youth were no more likely to have engaged in unprotected sex than control group.... In contrast to high levels of knowledge about the risks of unprotected sex, study youth are less knowledgeable about the potential health risks from STDs. (pp. viii–ix)

Why do you think such programs continue to be supported when there is no credible evidence to support their effectiveness?

Strategies for Addressing Resistance to Evaluation

One final area identified as a perennial issue in evaluation is that of overcoming resistance to evaluation. Some new evaluators are surprised when they encounter such resistance. After all, the evaluators think they are there to help an organization improve, and who could be against that? Yet, if we place ourselves in the shoes of the stakeholders and think about the possibility of somewhat public criticism that can have serious implications for those individuals (e.g., reduced program funding or actual job loss), it is easier to appreciate resistance. Some staff members may view evaluation as an unnecessary drain of resources that would be better put toward supporting program activities. This does raise the question of the cost-effectiveness of evaluations themselves. An evaluation should provide sufficient benefit to justify the expenditure of funds, rather than draining resources in an already cash-strapped project.

    Also, staffers in some organizations may have the attitude that they got along fine without evaluation before and may resent the intrusion of these outsiders (or even internal evaluators) telling them what they should or should not do. Of course, as evaluators, we know that our jobs are not to tell people what to do. Rather, we collect data to improve the process of decision making. However, individuals who do not have a positive and productive history of working with evaluators may dig in their heels and either refuse to participate or engage in passive–aggressive behaviors that only superficially respond to the evaluators' requests. As a bit of humor, Box 15.2 lists some of the reasons for not evaluating that were posted on the UNESCO website over 20 years ago. The UNESCO list was brought to our attention in a blog post written by Patricia Rogers and Jane Davidson (2010). Rogers and Davidson suggest that a review of these reasons will save new evaluators a lot of time, because they can anticipate these excuses and develop responses to them. (However, if project directors find this list, they will have a ready set of excuses. So treat it with discretion.) Evaluators should also be aware that project directors will sometimes use a combination of two or three of these reasons to bolster their case that evaluation should not be applied to their projects.

Many of the strategies discussed in earlier chapters for working with stakeholders and for building partnerships and relationships can be used to overcome resistance to evaluation. The James Irving Foundation (2009) developed a guide for its board of trustees on strategies to overcome resistance to evaluation, focused on four commonly given excuses for not paying attention to evaluation at the highest decision-making levels (see Box 15.3).

Many of these suggestions could be transferred to other stakeholder groups as well.

Finally, practicing evaluators all have stories to tell about forms of resistance and strategies for overcoming resistance. Two evaluators' stories appear in Box 15.4.

Emerging Issues: From Here to Eternity

This chapter could go on without end, because evaluation is a dynamic and evolving discipline (transdiscipline). Involvement of evaluators with stakeholders in a variety of contexts; building linkages with policy makers; developing and refining new strategies for planning, implementing, and using evaluations—there is an unending list of emerging issues. For example, just in the area of using visual data, many exciting developments provide opportunities to present findings in ways that heretofore have not been commonly present in evaluation work (e.g., geographical information systems, or web-based visualizations that can include video and pictures). Such developments are exciting because they can increase our ability to accurately capture and represent experiences of stakeholders. They can also be fruitful ground for additional research into the effectiveness of evaluations. Yet they can also raise issues of privacy and ethics that need critical examination.

Other topics that could have been addressed in this chapter include the implications of discipline-specific knowledge for evaluators. To what extent do evaluators need to be experts in a field before they are capable of conducting a high-quality evaluation? I find that having background knowledge is a real asset, because it provides the contextual base for identifying issues and asking questions. However, on occasion, I have accepted evaluation contracts for topics for which my personal experience and knowledge base were more limited, such as the accessibility of courts for deaf and hard-of-hearing people. I know about deafness and hearing loss from having spent many years in the deaf community as a professor at Gallaudet. However, my knowledge of issues in court access was limited. As mentioned in a previous chapter, the project was established with an advisory board that had expertise in court access. We agreed to work in partnership: I would supply knowledge about evaluation and deafness, and the board would provide knowledge about deafness, hard-of-hearing people, and court access.

Box 15.2. Reasons for Avoiding Evaluation in the United Nations System

- Our project is different.
- It would cost too much.
- We don't have the time.
- The project/activity is too limited.
- It doesn't figure in the work plan.
- We've never done it before.
- The government/organization wouldn't like it.
- Give me the funds.
- It's not my responsibility.
- An evaluation isn't necessary.
- It's too theoretical an exercise.
- Let's be realistic.
- It's none of our business.
- It works, so why change it?
- We're not ready for it yet.
- It's not included in the budget.
- We've never done this before.
- There must be some ulterior motive.
- Is somebody trying to teach me my job?
- It might work in any other organization (region/country/technical domain) but it will never work here.
- I'm not convinced that it would be useful.
- It's a trap!
- We've always worked like this.
- We've done what we said we'd do.
- We've done what was in the project document.
- We've already been evaluated.
- We don't have any problems.
- The equipment hasn't been installed yet.
- The institutional framework hasn't been worked out yet.
- We can't find the original work plan.
- The programme specialist in charge at the beginning of the project was somebody else.

(cont.)

Box 15.2 (*cont.*)

- The government was happy with the project.

- The government hasn't given its contribution yet.

- The project isn't ready for evaluation yet.

- We don't have all the data.

- The project document is too vague.

- It's a national holiday.

- It's the rainy season.

- Let the Inspection Unit take care of it.

- Outsiders won't understand the complexities.

- We are constantly evaluating ourselves.

- I have to take my annual leave.

- Another donor agency might want to evaluate us at the same time.

Source: Rogers and Davidson (2010), from a UNESCO list of January 1991.

Postings on the AEA EvalTalk listserv are frequently questions about conducting evaluations within specific contexts. For example, one evaluator asked about evaluating academic uses of technology. Members of the listserv responded by identifying resources such as a website with specific references for evaluation in that context (***bit.ly/Flashlight-Approach***). Another evaluator asked about the specifics of evaluating projects related to environmental projects. The answers provided by list members included these:

- EPE Week: A. Rowe on Getting the Evaluand Right for Environmental, Conservation & Resource Initiatives (***aea365.org/blog/?p=606***).

- EPE Week: J. Peters on Engagement in the Field of Energy Evaluation (***aea365.org/blog/?p=602***).

The possibilities of specific contextual evaluation issues are as long as the profession is wide.

Fortunately for novice and experienced evaluators alike, there are many web-based resources that can provide answers to these types of questions. In addition to the Eval-Talk listserv, AEA has an electronic resource library and the Tip-A-Day blog, which are available through its website and are searchable databases. Evaluators around the world can access AEA's resources at its website (some are limited to members only). In addition, many other nations host evaluation organizations and have resources and listservs for their members (e.g., AfrEA, EES, and the Australasian Evaluation Society). So, when faced with new challenges that make your life as an evaluator exciting, you can find many

Box 15.3. Excuses Not to Engage with Evaluation Data, and Strategies to Address These Excuses

Excuse	Strategies
There isn't enough time to discuss evaluation results.	■ Consider having one meeting a year or a retreat that is specifically focused on examining evaluation results.
	■ Restructure board meetings so evaluation data can be integrated into discussions that allow the board members to learn from past experiences.
	■ Form a subcommittee of the board that is responsible for reviewing evaluation results and reporting them to the full board.
Evaluation results are not actionable.	■ Synthesize evaluation results so you can get to the point quickly.
	■ Anticipate decision points: When does the board make decisions about continuation or awards of new funding?
	■ Be sure evaluation is included in the plan for a project before it is funded.
	■ Develop a specific agenda for what can be learned from an evaluation.
Information isn't presented in a format that is helpful for trustees.	■ Tailor your presentation to the decisions that need to be made. This can include a short summary shared for the board to read before the presentation. Give the board members information at different levels of depth, depending on their interest in delving into the evaluation beyond what can be said in a brief presentation.
	■ Because foundations generally are in the business of giving money, they will appreciate having evaluation reports that show charts, trends, risks, etc.
	■ Prior to the presentation, share the information with another colleague who has a critical eye. Consider having communications experts consult with you and professional narrators give the report.
	■ Make the presentation in a manner that facilitates dialogue, rather than a straight lecture format.
Trustees don't see the value in evaluation.	■ Realize that not all trustees are familiar with the potential contribution evaluation has to offer. Capacity building even at this level may be necessary to explain what they can gain by paying attention to evaluation.
	■ Development of an overall evaluation plan for the foundation would go a long way towards creating the culture of learning that organizations need to benefit from evaluation activities.
	■ External consultants who are experts in evaluation can be used as part of the educative process for board members.

Source: Based on James Irving Foundation (2009).

Box 15.4. Practicing Evaluators' Reflections on Overcoming Resistance

Evaluations are sometime resisted by stakeholders because evaluation is perceived as a threat, particularly if there are high stakes linked to evaluation results. For example, project managers may fear an evaluation of their project if funding decisions will be made on the basis of the evaluation results. Evaluation may be resisted if stakeholders are concerned that the evaluation may show the stakeholders are not effective in their job responsibilities. Sometimes evaluation stakeholders want to control information and are concerned about the loss of control of information if their program, project, or department must submit to an evaluation.

Evaluation may be resisted if a stakeholder does not believe the evaluation will bring value. Sometimes stakeholders believe money is better spent on program or project activities than on evaluating the program or project. Also, stakeholders might be resistant to a particular evaluation methodology, because of biases [against that methodology or toward another] methodology.

Even if an evaluation won't be used for high-stakes decisions, stakeholders sometimes resist participating in an evaluation because participation may create additional work for them, or they may view the evaluation as nothing more than an additional bureaucratic process. For example, schools may resist hosting evaluation site visitors because there are so many other important things going on, or they may resist data collection in a school because they believe it detracts from student education.

Evaluation resistance can be overcome by engaging in and understanding the social and political contexts in which an evaluation is conducted. Evaluation planning with stakeholders gives an evaluator good opportunities to build relationships with stakeholders and to figure out who has the most at stake from the outcome of an evaluation and who might perceive a particular evaluation as a threat. An evaluator should work with the evaluation commissioners (clients), by establishing consensus about the purpose and use of evaluation, and learning in what social and political contexts the proposed evaluation would take place. Evaluators may also provide support to clients and key stakeholders who might be crucial for facilitating support for evaluation about how they might want to communicate with other stakeholders about the scope and purpose of evaluation, roles, and consequences of evaluation.

Evaluators need to know who can deal with evaluation resistance and what role evaluators and evaluation commissioners can play in a particular evaluation project. Once an evaluator knows who has a stake in the evaluation results or perceives evaluation as a threat, it is possible to deal with those concerns with evaluation commissioners. Sometimes framing the evaluation early on as a way [to help] the stakeholders, rather than [to pass] judgment on a program or project, can create buy-in.

Source: Mika Yamashita and Bryan Yoder (personal communication, May 25, 2010).

kindred spirits who are willing to share their experiences and insights. It is a good time to be an evaluator.

Think about the water metaphor of evaluation branches that we have presented throughout this text. The future of evaluation may well lie in the swirling waters that combine thinking from four different paradigms and the branches of evaluation associated with them. Because evaluation is an ever-developing field, it presents multiple opportunities for all of us who are involved in it to contribute to furthering its excellence in theory and practice.

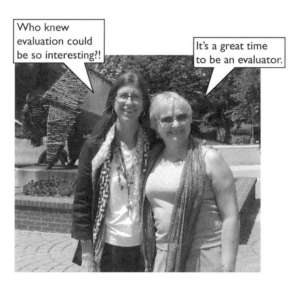

Notes

1. This prioritization was not limited to the NCLB Act. Similar language subsequently appeared in many other pieces of U.S. legislation (e.g., the Reading Excellence Act required that "grant funds be used to help schools adopt those programs that incorporate 'scientifically based principles' of reading instruction" [Borman et al., 2005, p. 2]). The strict definition of SBR, with the experimental design requirement, also began to appear in other countries around the world. These requirements were not restricted to legislative initiatives; they also encompassed many foundations and other donor agencies.

2. It should also be noted that Scriven developed the goal-free evaluation method, which calls for evaluators to conduct their work without reference to the stated project goals. The assumption is that if the effects are strong enough, they will emerge without direct inquiry about them.

3. One exception should be noted: The transformative ontological assumption interrogates versions of reality to expose those that have the potential to further oppress or enhance human rights for people who have been marginalized (Mertens, 2009).

4. The lack of attention to the Social Justice Branch might be attributed to the lack of persons from underserved communities in the list of contributing authors.

Glossary

Anonymity: An evaluation condition in which the researchers do not request any identifying materials that could link the persons from whom they collect data with the collected data.

Concurrent mixed methods design: Evaluation design in which qualitative and quantitative methods are both used in the same time frame.

Confidentiality: An evaluation condition in which the researchers collect data in such a way that only they are able to identify the persons responding to interviews, surveys, observations, or document reviews.

Connoisseurship: Eisner's model of evaluation, in which researchers are connoisseurs—able to see the unique qualities in complex settings, and then to evaluate the collected data in a holistic manner, using multiple perspectives.

Constructivist paradigm: The belief that knowledge is socially constructed by people active in the research process, and that researchers should attempt to understand the complex world of lived experience from the point of view of those who live it. Focuses primarily on identifying multiple values and perspectives through qualitative methods.

Context evaluation: Examining and describing the values, goals, mission, objectives, and priorities of a program; assessing needs; and determining whether the defined objectives will be responsive to the identified needs.

Context, input, process, product (CIPP) model: Stufflebeam's four-part model of evaluation. The context evaluation prioritizes goals; the input evaluation assesses different approaches; the process evaluation assesses the implementation of plans; and the product evaluation assesses both the intended and unintended outcomes.

Control group: The group in an experiment that does not receive the "treatment" or the independent variable.

Convenience sampling: Selection of easily obtainable participants for a sample group; usually the cheapest and fastest way of obtaining a sample group.

Cost analysis: An evaluation's determination of whether a program's effect was worth its cost.

Country-led evaluation (CLE): A type of evaluation in which an individual country implements the evaluation, guides its process, determines the policy or program to be evaluated, chooses the methodology and analytical approach, and decides how the resulting data will be disseminated and ultimately used.

Critical race theory (CRT): Theoretical framework that allows researchers to interrogate social, educational, and political issues by prioritizing the voices of participants of color and respecting the multiple roles played by scholars of color.

Culturally responsive evaluation: Type of evaluation in which the focus is on understanding the cultural and historical context of the programs and implementing all aspects of the evaluation to fit the needs of the community (language, tools, cultural practices, etc.).

Deliberative democratic evaluation (DDE): Type of evaluation that uses reflective reasoning about relevant issues (including preferences and values) with appropriate parties. There is intentional deliberation about the results, an inclusion of all relevant interests, and dialogue so that the interests of various stakeholders are accurately ascertained; thus power relations are equalized when evaluative judgments are made.

Dependent variable: The observed result of the independent variable being manipulated.

Design evaluation: An evaluation that uses the data collected before a program begins. Examples include pilot projects, baseline surveys, and feasibility studies.

Dialectical approach: Evaluation approach in which both quantitative and qualitative designs are implemented independently and during various points of a study; the qualitative and quantitative evaluators share their findings to reveal similarities and differences between the results obtained with the two methodologies.

Dialectical mixed methods design: Research design in which both qualitative and quantitative data are collected at the same time during the study, and then a dialogue occurs between the qualitative and quantitative evaluators.

Disability- and deaf-rights-based evaluation: Evaluation approaches in which evaluators accommodate the linguistic, physical, cognitive, and psychological differences of the stakeholders (e.g., use of sign language interpreters, audio surveys) and are responsive to other characteristics, such as gender and ethnicity.

Educational criticism: Eisner's recommendation that when evaluating as a "connoisseur," the researcher should describe, interpret, evaluate, and identify dominant themes and qualities in a manner that is understood by all stakeholders.

Embedded mixed methods design: Design in which one data set (such as qualitative data) is collected to support the larger data set in a study (such as quantitative data).

Emergent evaluation: An evaluation that is allowed to evolve throughout the course of the project. Examples include participatory, qualitative, critical, hermeneutical, bottom-up, collaborative, and transdisciplinary approaches.

Empowerment evaluation: An evaluation in which the program staff is in charge of the direction and execution, while the evaluator serves as a critical friend, coach, advisor, or guide.

Evaluand: The entity that is to be evaluated, such as a project, program, policy, or product.

Evaluation theory: Any type of theory that identifies the paradigms within which evaluators gather data and explains the conceptual framework within which they construct knowledge in order to evaluate programs.

Experimental group: The group in an experiment that receives the "treatment" or the independent variable.

External evaluation: An evaluation conducted by an evaluator who is not an employee of the organization that houses the object of the evaluation (e.g., program).

External validity: The ability to generalize the results of a study to other people or other situations (e.g., tutoring that helps improve students' test scores at one school does the same at the other schools in the county).

Feminist evaluation: Evaluation approach that focuses on gender inequities and women's realities; a program's context is understood from a feminist perspective, and the findings are used to advocate for rights and justice for all.

Formative evaluation: An evaluation conducted during the development or delivery of a program or product, with the intention of providing feedback to improve the evaluand; it may also focus on program plans or designs.

Fourth-generation evaluation: A qualitative methodology that includes intensive involvement with stakeholders in the design, conduct, and building of meaning based on the collected evaluation data.

Gender analysis: An analysis of the different effects that a project or program may have on women, girls, men, and boys, and on the economic and social relationships between and among these groups.

Goal-free evaluation: Scriven's method of evaluating programs, in which a researcher intentionally remains unaware of a program's goals and searches for its effects regardless of the program's objectives.

Hermeneutic process: The construction of reality by the research participants through conversational interaction with the researcher; multiple meanings are constructed and analyzed.

Homogeneous sampling: A qualitative research sampling approach that focuses on studying cases with similar characteristics, in order to develop an in-depth analysis of a particular category.

Impact evaluation: An evaluation that assesses a program's effects and the extent to which the program's goals were achieved.

Impact study: An evaluation that establishes causal links between an independent variable (the intervention) and a dependent variable (the anticipated change), and identifies the independent variable's effects.

Independent variable: The variable being manipulated or changed.

Indigenous evaluation: An evaluation that is respectful of the indigenous culture and is carried out based on the values of the indigenous stakeholders.

Informed consent: An ethical requirement that educates research participants about what their rights during a study are, what the study consists of, what will happen to the data that they contribute, and whether there are any negative or positive consequences of their participation.

Input evaluation: A needs assessment that determines what can be achieved based on the given set of goals in terms of scheduling, staffing, and budget.

Internal evaluation: The use by an organization of evaluators who are employees of that organization to evaluate the organization's own programs.

Internal validity: Evidence that the independent variable in a study does affect the dependent variable (e.g., tutoring in a school helps improve the students' test scores).

Logical framework or log frame: A tool for planning and managing development projects; it looks like a table and structures components of a project in a clear, concise, organized, and logical way.

Logic model: A model that displays the sequence of actions in a program, describes what the program is and will do, and describes how investments will be linked to results.

Merit: The absolute or relative quality of something, either overall or in regard to a particular criterion (as opposed to **worth,** which is determined by a particular context).

Meta-evaluation: The study of the quality of the evaluation.

Mixed methods: A combination of qualitative and quantitative approaches in the study and/or data collection.

Monitoring: A term used in the field of international development; the parallel term in the wider evaluation community is **process evaluation.**

Myth of homogeneity: The assumption that all people within a particular subgroup are similar to each other in terms of their other background characteristics, or similar enough where differences are not identified.

Naturalistic evaluation: Observation of a program in its natural state without a defined hypothesis (as opposed to the experimental approach, where the independent and dependent variables are carefully defined and controlled before the study begins).

Paradigms: Broad metaphysical constructs that include sets of logically related philosophical assumptions.

Postpositivist paradigm: The belief that the social world can be studied in the same way as the natural world, that there is a value-free method for studying the social world, and that explanations of a causal nature can be provided. Focuses primarily on quantitative designs and data.

Practical participatory evaluation: An evaluation in which decision makers are end users of a formative, improvement- or utilization-oriented final evaluation (as opposed to **transformative participatory evaluation**).

Pragmatic paradigm: The belief that reality is individually interpreted and that the methodological choices will be determined by the evaluation questions. Focuses primarily on data that are found to be useful by stakeholders, and advocates for the use of mixed methods.

Probability-based sampling: The selection of a sample from a population in a way that allows for an estimation of the amount of possible bias and sampling error.

Process evaluation: An evaluation that continually informs the management and main stakeholders of an ongoing intervention about early indications of progress (or lack of progress) in achieving results of a project or program, or other kind of support to an outcome.

Product evaluation: An evaluation that measures, interprets, and judges the achievements of a program in attaining its overall goals.

Program theory: A set of beliefs about how a program works or why a problem occurs.

Purposeful sampling or theoretical sampling: Selection of participants for a sample according to specific criteria established by the researcher that are aligned with the research purpose.

Quantitative research: Research focused on gathering information that deals with numbers and is measurable.

Quasi-experimental method: Selection method in which participants are not randomly chosen or randomly assigned to the experimental and control groups.

Qualitative research: Research focused on an interpretive, naturalistic approach to its subject, searching for the meanings that people bring to the study.

Random purposeful sampling: Random selection from a sample of participants who share a common characteristic.

Random sampling: Selection method in which a participant in a defined population has an equal and independent chance of being chosen for the sample.

Randomized control trials: Trials in which participants are randomly selected and then randomly divided into treatment and control groups.

Rapid evaluation and assessment methods (REAM): Methods used to gather data in an emergency response situation in order to share information in real time.

Responsive evaluation: Stake's evaluation model, which includes engagement with various stakeholders in a program to determine the merits or shortcomings of a program's responsiveness to the stakeholders.

Sampling error: A type of error in which the sample represents the characteristics of just one part of the population and does not represent the whole population.

Sequential mixed methods design: Research design in which one type of data (qualitative or quantitative) are collected first, and then new questions based on these findings are generated for collection of the other type of data.

Snowball sampling: A qualitative sampling approach in which the evaluator asks participants for names of others who can provide further information.

Social science theory: A set of principles organized into a conceptual framework that allows the evaluator to explain the dynamics of the phenomenon being studied. Examples of social science theories include theories of motivation and human development.

Stakeholders: People who have a stake or a vested interest in the program, policy, or product being evaluated, and also have a stake in the evaluation.

Stratified sampling: Assigning participants to a particular category or stratum, and then sampling randomly within each stratum.

Summative evaluation: An evaluation done at the end of or on completion of a program.

Thick description: A robust description of the context in which qualitative research is conducted; it is called "thick" because of its detailed nature.

Transformative cyclical mixed method design: Subtype of transformative mixed method design (see below) in which an evaluation cycles through several phases. For example, information is initially gathered through a document review; this leads to a second phase of observations and interviews, which will prepare the evaluators for richer data collection and for creating web-based surveys or further interviews with other stakeholders; the final phase consists of analysis, dissemination, and monitoring of social channels. Particular responsiveness to diversity and cultural issues is prominent.

Transformative mixed method design: Any research design that uses both quantitative and qualitative collection methods (either sequentially or concurrently) with the goal of social change at levels ranging from the personal to the political.

Transformative paradigm: The belief that the lives and experiences of diverse groups of people are of central importance in the evaluation to address issues of power and justice. Focuses primarily on viewpoints of marginalized groups and interrogating systemic power structures through mixed methods to further social justice and human rights.

Transformative participatory evaluation: An evaluation in which the focus is on engaging all stakeholders, especially those who have traditionally been excluded from evaluations and from the decisions associated with evaluation studies.

Triangulation: The use of multiple data sources and different data collection strategies to strengthen the credibility of the findings of an evaluation.

Typical case sampling: Sampling of subjects according to what is typical, normal, or average in a population.

Universal design: Designing products, communications, and the built environment so that they can be used by all people, regardless of their differences.

Utilization-focused evaluation (UFE): An evaluation approach developed by Patton, in which an evaluation is carried out for and with intended primary users that provides information to specific intended users.

Variable: A measurable aspect or characteristic.

Worth: The value of the evaluand in a particular context (as opposed to the evaluand's intrinsic value, which is its **merit**).

References

Aaron, P., Joshi, R. M., Gooden, R., & Bentum, K. (2008). Diagnosis and treatment of reading disabilities based on the component model of reading: An alternative to the discrepancy model of LD. *Journal of Learning Disabilities, 41*(67), 67–84.

Abes, E. S., & Kasch, D. (2007). Using queer theory to explore lesbian college students' multiple dimensions of identity. *Journal of College Student Development, 48*, 619–636.

Abma, T. A. (2005). Responsive evaluation: Its value and special contribution to health promotion. *Evaluation and Program Planning, 28*, 279–289.

Abma, T. A. (2006). The practice and politics of responsive evaluation. *American Journal of Evaluation, 27*, 31–43.

Abma, T. A., & Widdershoven, G. A. M. (2008). Evaluation and/as social relation. *Evaluation, 14*, 209–225.

African Evaluation Association (AfrEA). (2000). *The African evaluation guidelines 2000.* Retrieved from *www.afrea.org/content/index.cfm?navID=5&itemID=204*

Ahsan, N. (2009). *Sustaining neighborhood change.* Baltimore, MD: Annie E. Casey Foundation.

Alkin, M. (2004). *Evaluation roots.* Thousand Oaks, CA: Sage.

Alkin, M. (2007, November). *Evaluation roots revisited.* Paper presented at the annual meeting of the American Evaluation Association, Baltimore.

Alkin, M., & Christie, C. A. (2004). An evaluation theory tree. In M. Alkin (Ed.), *Evaluation roots* (pp. 12–66). Thousand Oaks, CA: Sage.

Alkin, M. C. (1991). Evaluation theory development II. In M. McLaughlin & D. Phillips (Eds.), *Evaluation and education at quarter century* (pp. 91–112). Chicago: University of Chicago Press.

Alkin, M. C., Daillak, R., & White, P. (1979). *Using evaluation: Does evaluation make a difference?* Los Angeles, CA: The Center for the Study of Evaluation, University of California, Sage Library of Social Research, Vol. 76.

Alkire, S., & Deneulin S. (2009). A normative framework for development. In S. Deneulin & L. Shahuani (Eds.), *An introduction to the human development and capability approach* (pp. 3–21). London: Earthscan.

Alkire, S., & Foster, J. (2011). Counting and multidimensional poverty measurement. *Journal of Public Economics, 95*(6–7), 476–487.

Alkire, S., & Santos, M. E. (2010). *Acute multidimensional poverty: A new index for developing countries.* London: Oxford Poverty and Human Development Initiative, University of Oxford.

Altschuld, J. W., & Kumar, D. D. (2010). *Needs assessment.* Thousand Oaks, CA: Sage.

American Educational Research Association (AERA). (2004). *Guiding principles for evaluators.* Retrieved from *www.eval.org/Publications/GuidingPrinciples.asp*

American Educational Research Association (AERA), American Psychological Association (APA), & National Council on Research in Education. (1999). *Standards for educational and psychological testing.* Washington, DC: AERA.

American Evaluation Association (AEA). (2003). *Response to U.S. Department of Education's "Scientifically based evaluation methods: Studies capable of determining causality."* Retrieved from *www.eval. org/doestatement.htm*

American Evaluation Association (AEA). (2010). *Suggestions for presenters.* Retrieved from *www.eval. org/eval2010/10presenterguidelines.htm#Guidelines_for_serving_as_a_Presenter*

American Evaluation Association (AEA) Evaluation Policy Task Force. (2009). *An evaluation roadmap for a more effective government.* Retrieved from *www.eval.org/aea09.eptf.eval.roadmapF.pdf*

American Psychiatric Association. (2009). *Psychiatric advance directives.* Retrieved from *www.psych. org/Departments/EDU/Library/APAOfficialDocumentsandRelated/ResourceDocuments/200906. aspx*

American Psychological Association (APA) Joint Task Force of Divisions 17 and 45. (2002). *Guidelines on multicultural education, training, research, practice, and organizational change for psychologists.* Washington, DC: Author.

Amsden, J., & VanWynsberghe, R. (2005). Community mapping as a research tool with youth. *Action Research, 3*(4), 353–377.

Anderson, N. (2011, January 10). Schools prepare for national standards. *The Washington Post,* p. B01. (Also available at *www.washingtonpost.com/wp-dyn/content/article/2011/01/09/ AR2011010904382_pf.html*)

Anderson-Butcher, D., Iachini, A., & Amorose, A. (2008). Initial reliability and validity of the Perceived Social Competence Scale. *Research on Social Work Practice, 18*(1), 47–54.

Arango, L. L., Kurtines, W. M., Montgomery, M. J., & Ritchie, R. (2008). A multi-stage longitudinal comparative design Stage II evaluation of the Changing Lives Program: The Life Course Interview (RDA-LCI). *Journal of Adolescent Research, 23,* 310–341.

Asante, M. K. (1987). *The Afrocentric idea.* Philadelphia: Temple University Press.

Asante, M. K. (1988). *Afrocentricity.* Trenton, NJ: Africa World Press.

Asante, M. K. (1992). *Kemet, Afrocentricity and knowledge.* Trenton, NJ: Africa World Press.

Asian Development Bank. (2010). *Independent evaluation. Project/program performance evaluations.* Retrieved from *www.adb.org/Evaluation/reports.asp?s=1&type=0&p=evalpppe*

Australasian Evaluation Society. (2006). *AES ethics committee.* Retrieved from *www.aes.asn.au/about*

Bailey, D. B., Bruder, M. B., Hebbeler, K., Carta, J., Defosset, M., Greenwood, C., et al. (2006). Recommended outcomes for families of young children with disabilities. *Journal of Early Intervention, 28,* 227–251.

Baizerman, M., & Compton, D. W. (2009a). A perspective on managing evaluation. *New Directions for Evaluation, 121,* 7–15.

Baizerman, M., & Compton, D. W. (2009b). What did we learn from the case studies about managing evaluation? *New Directions for Evaluation, 121,* 79–86.

Baker, J. L. (2000). *Evaluating the impact of development projects on poverty: A handbook for practitioners.* Washington DC: The World Bank.

Bakri, N. (2009, May 24). For displaced Iraquis, "No life." *The Washington Post,* p. A14.

Balde, M., Crisp, J., Macleod, E., & Tennat, V. (2011, June). *Shelter from the storm: A real time evaluation of UNHCR's response to the emergency in Cote Ivoire and Liberia.* Geneva: United Nations High Commissioner for Refugees. Retrieved August 9, 2011 from *reliefweb.int/sites/reliefweb.int/files/ resources/Full_Report_1464.pdf*

Banks, J. (2008). *An introduction to multicultural education* (4th ed.). Boston: Allyn & Bacon.

Bardwell, G., Morton, C., Chester, A., Pancoska, P., Buch, S., Cecchetti, A., et al. (2009). Feasibility of adolescents to conduct community-based participatory research on obesity and diabetes in rural Appalachia. *Clinical and Translational Science 2*(5), 340–349. (Also available at *www3. interscience.wiley.com/cgi-bin/fulltext/122664033/HTMLSTART*)

Barela, E. (2008). Title I Achieving Schools study. *American Journal of Evaluation, 29*(4), 531–533.

Barker, J., & Weller, S. W. (2003). "Never work with children?": The geography of methodological issues in research with children. *Qualitative Research, 3*(2), 207–227.

Barker, M. (2003). *Satanic subcultures?: A discourse analysis of the self-perceptions of young goths and pagans.* In T. Waddell (Ed.), *Cultural expressions of evil and wickedness: wrath, sex, and crime.* Amsterdam: Rodopi.

Barnett, S. W. (1993). Economic evaluation of home visiting programs. *The Future of Children, 3,* 93–112.

Barrington, G. (2005). External evaluation. In S. Mathison (Ed.), *Encyclopedia of evaluation* (pp. 150–156). Thousand Oaks, CA: Sage.

Bassey, M. O. (2007). What is Africana critical theory or black existential philosophy? *Journal of Black Studies, 37,* 914–935.

Batsche, G., Elliott, J., Graden, J., Grimes, J., Kovaleski, J., Prasse, D., et al. (2005). *Response to intervention policy considerations and implementation.* Reston, VA: National Association of State Directors of Special Education.

Battiste, M. (Ed.). (2000). *Reclaiming indigenous voice and vision.* Vancouver: University of British Columbia Press.

Bazeley, P. (2006). The contribution of computer software to integrating qualitative and quantitative data and analyses. *Research in the Schools, 13*(1), 64–74.

Bazeley, P. (2009a). Editorial: Integrating data analysis in mixed methods research. *Journal of Mixed Methods Research, 3,* 203–209.

Bazeley, P. (2009b). Mixed methods data analysis. In S. Andrew & E. Halcomb (Eds.), *Mixed methods research for nursing and the health sciences* (pp. 84–118). Chichester, UK: Wiley-Blackwell.

Bell, J. B. (2004). Managing evaluation projects. In J. S. Wholey, H. P. Hatry, & K. E. Newcomer (Eds.), *Handbook of practical program evaluation* (2nd ed., pp. 571–603). San Francisco: Jossey-Bass.

Benjamin, L. M., & Greene, J. C. (2009). From program to network: The evaluator's role in today's problem solving environment. *American Journal of Evaluation, 30,* 296–309.

Berman, G., & Fox, A. (2009). *Lessons from the battles over D.A.R.E.* Washington, DC: Bureau of Juvenile Justice.

Beutler, L. E. (1991). Have all won and must all have prizes?: Revisiting Luborsky et al.'s verdict. *Journal of Consulting and Clinical Psychology, 59*(2), 226–232.

Bewaji, J. A. I. (1995). Critical comments on Pearce, African philosophy, and the sociological thesis. *Philosophy of the Social Sciences, 25,* 99–119.

Bickman, L. (2009, November). *The influence of context on choices in the evaluations of the Fort Bragg and Stark County Systems of Care for Children and Adolescents.* Paper presented at the annual meeting of the American Evaluation Association, Orlando, FL.

BioMed Central. (2008, February 1). *iPods do not interfere with cardiac pacemakers, study shows. Science Daily.* Retrieved from *www.sciencedaily.com/releases/2008/01/080131214602.htm*

Bledsoe, K. (2009, November). *The influence of context on choices in the evaluation of the Fun with Books program.* Paper presented at the annual meeting of the American Evaluation Association, Orlando, FL.

Bledsoe, K. L., & Graham, J. A. (2005). The use of multiple evaluation approaches in program evaluation. *American Journal of Evaluation, 26*(3), 302–319.

Bloom, H. S., & Riccio, J. A. (2005, May). Using place-based assignment and comparative interrupted time-series analysis for the Jobs-Plus Employment Program for Public Housing Residents. *Annals of the American Academy of Political and Social Science, 599,* 19–51.

Borman, G. D., Slavin, R. E., Cheung, A., Chamberlain, A. M., Madden, N. A., & Chambers, B. (2005). Success for all: First-year results from the national randomized field trial. *Educational Evaluation and Policy Analysis, 27*(1), 1–22.

Borman, G. D., Slavin, R. E., Cheung, A., Chamberlain, A. M., Madden, N. A., & Chambers, B. (2007). Final reading outcomes of the national randomized field trial of Success for All. *American Educational Research Journal, 44*(3), 701–731.

Boruch, R. (1997). *Randomized experiments for planning and evaluation.* Thousand Oaks, CA: Sage.

Boruch, R. F. (2007). Encouraging the flight of error: Ethical standards, evidence standards, and randomized trials. *New Directions for Evaluation, 113*, 55–73.

Bowman, M. (2005). Retrieved from *www.bpcwi.com/nativeamerican.html*

Brabeck, M. M., & Brabeck, K. M. (2009). Feminist perspectives on research ethics. In D. M. Mertens & P. E. Ginsberg (Eds.), *Handbook of social research ethics* (pp. 39–53). Thousand Oaks, CA: Sage.

Bradbury, H., & Reason, P. (2001). Conclusion: Broadening the bandwidth of validity—Issues and choice points for improving the quality of action research. In P. Reason & H. Bradbury (Eds.), *Handbook of action research* (pp. 447–455). London: Sage.

Bradbury, M., Hofmann, C. A., Maxwell, S., Venekamp, D., & Montani, A. (2003). *Measuring humanitarian needs*. London: Humanitarian Policy Group.

Bradshaw, S. (2000). *Socio-economic impacts of natural disasters: A gender analysis*. Santiago, Chile: Sustainable Development and Human Settlements Division, Women and Development Unit.

Brady, B., & O'Regan, C. (2009). Meeting the challenge of doing an RCT evaluation of youth mentoring in Ireland: A journey in mixed methods. *Journal of Mixed Methods Research, 3*, 265–280.

Brandon, P. R., & Singh, M. (2009). The strength of the methodological warrants for the findings of research on program evaluation use. *American Journal of Evaluation, 30*, 123–157.

Brinkerhoff, R. O. (2003). *The success case method: Find out quickly what's working and what's not*. San Francisco: Berret-Koehler.

Brugge, D., & Missaghian, M. (2006). Research ethics and environmental health: Protecting the Navajo people through tribal regulation of research. *Science and Engineering Ethics, 12*, 491–507.

Brydon-Miller, M. (2009). Participatory action research: Contributions to the development of practitioner inquiry in education. *Educational Action Research, 17*(1), 79–93.

Brydon-Miller, M., Maguire, P., & McIntyre, A. (Eds.). (2004). *Traveling companions: Feminism, teaching, and action research*. Westport, CT: Praeger.

Burbules, N. (2009). Privacy and new technologies: The limits of traditional research ethics. In D. M. Mertens & P. E. Ginsberg (Eds.), *Handbook of social research ethics* (pp. 547–549). Thousand Oaks, CA: Sage.

Busch, J. R., O'Brien, T. P., & Spangler, W. D. (2005). Increasing the quantity and quality of school leadership candidates through formation experiences. *Journal of Leadership and Organizational Studies, 11*, 95–108.

Buskens, I., & Earl, S. (2008). Research for change: Outcome mapping's contribution to emancipatory action research in Africa. *Action Research, 6*, 171–192.

Cajete, G. (2000). *Native science: Natural laws of interdependence*. Santa Fe, NM: Clear Light.

Caldwell, J. Y., Davis, J. D., Du Bois, B., Echo-Hawk, H., Erickson, J. S., Goins, R. T., et al. (2005). Culturally competent research with American Indians and Alaska Natives: Findings and recommendations of the first symposium of the work group on American Indian research and program evaluation methodology. *Journal of the National Centre, 12*, 1–21.

Campbell, D., & Stanley, J. (1963). *Experimental and quasi-experimental designs for research*. Chicago, IL: Rand-McNally.

Campbell, D. T. (1969). Reforms as experiments. *American Psychologist, 24*, 409–429.

Campbell, D. T. (1991). Methods for the experimenting society. *American Journal of Evaluation, 12*, 223–260.

Canadian International Development Agency. (1999). *Gender equality policy and tools*. Gatineau, Quebec, Canada: Author.

Caracelli, V., & Greene, J. (1993). Data analysis strategies for mixed-method evaluation designs. *Educational Evaluation and Policy Analysis, 15*(2), 195–207.

Cardoza Clayson, Z., Castañeda, X., Sanchez, E., & Brindis, C. (2002). Unequal power—changing landscapes: Negotiations between evaluation stakeholders in Latino communities. *American Journal of Evaluation, 23*(1), 33–44.

Carter, J. (2009). Evaluate experiences: A qualitative technique to complement quantitative impact assessments. *Journal of Development Effectiveness, 1*(1), 86–102.

Catholic Relief Services. (n.d.). *What is a lesson learnt?* Washington, DC: Author.

Catsambas, T., & Webb, L. (2003). Using appreciative inquiry to guide an evaluation of the international women's media foundation Africa program. *New Directions for Evaluation, 100,* 41–52.

Center for Family, Work and Community at the University of Massachusetts, Lowell. (2004). *Research ethics tip sheets.* Retrieved from *www.uml.edu/centers/cfwc/Community_Tips/Research Ethics/Research_Ethics.html*

Center for Substance Abuse Prevention (CSAP). (2008, November). Engaging community representatives for health prevention projects. Retrieved from *captus.samhsa.gov/prevention-practice/strategic-prevention-framework*

Center for Universal Design. (1997). *What is universal design?* Retrieved from *www.design.ncsu.edu/cud/univ_design/ud.htm*

Centers for Disease Control and Prevention (CDC). (1999). *Selected uses for evaluation in public health practice.* Retrieved from *www.cdc.gov/mmwr/preview/mmwrhtml/rr4811a1.htm*

Cenziper, D. (2009, October 18). Staggering need, striking neglect. *The Washington Post.* Retrieved from *www.washingtonpost.com/wp-dyn/content/article/2009/10/17/AR2009101701984.html*

Chambers, R. (2005). *Ideas for development.* London: Earthscan.

Chandler, M. A. (2009, May 7). It's not for everyone. *The Washington Post.* Retrieved from *www.washingtonpost.com/wp-dyn/content/article/2009/05/05/AR2009050504406.html*

Charmaz, K. (2006). *Constructing grounded theory: A practical guide through qualitative analysis.* Thousand Oaks, CA: Sage.

Charmaz, K. (2007). Grounded theory. In G. Ritzer (Ed.), *Blackwell encyclopedia of sociology.* Oxford, UK: Blackwell.

Chatterji, M. (2005). Evidence on "what works": An argument for extended-term mixed-method (ETMM) evaluation designs. *Educational Researcher, 34,* 14–24.

Cheek, J. (2004). At the margins?: Discourse analysis and qualitative research. *Qualitative Health Research, 14,* 1040–1050.

Chen, H.-T. (1994). Theory-driven evaluations: Need, difficulties, and options. *American Journal of Evaluation, 15,* 79–82.

Chen, H.-T. (2005). *Practical program evaluation: Assessing and improving planning, implementation, and effectiveness.* Thousand Oaks, CA: Sage.

Chen, H.-T., & Rossi, P. H. (1980). The multi-goal, theory-driven approach to evaluation: A model linking basic and applied social science. *Social Forces, 59*(1), 106–122.

Chen, H.-T., & Rossi, P. H. (1983). Evaluating with sense: The theory-driven approach. *Evaluation Review, 7*(3), 283–302.

Chi, B., Jastrzab, J., & Melchior, A. (2006). *Developing indicators and measures of civic outcomes for elementary school students.* Medford, MA: Center for Information & Research on Civic Learning and Engagement.

Chianca, T. (2008). The OECS/DAC criteria for international development evaluations: As assessment and ideas for improvement. *Journal of MultiDisciplinary Evaluation, 5*(9), 41–51.

Chilisa, B. (2005). Educational research within postcolonial Africa: A critique of HIV/AIDS research in Botswana. *International Journal of Qualitative Studies in Education, 18,* 659–684.

Chilisa, B. (2009). Indigenous African-centered ethics: Contesting and complementing dominant models. In D. M. Mertens & P. Ginsberg (Eds.), *Handbook of social research ethics* (pp. 407–425). Thousand Oaks, CA: Sage.

Chilisa, B. (2011). *Indigenous research methodologies.* Thousand Oaks, CA: Sage.

Chilisa, B., & Preece, J. (2005). *Research methods for adult educators in Africa.* Cape Town, South Africa: Pearson.

Chinman, M., Imm, P., & Wandersman, A. (2004). *Getting to outcomes.* Atlanta, GA: Centers for

Disease Control and Prevention. (Also available at *www.rand.org/pubs/technical_reports/TR101/index.html*)

Chiu, L. F. (2003). Transformational potential of focus group practice in participatory action research. *Action Research, 1*(2), 165–183.

Christians, C. G. (2005). Ethics and politics in qualitative research. In N. K. Denzin & Y. S. Lincoln (Eds.), *The Sage handbook of qualitative research* (3rd ed., pp. 139–164). Thousand Oaks, CA: Sage.

Christie, C. A. (2007). Reported Influence of Evaluation Data on Decision Makers' Actions: An Empirical Examination. *American Journal of Evaluation* 2007; 28; 8–25.

Christie, C. A. (2008). Interview with Eric Barela. *American Journal of Evaluation, 29*, 534–546.

Christie, C. A., & Fleischer, D. N. (2009). Social inquiry paradigms as a frame for the debate on credible evidence. In S. I. Donaldson, C. A. Christie, & M. M. Mark (Eds.), *What counts as credible evidence in applied research and evaluation practice?* (pp. 19–30). Thousand Oaks, CA: Sage.

CIA Factbook. (2010). *Field listing: Languages.* Retrieved from *www.cia.gov/library/publications/the-world-factbook/geos/sf.html*

Coady, D., Wang, L., & Dai, X. (2001). *Community programs and women's participation: The Chinese experience* (Policy Research Working Paper No. 2622). Washington, DC: World Bank, Development Economics Research Group.

Coetzee, P. H., & Roux, A. P. J. (Eds.). (1998). *The African philosophy reader.* London: Routledge.

Coghlan, A. T., Preskill, H., Catsambas, T. T. (2003). An overview of appreciative inquiry in evaluation. *New Directions for Evaluation, 100*, 5–22.

Collins, S. B. (2005). An understanding of poverty from those who are poor. *Action Research, 3*(1), 9–31.

Collins, K. M. T., Onwuegbuzie, A. J., & Jiao, Q. G. (2007). Mixed methods investigation of mixed methods sampling designs in social and health science research. *Journal of Mixed Methods Research, 1*(3), 267–294.

Colorado State University. (2008). *Best practices through universal design for learning.* Retrieved from *accessproject.colostate.edu/udl*

Compton, D. W. (2009). Where is the literature in evaluation on managing studies, evaluators, and evaluation units? *New Directions for Evaluation, 121*, 17–25.

Conlin, S., & Stirrat, R. L. (2008). Current challenges in development evaluation. *Evaluation, 14*, 193–208.

Cook, T. D., & Campbell, D. T. (1979). *Quasi-experimentation: Design and analysis issues for field settings.* Boston: Houghton Mifflin.

Cook, T. D., Murphy, R. F., & Hunt, H. D. (2000). Comer's school development program in Chicago: A theory-based evaluation. *American Educational Research Journal, 37*, 535–597.

Cooksy, L. J., & Caracelli, V. J. (2009). Metaevaluation in practice: Selection and application of criteria. *Journal of MultiDisciplinary Evaluation, 6*(11), 1–15.

Corbin, J., & Morse, J. M. (2003). The unstructured interactive interview: Issues of reciprocity and risks when dealing with sensitive topics. *Qualitative Inquiry, 9*(3), 335–354.

Corbin, J., & Strauss, A. (2008). *Basics of qualitative research* (3rd ed.). Los Angeles: Sage.

Coryn, C. L. S., Schröter, E. C., & Hanssen, C. E. (2009). Adding a time-series design element to the success case method to improve methodological rigor: An Application for Nonprofit Program Evaluation. *American Journal of Evaluation 30*, 80–92.

Costantino, T. E., & Greene, J. C. (2003). Reflections on the use of narrative in evaluation. *American Journal of Evaluation, 24*, 35–49.

Costner, H. L. (1989). The validity of conclusions in evaluation research: A further development of Chen and Rossi's theory-driven approach. *Evaluation and Program Planning, 12*, 345–353.

Cousins, J. B., & Earl, L. E. (1995). *Participatory evaluation in education.* London: Falmer Press.

Cousins, J. B., Goh, S., & Lee, L. (2003). *The learning capacity of schools as a function of evaluative inquiry: An empirical study.* Paper presented at the Learning Conference, Institute of Education, University of London.

Cousins, J. B., & Whitmore, E. (1998). Framing participatory evaluation. *New Directions for Evaluation, 80,* 5–23.

Cram, F. (2009). Maintaining indigenous voices. In D. M. Mertens & P. E. Ginsberg (Eds.), *Handbook of social research ethics* (pp. 308–322). Thousand Oaks, CA: Sage.

Cram, F., Ormond, A., & Carter, L. (2006). Researching our relations: Reflections on ethics and marginalization. *Ngā Pae o te Māramatanga, 2*(1), 180–198.

Creswell, J. W. (2009). *Research design: Qualitative, quantitative, and mixed methods approaches* (3rd ed.). Thousand Oaks, CA: Sage.

Creswell, J. W., & Plano Clark, V. L. (2007). *Designing and conducting mixed methods research.* Thousand Oaks, CA: Sage.

Cronbach, L. J., Ambron, S. R., Dornbusch, S. M., Hess, R. D., Hornik, R. C., Phillips, R. C., et al. (1980). *Toward reform of program evaluation.* San Francisco: Jossey-Bass.

Cross, J. E., Dickmann, E., Newman-Gonchar, R., & Fagan, J. M. (2009). Using mixed-method design and network analysis to measure development of interagency collaboration. *American Journal of Evaluation, 30,* 310–329.

Cross, T. L., Earle, K., Echo-Hawk Solie, K. E., & Manness, K. (2000). *Cultural strengths and challenges in implementing a system of care model in American Indian communities.* Portland, OR: National Indian Child Welfare Association.

Danish International Development Agency (DANIDA). (2006). *Gender-sensitive monitoring and indicators.* Copenhagen: Ministry of Foreign Affairs of Denmark.

Dart, J. J. (2008, September). *Report on outcomes and get everyone involved: The participatory performance story reporting technique.* Paper presented at the annual conference of the Australasian Evaluation Society, Perth, Australia.

Dart, J. J., & Davies, R. J. (2003). A dialogical story-based evaluation tool: The most significant change technique. *American Journal of Evaluation, 24,* 137–155.

Davidson, E. J. (2005). *Evaluation methodology basics: The nuts and bolts of sound evaluation.* Thousand Oaks, CA: Sage.

Davies, R. (2004). Scale, complexity and the representation of theories of change. *Evaluation, 10*(1), 101–121.

Davies, R. (2005). Scale, complexity and the representation of theories of change: Part II. *Evaluation, 11*(2), 133–149.

Davies, Randall. (2009, November). *Proven and creative strategies and techniques for teaching evaluation.* Paper presented at the annual meeting of the American Evaluation Association, Orlando, FL.

Davies, Rick. (2009a). *Expectations about identifying and documenting lessons learned?* Retrieved from *mande.co.uk/blog/wp-content/uploads/2009/08/Guidance-on-identifying-and-documenting-LL-vs21.pdf*

Davies, Rick. (2009b). *Monitoring and evaluation news. Identifying and documenting "lessons learned": A list of references.* Retrieved from *mande.co.uk/?s=lessons+learned*

Davis, S. (2008). Centering the folder: What if? In M. Morris (Ed.), *Evaluation ethics for best practice: Cases and commentaries* (pp. 100–111). New York: Guilford Press.

Davis, S. P., Arnette, N. C., Kafi, B. S., Graves, K. N., Rhodes, M. N., Harp, S. E., et al. (2009). The Grady Nia Project: A culturally competent intervention for low-income, abused, and suicidal African American women. *Professional Psychology: Research and Practice, 40*(2), 141–147.

Delay, P. (2004). Gender and monitoring the response to HIV/AIDS pandemic. *Emerging Infectious Diseases, 10*(11), 1979–1983.

Delgado Bernal, D. (1998). Using a Chicana feminist epistemology in educational research. *Harvard Educational Review, 68,* 555–579.

Denzin, N., & Lincoln, Y. S. (2005). *The SAGE handbook of qualitative research* (3rd ed.). Thousand Oaks, CA: Sage.

Dillard, C. (2000a). The substance of things hoped for, the evidence of things not seen: Examining an endarkened feminist epistemology in educational research and leadership. *Qualitative Studies in Education, 13*(6), 661–681.

Dillard, C. (2000b). *Cultural considerations in paradigm proliferation.* Paper presented at the annual meeting of the American Educational Research Association, New Orleans, LA.

Dodd, S. J. (2009). LGBTQ: Protecting vulnerable subjects in all studies. In D. M. Mertens & P. E. Ginsberg (Eds.), *Handbook of social research ethics* (pp. 474–488). Thousand Oaks, CA: Sage.

Donaldson, S. (2007). *Program theory driven evaluation science: Strategies and applications.* Mahwah, NJ: Erlbaum.

Donaldson, S., & Gooler, L. E. (2002). Theory-driven evaluation of the work and health initiative: A focus on winning new jobs. *American Journal of Evaluation, 23,* 341–346.

Donaldson, S. I., Christie, C. A., & Mark, M. M. (Eds.). (2009). *What counts as credible evidence in applied research and evaluation practice?* Thousand Oaks, CA: Sage.

Donaldson, S. I., & Lipsey, M. W. (2006). Roles for theory in contemporary evaluation practice. In I. Shaw, J. Greene, & M. Mark (Eds.), *Handbook of evaluation* (pp. 56–75). London: Sage.

Donaldson, S. I., Patton, M. Q., Fetterman, D. M., & Scriven, M. (2010). The 2009 Claremont debates: The promises and pitfalls of utilization-focused and empowerment evaluation. *Journal of MultiDisciplinary Evaluation, 6*(13), 15–57.

Donnelly-Wijting, K. (2007). *HIV/AIDS prevention for deaf youth in South Africa.* Unpublished manuscript, Gallaudet University.

Duarte, N. (2008). *The art and science of creating great presentations.* Sebastopol, CA: O'Reilly Media.

Du Bois, W. E. B. (1989). *The souls of black folk.* New York: Penguin Books. (Original work published 1903)

Du Bois, D. L., & Karcher, M. J. (Eds.). (2005). *Handbook of youth mentoring.* Thousand Oaks, CA: Sage.

Dubose, M. (2008). *Selecting the right independent grant evaluator: What you need to know. Finding an evaluator.* Retrieved from *findgrantevaluators.com/Finding_The_Right_Evaluator.php*

Durland, M. (2005). Exploring and understanding relationship. *New Directions for Evaluation, 54*(4), 25–40.

Duwe, G., & Kerschner, D. (2008). Removing a nail from the boot camp coffin: An outcome evaluation of Minnesota's Challenge Incarceration program. *Crime Delinquency, 54,* 614–643.

Easterly, W. (2006). *The white man's burden.* New York: Penguin.

Eisner, E. W. (1976a). Educational connoisseurship and educational criticism, their form and function in educational evaluation. *Journal of Aesthetic Education, 10*(3–4), 135–150.

Eisner, E. W. (1976b). Reading and the creation of meaning. *Claremont Reading Conference, 40th Yearbook, 1,* 1–15.

Eisner, E. W. (1977). Use of educational connoisseurship and educational criticism for evaluating classroom life. *Teachers College Record, 78*(3), 345–358.

Eisner, E. W. (1978). The impoverished mind. *Educational Leadership, 35*(8), 617–623.

Eisner, E. W. (1979a). *The educational imagination: On the design and evaluation of school programs.* New York: MacMillan.

Eisner, E. W. (1979b). The use of qualitative forms of evaluation for improving educational practice. *Educational Evaluation and Policy Analysis, 1,* 11–19.

Eisner, E. W. (1991). *The enlightened eye: Qualitative inquiry and the enhancement of educational practice.* New York: Macmillan.

Endo, T., Joh, T., & Yu, H. C. (2003). *Voices from the field: Health and evaluation leaders on multicultural evaluation.* Oakland, CA: Social Policy Research Associates.

Erickson, F., & Gutierrez, K. (2002). Comment: Culture, rigor, and science in educational research. *Educational Researcher, 31,* 21–24.

European Evaluation Society (EES). (2007). EES statement: The importance of a methodologically diverse approach to impact evaluation—specifically with respect to development aid and development interventions. Retrieved from *www.europeanevaluation.org.*

Eze, E. (1998). *African philosophy: An anthology*. Oxford, UK: Blackwell.

Fals Borda, O. (2001). Participatory (action) research in social theory: Origins and challenges. In P. Reason & H. Bradbury (Eds.), *Handbook of action research* (pp. 27–37). London: Sage.

Fals-Stewart, W., Yates, B. T., & Klostermann, K. (2005). Assessing the costs, benefits, cost-benefit ratio, and cost-effectiveness of marital and family treatments: Why we should and how we can. *Journal of Family Psychology, 19*(1), 28–39.

Fernandez, L. (2002). Telling stories about school: Using critical race and Latino critical theories to document Latina/Latino education and resistance. *Qualitative Inquiry, 8*(1), 45–65.

Fetterman, D., & Wandersman, A. (2007). Empowerment evaluation: Yesterday, today, and tomorrow. *American Journal of Evaluation, 28*, 179–198.

Fetterman, D. M. (1994). Empowerment evaluation. *American Journal of Evaluation, 15*, 1–15.

Fetterman, D. M. (2001). *Foundations of empowerment evaluation*. Thousand Oaks, CA: Sage.

Fetterman, D. M. (2009). Empowerment evaluation at the Stanford University School of Medicine: Using a critical friend to improve the clerkship experience. *Ensaio: Avaliação e Políticas Públicas em Educação, 17*(63), 197–204.

Fetterman, D. M., & Wandersman, A. (2005). *Empowerment evaluation principles in practice*. New York: Guilford Press.

Fielding, N. G. (2009). Going out on a limb: Postmodernism and multiple method research. *Current Sociology, 57*, 427–447.

Fierro, R. S. (2006). *African American agency within welfare agencies: A critical study of African American mothers with transitional custody*. Unpublished doctoral dissertation, Temple University.

Finney, J. W., & Moos, R. H. (1984). Theory and method in treatment evaluation. *Evaluation and Program Planning, 12*, 307–316.

Fitzpatrick, J. L., Sanders, J. R., & Worthen, B. R. (2004). *Program evaluation: Alternative approaches and practical guidelines*. Upper Saddle River, NJ: Pearson/Allyn & Bacon.

Fixsen, D., Panzano, P., Naoom, S., & Blasé, K. (2008). *Measures of implementation components of the National Implementation Research Network Frameworks*. Chapel Hill, NC: National Implementation Research Network.

Fixsen, D. L., Naoom, S. F., Blasé, K. A., Friedman, R. M., & Wallace, F. (2005). *Implementation research: A synthesis of the literature* (FMHI Publication No. 231). Tampa: University of South Florida, Louis de la Parte Florida Mental Health Institute, The National Implementation Research Network.

Ford Foundation. (2010). *How we make grants*. Retrieved from *www.fordfoundation.org/pdfs/grants/grant-application-guide.pdf*

Foster, J. E., Horowitz, A. W., & Méndez, F. (2009, May). *An axiomatic approach to the measurement of corruption: Theory and applications* (OPHI Working Paper No. 29). Retrieved from *www.ophi.org.uk/working-paper-number-29*

Fournier, D. M. (2005). Evaluation. In S. Mathison (Ed.), *Encyclopedia of evaluation* (pp. 139–140). Thousand Oaks, CA: Sage.

Fox, R., & Fox, J. (2002). The power-discourse relationship in a Croatian higher education setting. *Education Policy Analysis Archives, 10*(5), 1–16.

Franklin, J., & Bloor, M. (1999). Some issues arising in the systematic analysis of focus group materials. In R. S. Barbour & J. Kitzinger (Eds.), *Developing focus group research* (pp. 144–155). Thousand Oaks, CA: Sage.

Fredericks, K. A., Deegan, M., & Carman, J. G. (2008). Using system dynamics as an evaluation tool: Experience from a demonstration program. *American Journal of Evaluation, 29*, 251–267.

Freire, P. (1970). *Pedagogy of the oppressed*. New York: Seabury.

French, M. T., Salome, H. J., Krupski, A., McKay, J. R., Donovan, D. M., McLellan, A. T., & Durell, J. (2000). Benefit–cost analysis of residential and outpatient addiction treatment in the state of Washington. *Evaluation Review, 24*(6), 609–634.

Frierson, H. T., Hood, S., & Hughes, G. B. (2002). A guide to conducting culturally responsive evaluations. In *The 2002 user-friendly handbook for project evaluation.* Arlington, VA: National Science Foundation.

Frohmann, L. (2005). The Framing Safety Project: Photographs and narratives by battered women. *Violence against Women, 11,* 1396–1419.

Furrobo, J.-E., Rist, R., & Sandahl, R. (Eds.). (2002). *International atlas of evaluation.* New Brunswick, NJ: Transaction.

Gall, M., Gall, J., & Borg, W. (2007). *Educational research: An introduction* (8th ed.). Boston: A & B.

Gangopadhyay, P. (2002). Making Evaluation Meaningful to All Education Stakeholders: Evaluation Checklists Project. Retrieved from the Western Michigan University Evaluation Center website: *www.wmich.edu/evalctr/archive_checklists/makingevalmeaningful.pdf*

Gantt, H. L. (1974). *Work, wages and profits.* Easton, PA: Hive. (Original work published 1910)

Garbarino, S., & Holland, J. (2009). *Quantitative and qualitative methods in impact evaluation and measuring results.* Birmingham, UK: Governance and Social Development Researcher Centre.

Gee, J. P. (2005). *An introduction to discourse analysis: Theory and method.* London: Routledge.

Ghertner, D. A. (2006). Technology and tricks: Intra-household technologies implementation and gender struggles. *Gender, Technology and Development, 10,* 281–311.

Ginsberg, P. E., & Mertens, D. M. (2009). Frontiers of social research ethics: Fertile ground for evolution. In D. M. Mertens & P. E. Ginsberg (Eds.), *Handbook of social research ethics* (pp. 580–613). Thousand Oaks, CA: Sage.

Ginsburg, A., & Rhett, N. (2003). Building a better body of evidence: New opportunities to strengthen evaluation utilization. *American Journal of Evaluation, 24,* 489–498.

Glaser, B. G., & Strauss, A. L. (1967). *The discovery of grounded theory.* Chicago: Aldine.

Goode, E. (1996). Gender and courtship entitlement: Responses to personal ads. *Sex Roles, 34,* 141–169.

Goodman, L. A., Liang, B., Helms, J. E., Latta, R. E. Sparks, E., & Weintraub, S. R. (2004). Training counseling psychologists as social justice agents: Feminist and multicultural principles in action. *Counseling Psychologist, 32*(6), 793–837.

Gordon, L. R. (1997). Introduction. In L. R. Gordon (Ed.), *Existence in black: An anthology of black existential philosophy* (pp. 1–9). New York: Routledge.

Green, J., & Lee, C. D. (2005). Making visible the invisible logic of inquiry: Uncovering multiple challenges (Essay book review of *Discourse analysis and the study of classroom language and literacy events). Reading Research Quarterly, 41*(1).

Greene, C., & McClintock, C. (1991). The evolution of evaluation methodology. *Theory into Practice, 30*(1), 13–21.

Greene, J. (2005). Stakeholders. In S. Mathison (Ed.), *Encyclopedia of evaluation* (pp. 397–398). Thousand Oaks, CA: Sage.

Greene, J., & Lee, J.-H. (2006). Quieting educational reform … with educational reform. *American Journal of Evaluation, 27*(3), 337–352.

Greene, J. C. (2000). Understanding social programs through evaluation. In N. K. Denzin & Y. S. Lincoln (Eds.), *Handbook of qualitative research* (2nd ed., pp. 981–999). Thousand Oaks, CA: Sage.

Greene, J. C. (2003). War and peace … and evaluation. In O. Karlsson (Ed.), *Studies in educational policy and educational philosophy* (Vol. 2). Uppsala, Sweden: Uppsala University.

Greene, J. C. (2006). Evaluation, democracy, and social change. In I. Shaw, J. C. Greene, & M. Mark (Eds.), *Handbook of evaluation* (pp. 118–140). Thousand Oaks, CA: Sage.

Greene, J. C. (2007). *Mixed methods in social inquiry.* San Francisco: Jossey-Bass.

Greene, J. C. (2009). Evidence as "proof" and evidence as "inkling." In S. I. Donaldson, C. A. Christie, & M. M. Mark (Eds.), *What counts as credible evidence in applied research and evaluation practice?* (pp. 153–167). Thousand Oaks CA: Sage.

Greene, J. C., Kreider, H., & Mayer, E. (2005). Combining qualitative and quantitative methods in social inquiry. In B. Somekh & C. Lewin (Eds.), *Research methods in the social sciences* (pp. 274–281). London: Sage.

Greenwood, D. J., Brydon-Miller, M., & Shafer, C. (2006). Intellectual property and action research. *Action Research, 4*(1), 81–95.

Grigg-Saito, D., Och, S., Liang, S., Toof, R., & Silka, L. (2008). Building on the strengths of a Cambodian refugee community through community-based outreach. *Health Promotion Practice, 9*, 415–425.

Guba, E. G. (1978). *Toward a methodology of naturalistic inquiry in educational evaluation.* Los Angeles: University of California.

Guba, E. G. (1990). The alternative paradigm dialog. In E. G. Guba (Ed.), *The paradigm dialog* (pp. 17–30). Newbury Park, CA: Sage.

Guba, E. G., & Lincoln, Y. S. (1981). *Effective evaluation: Improving the usefulness of evaluation results through responsive and naturalistic approaches.* San Francisco: Jossey-Bass.

Guba, E. G., & Lincoln, Y. S. (1989). *Fourth generation evaluation.* Newbury Park, CA: Sage.

Guba, E. G., & Lincoln, Y. S. (Eds.). (2005). *Handbook of qualitative research.* Thousand Oaks, CA: Sage.

Gubrium, J. F., & Holstein, J. A. (Eds.). (2002). *Handbook of interview research: Context and method.* Thousand Oaks, CA: Sage.

Gueron, J. M. (2007). Building evidence: What it takes and what it yields. *Research on Social Work Practice, 17*, 134–142.

Gullickson, A., & Stufflebeam, D. (2001). Feedback Workshop Checklist: Evaluation Checklists Project. Retrieved from the Western Michigan University Evaluation Center website: *www.wmich. edu/evalctr/archive_checklists/feedbackworkshop.pdf*

Gupton, C., Kelley, M. B., Lensmire, T., Ngo, B., & Goh, M. (2009). *Teacher Education Redesign Initiative: Race, Culture, Class, and Gender Task Group final report.* Minneapolis: University of Minnesota.

Gurin, P., Dey, E. L., Hurtado, S., & Gurin, G. (2002). Diversity and higher education: Theory and impact on educational outcomes. *Harvard Educational Review, 72*(3), 1–32.

Gyekye, K. (1995). *An essay on African philosophical thought: The Akan conceptual scheme.* Philadelphia: Temple University Press.

Gysen, J., Bruyninckx, H., & Bachus, K. (2006). The modus narrandi: A methodology for evaluating effects of environmental policy. *Evaluation, 12*(1), 95–118.

Habermas, J. (1971). *Knowledge and human interests* (J. Shapiro, Trans.). Boston: Beacon Press.

Hall, M. E., Sedlacek, A. R., Berenback, J. A. R., & Dieckman, N. G. (2007). Military sexual trauma services for women veterans in the Veterans Health Administration: The patient-care practice environment and perceived organizational support. *Psychological Services, 4*(4), 229–238.

Hanberger, A. (2001). Policy and program evaluation, civil society, and democracy. *American Journal of Evaluation, 22*(2), 211–228.

Hanssen, C. E., Lawrenz, F., & Dunet, D. O. (2008). Concurrent meta-evaluation: A critique. *American Journal of Evaluation, 29*, 572–582.

Harris, R., Holmes, H., & Mertens, D. M. (2009). Research ethics in sign language communities. *Sign Language Studies, 9*(2), 104–131.

Hedler, H. C., & Gibram, N. (2009). The contribution of metaevaluation to program evaluation: Proposition of a model. *Journal of MultiDisciplinary Evaluation, 6*(12), 210–223.

Hegel, G. W. F. (1929). *Science of logic* (W. H. Johnston & L. G. Struthers, Trans.). London: George Allen & Unwin. (Original work published 1812)

Helga, H., & Ribeiro, N. G. (2009). The contribution of meta-evaluation to program evaluation: Proposition of a model. *Journal of MultiDisciplinary Evaluation, 6*(12), 210–223.

Hendricks, M. (2008). Hold 'em or fold(er) 'em: What's an evaluator to do? In M. Morris (Ed.), *Evaluation ethics for best practice* (pp. 89–99). New York: Guilford Press.

Hennekens, C. H., & Buring, J. E. (1989). Methodological considerations in the design and conduct of randomized trials: The U.S. Physicians' Health Study. *Controlled Clinical Trials, 10*, 142S–150S.

Henry, E., & Pene, H. (2001). *Kaupapa Māori*: Locating indigenous ontology, epistemology and methodology in the academy. *Organization, 8*(2), 234–242.

Henry, G., Julnes, J., & Mark, M. (1998). Realist evaluation: An emerging theory in support of practice. *New Directions for Evaluation, 78.*

Henry, G. T. (2005, Summer). Evaluation methodology: A conversation with Gary Henry. *The Evaluation Exchange, 11*(2). Retrieved from *www.hfrp.org/evaluation/the-evaluation-exchange/issue-archive/evaluation-methodology/a-conversation-with-gary-henry*

Henry, G. T., & Mark, M. M. (2003). Beyond use: Understanding evaluation's influence on attitudes and actions. *American Journal of Evaluation, 24,* 293–314.

Heron, J., & Reason, P. (2006). The practice of co-operative inquiry: Research "with" rather than "on" people. In P. Reason & H. Bradbury (Eds.), *Handbook of action research* (pp. 144–154). London: Sage.

Hesperian Foundation. (2010a). *About Hesperian.* Retrieved from *www.hesperian.org/about.php*

Hesperian Foundation. (2010b). *Gratis Fund.* Retrieved from *www.hesperian.org/gratis*

Hesse-Biber, S., & Leavy, P. (2006). *The practice of qualitative research.* Thousand Oaks, CA: Sage.

Hood, S., & Hopson, R. K. (2008). Evaluation roots reconsidered: Asa Hilliard, a fallen hero in the "Nobody Knows My Name" project, and African educational excellence. *Review of Educational Research, 78,* 410–426.

Hood, S., Hopson, R. K., & Frierson, H. T. (Eds.). (2005a). *The role of culture and cultural context: A mandate for inclusion, the discovery of truth and understanding in evaluative theory and practice.* Charlotte, NC: Information Age.

Hood, S., Hopson, R. K., & Frierson, H. T. (2005b). Introduction: This is where we stand. In S. Hood, R. K. Hopson, & H. T. Frierson (Eds.), *The role of culture and cultural context* (pp. 1–6). Greenwich, CT: Information Age.

Hopkins, C. Q., & Koss, M. P. (2005). Incorporating feminist theory and insights into a restorative justice response to sex offenses. *Violence against Women, 11,* 693–723.

Hopson, R. (2001). Global and local conversations on culture, diversity, and social justice in evaluation: Issues to consider in a 9/11 era. *American Journal of Evaluation, 22,* 375–380.

Hopson, R. (2002). Room at the evaluation table for ethnography: Contributions to the responsive constructivist generation. In K. Ryan & T. Schwandt (Eds.), *Exploring evaluator role and identity.* Scottsdale, AZ: Information Age.

Hopson, R., Lucas, K. J., & Peterson, J. A. (2000). HIV/AIDS talk: Implications for prevention intervention and evaluation. *New Directions for Evaluation, 86,* 29–42.

Hopson, R. K., & Hood, S. (2005). An untold story in evaluation roots: Reid E. Jackson and his contributions towards culturally responsive evaluation at 3/4 century. In S. Hood, R. K. Hopson, & H. T. Frierson (Eds.), *The role of culture and cultural context: A mandate for inclusion, the discovery of truth and understanding in evaluative theory and practice* (pp. 85–102). Charlotte, NC: Information Age.

Horkheimer, M. (1972). *Critical theory.* New York: Seabury Press.

Horn, J. (2001). A Checklist for Developing and Evaluating Budgets: Evaluation Checklists Project. Retrieved from the Western Michigan University Evaluation Center website: *www.wmich.edu/evalctr/archive_checklists/evaluationbudgets.pdf*

Horn, K., McCracken, L., Dino, G., & Brayboy, M. (2008). Applying community-based participatory research principles to the development of a smoking-cessation program for American Indian teens: "Telling our story." *Health Education and Behavior, 35*(1), 44–69.

House, E. (1990). Research news and comment: Trends in evaluation. *Educational Researcher, 19,* 24–28.

House, E. R. (2003). Bush's neo-fundamentalism and the new politics of evaluation. In O. Karlsson (Ed.), *Studies in educational policy and educational philosophy* (Vol. 2). Uppsala, Sweden: Uppsala University.

House, E. R. (2004, October 2). *Democracy and evaluation.* Paper presented at the annual meeting of the European Evaluation Society, Berlin. Retrieved from *www.informat.org/publications/ernest-r-house.html*

House, E. R., & Howe, K. R. (1999). *Values in evaluation and social research.* Thousand Oaks, CA: Sage.

Hovey, J. D., Booker, V., & Seligman, L. (2007). Using theatrical presentations as a means of disseminating knowledge of HIV/AIDS risk factors to immigrant farmworkers: An evaluation of the effectiveness of the Infómate program. *Journal of Immigrant and Minority Health, 9*(2), 147–156.

Hruschka, D., Schwartz, D., St. John, D., Picone-Decaro, E., Jenkins, R., & Carey, J. (2004). Reliability in coding open-ended data: Lessons learned from HIV behavioral research. *Field Methods, 16*, 307–331.

Huffman, D., Thomas, K., & Lawrenz, F. (2008). A collaborative immersion approach to evaluation capacity building. *American Journal of Evaluation, 29*, 358–368.

Hummel-Rossi, B., & Ashdown, J. (2002). The state of cost–benefit and cost-effectiveness analyses in education. *Review of Educational Research, 72*, 1–30.

Husserl, E. (1970). *The crisis of European sciences and transcendental phenomenology* (D. Carr, Trans.). Evanston, IL: Northwestern University Press. (Original work published 1936)

Imbo, S. O. (2002). *Oral traditions as philosophy: Okot p'Bitek's legacy for African philosophy.* Lanham, MD: Rowman & Littlefield.

Interagency Coalition on AIDS and Development. (2007). *Gender analysis for project planners.* Ottawa, Ontario, Canada: Author.

International Fund for Agricultural Development (IFAD). (2003). *A methodological framework for project evaluation: Main criteria and key questions for project evaluation.* Rome: Author.

International Fund for Agricultural Development (IFAD) Office of Evaluation. (2009). *Evaluation manual: Methodology and processes.* Rome: Author.

International Network for Social Network Analysis (INSNA). (2008). *What is INSNA?* Retrieved from *www.insna.org/insna_what.html*

Israel, G. (2009). *Determining sample size.* Retrieved from the Institute of Food and Agricultural Sciences, University of Florida website: *www.edis.ifas.ufl.edu/pd006*

Jacob, S. (2008). Cross-disciplinarization: A new talisman for evaluation? *American Journal of Evaluation, 29*, 175–194.

Jacobs, N. (2005). Educating children with visual impairments in rural South India: Examining maternal belief profiles. *Disability and Society, 20*(3), 277–291.

Jacobsgaard, M. (2003). Using appreciative inquiry to evaluate project activities of a nongovernmental organization supporting victims of trauma in Sri Lanka. *New Directions for Evaluation, 100*, 53–62.

James Irvine Foundation. (2009). *Let's make evaluation work.* Retrieved from *www.irvine.org/publications/publications-by-topic/philanthropyandthenonprofitsector#phil5*

Jang, E. E., McDougall, D. E., Pollon, D., Herbert, M., & Russell, P. (2008). Integrative mixed methods data analytic strategies in research on school success in challenging circumstances. *Journal of Mixed Methods Research, 2*, 221–247.

Johnson, B., & Christensen, L. (2008). *Educational research: Quantitative, qualitative, and mixed approaches.* Thousand Oaks, CA: Sage.

Johnson, E. (2005). The use of contextually relevant evaluation practices with programs designed to increase participation of minorities in science, technology, engineering and mathematics (STEM) education. In S. Hood, R. Hopson, & H. Frierson (Eds.), *The role of culture and cultural context* (pp. 217–229). Greenwich, CT: Information Age.

Johnson, K., Greenseid, L. O., Toal, S. A., King, J. A., Lawrenz, F., & Volkov, B. (2009). Research on evaluation use: A review of the empirical literature from 1986 to 2005. *American Journal of Evaluation, 30*, 377–410.

Johnson, K. W., Young, L. C., Suresh, G., & Berbaum, M. L. (2002). Drug abuse treatment training in Peru: A social policy experiment. *Evaluation Review, 26*, 480–519.

Johnson, R. L., McDaniel, F., II, & Willeke, M. J. (2000). Using portfolios in program evaluation: An investigation of interrater reliability. *American Journal of Evaluation, 21*, 65–80.

Joint Committee on Standards for Educational Evaluation. (1994). *The program evaluation standards* (2nd ed.). Thousand Oaks, CA: Sage.

Joint Committee on Standards for Educational Evaluation. (2011). *The program evaluation standards* (3rd ed.). Thousand Oaks, CA: Sage.

Joint United Nations Programme on HIV/AIDS. (2005). *Operational guide on gender and HIV/AIDS: A rights based approach.* Retrieved from *www.unfpa.org/hiv/docs/rp/op-guide.pdf*

Joint United Nations Programme on HIV/AIDS. (2009). *Children and AIDS: Fourth stocktaking report.* New York: Author.

Kadushin, C., Hecht, S., Sasson, T., & Saxe, L. (2008). Triangulation and mixed methods designs: Practicing what we preach in the evaluation of an Israel experience educational program. *Field Methods, 20*, 46–65.

Kant, I. (1966). *Critique of pure reason.* Garden City, NY: Doubleday. (Original work published 1781)

Karlsson, O. (1996). A critical dialogue in evaluation: How can interaction between evaluation and politics be tackled? *Evaluation, 2*, 405–416.

Karlsson, O. (2003). Evaluation politics in Europe: Trends and tendencies. In O. Karlsson (Ed.), *Studies in educational policy and educational philosophy* (Vol. 1). Uppsala, Sweden: Uppsala University.

Kee, J. E. (1999). At what price?: Benefit–cost analysis and cost-effectiveness in program evaluation. *Evaluation Exchange, 5*(2–3), 4–5.

Kemmis, S., & McTaggart, R. (2000). Participatory action research. In N. Denzin & Y. Lincoln (Eds.), *Handbook of qualitative research* (2nd ed., pp. 567–605). Beverly Hills, CA: Sage.

Kemmis, S., & McTaggart, R. (2005). Participatory action research. In N. Denzin & Y. S. Lincoln (Eds.), *The Sage handbook of qualitative research* (3rd ed, pp. 271–330.), Thousand Oaks, CA: Sage.

Kendall, F. E. (2006). *Understanding white privilege.* New York: Routledge.

Ketterlin-Geller, L. R. (2005). Knowing what all students know: Procedures for developing universally designed assessments. *Journal of Technology, Learning, and Assessment, 4*(2), 2–22.

Kincheloe, J. L., & McLaren, P. (2002). Rethinking critical theory and qualitative research. In Y. Zou & E. T. Tur (Eds.), *Qualitative approaches to the study of education* (pp. 87–113). Lanham, MD: Rowman & Littlefield.

Kincheloe, J. L., & McLaren, P. (2005). Rethinking critical theory and qualitative research. In N. Denzin & Y. S. Lincoln (Eds.), *The Sage handbook of qualitative research* (3rd ed., pp. 303–342). Thousand Oaks, CA: Sage.

King, J. (2007). Developing evaluation capacity through process use. *New Directions for Evaluation, 116*, 45–59.

King, J. A. (1998). Making sense of participatory evaluation. *New Directions for Evaluation, 80*, 57–67.

King, J. A. (2005). A proposal to build evaluation capacity at the Bunche–Da Vinci Learning Partnership Academy. *New Directions for Evaluation, 106*, 85–97.

King, J. A., & Thompson, B. (1983). Research on school use of program evaluation: A literature review and research agenda. *Studies in Educational Evaluation, 9*, 5–21.

Kingsbury, N., Shipman, S., & Caracelli, V. (2009). *Program evaluation: A variety of rigorous methods can help identify effective interventions* (Publication No. GAO-10-30). Washington, DC: U.S. General Accounting Office.

Kirkhart, K. (1995). Seeking multicultural validity: A postcard from the road. *Evaluation Practice, 16*(1), 1–12.

Kirkhart, K. (2005). Through a cultural lens: Reflections on validity and theory in evaluation. In S. Hood, R. Hopson, & H. Frierson (Eds.), *The role of culture and cultural context* (pp. 21–38). Greenwich, CT: Information Age.

Kirkpatrick, D. L. (Ed.). (1975). *Evaluating training programs.* Madison, WI: American Society for Training and Development.

Kirkpatrick, D. L. (1998). *Evaluating training programs: The four levels.* San Francisco: Berrett-Koehler.

Kretzmann, J. P., & McKnight, J. L. (2005). *Discovering community power: A guide to mobilizing local assets and your organization's capacity.* Evanston, IL: Northwestern University, Asset-Based Community Development Institute.

Krogstrup, H. K. (2003) User participation in evaluation: Top-down and bottom-up perspectives. In O. Karlsson (Ed.), *Studies in educational policy and educational philosophy* (Vol. 1). Uppsala, Sweden: Uppsala University.

Krueger, R. A. (2000). *Focus groups: A practical guide for applied research* (3rd ed.). Thousand Oaks, CA: Sage.

Kuhn, T. (1962). *The structure of scientific revolutions.* Chicago: University of Chicago Press.

Kummerer, S. E., & Lopez-Reyna, N. E. (2009). Engaging Mexican immigrant families in language and literacy interventions: Three case studies. *Remedial and Special Education, 30,* 330–343.

Kushner, S. (2000). *Personalizing evaluation.* London: Sage.

Kushner, S. (2005). Democratic theorizing: From noun to participle. *American Journal of Evaluation, 26,* 579–581.

Ladd, P. (2003). *Understanding deaf culture: In search of deafhood.* Tonawanda, NY: Multilingual Matters.

Ladson-Billings, G. (2000). Racialized discourses and ethnic epistemologies. In N. Denzin & Y. Lincoln (Eds.), *Handbook of qualitative research* (2nd ed., pp. 257–277). Thousand Oaks: Sage.

LaFrance, J., & Crazy Bull, C. (2009). Researching ourselves back to life: Taking control of the research agenda in Indian country. In D. M. Mertens & P. E. Ginsberg (Eds.), *Handbook of social research ethics* (pp. 135–149). Thousand Oaks, CA: Sage.

Lai, M. K. (2009). *Statistical significance testing as widely practiced and published: An illogical procedure in educational research.* Paper presented at the annual meeting of the Hawai'i Educational Research Association, Honolulu, HI.

Langan, D., & Morton, M. (2009). Reflecting on community/academic "collaboration": The challenge of "doing" feminist participatory action research. *Action Research, 7,* 165–184.

Lawless, K. A., & Pellegrino, J. W. (2007). Professional development in integrating technology into teacher learning: Knowns, unknowns, and ways to purse better questions and answers. *Review of Educational Research, 77,* 575–614.

Lipsey, M. W. (1993). A big chapter about small theories. Theories as method: Small theories of treatments. *New Directions for Evaluation, 114*(Summer), 27–62.

Lee, C. D. (2003). "Race" and "ethnicity" in biomedical research: How do scientists construct and explain differences in health? *Social Science and Medicine, 68*(6), 1183–1190.

Lee, K. (2003). Understanding culture, social organization, and leadership to enhance engagement. In *Community tool box.* Retrieved from the University of Kansas, Work Group for Community Health and Development website: *ctb.ku.edu/en/tablecontents/section_1879.aspx*

Lee, K. (2009). *The importance of culture in evaluation: A practical guide for evaluators.* Denver: The Colorado Trust. Retrieved from *www.coloradotrust.org*

Leech, N. L., Dellinger, A., Brannagan, K. B., & Tanaka, H. (2010). Evaluating mixed methods research studies: A mixed methods approach. *Journal of Mixed Methods Research, 4,* 17–31.

Leech, N. L., & Onwuegbuzie, A. J. (2007). An array of qualitative data analysis tools: A call for qualitative data analysis triangulation. *School Psychology Quarterly, 22,* 557–584.

Leech, N. L., & Onwuegbuzie, A. J. (2008). Qualitative data analysis: A compendium of techniques and a framework for selection for school psychology research and beyond. *School Psychology Quarterly, 23*(4), 587–604.

Legovini, A. (2010). *Development impact evaluation initiative: A World Bank-wide strategic approach to enhance developmental effectiveness.* Washington, DC: World Bank.

Levin, H. M. (1983). *Cost-effectiveness: A primer.* Beverly Hills, CA: Sage.

Levine, R. (2010, June). *Remarks by Ruth Levine.* Paper presented at the annual meeting of InterAction Forum, Washington, DC.

Leviton, L. (2003). Evaluation use: Advances, challenges and applications. *American Journal of Evaluation, 24*(4), 525–535.

Lewins, A., Taylor, C., & Gibbs, G. R. (2005). *What is qualitative data analysis?* Retrieved from *onlineqda.hud.ac.uk/Intro_QDA/what_is_qda.php*

Lincoln, Y. S. (1991). The arts and sciences of program evaluation: A moral tale for practitioners. *Evaluation Practice, 12*(1), 1–7.

Lincoln, Y. S. (1995). Emerging criteria for quality in qualitative and interpretive research. *Qualitative Inquiry, 1*, 275–289.

Lincoln, Y. S. (2009). Ethical practices in qualitative research. In D. M. Mertens & P. E. Ginsberg (Eds.), *Handbook of social research ethics* (pp. 150–169). Thousand Oaks, CA: Sage.

Lincoln, Y. S. (2010). "What a long, strange trip it's been": Twenty-five years of qualitative and new paradigm research. *Qualitative Inquiry, 16*(1), 3–9.

Lincoln, Y. S., & Guba, E. G. (1980). The distinction between merit and worth in evaluation. *Educational Evaluation and Policy Analysis, 2*, 61–71.

Lincoln, Y. S., & Guba, E. G. (1985). *Naturalistic inquiry.* Beverly Hills, CA: Sage.

Lincoln, Y. S., & Guba, E. G. (2000). Paradigmatic controversies, contradictions and emerging confluences. In N. K. Denzin & Y. S. Lincoln (Eds.), *Handbook of qualitative research* (2nd ed., pp. 163–188). Thousand Oaks, CA: Sage.

Lindsay, A. C. (2002). Integrating quantitative and qualitative methods to assess the impact of child survival programs in developing countries: The case of a program evaluation in Ceara, Northeast Brazil. *Health Education Behavior, 29*, 570–584.

Lindsay, A. C., Machado, M., Sussner, K., Hardwick, C., Kerr, R., & Peterson, K. (2009). Brazilian mothers' beliefs, attitudes and practices related to child weight status and early feeding within the context of nutrition transition. *Journal of Biosocial Science, 41*, 21–37.

Linton, D. G., Khajenoori, S., Heileman, M. D., Van Bullington, J., Cat, H., Halder, K., et al. (1994). Reporter object: An analysis module which aids in verifying, validating and graphically displaying results of simulation models. *Simulation, 62*, 313–328.

Lipsey, M. K. (1990). *Design sensitivity.* Newbury Park, CA: Sage.

Lipsey, M. W. (1988). Reports on topic areas: Practice and malpractice in evaluation research. *American Journal of Evaluation, 9*, 5–24.

Lipsey, M. W. (2007). Peter H. Rossi: Formative for program evaluation. *American Journal of Evaluation, 28*, 199–202.

Luke, A. (1995/1996). Text and discourse in education: An introduction to critical discourse analysis. *Review of Research in Education, 21*, 3–48.

MacDonald, B. (1976). Evaluation and the control of education. In D. Tawney (Ed.), *Curriculum evaluation today: Trends and implications* (pp. 125–134). London: Macmillan Education.

MacDonald, B. (1977). A political classification of evaluation studies. In D. Hamilton, D. Jenkins, C. King, B. MacDonald, & M. Parlett (Eds.), *Beyond the numbers game.* London: Macmillan.

MacDonald, B., & Kushner, S. (2005). Democratic evaluation. In S. Mathison (Ed.), *Encyclopedia of evaluation* (pp. 109–113). Thousand Oaks, CA: Sage.

Malcolm X. (1992). *The final speeches* (S. Clark, Ed.). New York: Pathfinder.

Marcus, G. E. (1998). *Ethnography through thick and thin.* Princeton, NJ: Princeton University Press.

Mareschal, P. M., McKee, W. L., Jackson, S. E., & Hanson, K. L. (2007). Technology-based approaches to preventing youth violence: Formative evaluation of program development and implementation in four communities. *Youth Violence and Juvenile Justice, 5*, 168–187.

Mark, M. M. (2002). Toward better understanding of alternative evaluator roles. In K. E. Ryan & T. A. Schwandt (Eds.), *Exploring evaluator role and identity* (pp. 17–36). Greenwich, CT: Information Age.

Mark, M. M., & Gamble, C. (2009). Experiments, quasi-experiments and ethics. In D. M. Mertens & P. Ginsburg (Eds.), *Handbook of social research ethics* (pp. 198–213). Thousand Oaks, CA: Sage.

Mark, M. M., Greene, J. C., & Shaw, I. E. (2006). The evaluation of policies, programs, and practices. In I. E. Shaw, J. C. Greene, & M. M. Mark (Eds.), *The Sage handbook of evaluation* (pp. 3–32). Thousand Oaks, CA: Sage.

Mark, M. M., & Henry, G. T. (2004). The mechanisms and outcomes of evaluation influence. *Evaluation, 10*, 35–57.

Mark, M. M., & Henry, G. T. (2006). Methods for policy-making and knowledge development evaluations. In I. E. Shaw, J. C. Greene, & M. M. Mark (Eds.), *The Sage handbook of evaluation* (pp. 317–339). Thousand Oaks, CA: Sage.

Mark, M. M., Henry, G. T., & Julnes, G. (2000). *Evaluation*. San Francisco: Jossey-Bass.

Marra, M. (2000). How much does evaluation matter?: Some examples of the utilization of the evaluation of the World Bank's anti-corruption activities. *Evaluation, 6*, 22–36.

Marson, S. M., Wei, G., & Wasserman, D. (2009). A reliability analysis of goal attainment scaling (GAS) weights. *American Journal of Evaluation, 30*, 203–216.

Marx, K. (1978). Economic and philosophical manuscripts of 1844. In R. C. Tucker (Ed.), *The Marx–Engles reader* (2nd ed., pp. 52–103). New York: Norton.

Mathison, S. (Ed.). (2005). *Encyclopedia of evaluation*. Thousand Oaks, CA: Sage.

Mathison, S. (2008). What is the difference between evaluation and research—and why do we care? In N. L. Smith & P. R. Brandon (Eds.), *Fundamental issues in evaluation* (pp. 183–196). New York: Guilford Press.

Maxcy, S. (2003). Pragmatic threads in mixed methods research in the social sciences: The search for multiple modes of inquiry and the end of the philosophy of formalism. In A. Tashakkori & C. Teddlie (Eds.), *Handbook of mixed methods in social and behavioral research* (2nd ed., pp. 51–90). Thousand Oaks, CA: Sage.

Maxwell, J. A. (2004). Using qualitative methods for causal explanation. *Field Methods, 16*, 243–264.

May, G. E., & Raske, M. B. (2005). *Ending disability discrimination: Strategies for social workers*. Boston: Pearson Education/Allyn & Bacon.

Mbiti, J. S. (1970). *African religions and philosophy*. Garden City, NY: Anchor Books.

McDonald, K. E., & Myrick, S. E. (2008). Principles, promises, and a personal plea: What is an evaluator to do? *American Journal of Evaluation, 29*, 343–351.

McDuffie, K., & Scruggs, T. (2008). The contributions of qualitative research to discussions of evidence-based practice in special education. *Intervention in School and Clinic, 44*, 91–97.

McNall, M., & Foster-Fishman, P. G. (2007). Methods of rapid evaluation, assessment and appraisal mixed methods in intervention research. *American Journal of Evaluation, 28*, 151–168.

Meadow-Orlans, K., Mertens, D., & Sass-Lehrer, M. (2003). *Parents and their deaf children: The early years*. Washington, DC: Gallaudet University.

Meekosha, H., & Shuttleworth, R. (2009). "What's so critical about Critical Disability Studies?" *Australian Journal of Human Rights, 15*(1), 47–75.

Mercado, F. J., & Hernández, E. (2007). Las enfermedades crónicas desde la mirada de los enfermos y los profesionales de la salud: Un estudio cualitativo en México [Chronic illness from the perspective of patients and health professionals: A qualitative study in Mexico]. *Cadernos Saude Publica, 23*(9), 2178–2186.

Mercado-Martinez, F. J., Tejada-Tayabas, L. M., & Springett, J. (2008). Methodological issues in emergent evaluations of health programs: Lessons from Iberoamerica. *Qualitative Health Research, 18*, 1277–1288.

Merriam, S. (2001). *Qualitative research: A guide to design and implementation*. San Francisco: Jossey-Bass.

Mertens, D. M. (2000). Deaf and hard of hearing people in court: Using an emancipatory perspective to determine their needs. In C. Truman, D. M. Mertens, & B. Humphries (Eds.), *Research and inequality* (pp. 111–125). London: Taylor & Francis.

Mertens, D. M. (2002). The evaluator's role in the transformative context. In K. Ryan & T. Schwandt (Eds.), *Exploring evaluator role and identity* (pp. 103–117). Scottsdale, AZ: Information Age.

Mertens, D. M. (2003). The inclusive view of evaluation: Visions for the new millennium. In S. I. Donaldson & M. Scriven (Eds.), *Evaluating social programs and problems: Visions for the new millennium* (pp. 91–108). Mahwah, NJ: Erlbaum.

Mertens, D. M. (2005). The inauguration of the International Organization for Cooperation in Evaluation. *American Journal of Evaluation, 26*(1), 124–130.

Mertens, D. M. (2009). *Transformative research and evaluation*. New York: Guilford Press.

Mertens, D. M. (2010). *Research and evaluation in education and psychology: Integrating diversity with quantitative, qualitative, and mixed methods* (3rd ed.). Thousand Oaks, CA: Sage.

Mertens, D. M., Bledsoe, K., Sullivan, M. J., & Wilson, A. (2010). Utilization of mixed methods for transformative purposes. In A. Tashakkori & C. Teddlie (Eds.), *Handbook of mixed methods in social and behavioral research* (2nd ed., pp. 193–214). Thousand Oaks, CA: Sage.

Mertens, D. M., Fraser, J., & Heimlich, J. E. (2008). M or F?: Gender, identity and the transformative research paradigm. *Museums and Social Issues, 3*(1), 81–92.

Mertens, D. M., & Ginsberg, P. E. (2008). Deep in ethical waters: Transformative perspectives for qualitative social work research. *Qualitative Social Work, 7*(4), 484–503.

Mertens, D. M., & Ginsberg, P. E. (Eds.). (2009). *Handbook of social research ethics*. Thousand Oaks, CA: Sage.

Mertens, D. M., Harris, R., Holmes, H., & Brandt, S. (2007). *Project SUCCESS Summative Evaluation Report*. Washington, DC: Gallaudet University.

Mertens, D. M., Holmes, H. M., & Harris, R. L. (2009). Transformative research and ethics. In D. M. Mertens & P. E. Ginsberg (Eds.), *Handbook of social research ethics* (pp. 85–102). Thousand Oaks, CA: Sage.

Mertens, D. M., & McLaughlin, J. (2004). *Research and evaluation methods in special education*. Thousand Oaks, CA: Corwin Press.

Mertens, D. M., Sullivan, M., & Stace, H. (2011). Disability communities: Transformative research and social justice. In N. K. Denzin & Y. S. Lincoln (Eds.), *Handbook of qualitative research* (4th ed., pp. 227–242). Thousand Oaks, CA: Sage.

Mertens, D. M., & Yamashita, M. (2010). *Mission statement for the American Evaluation Association's Topical Interest Group: Mixed methods in evaluation*. Washington, DC: Author.

Messick, S. (1989). Meaning and values in test validation: The science and ethics of assessment. *Educational Researcher, 18*, 5–11.

Messick, S. (1996). Test validity: A matter of consequence. *Social Indicators Research, 45*(1), 35–44.

Mettrick, H. (2004). *Oxenisation in the Gambia*. Retrieved from the U.S. Department for International Development website: *webarchive.nationalarchives.gov.uk/+/http://www.dfid.gov.uk/Documents/publications/evaluation/ev014s.pdf*

Mienczakowski, J. (2000). People like us: Ethnography in the form of theatre with emancipatory intentions. In C. Truman, D. M. Mertens, & B. Humphries (Eds.), *Research and inequality* (pp. 126–142). London: Taylor & Francis.

Mienczakowski, J., & Morgan, S. (2001). Ethnodrama: Constructing participatory, experiential and compelling action research through performance. In P. Reason & H. Bradbury (Eds.), *Handbook of action research* (pp. 176–184). London: Sage.

Mi'kmaq College Institute. (2006). *Research principles and protocols: Mi'kmaw ethics watch*. Retrieved from *www.cbu.ca/mrc/ethics-watch*

Miles, M. B., & Huberman, A. M. (1994). *Qualitative data analysis: An expanded sourcebook*. Thousand Oaks, CA: Sage.

Miller, C., & Albert, B. (2005). *Mainstreaming disability in development: Lessons from gender main-*

streaming. London: Department for International Development (DFID), Disability Knowledge and Research.

Miller, R. L., & Campbell, R. (2006). Taking stock of empowerment evaluation: An empirical review. *American Journal of Evaluation, 27*, 296–319.

Milstein, B., Chapel, T. J., Wetterhall, S. F., & Cotton, D. A. (2002). Building capacity for program evaluation at the Centers for Disease Control and Prevention. *New Directions for Evaluation, 93*, 27–46.

Miron, G. (2004). *Evaluation Report Checklist: Evaluation Checklists Project*. Retrieved from the Western Michigan University Evaluation Center website: *www.wmich.edu/evalctr/archive_checklists/reports.xls*

Moewaka Barnes, H., & Te Ropu Whariki. (2009). *The evaluation hikoi: A Māori overview of programme evaluation*. Auckland: Te Ropu Whariki, Massey University. Retrieved from *www.whariki.ac.nz*

Morgan, D. L. (2007). Paradigms lost and pragmatism regained: Methodological implications of combining qualitative and quantitative methods. *Journal of Mixed Methods Research, 1*, 48–76.

Morris, M. (Ed.). (2008). *Evaluation ethics for best practice: Cases and commentaries*. New York: Guilford Press.

Morrow, S. L. (2007). Qualitative research in counseling psychology: Conceptual foundations. *The Counseling Psychologist, 35*, 209–235.

Morse, J. M. (2000). Determining sample size. *Qualitative Health Research, 10*(1), 3–5.

Moser, C. O. (1996). *Confronting crisis: A comparative study of household responses to poverty and vulnerability in four poor urban communities* (Environmentally Sustainable Development Studies and Monograph Series No. 8). Washington, DC: World Bank.

Moss, B. G., & Yeaton, Y. H. (2006). Shaping policies related to developmental education: An evaluation using regression–discontinuity design. *Educational Evaluation and Policy Analysis, 28*, 215–229.

Moss, P. A., Phillips, D. C., Erickson, F. D., Floden, R. E., Lather, P. A., & Schneider, B. L. (2009). Learning from our differences: A dialogue across perspectives on quality in education research. *Educational Researcher, 38*, 501–517.

Mukoma, W., Fisher, A. J., Helleve, A., Aaro, L. E., Mathews, C., Kaaya, S., et al. (2009). Development and test retest reliability of a research instrument designed to evaluation school-based HIV/AIDS interventions in South Africa and Tanzania. *Scandinavian Journal of Public Health, 37*, 7–15.

Murray, M. (2008). Narrative psychology. In J. A. Smith (Ed.), *Qualitative psychology: A practical guide to research methods* (pp. 11–131). London: Sage.

Murray, R. (2002). Citizens' control of evaluations. *Evaluation, 8*(1), 81–100.

Nastasi, B. K., Hitchcock, J., Sarkar, S., Burkholder, G., Varjas, K., & Jayasena, A. (2007). Mixed methods in intervention research: Theory to adaptation. *Journal of Mixed Methods Research, 1*, 164–182.

National AIDS Control Council. (2002). *Mainstreaming gender into the Kenya National HIV/AIDS Strategic Plan: 2000–2005*. Nairobi: Gender and HIV/AIDS Technical Sub-Committee of the National AIDS Control Council.

National Commission for the Protection of Human Subjects of Biomedical and Behavioral Research. (1979, April 18). *The Belmont report: Ethical principles and guidelines for the protection of human subjects of research*. Washington, DC: U.S. Department of Health, Education and Welfare. Retrieved from *ohsr.od.nih.gov/guidelines/belmont.html*

National Oceanic and Atmospheric Administration (NOAA). (2009). *Ocean service education*. Washington, DC: U.S. Department of Commerce. Retrieved from *oceanservice.noaa.gov/education/kits/currents/welcome.html*

National Registry of Evidence-Based Programs and Practices (NREPP). (n.d.). *Intervention summary: Project Alert*. Retrieved from *www.promoteprevent.org/publications/ebi-factsheets/project-alert*

National Research Council. (2002). *Scientific research in education*. Washington, DC: National Academy Press.

National Research Council. (2004). *On evaluating curricular effectiveness: Judging the quality of K–12 mathematics evaluations*. Washington, DC: National Academies Press.

Neely, C. L. (2001, November). *Priorities of stakeholder decision makers*. Retrieved from *sanrem.cals.vt.edu/1027/Neely.pdf*

Nichols, L. A. (2004). The infant caring process of Cherokee mothers. *Journal of Holistic Nursing, 22,* 226–253.

Nickols, R. W. (2005). Why a stakeholder approach to evaluating training? *Advances in Developing Human Resources, 7* 121–134.

Nielsen, S. B., & Ejler, N. (2008). Improving performance?: Exploring the complementarities between evaluation and performance management. *Evaluation, 14,* 171–192.

No Child Left Behind (NCLB) Act of 2001, Pub. L. 107-110, 115 Stat. 1425 (January 8, 2002).

Ntseane, P. G. (2009). The ethics of the researcher–subject relationship: Experiences from the field. In D. M. Mertens & P. E. Ginsberg (Eds.), *Handbook of social research ethics* (pp. 295–307). Thousand Oaks, CA: Sage.

Oakley, A. (2000). *Experiments in knowing: Gender and method in the social sciences.* Cambridge, UK: Polity Press.

Onwuegbuzie, A. J., Jiao, Q. G., & Bostick, S. L. (2004). *Library anxiety: Theory, research, and applications.* Lanham, MD: Scarecrow.

Opfer, V. D. (2006). Equity: A framework for understanding action and inaction on social justice. *Educational Policy, 20,* 271–290.

Oral History Project Team. (2005) The oral history of evaluation, Part 3: The professional evolution of Michael Scriven. *American Journal of Evaluation, 26,* 378–388.

Oral History Project Team. (2007). The oral history of evaluation, Part 5: An interview with Michael Quinn Patton. *American Journal of Evaluation, 28,* 102–114.

Oral History Project Team. (2009). The oral history of evaluation: The professional development of Eleanor Chelimsky. *American Journal of Evaluation, 30,* 232–244.

Organisation for Economic Co-operation and Development (OECD). (2005). *The Paris Declaration and Accra Agenda for Action.* Retrieved from *www.oecd.org/document/18/0,3343,en_2649_323639 8_35401554_1_1_1,00.html#Paris*

Organisation for Economic Co-operation and Development (OECD) Development Assistance Committee (DAC). (2006a). *Evaluation quality standards.* Paris: Author, Network on Development Evaluation.

Organisation for Economic Co-operation and Development (OECD) Development Assistance Committee (DAC). (2006b). *Guidance for managing joint evaluations.* Retrieved from *www.oecd.org/dac/evaluation*

Organisation for Economic Co-operation and Development (OECD). (2008). *Better aid: 2008 survey on monitoring the Paris Declaration–Making aid more effective by 2010.* Paris: Author. Retrieved from *www.oecd.org/dataoecd/58/41/41202121.pdf*

Organisation for Economic Co-operation and Development (OECD) Development Assistance Committee (DAC). (n.d.). *Glossary of terms in evaluation and results based management.* Paris: Author, Working Party on Aid Evaluation.

Osborne, R., & McPhee, R. (2000, December). *Indigenous terms of reference (ITR).* Paper presented at the 6th UNESCO-ACEID International Conference on Education, Bangkok.

O'Toole, S. (2009, August). Kirkpatrick on evaluation: Not crazy after all these years. *Training and Development in Australia, 36*(4), 23–25.

Owen, J. M. (2006). *Program evaluation: Forms and approaches* (3rd ed.), New York: Guilford Press.

Owen, J. M., & Rogers, P. (1999). *Program evaluation: Forms and approaches.* Thousand Oaks, CA: Sage.

Parlett, M., & Hamilton, D. (1972). Evaluation as illumination: A new approach to the study of innovatory programs. In G. Glass (Ed.), *Evaluation review studies annual* (Vol. 1, pp. 140–157). Beverly Hills, CA: Sage.

Parry, C., & Berdie, J. (1999). *Training evaluation in the human services.* Washington, DC: American Public Human Services Association.

Patton, M. Q. (1987). Evaluation's political inherency: Practical implications for design and use. In D. J. Palumbo (Ed.), *The politics of program evaluation* (pp. 100–145). Newbury Park, CA: Sage.

Patton, M. Q. (2002a). A vision of evaluation that strengthens democracy. *Evaluation, 8*(1), 125–139.

Patton, M. Q. (2002b). *Utilization-focused evaluation* (2nd ed.). Thousand Oaks, CA: Sage.

Patton, M. Q. (2004). *The roots of utilization focused evaluation.* In M. Alkin (Ed.), *Evaluation roots* (pp. 276–292). Thousand Oaks, CA: Sage.

Patton, M. Q. (2005). Toward distinguishing empowerment evaluation and placing it in a larger context: Take two. *American Journal of Evaluation, 26*(3), 408–414.

Patton, M. Q. (2008). *Utilization focused evaluation.* Thousand Oaks, CA: Sage.

Patton, M. Q. (2010). *Developmental evaluation: Applying complexity concepts to enhance innovation and use.* New York: Guilford.

Paul, J. L., & Marfo, K. (2001). Preparation of educational researchers in philosophical foundations of inquiry. *Review of Educational Research, 71,* 525–547.

Pawson, R., & Tilley, N. (1997). *Realistic evaluation.* London: Sage.

Payne, C. (1998). *Overview of the Chicago Comer Ethnography.* Unpublished manuscript, Northwestern University.

Pear, R. (2004, February 22). Taking spin out of report that made bad into good health. *The New York Times.*

Pennarz, J., Holicek, R. A. M., Rasidagic, E. K., & Rogers, D. (2007). *Joint country-led evaluation of child-focused policies within the social protection sector in Bosnia and Herzegovina.* Hove, UK: ITAD.

Perry, K. M. (2008). A reaction to and mental metaevaluation of the experiential learning evaluation project. *American Journal of Evaluation, 29*(3), 352–357.

Phillips, J. J. (1997). *Handbook of training evaluation and measurement methods* (3rd ed.). Houston, TX: Gulf.

Picciotto, R. (2007). The new environment for development evaluation. *American Journal of Evaluation, 28,* 509–521.

Picciotto, R. (2009). Evaluating development: Is the country the right unity of account? In M. Segone (Ed.), *Country-led monitoring and evaluation systems.* Geneva, Switzerland: UNICEF.

Pink, S. (2007). *Doing visual ethnography* (2nd ed.). Thousand Oaks, CA: Sage.

Planty, M., Hussar, W., Snyder, T., Kena, G., Kewal Ramani, A., Kemp, J., et al. (2009). *The condition of education 2009* (NCES Publication No. 2009-081). Washington, DC: U.S. Department of Education, National Center for Education Statistics. (Available at *nces.ed.gov/pubs2009/2009081. pdf*)

Platt, I. (1996). *Review of participatory monitoring and evaluation.* London: Concern.

Plummer, K. (2005). Critical humanism and queer theory: Living with the tensions. In N. Denzin & Y. S. Lincoln (Eds.), *The Sage handbook of qualitative research* (3rd ed.). Thousand Oaks, CA: Sage.

Pon, G. (2009). Cultural competency as new racism: An ontology of forgetting. *Journal of Progressive Human Services, 20*(1), 59–71.

Ponterotto, J. G. (2005). Qualitative research in counseling psychology: A primer on research paradigms and philosophy of science. *Journal of Counseling Psychology, 52*(2), 126–136.

Porter, G. (1995). "Third World" research by "First World" geographers: An Africanist perspective. *Area, 27*(2), 139–141.

Powell, K. (2007). *The SARD [Sustainable Agriculture and Rural Development] Project toolkit.* New York: United Nations Food and Agriculture Organization.

Prell, C., Hubacek, K., & Reed, M. (2007). *Stakeholder analysis and social network analysis in natural resource management*. Leeds, UK: University of Leeds, Sustainability Research Institute.

Preskill, H. (1984). *Evaluation use in the management/supervisory training programs*. Unpublished doctoral dissertation, University of Illinois at Urbana–Champaign.

Preskill, H., & Torres, R. (2001). The Readiness for Organizational Learning and Evaluation instrument (ROLE). In D. Russ-Eft & H. Preskill (Eds.), *Evaluation in organizations: A systematic approach to enhancing learning, performance, and change*. New York: Basic Books.

Preskill, H., & Torres, R. T. (1999). *Evaluative inquiry for learning in organizations*. Thousand Oaks, CA: Sage.

Pron, N., Oswalt, K., Segone, M., & Sakvarelidze, G. (2009). Strengthening country data dissemination systems. Good practices in using DevInfo. In M. Segone (Ed.), *Country-led monitoring and evaluation systems*. New York: UNICEF.

Public Broadcasting Service (PBS). (2010). *Bhutan: The last place 2002*. Retrieved from *www.pbs.org/frontlineworld/stories/bhutan/map.html*

Quigley, D. (2006). A review of improved ethical practices in environmental and public health research: Case examples from native communities. *Health Education and Behavior 33*, 130–147.

Randall, R., Cox, T., & Griffiths, A. (2007). Participants' accounts of a stress management intervention. *Human Relations, 69*(8), 11181–1209.

Reason, P., & Bradbury, H. (2008). *Handbook of action research: Participative inquiry and practice* (2nd ed.). London: Sage.

Renn, K. Q. (2010). LGBT and queer research in higher education: The state and status of the field. *Educational Researcher, 39*, 132–141.

Reynolds, G. (2008). *Presentation Zen: Simple ideas on presentation design and delivery*. Berkeley, CA: New Riders.

Rietbergen-McCraken, J., & Narayan-Parker, D. (1998). *Participation and social assessment: Tools and techniques*. Washington, DC: World Bank.

Roeber, E. (2002). *Setting standards in alternate assessments* (NCEO Synthesis Report 42). Minneapolis: University of Minnesota, National Center on Educational Outcomes.

Roethlisberger, F. J., & Dickson, W. J. (1939). *Management and the worker*. Cambridge, MA: Harvard University Press.

Rog, D. J. (2009). [Letter to the membership of the American Evaluation Association]. Unpublished letter.

Rogers, P. J., & Davidson, E. J. (2010, April 2). The Friday funny: 62 (good) reasons for avoiding evaluation in the United Nations system [Web log post]. Retrieved from *genuineevaluation.com/the-friday-funny-62-good-reasons-for-avoiding-evaluation-in-the-united-nations-system*

Rogers, P. J., & Williams, B. (2008). *Sustainability of services for young children and their families: What works?* Melbourne, Australia: Royal Melbourne Institute of Technology.

Rogers, R., Malancharuvil-Berkes, E., Mosley, M., Hui, D., & Joseph, G. O. (2005). Critical discourse analysis in education: A review of the literature. *Review of Educational Research, 75*, 365–416.

Rooke, A., & Limbu, M. (2009). *Gender toolkit for international finance-watchers*. Washington, DC: GenderAction.

Rose, G. (2007). *Visual methodologies* (2nd ed.). Thousand Oaks, CA: Sage.

Rosenstein, B., & Ganem, G. (2008). *Kindergarten teachers as parent group leaders*. Tel Aviv, Israel: Author.

Rossi, P., Lipsey, M. W., & Freeman, H. E. (2004). *Evaluation: A systematic approach* (7th ed.). Thousand Oaks, CA: Sage.

Roulston, K., deMarrais, K., & Lewis, J. B. (2003). Learning to interview in the social sciences. *Qualitative Inquiry, 9*(4), 643–668.

Russ-Eft, D. F., & Preskill, H. S. (2001). *Evaluation in organizations: A systematic approach to enhancing learning, performance, and change*. Cambridge, MA: Perseus.

Russ-Eft, D. F., & Preskill, H. S. (2005). In search of the Holy Grail: Return on investment evaluation in human resource development. *Advances in Developing Human Resources, 7,* 71–85.

Ryan, K., & Schwandt, T. (2002). *Exploring evaluator role and identity.* Scottsdale, AZ: Information Age.

Ryan, K. E. (2005). Making educational accountability more democratic. *American Journal of Evaluation, 26,* 532–543.

Ryan, K. E., & DeStefano, L. (Eds.). (2000). Evaluation as a democratic process: Promoting inclusion, dialogue, and deliberation. *New Directions for Evaluation, 85.*

Saulnier, C. F. (2000). Groups as data collection method and data analysis technique: Multiple perspectives on urban social work education. *Small Group Research, 31,* 607–627.

Savaya, S., Elsworth G., & Rogers, P. J. (2009). Projected sustainability of innovative social programs. *Evaluation Review, 33*(2), 189–205.

Savaya, R., Spiro, S., & Elran-Barak, R. (2008). Sustainability of social programs: A comparative case study analysis. *American Journal of Evaluation 29,* 478–492.

Scheirer, M. A. (2005). Is sustainability possible?: A review and commentary on empirical studies of program sustainability. *American Journal of Evaluation, 26,* 320–347.

Scherr, S. J. (1999, January). *Poverty–environment interactions in agriculture: Key factors and policy implications.* Paper presented at the UNDP/EC Expert Workshop on Poverty and the Environment, Brussels.

Scheurich, J. (1996). The masks of validity: A deconstructive investigation. *Qualitative Studies in Education, 9*(1), 49–60.

Schmidt, P. (2009, December 2). U of Minnesota takes heat for proposal to gauge future teachers' sensitivity. *The Chronicle of Higher Education.* Retrieved from *chronicle.com/article/U-of-Minnesota-Takes-Heat-for/49313/?sid*

Schochet, P. Z. (2009). Evaluations statistical power for regression discontinuity designs in education. *Journal of Educational and Behavioral Statistics, 34,* 238–266.

Schwab, J. (1969). The practical: A language for curriculum. *School Review, 78*(1), 1–23.

Schwandt, T. A. (1989). The politics of verifying trustworthiness in evaluation auditing. *American Journal of Evaluation, 10*(4), 33–40.

Schwandt, T. A. (2000). Three epistemological stances for qualitative inquiry: Interpretivism, hermeneutics, and social constructionism. In N. K. Denzin & Y. S. Lincoln (Eds.), *Handbook of qualitative research* (2nd ed., pp. 189–213). Thousand Oaks, CA: Sage.

Schwandt, T. A. (2001). Responsiveness and everyday life. *New Directions for Evaluation, 92,* 73–88.

Schwandt, T. A. (2003). In search of political morality of evaluation practice. In O. Karlsson (Ed.), *Studies in educational policy and educational philosophy* (Vol. 2, pp. 1–6). Uppsala, Sweden: Uppsala University.

Schwandt, T. A. (2008). Educating for intelligent belief in evaluation. *American Journal of Evaluation, 29,* 139–150.

Schwandt, T. A. (2009). Recapturing moral discourse in evaluation. *Educational Researcher, 18*(8), 11–16, 34.

Scott, A. G., & Sechrest, L. (1989). Strength of theory and theory of strength. *Evaluation and Program Planning, 12,* 329–336.

Scriven, M. (1967a). The logic of evaluation. In R. W. Tyler, R. M. Gagne, & M. Scriven (Eds.), *Perspectives of curriculum evaluation.* (AERA Monograph Series—Curriculum Evaluation). Chicago: Rand McNally.

Scriven, M. (1967b). The methodology of evaluation. In R. W. Tyler, R. M. Gagne, & M. Scriven (Eds.), *Perspectives of curriculum evaluation* (AERA Monograph Series—Curriculum Evaluation). Chicago: Rand McNally.

Scriven, M. (1969), An introduction to meta-evaluation. *Educational Product Report, 2,* 36–38.

Scriven, M. (1980). *The logic of evaluation.* Inverness, CA: Edgepress.

Scriven, M. (1991). Pros and cons about goal free evaluation. *Evaluation Practice, 2*(1), 55–76. (Original work published 1972)

Scriven, M. (1998). Minimalist theory: The least theory that evaluation practice requires. *American Journal of Evaluation, 19*(1), 57–70.

Scriven, M. (2003). Evaluation in the new millennium: The transdisciplinary vision. In S. I. Donaldson & M. Scriven (Eds.), *Evaluating social programs and problems* (pp. 19–41). Mahwah, NJ: Erlbaum.

Scriven, M. (2005). Empowerment evaluation principles in practice. *American Journal of Evaluation, 26*(3), 415–417.

Scriven, M. (2007). *Key Evaluation Checklist*. Retrieved from the Western Michigan University Evaluation Center website: *www.wmich.edu/evalctr/archive_checklists/kec_feb07.pdf*

Scriven, M. (2009). Meta-evaluation revisited. *Journal of Multidisciplinary Evaluation, 6*(11), iii–viii.

Sechrest, L. E. (1997). Empowerment evaluation: Knowledge and tools for self-assessment and accountability. *Environment and Behavior, 29*(3), 422–426.

Segerholm, C. (2003). To govern in silence: An essay on the political in national evaluations of the public schools in Sweden. In O. Karlsson (Ed.). *Studies in educational policy and educational philosophy* (Vol. 2). Uppsala, Sweden: Uppsala University.

Segone, M. (2006). *New trends in development evaluation*. Geneva, Switzerland: UNICEF Regional Office.

Segone, M. (2009). *Country-led monitoring and evaluation systems*. Geneva: UNICEF.

Seigart, D. (2007, November). *Gender and healthcare: Why Australian men can't get vasectomies*. Paper presented at the annual meeting of the American Evaluation Association, Baltimore, MD.

SenGupta, S., Hopson, R., & Thompson-Robinson, M. (2004). Cultural competence in evaluation: An overview. *New Directions for Evaluation, 102*, 5–19.

Shadish, W. R. (1998). Evaluation theory is who we are. *American Journal of Evaluation, 19*, 1–19.

Shadish, W. R., & Cook, T. D. (1998). Donald Campbell and evaluation theory. *American Journal of Evaluation, 19* 417–422.

Shadish, W. R., Cook, T. D., & Leviton, L. C. (1991). *Foundations of program evaluation*. Thousand Oaks, CA: Sage.

Sharma, M., & Deepak, S. (2001). A participatory evaluation of community-based rehabilitation programme in North Central Vietnam. *Disability and Rehabilitation, 23*(8), 352–358.

Shavelson, R. J. (2002). Lee J. Cronbach, 1916–2001. *Educational Researcher, 31*, 37–39.

Shaw, I. (1999). *Qualitative evaluation*. London: Sage.

Shen, J., Yang, H., Cao, H., & Warfield, C. (2008). The fidelity adaptation relationship in non-evidence-based programs and its implications for program evaluation. *Evaluation, 14*, 467–481.

Sherow, M. S. (2000, Spring). Adult and family literacy adaptations of goal attainment scaling. *Adult Basic Education, 10*(1), 30–39.

Sidani, S., & Sechrest, L. (1999). Putting program theory into operation. *American Journal of Evaluation, 20*, 227–238.

Sieber, J. E. (1992). *Planning ethically responsible research: A guide for students and internal review boards*. Newbury Park, CA: Sage.

Sielbeck-Bowen, K. A., Brisolara, S., Seigart, D., Tischler, C., & Whitmore, E. (2002). Exploring feminist evaluation: The ground from which we rise. *New Directions for Evaluation, 96*, 3–8.

Silka, L. (2005, August). *Building culturally competent research partnerships*. Paper presented at the annual meeting of the American Psychological Association, Washington, DC.

Simons, H. (1987). *Getting to know schools in a democracy*. London: Falmer.

Sireci, S. (2007). On validity and test evaluation. *Educational Researcher, 36*(8), 477–481.

Sirotnik, K. A., & Oakes, J. (1990). Evaluation as critical inquiry: School improvement as a case in point. *New Directions for Program Evaluation, 45*, 37–59.

Skolits, G. J., Morrow, J. A., & Burr, E. M. (2009). Reconceptualizing evaluator roles. *American Journal of Evaluation, 30*, 275–295.

Smart, D., & Mann, M. (2003, winter). Incorporating appreciative inquiry methods to evaluate a youth development program. *New Directions for Evaluation* (No. 100), 63–74.

Smith, E. R., & Tyler, R. W. (1942). *Appraising and recording student progress.* New York: HarperCollins.

Smith, L. T. (1999). *Decolonizing methodologies: Research and indigenous peoples.* London: Zed Books.

Smith, L. T. (2004). *Researching in the margins: Issues for Māori researchers.* Unpublished manuscript.

Smith, L. T. (2005). On tricky ground: Researching the native in the age of uncertainty. In N. K. Denzin & Y. S. Lincoln (Eds.), *The Sage handbook of qualitative research* (3rd ed., pp. 85–108). Thousand Oaks, CA: Sage.

Smith, N. L. (2008). Fundamental issues in evaluation. In N. L. Smith & P. R. Brandon (Eds.), *Fundamental issues in evaluation* (pp. 159–166). New York: Guilford Press.

Smith, N. L., & Brandon, P. R. (Eds.). (2008). *Fundamental issues in evaluation.* New York: Guilford Press.

Society for Prevention Research. (2004). *Standards of evidence: Criteria for efficacy, effectiveness and dissemination.* Retrieved from *www.preventionscience.org/StandardsofEvidencebook.pdf*

Solorzano, D. G. (1997). Images and words that wound: Critical race theory, racial stereotyping and teacher education. *Teacher Education Quarterly, 24*, 5–19.

Solorzano, D. G., & Delgado Bernal, D. (2001). Examining transformational resistance through a critical race and latcrit theory framework: Chicana and Chicano students in an urban context. *Urban Education, 36*, 308–342.

Solorzano, D. G., & Yosso, T. J. (2001). Critical race and LatCrit theory and method: Counterstorytelling Chicana and Chicano graduate school experiences. *International Journal of Qualitative Studies in Education, 14*, 471–495.

Spilsbury, M. J., Perch, C., Norgbey, S., Rauniyar, G., & Battaglino, C. (2007). *Lessons learned from evaluation: A platform for sharing knowledge.* New York: United Nations Environment Programme.

Squire, P. (1988). Why the 1936 *Literary Digest* poll failed. *Public Opinion Quarterly, 52*(1), 125–133.

Stake, R. E. (Ed.). (1975a). *Evaluating the arts in education: A responsive approach.* Columbus, OH: Merrill.

Stake, R. E. (1975b). To evaluate an arts program. In R. E. Stake (Ed.), *Evaluating the arts in education: A responsive approach* (pp. 13–31). Columbus, OH: Merrill.

Stake, R. E. (1976a). *Evaluating educational programmes: The need and the response.* Washington, DC: Organisation for Economic Co-operation and Development.

Stake, R. E. (1976b). *Negotiating agreements: Evaluation Checklists Project.* Retrieved from the Western Michigan University Evaluation Center website: *www.wmich.edu/evalctr/archive_checklists/plans_operations.pdf*

Stake, R. E. (1978). The case study method in social inquiry. *Educational Researcher, 7*, 5–8.

Stake, R. E. (1981). *Case study methodology.* Newbury Park, CA: Sage.

Stake, R. E. (1983). The case study method in social inquiry. In G. F. Madaus, M. Scriven, & D. L. Stufflebeam (Eds.), *Evaluation models* (pp. 279–286). Boston: Kluwer-Nijhoff.

Stake, R. E. (1991). Excerpts from "Program evaluation, particularly responsive evaluation." *American Journal of Evaluation, 12*, 63–76.

Stake, R. E. (2004). *Standards-based and responsive evaluation.* Thousand Oaks, CA: Sage.

Stake, R. E., & Abma, T. A. (2005). Responsive evaluation. In S. Mathison (Ed.), *Encyclopedia of evaluation* (pp. 376–379). Thousand Oaks, CA: Sage.

Stake, R. E., & Rizvi, F. (2009). Research ethics in transnational spaces. In D. M. Mertens & P. E. Ginsberg (Eds.), *The handbook of social research ethics* (pp. 521–536). Thousand Oaks, CA: Sage.

Stanczak, G. C. (Ed.). (2007). *Visual research methods.* Thousand Oaks, CA: Sage.

Stein, J. G. (2001). *The cult of efficiency.* Toronto, Ontario, Canada: Anansi.

Stewart, D., & Shamdasani, P. (1990). *Focus groups: Theory and practice.* Newbury Park, CA: Sage.

Strauss, V. (2010, September 9). The elephant that Obama and Lauer ignored: Poverty and student achievement. *The Washington Post.* Retrieved from *voices.washingtonpost.com/answer-sheet/race-to-the-top/the-elephant-obama-lauer-ignor.html*

Stufflebeam, D. L. (1968, January). *Evaluation as enlightenment for decision-making.* Paper presented at the Association for Supervision and Curriculum Development Conference on Assessment Theory, Sarasota, FL.

Stufflebeam, D. L. (1980). Interview: An EEPA interview with Daniel L. Stufflebeam. *Educational Evaluation and Policy Analysis, 2,* 85–90.

Stufflebeam, D. L. (1982). A review of progress in educational evaluation. *American Journal of Evaluation, 3,* 15–27.

Stufflebeam, D. L. (1994). Empowerment evaluation, objectivist evaluation, and evaluation standards: Where the future of evaluation should not go and where it needs to go. *American Journal of Evaluation, 15,* 321–338.

Stufflebeam, D. L. (1999a). Evaluation Contracts Checklist: Evaluation Checklists Project. Retrieved from the Western Michigan University Evaluation Center website: *www.wmich.edu/evalctr/archive_checklists/contracts.pdf*

Stufflebeam, D. L. (1999b). Evaluation Plans and Operations Checklist: Evaluation Checklists Project. Retrieved from the Western Michigan University Evaluation Center website: *www.wmich.edu/evalctr/archive_checklists/plans_operations.pdf*

Stufflebeam, D. L. (1999c). Program Evaluations Metaevaluation Checklist. Retrieved from the Western Michigan University Evaluation Center website: *www.wmich.edu/evalctr/archive_checklists/metaevaluation*

Stufflebeam, D. L. (2002, June). *CIPP Evaluation Model Checklist: A tool for applying the fifth installment of the CIPP model to assess long-term enterprises, intended for use by evaluators and evaluation clients/stakeholders.* Retrieved from the Western Michigan University Evaluation Center website: *www.wmich.edu/evalctr/archive_checklists/cippchecklist.pdf*

Stufflebeam, D. L. (2003). *The CIPP evaluation model.* Paper presented at the annual conference of the Oregon Program Evaluators Network, Portland, OR.

Stufflebeam, D. L. (2004). Evaluation Design Checklist: Evaluation Checklists Project. Retrieved from the Western Michigan University Evaluation Center website: *www.wmich.edu/evalctr/archive_checklists/evaldesign.pdf*

Stufflebeam, D. L. (2007). *The CIPP Evaluation Model Checklist.* Retrieved from the Western Michigan University Evaluation website: *www.wmich.edu/evalctr/archive_checklists/cippchecklist_mar07.pdf*

Stufflebeam, D. L. (2008). Egon Guba's conceptual journey to constructivist evaluation: A tribute. *Qualitative Inquiry, 14,* 1386–1400.

Stufflebeam, D. L., Foley, W. J., Gephart, W. J., Guba, E. G., Hammong, R. L., Merriman, H. O., et al. (1971). *Educational evaluation and decision making.* Itasca, IL: Peacock.

Stufflebeam, D. L., Gullickson, A., & Wingate, L. (2002). *The spirit of Consuelo: An evaluation of Ke Aka Ho'ona.* Retrieved from the Western Michigan University Evaluation Center website: *www.wmich.edu/evalctr*

Stufflebeam, D. L., Madaus, G. F., & Kellaghan, T. (2000). *Evaluation models.* Boston: Kluwer Academic.

Stufflebeam, D. L., & Shinkfield, A. J. (2007). *Evaluation theory, models, and applications.* San Francisco: Jossey-Bass.

Suarez-Balcazar, Y., Harper, G. W., & Lewis, R. (2005). An interactive and contextual model of community–university collaborations for research and action. *Health Education and Behavior, 32,* 84–101.

Sullivan, M. (2009). Philosophy, ethics, and the disability community. In D. M. Mertens & P. E. Gins-berg (Eds.), *Handbook of social research ethics* (pp. 69–84). Thousand Oaks, CA: Sage.

Sutherland, S. (2004). Creating a culture of data use for continuous improvement: A case study of an Edison Project school. *American Journal of Evaluation, 25,* 277–293.

Symonette, H. (2004). Walking pathways toward becoming a culturally competent evaluator: Bound-aries, borderlands, and border crossings. *New Directions for Evaluation, 102,* 95–109.

Szala-Meneok, K. (2009). Ethical research with older adults. In D. M. Mertens & P. E. Ginsberg (Eds.), *Handbook of social research ethics* (pp. 507–581). Thousand Oaks, CA: Sage.

Tall, O. B. (2009). Preface. In S. Segone (Ed.), *From policies to results: Developing capacities for country monitoring and evaluation systems* (pp. 10–11). New York: UNICEF.

Tarsilla, M. (2010a). Being blind in a world of multiple perspectives: The evaluator's dilemma between the hope of becoming a team player and the fear of becoming a critical friend with no friends. *Journal of MultiDisciplinary Evaluation, 6*(13), 200–205.

Tarsilla, M. (2010b). Theorists' theories of evaluation: A conversation with Jennifer Greene. *Journal of MultiDisciplinary Evaluation, 6*(13), 209–219.

Tashakkori, A., & Teddlie, C. (1998). Mixed methodology: Combining qualitative and quantita-tive approaches. In *Applied Social Research Methods* (Vol. 46, pp. 3–50). Thousand Oaks, CA: Sage.

Tashakkori, A., & Teddlie, C. (2003). Major issues and controversies in the use of mixed methods in the social and behavioral sciences. In A. Tashakorri & C. Teddlie (Eds.), *Handbook of mixed methods in social and behavioral research* (pp. 3–50). Thousand Oaks, CA: Sage.

Taut, S. (2007). Studying self-evaluation capacity building in a large international development organization. *American Journal of Evaluation, 28,* 45–59.

Teddlie, C., & Tashakkori, A. (2009). *Foundations of mixed methods research.* Thousand Oaks, CA: Sage.

Teddlie, C., & Yu, F. (2007). Mixed methods sampling: A typology with examples. *Journal of Mixed Methods Research, 1,* 77–100.

Theobald, S., Simwaka, B. N., & Klugman, B. (2006). Gender, health and development III: Engen-dering health research. *Progress in Development Studies, 6,* 337–342.

Thomas, V. G. (2009). Critical race theory: Ethics and dimensions of diversity in research. In D. M. Mertens & P. E. Ginsberg (Eds.), *Handbook of social research ethics* (pp. 54–68). Thousand Oaks, CA: Sage.

Thompson, B. (2002). What future quantitative social science research could look like: Confidence intervals for effect sizes. *Educational Researcher, 31*(3), 25–32.

Thompson, S. J., Thurlow, M. L. L., Quenemoen, R. F., & Lehr, C. A. (2002). *Access to computer-based testing for students with disabilities.* Minneapolis: University of Minnesota, National Center on Educational Outcomes.

Tikare, S., Youssef, D., Donnelly-Roark, P., & Shah, P. (2001). *Organizing participatory processes in the PRSP.* Washington, DC: World Bank.

Todahl, J. L., Linville, D., Bustin, A., Wheeler, J., & Gau, J. (2009). Sexual assault support services and community systems: Understanding critical issues and needs in the LGBTQ community. *Violence against Women, 15,* 952–976.

Trenholm, C., Devaney, B., Fortson, K., Clark, M., Quay, L., & Wheeler, J. (2008). Impacts of absti-nence education on teen sexual activity, risk of pregnancy, and risk of sexually transmitted diseases. *Journal of Policy Analysis and Management, 27*(2), 255–276.

Trochim, W. (1989). An introduction to concept mapping for planning and evaluation. *Evaluation and Program Planning, 12,* 1–16.

Trochim, W. (1990). The regression-discontinuity design. In L. Sechrest, E. Perrin, & J. Bunker (Eds.), *Research methodology: Strengthening causal interpretations of nonexperimental data* (DHHS Publication No. 90-3454) (pp. 141–143). Washington, DC: U.S. Department of Health and Human Services.

Trochim, W. (1998). An evaluation of Michael Scriven's "Minimalist theory: The least theory that practice requires." *American Journal of Evaluation, 19*(2), 243–249.

Trochim, W. (2006). *The research methods knowledge base* (2nd ed.). Ithaca, NY: Author.

Trochim, W. M., Marcus, S. E., Mâsse, L. C., Moser, R. P., & Weld, P. C. (2008). The evaluation of large research initiatives: A participatory integrative mixed-methods approach. *American Journal of Evaluation, 29*, 8–28.

Trochim, W. M., Milstein, B., Wood, B. J., Jackson, S., & Pressler, V. (2004). Setting objectives for community and systems change: An application of concept mapping for planning a statewide health improvement initiative. *Health Promotion Practice, 5*, 8–19.

Trotman, D. (2006). Interpreting imaginative lifeworlds: Phenomenological approaches in imagination and the evaluation of educational practice. *Qualitative Research, 6*, 245–265.

Tufte, E. (2001). *The visual display of quantitative information* (2nd ed.). Cheshire, CT: Graphics Press.

Turner, J. H. (2001). The origins of positivism: The contributions of Auguste Comte and Herbert Spencer. In G. Ritzer & B. Smart (Eds.), *Handbook of social theory*. Thousand Oaks, CA: Sage.

Twesigye, E. K. (2005). Book review: *Oral traditions as philosophy: Okot p'Bitek's legacy for African philosophy. Journal of Asian and African Studies, 40*, 237–239.

Unger, Z. M. (2009, November). *Pricing evaluation*. PowerPoint presentation at the annual meeting of the American Evaluation Association, Orlando, FL.

United Nations. (2006). *The Millennium Development Goals Report 2006*. New York: Author.

United Nations. (2009). *Making data meaningful: Part 2. A guide to presenting statistics*. New York: Author.

United Nations Children's Fund (UNICEF). (2009a). *Selected lessons learned from UNICEF programme cooperation 2007*. Retrieved from *www.unicef.org/evaluation/files/11compexternal2007_17feb09. pdf*

United Nations Children's Fund (UNICEF). (2009b). Evaluation and lessons learned. Retrieved from *www.unicef.org/evaluation/index_49082.html*

United Nations Development Fund for Women (UNIFEM). (2009, July). *EU gender politics in an international context–Gender perspectives and gender indicators*. Report from the international WOMNET conference, Berlin, Germany.

United Nations Development Fund for Women (UNIFEM). (2010). *Guide to integration of gender in policy for poverty reduction strategies*. New York: Author.

United Nations Development Programme (UNDP). (2007). *Inter-agency programme for the promotion of gender and ethnic–racial equality in Public Policies in Brazil*. Retrieved from *www.mdgfund.org/ program/interagencyprogrammepromotiongenderandethnicracialequality*

United Nations Foundation–Vodafone Foundation Partnership. (2009). *Health for development: The opportunity of mobile technology for healthcare in the developing world*. Retrieved from *www. globalproblems-globalsolutions-files.org/unf_website/assets/publications/technology/mhealth/ mHealth_for_Development_full.pdf*

United Nations Office of the High Commissioner for Human Rights. (2006). *United Nations convention on the rights of persons with disabilities*. Retrieved from *www2.ohchr.org/english/law/ disabilities-convention.htm*

United Nations Population Fund (UNFPA), Joint United Nations Programme on HIV/AIDS (UNAIDS), and United Nations Development Fund for Women (UNIFEM). (n.d.) *Women: Meeting the challenges of HIV/AIDS* [Brochure]. New York: Authors. (Available at *www.unfpa.org/hiv/ docs/women-aids.pdf*)

Ura, K. (2010). *Explanation of GNH index*. Retrieved from *www.icyte.com/system/snapshots/fs1/5/7/5/8 /5758e053fc39f0a4c8d73a45a57976e71518be58/index.html*

Ura, K., & Galay, K. (2004). Preface. *Gross national happiness and development*: *Proceedings of the First International Seminar on Operationalization of Gross National Happiness*. The Centre for Bhutan Studies, Bhutan.

U.S. Agency for International Development (USAID). (2009). *Performance monitoring and assessment.* Retrieved from *fa.usaidallnet.gov/fa-pme/viewhome.html*

U.S. Department of Education, Office of Special Education and Rehabilitative Services, Office of Special Education Programs. (2009). *28th annual report to Congress on the implementation of the Individuals with Disabilities Education Act.* Washington, DC: Author.

U.S. Department of Health and Human Services. (1996). *Cost-effectiveness in health and medicine: Report to the U.S. Public Health Service.* Washington, DC: U.S. Government Printing Office.

U.S. Department of Health and Human Services. (2005). *Selecting an evaluation consultant.* Washington, DC: U.S. Government Printing Office.

U.S. Department of Justice. (2009). *OJJDP FY 09 Gang Prevention Youth Mentoring Program.* Retrieved from *www.ojjdp.gov/grants/solicitations/FY2009/TYP.pdf*

U.S. Government Accountability Office (GAO). (2009, November). *Program evaluation: A variety of rigorous methods can help identify effective interventions.* Washington, DC: Author.

Valdes, F. (1996). Foreword: Latina/o ethnicities, critical race theory and post-identity politics in postmodern legal culture: From practices to possibilities. *La Raza Law Journal, 9,* 1–31.

Valdes, F. (1998). Under construction: LatCrit consciousness, community and theory. *La Raza Law Journal, 10,* 3–6.

Vargas, L. A., & Montoya, M. E. (2009). Involving minors in research: Ethics and law within multicultural settings. In D. M. Mertens & P. E. Ginsberg (Eds.), *Handbook of social research ethics* (pp. 489–506). Thousand Oaks, CA: Sage.

Velazquez, T. (2009, May 24). The wrong way to fight gang crime. *The Washington Post,* p. C7.

Vlado Networks. (n.d.). *Networks/Pajek.* Retrieved from *vlado.fmf.uni-lj.si/pub/networks/pajek/pics/examples.htm*

Walden, V. M., & Baxter, D. (2001). The comprehensive approach: An evaluation model to assess HIV/AIDS-related behavior change in developing countries. *Evaluation, 7*(4), 439–452.

Walker, R., & Wiseman, M. (2006). Managing evaluations. In I. Shaw, J. Greene, & M. Mark (Eds.), *Handbook of policy evaluation* (pp. 360–383). London: Sage.

Wandersman, A. (2009, May). *Evaluation as an intervention to help you achieve results: Empowerment evaluation.* Paper presented at the Administration for Children and Families Evaluation Summit, Washington, DC.

Wehipeihana, N., Davidson, E. J., McKegg, K., & Shanker, V. (2010). What does it take to do evaluation in communities and cultural contexts other than our own? *Journal of MultiDisciplinary Evaluation, 6*(13), 182–192.

Wehipeihana, N., & Oakden, J. (2009). *Evaluation of the Rotura trial of the Reading Together programme: A focus on whānau engagement.* Wellington: New Zealand Ministry of Education.

Wehipeihana, N., & Pipi, K. (2008). *Working for families tax credit: Barriers to take-up from potentially eligible families.* Unpublished report, Research Evaluation Consultancy Limited.

Weiss, C. H. (1972). *Evaluation research: Methods of assessing program effectiveness.* Englewood Cliffs, NJ: Prentice-Hall.

Weiss, C. H. (1987). Where politics and evaluation research meet. In D. J. Palumbo (Ed.), *The politics of program evaluation* (pp. 47–70). Newbury Park, CA: Sage.

Weiss, C. H. (1998). *Evaluation research: Methods for studying programs and policies* (2nd ed.). Upper Saddle River, NJ: Prentice Hall.

Weiss, C. H. (2004). Rooting for evaluation: A Cliff Notes version of my work. In M. C. Alkin (Ed.), *Evaluation roots: Tracing theorists' views and influences* (pp. 153–168). Thousand Oaks, CA: Sage.

Werner, D., & Bower, B. (1995). *Helping health workers learn.* Berkeley, CA: Hesperian Foundation.

Wertz, F. J. (1999). Multiple methods in psychology: Epistemological Grounding and the Possibility of Unity. *Journal of Theoretical and Philosophical Psychology, 19*(2), 131–166.

Wertz, F. J. (2005). Phenomenological research methods for counseling psychology. *Journal of Counseling Psychology, 52*(2), 167–177.

White, H. (2008). *Of probits and participation: The use of mixed methods in quantitative impact evaluation* (Working Paper No. 6, Network of Networks on Impact Evaluation [NONIE]. Retrieved from *www.worldbank.org/ieg/nonie/docs/WP7_White.pdf*

Whitmore, E. (Ed.). (1998). Understanding and practicing participatory evaluation. *New Directions for Evaluation, 80.*

Whitmore, E., Gujit, I., Mertens, D. M., Imm, P. S., Chinman, M., & Wandersman, A. (2006). Embedding improvements, lived experience, and social justice in evaluation practice. In I. Shaw, J. Greene, & M. Mark (Eds.), *The Sage handbook of evaluation* (pp. 340–359). Thousand Oaks, CA: Sage.

Wholey, J. (2001). Defining, improving, and communicating program quality. In P. Alexis, D. Benson, D. Michelle Hinn, & C. Lloyd (Eds.), *Vision of quality: How evaluators define, understand and represent program quality* (Advances in Program Evaluation, Vol. 7, pp. 201–216). Bingley, UK: Emerald Group.

Wiles, R., Crow, G., Heath, S., & Charles, V. (2006, July). *Anonymity and confidentiality.* Paper presented at the ESRC Research Methods Festival, University of Oxford, Oxford, UK.

Wilson, A. (2005). The effectiveness of international development assistance from American organizations to deaf communities in Jamaica. *American Annals of the Deaf, 150*(3), 292–304.

Wilson, A. (2007, October). *Ten-country evaluation: A study of Hilton/Perkins international programs.* Los Angeles: Conrad N. Hilton Foundation.

Wilson, A. (2008, September). *Female condom use in the GLBT community.* Paper presented at the Whitman Walker Clinic, Washington, DC.

Winegrad, G. W., & Ernst, H. (2009, May 24). A bay full of broken promises. *The Washington Post,* p. C7.

W.K. Kellogg Foundation (WKKF). (1998). *Evaluation handbook.* Battle Creek, MI: Author.

W.K. Kellogg Foundation (WKKF). (2004). *Logic model development guide.* Retrieved from *www.wkkf. org/knowledge-center/resources/2006/02/WK-Kellogg-Foundation-Logic-Model-Development-Guide. aspx*

Wood, B., Betts, J., Etta, F., Gayfer, J., Kabell, D., Ngwira, N., Sagasti, F., & Samaranayake, M. (2011, May). *The evaluation of the Paris Declaration, final report.* Copenhagen.

World Bank. (n.d.). *Methodologies and tools: Modeling to monitor the MDGs.* Retrieved from *go.worldbank. org/QJNBFDJ7S0*

World Bank Independent Evaluation Group. (2009). *Country assistance evaluations (CAEs).* Retrieved from *www.worldbank.org/ieg/countries/cae/featured/cae_retrospective.html#issues*

World Health Organization (WHO). (2002). *Gender analysis in health.* Geneva, Switzerland: Author.

World Health Organization (WHO). (2003). *Mainstreaming Gender in Health: A WHO manual for health managers.* Geneva, Switzerland: Author.

World Health Organization (WHO). (2010). *Antiretroviral drugs for treating pregnant women and preventing HIV infection in infants.* Retrieved from the WHO website: *www.who.int/hiv/pub/mtct/ guidelines/en*

World Medical Association. (2008, October 20). WMA Declaration of Helsinki–Ethical principles or medical research involving human subjects. Retrieved from *www.wma.net/ en/30publication/10policies/b3/index.html*

Wright, H. K. (2003). An endarkened feminist epistemology?: Identity difference and the politics of representation in education research. *Qualitative Studies in Education, 16*(2), 197–214.

Yin, R. (2003). Case study research: Design and methods. *Applied Social Research Methods, 5.*

Yin, R. (2009). *Case study research* (4th ed.). Thousand Oaks, CA: Sage.

Yoshikawa, H., Weisner, T., Kalil, A., & Way, N. (2008). Qualitative and quantitative research in developmental science: Uses and methodological considerations. *Developmental Psychology, 44*(2), 344–354.

Zulli, R. A., & Frierson, H. T. (2004). Evaluating an Upward Bound Program. *New Directions for Evaluation, 102,* 81–93.

Author Index

Subject Index

About the Authors

Donna M. Mertens, PhD, is Professor in the Department of Educational Foundations and Research at Gallaudet University, where she teaches advanced research methods and program evaluation to deaf and hearing students. She received the Distinguished Faculty Award from Gallaudet in 2007. The primary focus of her work is transformative mixed methods inquiry in diverse communities, with priority given to the ethical implications of research in pursuit of social justice. A past president of the American Evaluation Association (AEA), Dr. Mertens provided leadership in the development of the International Organization for Cooperation in Evaluation and the establishment of the AEA Diversity Internship Program with Duquesne University. She has received AEA's highest honors for service to the organization and the field, as well as for her contributions to evaluation theory. She is the author of several books and is widely published in major professional journals (e.g., the *Journal of Mixed Methods Research, American Journal of Evaluation*, and *American Annals of the Deaf*). Dr. Mertens conducts and consults on evaluations in many countries, including Egypt, India, South Africa, Botswana, Israel, Australia, New Zealand, and Costa Rica.

Amy T. Wilson, PhD, is Associate Professor in the Department of Educational Foundations and Research at Gallaudet University. After living in developing countries and noting the poor assistance people with disabilities were receiving from U.S. development organizations, she developed Gallaudet's MA degree in International Development. The degree, which is the only one of its kind in the United States, focuses on the inclusion of people with disabilities in development assistance programs and in nongovernmental, federal, and faith-based development organizations both in the United States and overseas. Dr. Wilson is Program Director of the International Development Program; she also teaches deaf and hearing students research and evaluation, theory and practice of international development, micropolitics, community development with people with disabilities, multicultural education, and gender disability and development. Dr. Wilson evaluates and advises development organizations and agencies (e.g., U.S. Agency for International Development [USAID], the InterAmerican Development Bank, the World Bank, and the Peace Corps) about the inclusiveness of their programs, as well as their effectiveness with various disability communities.